Cytokines and Autoimmune Diseases

Cytokines and Autoimmune Diseases

Edited by

Vijay K. Kuchroo, DVM, PhD

*Center for Neurologic Diseases, Brigham and Women's Hospital,
Harvard Medical School, Boston, MA*

Nora Sarvetnick, PhD

*Department of Immunology, Scripps Research Institute,
La Jolla, CA*

David A. Hafler, MD

*Center for Neurologic Diseases, Brigham and Women's Hospital,
Harvard Medical School, Boston, MA*

Lindsay B. Nicholson, PhD, MB

*Center for Neurologic Diseases, Brigham and Women's Hospital,
Harvard Medical School, Boston, MA*

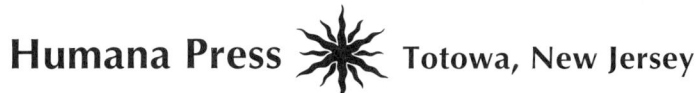

Humana Press Totowa, New Jersey

Cover illustration: Fig. 2 from Chapter 9, "The Role of Cytokines in Induction and Regulation of Autoimmune Uveitis," by Rachel R. Caspi.

Production Editor: Jessica Jannicelli.
Cover design by Patricia F. Cleary.

For additional copies, pricing for bulk purchases, and/or information about other Humana titles, contact Humana at the above address or at any of the following numbers: Tel.: 973-256-1699; Fax: 973-256-8341; E-mail: humana@humanapr.com or visit our Web site: humanapress.com

Library of Congress Cataloging in Publication Data
Cytokines and autoimmune diseases / edited by Vijay K. Kuchroo ... [et al.].
    p. ; cm.
  Includes bibliographical references and index.
  ISBN 0-89603-856-4 (alk. paper)
    1. Cytokines. 2. Autoimmunity. I. Kuchroo, Vijay K.
    [DNLM: 1. Autoimmune Diseases--physiopathology. 2. Autoimmune
  Diseases--etiology. 3. Autoimmune Diseases--immunology. 4. Cytokines--immunology.
    5. Cytokines--physiology. WD 305 C9965 2001]
    QR185.8.C95 C958 2001
    616.97'8--dc21
                                                                            2001016934

Preface

Cytokines, produced by immune cells, are soluble molecules by which the immune system communicates with other cell types within or outside the immune system. Cytokines form a central coordinating network of soluble effector molecules that plays a crucial role at every step of the development of autoimmune disease: in the generation of pathogenic or protective effector cells, in the trafficking of pathogenic cells to the target organ, and in mediating tissue damage or tissue tolerance in the target organ.

Upon activation, naive autoreactive T cells differentiate into cells that produce proinflammatory or anti-inflammatory cytokines. Cells producing proinflammatory cytokines are pathogenic and induce organ-specific autoimmune diseases, whereas autoreactive cells producing anti-inflammatory cytokines may inhibit autoimmune diseases, although they do not always do so. Thus, interventions targeted to inhibit the secretion of proinflammatory cytokines or the differentiation of cells to a proinflammatory phenotype, or alternatively to enhance anti-inflammatory cytokines or the differentiation of cells to an anti-inflammatory phenotype, may inhibit and/or reverse an autoimmune disease. This highlights the enormous therapeutic potential of cytokine modulation in the treatment of autoimmune diseases.

Over 18 different cytokines with both overlapping and distinct functions in the activation, expansion, and differentiation of other cell types in the immune system have been discovered. In addition there are over 20 different chemokines, molecules that are chemotactic and affect the accumulation of different types of cells at the sites of inflammation and tissue injury. In an immune response there is a complex interplay between these various cytokines and chemokines that determines the outcome of inflammation and the probability of developing autoimmune disease.

The current literature contains a large amount of primary data on the role of various cytokines in the induction and regulation of autoimmunity; however, there is no clear consensus. *Cytokines and Autoimmune*

Diseases aims to synthesize the available information on this single topic, the role of cytokines in autoimmunity, to help develop a clear understanding of how cytokines and chemokines are involved in the pathogenesis of autoimmune diseases.

Vijay K. Kuchroo, DVM, PhD

Contents

Contributors

ABUL K. ABBAS • *Department of Pathology, UCSF School of Medicine, San Francisco, CA*

ESTELLE BETTELLI • *Center for Neurologic Diseases, Brigham and Women's Hospital, Harvard Medical School, Boston, MA*

JANET E. BUHLMANN • *Immunology Division, Department of Pathology, Brigham and Women's Hospital, Harvard Medical School, Boston, MA*

RACHEL R. CASPI • *Section on Immunoregulation, Laboratory of Immunology, National Eye Institute, Bethesda, MD*

PREMKUMAR CHRISTADOSS • *Department of Microbiology and Immunology, University of Texas Medical Branch, Galveston, TX*

MARK EXLEY • *Beth Israel Deaconess Medical Center and Harvard Medical School, Boston, MA*

RONALD N. GERMAIN • *Laboratory of Immunology, National Institute of Allergy and Infectious Diseases, National Institutes of Health, Bethesda, MD*

LAURIE H. GLIMCHER • *Department of Immunology and Infectious Disease, Harvard School of Public Health, Boston, MA*

ELZBIETA GOLUSZKO • *Department of Microbiology and Immunology, University of Texas Medical Branch, Galveston, TX*

DAVID A. HAFLER • *Department of Neurology, Center for Neurologic Diseases, Brigham and Women's Hospital, Harvard Medical School, Boston, MA*

HELENA ERLANDSSON HARRIS • *Rheumatology Unit, Department of Medicine, Karolinska Institutet, Karolinska Hospital, Stockholm, Sweden*

ADELE F. HOLLOWAY • *Division of Biochemistry and Molecular Biology, John Curtin School of Medical Research, Australian National University, Canberra, Australia*

YASUSHI ITOH • *Laboratory of Immunology, National Institute of Allergy and Infectious Diseases, National Institutes of Health, Bethesda, MD*

WILLIAM J. KARPUS • *Department of Pathology, Northwestern University School of Medicine, Chicago, IL*

SALLY C. KENT • *Department of Neurology, Center for Neurologic Diseases, Brigham and Women's Hospital, and Harvard Medical School, Boston, MA*

LARS KLARESKOG • *Rheumatology Unit, Department of Medicine, Karolinska Institutet, Karolinska Hospital, Stockholm, Sweden*

VIJAY K. KUCHROO • *Center for Neurologic Diseases, Brigham and Women's Hospital, Harvard Medical School, Boston, MA*

PER LARSSON • *Rheumatology Unit, Department of Medicine, Karolinska Institutet, Karolinska Hospital, Stockholm, Sweden*

LINDSAY B. NICHOLSON • *Center for Neurologic Diseases, Brigham and Women's Hospital, Harvard Medical School, Boston, MA*

RICHARD M. RANSOHOFF • *Departments of Neurology and Neurosciences, Lerner Research Institute, Cleveland Clinic Foundation, Cleveland, OH*

JYOTHI RENGARAJAN • *Department of Immunology and Infectious Disease, Harvard School of Public Health, Boston, MA*

NORA SARVETNICK • *Department of Immunology, Scripps Research Institute, La Jolla, CA*

BENJAMIN M. SEGAL • *Departments of Neurology and Microbiology and Immunology, University of Rochester School of Medicine and Dentistry, Rochester, NY*

M. FRANCES SHANNON • *Division of Biochemistry and Molecular Biology, John Curtin School of Medical Research, Australian National University, Canberra, Australia*

ARLENE H. SHARPE • *Immunology Division, Department of Pathology, Brigham and Women's Hospital, Harvard Medical School, Boston, MA*

ETHAN M. SHEVACH • *Laboratory of Immunology, National Institute of Allergy and Infectious Diseases, National Institutes of Health, Bethesda, MD*

LUK VAN PARIJS • *Center for Cancer Research, Massachusetts Institute of Technology, Cambridge, MA*

VISSIA VIGLIETTA • *Department of Neurology, Center for Neurologic Diseases, Brigham and Women's Hospital, Harvard Medical School, Boston, MA*

MARIE WAHREN-HERLENIUS • *Rheumatology Unit, Department of Medicine, Karolinska Institutet, Karolinska Hospital, Stockholm, Sweden*

EDWARD K. WAKELAND • *Center for Immunology, University of Texas Southwestern Medical Center, Dallas, TX*

AMY E. WANDSTRAT • *Center for Immunology, University of Texas Southwestern Medical Center, Dallas, TX*

HOWARD L. WEINER • *Center for Neurologic Diseases, Brigham and Women's Hospital, Boston, WA*

S. BRIAN WILSON • *Cancer Immunology and AIDS, Dana Farber Cancer Institute, Boston, MA*

I

CYTOKINES: INDUCTION AND REGULATION

1

Transcriptional Regulation
of Cytokine Gene Expression in Th Subsets

Jyothi Rengarajan and Laurie H. Glimcher

1. INTRODUCTION

Cytokines are produced by a diverse array of cell types in response to antigenic stimulation and are instrumental in regulating the immune response. The expression of many key cytokines is controlled at the level of transcription. Because a considerable part of the experimental data pertaining to cytokine gene expression has been gathered in the context of studying the transcriptional regulation of CD4[+] T helper cells as they differentiate into cytokine-producing effector cells, this will serve as both an illustrative model and the focus of this chapter.

2. TH1/TH2 PARADIGM AND CYTOKINE REGULATION

T helper (Th) cells are classified into two distinct subtypes depending on the cytokines they secrete upon their activation and proliferation. Polarized Th1 cells produce interleukin-2 (IL-2), interferon-γ (IFN-γ), tumor necrosis factor (TNF)-α, and TNF-β while Th2 cells produce IL-4, IL-5, IL-6, IL-10, and IL-13 *(1–3)*. Th1 and Th2 subsets develop from a common T helper precursor (Thp). The cytokines themselves are the most potent inducers of subset development although the dose of antigen, strength of signal through the T cell receptor (TCR) and costimulation influence Th differentiation *(4–6)*. Naive Thp cells secrete IL-2 upon antigenic stimulation after which IL-12 is critical for IFN-γ production and Th1 differentiation and IL-4 for Th2 differentiation *(5)*. Thus, defining the molecular basis of Th-specific expression of these cytokines serves to elucidate cytokine gene regulation as well as lineage commitment of Th cells. We will summarize what is known about the transcriptional regulation of the *IL-2*, *IL-4*, and *IFN-γ* genes.

Early insights into transcriptional regulation were attained from studying regulatory DNA sequences in the promoter regions of cytokine genes (*cis-*

From: *Cytokines and Autoimmune Diseases*
Edited by: V. K. Kuchroo, et al. © Humana Press Inc., Totowa, NJ

acting elements) and sequence-specific DNA-binding proteins (*trans*-acting factors) such as transcription factors, that interact with these regulatory regions. More recently, Th subset-specific transcription factors have been identified that have shed light on the subset-restricted expression of some cytokines. We will discuss recent advances in the regulation of the *IL-2* , *IL-4* , and *IFN-* γ genes within the paradigm of naive Thp differentiation into Th1 and Th2 subsets. It has become increasingly evident that chromatin structure and chromosomal components greatly influence gene regulation and may confer stability on gene activity or inactivity. We will highlight what is known about the role of chromatin and the epigenetic control of cytokine gene transcription.

3. TRANSCRIPTION FACTORS IN CYTOKINE GENE EXPRESSION

Accurate transcriptional regulation requires the cooperative and synergistic action of multiple ubiquitous and sequence-specific *trans*-acting factors bound to multiple regulatory elements in the promoter *(7,8)*. Transcription factors adopt modular structures that contain various domains or motifs that represent activation (e.g., acidic residues), multimerization (e.g., leucine zippers), or DNA-binding domains (e.g., zinc fingers, helix-loop-helix proteins). Additional *cis*-elements such as enhancers and silencers provide further binding sites for such proteins and can function to enhance or repress transcription at large distances from promoter regions *(9)*. Furthermore, locus control regions (LCRs) are believed to have a more global role in keeping regions of the chromosome in an activated or repressed state *(9)*. The combinatorial effects of these protein-protein, protein-DNA contacts and their interactions with the basal-transcriptional machinery confer specificity and precision to the transcriptional process *(7,8)*. The resulting interaction surfaces, composed of transcription factors, coactivators/corepressors, architectural proteins and DNA, often assemble into stereo-specific enhanceosome complexes, the best-characterized example of which is the IFN-β enhanceosome. The activity of the IFN-β enhanceosome is distinct from that of the individual elements *(7)*. The context in which these elements are organized in three-dimensional space and their relative affinities to DNA thus provide another level of regulation. It is possible that similar mechanisms will prevail in the regulation of other cytokine genes.

3.1. IL-2

We will discuss IL-2 first because it is the cytokine produced earliest during Th differentiation by the naive Thp cell. Regulation of IL-2 expression is controlled almost completely at the level of transcription, although costimulation via signals transmitted through CD28 appears to also control IL-2 expression post-transcriptionally, by increasing the stability of *IL-2* mRNA *(10)*. *IL-2* is expressed exclusively in T cells and is rapidly induced upon activation through the TCR combined with costimulatory signals through CD28 *(11)*. TCR engagement activates the MAP kinase and Ca^{2+}-dependent signaling pathways. Both these pathways are essential for IL-2 expression and lead to the activation of several transcription factors including members of the Nuclear Factor of Activated T cells (NFAT) and Activator Protein 1 (AP-1) families *(12)*. In resting T cells, NFAT proteins are present in the cytoplasm in a phosphorylated state. They are rapidly dephosphorylated upon stimulation and translocate into the nucleus where, in combination with AP-1 proteins, they activate the transcription of several cytokine genes, including *IL-2 (12)*. The sensitivity of cytokine genes to the immunosuppressants cyclosporin A (CsA) and FK506 reflects the ability of these drugs to inhibit the phosphatase calcineurin, leading to inhibition of Ca^{2+}-mediated and hence NFAT-regulated pathways *(13)*.

Extensive studies on *IL-2* transcriptional regulation have delineated a 300-bp minimal promoter/enhancer region that is sufficient for tissue-specific inducibility of the *IL-2* gene in vitro. Multiple sites have been identified that are bound by distinct transcription factors, some of which are induced on stimulation, like NFAT, AP-1 (Jun and Fos), and NF-κB (p50, p65, c-Rel) family members and some of which are constitutive factors like Oct proteins *(12,14–16)* (Fig. 1). In addition, a CD28 response element has been shown to be recognized by NF-κB proteins, ATF-1, CREB2, and HMG I(Y) *(17–19)*. Point mutations at each of these sites severely reduce transcriptional activity *(14)*. In vivo footprinting of the *IL-2* locus in T cells demonstrated that each transcription factor does not bind autonomously but is dependent on the combinatorial interaction of multiple proteins on the *IL-2* promoter/enhancer, thus stabilizing the transcription complex *(11)*. However, none of these proteins individually specifies the T cell-restricted expression of *IL-2*. Therefore, T cell-specific expression of IL-2 may be mediated by a yet unidentified single factor or by the precise temporal and spatial combination of proteins at the transcription complex.

Although the 300-bp promoter/enhancer region is sufficient for *IL-2* transcription in vitro, evidence for additional regulatory regions is suggested by the inability to generate transgenic mice without including at least 600 bp of the *IL-2* promoter driving a reporter gene *(11)*. In addition, early DNase I hypersensitivity (HS) studies defined sites outside of this region *(20)*. DNase I HS sites are markers for alterations in chromatin structure and generally uncover important regulatory regions. Additional footprinting and DNase I HS studies have provided evidence for T cell-specific HS sites between –600

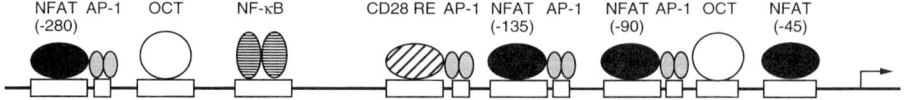

Fig. 1. The *IL-2* promoter. Adapted with permission from ref. *14*.

and –300 bp upstream of the transcriptional start site in resting T cells that increase in sensitivity on stimulation *(11,21)*. Additional HS sites between –400 and –300 bp are also revealed upon activation *(21)*. It will be important to determine which proteins bind to these regions in vivo. Thus the T cell lineage specificity of the *IL-2* locus may lie outside of the minimal promoter/enhancer region and influence chromatin accessibility and remodeling. Contact between distal and proximal regions of the promoter may occur to facilitate these processes.

Recent studies on *IL-2* gene regulation have generated interest in the unexpected possibility that *IL-2* transcription from a single cell may be monoallelic. Hollander et al. have reported that the *IL-2* gene appeared to be transcribed from a single, randomly chosen allele in the Th cell *(22)*. In contrast, other groups, using transgenic models with green fluorescent protein (GFP) "knocked in" at the *IL-2* locus or bearing a transgene that couples the murine *IL-2* promoter to a GFP reporter and the human *CD2* locus control regions, do not observe this *(23,24)*. These discrepancies may reflect alterations of regulatory regions in the transgenic systems. However, in the monoallelic studies, individual cells were analyzed early after activation and in limited numbers *(22)*. Therefore, early activation may lead to monoallelic expression of *IL-2* with biallelic expression occurring at later time points. This issue thus requires further study to be resolved. Moreover, the significance of monoallelic expression of cytokine genes in Th development remains to be elucidated, as will be discussed with respect to *IL-4* in Subheading 4.1.

3.2. IL-4

The production of *IL-4* is tightly regulated and expressed in only a subset of immune cells: αβ T cells, mast cells, natural killer (NK) T cells, γδ T cells, basophils, and eosinophils *(4)*. In this section, we describe what is known about the regulation of IL-4 in Th cells. Naive Thp cells transcribe detectable amounts of *IL-4* mRNA by 24 h following stimulation via the TCR; the levels peak at 48 h before declining *(25)*. In order to define the molecular basis for the inducible and Th2-specific expression of IL-4, several groups investigated the promoter region of the *IL-4* gene. The

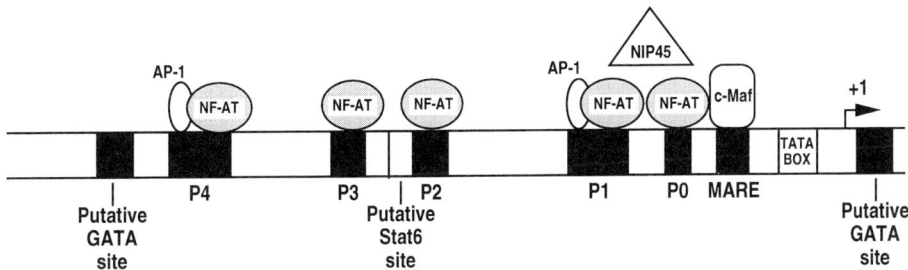

Fig. 2. The *IL-4* promoter. Adapted with permission from ref. *29.*

activity of the *IL-4* promoter is stimulated by phorbol esters and Ca^{2+} iono-phores (mimicking TCR-mediated activation) and inhibited by CsA *(26).*

Deletions of the murine *IL-4* 5' sequence in transient transfection assays delineated sequences within 87 bp of the transcription initiation site as sufficient for cell-specific and activation-dependent transcription in vitro *(27,28).* Extensive mutational analyses by many investigators have identified five sites, P0 through P4, within the proximal promoter, that are critical for inducible *IL-4* expression (reviewed in *29,30*) (Fig. 2). NFAT proteins were shown to bind to these sequences and mutations in each of these sites severely compromised promoter activity in vitro *(26,27,31,32).* P1 and P4 comprise composite NFAT/AP-1 sites to which AP-1 proteins such as Fra-1, Fra-2, JunB, and JunD bind in an NFAT-dependent manner *(33,34).* Although NFAT and AP-1 family proteins are important for inducible IL-4 transcription, they are functionally active in both Th1 and Th2 subsets and do not appear to account for the Th2-restricted expression of IL-4 *(32).*

The in vivo role for NFAT transcription factors in IL-4 transcription, however, appears to be more complex than was evident from in vitro experiments, which do not discern the precise physiologic functions of the three lymphoid-specific family members: NFATc1 (NFATc, NFAT2), NFATc2 (NFATp, NFAT1), and NFATc3 (NFAT4). Mice bearing a targeted disruption of the *NFATc2* gene have increased Th2 cytokines in the later phase of the immune response, whereas NFATc3-deficient mice do not display defects in cytokine production *(35–37).* Mice lacking both *NFATc2* and *NFATc3* have extremely high levels of IL-4 and other Th2 cytokines and highly elevated IgE titers *(38).* In contrast, RAG 2–/– mice reconstituted with *NFATc1* -deficient lymphoid cells, show a decrease in IL-4 levels *(39).* Thus, *NFATc 2* and *NFATc3* can exert a negative regulatory role in IL-4 expression whereas *NFATc1* is apparently a positive transactivator of the *IL-4* gene.

Whether this is directly at the level of transcription or indirect via the regulation of additional target genes in the IL-4 signaling pathway is still unknown. Thus, a balance between the different NFAT family members appears to be crucial in vivo. Specific combinations of NFAT proteins may control *IL-4* expression at multiple stages during Th2 differentiation.

3.2.1. Tissue-Specific Regulation of IL-4: c-maf and GATA3

The identification of transcription factors restricted to the Th2 subset was a substantial advance towards understanding Th2-specific expression of IL-4. The first such factor to be described was by Ho et al. who observed that the proto-oncogene c-maf was selectively upregulated, upon activation via the TCR, during the course of Th2 but not Th1 differentiation in vitro *(40)*. c-maf is a b-zip transcription factor belonging to the Maf subfamily of the AP-1 protein family and recognizes a Maf response element (MARE). A half MARE site is present in the *IL-4* promoter, adjacent to the P0 site, to which recombinant c-maf protein can bind *(40)*. c-maf strongly transactivates the *IL-4* promoter in vitro and synergizes with NFATc2 *(40)*. Enforced expression of c-maf, NFATc2 and the NFAT-interacting protein 45 (NIP45), can elicit endogenous IL-4 production in M12 B cell lymphoma cells, which do not normally produce IL-4 *(41)*. c-maf is specific for *IL-4* transcription and does not transactivate the *IL-5* and *IL-10* promoters *(42)*. Further, CD4+ T cells from mice lacking c-maf are deficient in IL-4 production and Th2 differentiation and can produce normal levels of IL-5, IL-10, and IL-13 when provided with exogenous IL-4 *(42)*. Thus, c-maf is critical for the high levels of *IL-4* transcription required for Th2 differentiation. Consistent with the aforementioned results, overexpression of c-maf in vivo resulted in preferential Th2 responses *(43)*. Th1 cells derived from c-maf transgenic mice were not, however, able to transcribe *IL-4 (43)*. Therefore, additional Th2-specific transcription factors are likely required for the initiation of IL-4-specific transcriptional events. In addition, Th1-specific factors may serve to repress *IL-4* transcription in Th1 cells. Interestingly, a silencer element has been characterized in transient transfection assays that functions only in Th1 cells *(44)*. Characterizing the molecular mechanism underlying the Th2-restricted expression of c-maf will be important in the further elucidation of tissue-specific IL-4 transcription.

A transcription factor that appears to have a more global role in controlling Th2 cytokine transcription is GATA3. GATA3 was isolated as a zinc-finger protein that binds the *TCR* -α gene enhancer via a WGATAR sequence *(45)*. Mice deficient for *GATA3* are embryonic lethal and the generation of *GATA3* -/- chimeras established its essential role in T cell development *(46,47)*. GATA3 was recently shown to be induced in developing Th2 cells and absent from Th1 cells *(48,49)*. Putative binding sites for GATA3 are present in the proximal promoter of *IL-4* . The ability of GATA3 to directly bind and transactivate the *IL-4* promoter via these sites, however, is not firmly established *(48,50)*. Genomic regions in the *IL-4/IL -13* locus containing consensus and nonconsensus GATA3 elements have been identified that significantly increase transactivation of the *IL-4* promoter by GATA3 *(50)*. Thus, GATA3 may function as an enhancer binding factor. Overexpression of GATA3 in vivo was reported to increase *IL-4* , *IL-5* , *IL-10* , and *IL-13* mRNA levels *(48)*. Transgenic mice expressing a dominant-negative form of GATA3 displayed significantly reduced levels of IL-4, IL-5, and IL-13, thereby implicating this factor in the regulation of all the Th2 cytokines *(51)*. GATA3 appears to play a more direct role in controlling IL-5 expression. It can activate endogenous IL-5 via a cAMP-dependent pathway in M12 cells *(52)*. Retroviral transduction of GATA3 into developing Th cells induced high levels of IL-5 but only low amounts of IL-4 (53). Importantly, GATA3 transduction into developing Th1, but not effector Th1 cells, resulted in repression of Th1 development and IFN-γ production, probably by repressing IL-12Rβ2 expression *(53)*. Thus, GATA3 appears to play an important role in balancing the generation of Th1 vs Th2 cytokines.

3.2.2. Stat6 and Bcl6

The transcription factor Stat6 (Signal Transducer and Activator of Transcription 6) is activated specifically by ligation of the IL-4 receptor by IL-4. Stat6 activation is required for Th2 differentiation as seen by the inability of Stat6-deficient lymphocytes to differentiate into Th2 cells *(54–56)*. It is not clear whether Stat6 has a direct role in *IL-4* transcription. Multimerization of a putative Stat6 site from the *IL-4* promoter led to a modest activation of the reporter construct by Stat6 in vitro *(25)*. The induction of GATA3 in Th2 cells appears to be dependent on Stat6 activation but this may be indirect *(53)*. Ectopic expression of activated Stat6 into developing Th1 cells induces c-maf and GATA3 leading to Th2-specific cytokine expression *(57)*. Bcl6, a transcriptional repressor, has been shown to negatively regulate Stat6 activity by competing for the Stat6 binding sites *(58)*. Consistent with these in vitro observations, mice lacking Bcl6 have increased levels of Th2 cytokines *(58)*. Mice doubly-deficient in Stat6 and Bcl6, however, continue to produce increased Th2 cytokines, revealing a Stat6-independent pathway for Th2 differentiation *(59)*. Supporting this, it was observed that Stat6-deficient mice contained a small number of IL-4-producing cells and that GATA3 expression was upregulated in these cells. These results suggest that IL-4 production can be independent of Stat6 *(60)*. In summary, although

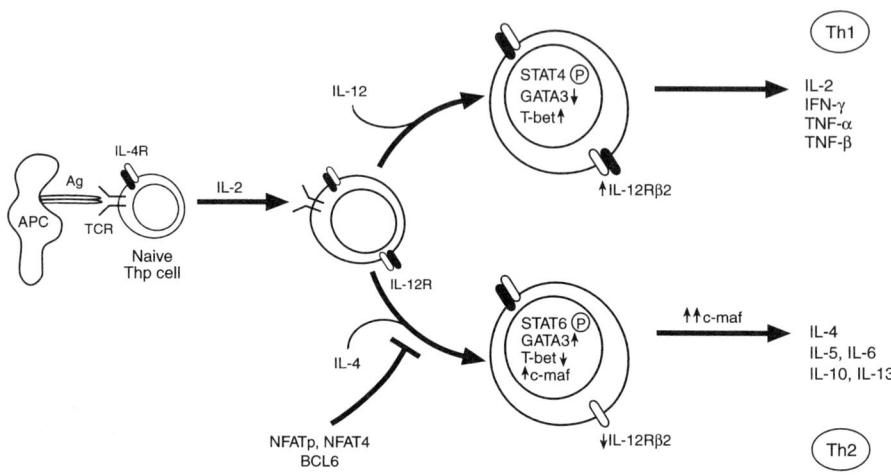

Fig. 3. Model of transcriptional regulation of T helper cell differentiation. A naive T helper cell precursor (Thp) is activated via the T cell receptor (TCR) when it encounters antigen (Ag) presented by an antigen-presenting cell (APC). The IL-4 receptor (IL-4R) is expressed on its cell surface at this stage. Upon activation, the Thp starts to proliferate and secrete IL-2 and and expresses the IL-12 receptor (IL-12R). On encountering IL-12 secreted by macrophages, a Th1 differentiation program is initiated. The IL-12Rβ2 chain is upregulated in the developing Th1 cell and ligation of the IL-12R by IL-12 leads to the activation of Stat4. Upregulation of T-bet and downregulation of GATA3 expression, which may be accompanied by chromatin remodeling of the IFN-γ locus, leads to IFN-γ production and Th1 differentiation. IL-4 produced intrinsically by the Thp and extrinsically by several cell types (*see* text) induces differentiation into the Th2 subset and downregulation of IL-12Rβ2 expression. Ligation of the IL-4R by IL-4 activates Stat6. This leads to the upregulation of GATA3, which may facilitate the transcription of IL-4 and other Th2 cytokines by remodeling the IL-4 locus, and perhaps other Th2 cytokine gene loci. The concomitant decrease in T-bet expression followed by high levels of c-maf expression lead to increased transcription of IL-4 and Th2 differentiation. NFAT/AP-1 and other transcription factors can then access their specific binding sites. Combinatorial interactions between the various factors thus promotes rapid transcription of Th1/Th2 cytokines upon restimulation.

Stat6 and Bcl6 clearly play important roles in Th2 differentiation, their direct effects on *IL-4* transcription remain poorly understood.

To summarize the role of transcription factors in Th2 differentiation, let us consider the following scenario (Fig. 3). A naive precursor Th cell is induced to differentiate along a Th2 pathway following signals delivered through the TCR and the production of IL-4 from extrinsic sources as well as from the Th cell itself. Activation of Stat6 induces GATA3 in the developing Th2 cell with the concomitant downregulation of the IL-12Rβ2 chain. The induction of c-maf by TCR signaling greatly augments the production of IL-4. The synergy of c-maf with NFAT and proteins like NIP45 leads to the establishment of the Th2 phenotype. We will further develop this model in Subheading 4.1. to incorporate the role of chromatin structure in cytokine regulation.

3.3. IFN-γ

IFN- γ expression is restricted to Th1 cells, CD8[+] cells, and NK cells and is upregulated by 24 h after stimulation of naïve cells *(25)*. Much less is known about the *cis-* and *trans*-acting elements required for tissue-specific regulation of *IFN* -γ compared to *IL-2* and *IL-4* . Early studies designated 8.6 kb as conferring T-cell-specific expression *(78)*. The Th1-specific regions within this sequence have not yet been delineated. Reporter constructs that contain 3 kb or 500 bp of upstream sequence are active in both Th1 and Th2 subsets *(63)*. The 500-bp promoter is induced by phorbol ester and ionomycin and is sensitive to CsA in vitro. Two essential regulatory elements were identified between –108 and –40 bp of the *IFN-γ* promoter that mirror the expression of the endogenous gene *(64)* (Fig. 4). Within this region, the distal element (–96 to 80 bp) contained a consensus GATA motif and GATA-3 was found to bind to this site in vitro *(64)*. The proximal regulatory element (–73 to –48 bp) when dimerized mimics inducibility and CsA sensitivity of *IFN-γ* in Jurkat T cells and in transgenic mice where it drives the expression of a luciferase reporter gene. In addition, this element was capable of binding CREB, ATF-1, ATF-2, c-jun, and Oct-1 proteins *(65)*. NF-κB proteins (c-Rel, p50, and p65) appear to bind to regions in the first intron of the *IFN-γ* gene and may cooperate with NFAT proteins, which may also recognize those sites *(66)*. Independent NFAT- binding sites have also been identified outside the proximal regulatory element and NFAT proteins transactivate and interact with these sites in vitro *(67,68)*. Ying-Yang 1 (YY1), can interact with a negative regulatory element and was thus thought to be a potential inhibitor of IFN-γ expression *(69)*. YY1 was, however, subsequently shown to also have a positive transactivating role by binding, in vitro, to an element between the two NFAT sites *(67)*. The transcription factors IRF-1 (Interferon Response Factor 1) and Stat4 have been implicated in Th1 differentiation. Mice deficient in each of these proteins fail to generate Th1 cells *(70–72)*. Recently, it has been demonstrated that IRF-1 may directly regulate transcription of the *IL-12* gene *(73)*. Thus these proteins likely function in the context of the IL-12 signaling pathway.

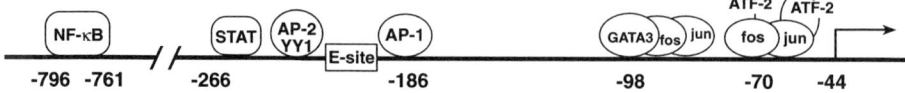

Fig. 4. The *IFN*-γ promoter.

3.3.1. Th1-Specific Transcription Factors

None of the aforementioned transcription factors explain the tissue-specificity of *IFN* -γ expression. Th1-restricted expression of IFN-γ may be, in part, attributable to Th1-restricted expression of transcription factors. The Ets family member, ERM, was reported to be expressed in Th1 but not in Th2 subsets. Its expression is induced by IL-12 in a Stat4-dependent manner but does not directly affect the production of Th1 cytokines *(74)*. *Egr3* is an early growth-response gene that is preferentially expressed in Th1 cells and controls the expression of FasL; its role in *IFN* -γ transcription is unknown *(75)*. A novel transcription factor, T-bet, has been recently isolated that plays an important role in *IFN* -γ expression and Th1 lineage commitment *(76)*.

T-bet (T-box expressed in T cells) is a member of the T-box family of transcription factors that regulate several developmental processes. The expression of T-bet strongly correlates with *IFN* -γ expression in Th1 and NK cells and when overexpressed in vitro, can significantly transactivate the *IFN* -γ promoter *(76)*. Putative binding sites for T-bet exist within the *IFN* -γ gene, but it is not yet known whether T-bet can bind to these sites. Thus, whether T-bet acts directly to transactivate the *IFN* -γ promoter or indirectly via the induction of other genes, remains an area of investigation. Nevertheless, T-bet clearly has a profound role in regulating IFN-γ production. Retroviral transduction of T-bet into primary, developing, and fully polarized Th2 cells induces IFN-γ secretion and represses IL-4 and IL-5 production *(76)*. This occurs even in the absence of IFN-γ receptor signaling *(76)*. Thus, T-bet appears to both initiate Th1 development as well as repress Th2 differentiation.

Understanding the molecular basis for T-bet function will be critical for the elucidation of *IFN*-γ transcription and Th1 development. Szabo et al. have proposed that T-bet may initiate IFN-γ production and repress the Th2 developmental program by inhibiting the expression of *GATA3*, while GATA3 may repress T-bet expression during Th2 development *(76)*. The relative predominance of T-bet and GATA3 may serve to control the fate of naive Th-cell commitment to specific subsets.

4. ROLE OF CHROMATIN AND EPIGENETIC CONTROL OF CYTOKINE TRANSCRIPTION

Genomic DNA is assembled into nucleosomes, which can form higher-order chromatin structures. Many cytokine genes including *IL-2* , *IL-4* , *IL-12* , *IL-13* , *IFN -γ*, and granulocyte-monocyte colony-stimulating factor (*GM-CSF*) are known to undergo regulated changes in chromatin structure. It has been proposed that these structures must be altered before transcription factors and RNA polymerase can access promoter regions. Distant control regions (e.g., enhancers, LCRs) may regulate accessibility to gene loci by regulating chromatin structure *(9)*.

Many such regulatory regions have been identified in cytokine genes using DNase I hypersensitivity assays, which provide a rough estimate of gene accessibility. Transcriptionally active chromatin is more accessible to nucleases like DNase I. Nucleosomal DNA is generally less accessible to to *trans*-acting factors. Thus, hypersensitivity to DNase I indicates that the region of DNA is free of nucleosomes, or that it is assembled into nucleosomes with remodeled structures *(77)*. DNase I HS assays have provided valuable information regarding long-range regulation of several cytokine genes *(78,79)*.

Changes in chromatin architecture can often be attributed to the activities of modifying enzymes (reviewed in *ref. 77*). The acetylation of histones by acetylases is known to facilitate access of *trans*-acting factors to DNA and is associated with transcriptionally active chromatin. Inactive genes appear to be hypoacetylated and the activity of histone deacetylases often correlates with repression. CpG methylation of genetic loci often corresponds to inactive chromatin regions. Demethylation of DNA during differentiation can parallel remodeling of chromatin leading to gene activation. The remodeling of chromatin is also reflected by changes in nucleosomal positioning. The regularity of the nucleosomal array can be disrupted by the binding of transcription factors in a manner that is dependent on the utilization of ATP.

We will summarize what is known about the role of chromatin remodeling in the regulation of the *IL-4* and *IFN-γ* loci, with emphasis on the *IL-4* gene.

4.1. Regulation of the IL-4 and IFN-γ Loci

IL-4 is tightly regulated during the development of a T helper cell. Multiple-transcription factors and associated proteins must be assembled in a cooperative manner leading to high levels of *IL-4* expression. Upon differentiating into a Th2 cell, an effector cell expresses *IL-4* more rapidly and at higher levels than a naive Th cell. Thus, the inefficiency of cytokine production in naive cells compared to effector cells appears to constitute a rate-limiting step in transcription (reviewed in *ref. 80*). Furthermore, activation of Th2 cells leads to a greater percentage of cells positive for IL-4, but the levels of IL-4 per cell appear to be the same *(81)*. These observations prompted several investigators to analyze the regulation of IL-4 at the level of chromatin structure. In addition, in vivo transgenic systems expressing varying lengths of the *IL-4* promoter suggested regulation of IL-4 beyond that of the promoter regions.

Transgenic models where segments of the *IL-4* promoter drive a reporter gene have shown that the proximal 800 bp of the promoter confer significant Th2-selective expression *(82)*. However, up to 3 kb of sequence are insufficient for transcription at levels equivalent to the endogenous *IL-4* gene, suggesting the necessity for additional elements for optimal expression *(26)*.

4.1.1. Evidence for Chromatin Remodeling

Changes in chromatin organization of regions within the *IL-4* locus were assessed by DNase I hypersensitivity assays and were shown to occur by 48 h following stimulation of naive T helper cells, implicating these regions in important regulatory functions *(83)*. These changes occurred during Th2 differentiation and were dependent on IL-4 and Stat6 *(83)*. Subsquently, it has been observed that GATA3 may induce the same changes when transduced into Stat6-deficient cells, indicating that GATA3 can induce remodeling at the *IL-4* locus downstream of Stat6 *(60)*. Decreased CpG methylation at the *IL-4* locus has been observed during Th2 but not Th1 differentiation *(84)*. Interestingly, when treated with trichostatin A and 5-azacytidine (histone deacetylase and methylase inhibitors respectively), naive cells display more rapid kinetics of IL-4 production *(84)*. Thus, alterations in chromatin components at the *IL-4* locus during T helper differentiation may contribute to the establishment of the Th2 phenotype.

Why is the chromatin configuration of the *IL-4* gene different in Th2 cells compared to Th1? (*see* Fig. 3) It has been proposed that Th2-specific transcription factors like c-maf and GATA3 may effect locus accessibility to TCR-induced factors by directly remodeling chromatin structure or indirectly, by recruiting modifying enzymes and necessary proteins *(79,83)*. Th1 cells do not express c-maf and GATA3 and would thus maintain a nonpermissive chromatin structure. The accessible chromatin environment created during Th2 differentiation could function to allow transcription factors like NFAT, which are induced on restimulation, to access their specific binding sites in the *IL-4* locus and promote rapid transcription of *IL-4* *(83)*. Complementary to this model, NFAT proteins may also alter chromatin configuration. Mice deficient in NFATc2 and NFATc3 show preferential Th2 differentiation and a highly allergic phenotype *(38)*. It is possible that NFAT proteins in combination with other proteins, may regulate the balance between the active/inactive state of the *IL-4/IL-5/IL-13* locus during the initiation of Th2 differentiation (Fig. 3). Controlling the levels of cytokine expression would be important for avoiding the deleterious effects of overproduction of Th2 cytokines.

Similar mechanisms may apply to the regulation of the *IFN*-γ gene. Although information regarding the *IFN*-γ locus is less detailed than that for the *IL-4* locus, DNase I HS regions have been identified in the first and third introns of the *IFN*-γ gene *(63,83)*. Several studies have analyzed methylation patterns of the *IFN*-γ locus during differentiation of T cells. Hypomethylation of the *IFN*-γ gene occurs in cells that transcribe IFN-γ, like Th1 cells and CD8⁺ cells *(63,85)*. The same locus is methylated in Th2 cytokine-expressing cells. The demethylation of the *IFN*-γ locus appears to be a stable, long term, inheritable trait *(85)*. DNase I HS assays have also provided evidence for alterations of the *IFN*-γ locus in naive Th1 cells compared to Th2 cells *(83)*. Transcription factors may cooperate to transcribe the *IFN*-γ gene through combinatorial interactions that affect chromatin structure. The assembly of Th1-specific transcription factors may maintain the chromatin in a configuration that allows other transcription factors necessary for IFN-γ transcription to bind. It will be interesting to determine whether T-bet is involved in the remodeling of the *IFN*-γ locus during Th1 differentiation.

4.1.2. DNA Replication and Monoallelic Expression

DNA replication may be necessary for remodeling the *IL-4* and *IFN*-γ genes. Naive cells were reported by Bird et al. to require three cell divisions before producing IL-4 in vitro, while Richter et al. observe in their system that entry into the S phase is required in order for cells to express IL-4 upon restimulation *(84,86)*. Both results, however, point to a role for cell division in the initiation and maintenance of *IL-4* gene transcription. The expression of IFN-γ also appears to be dependent on the cell cycle. CD4⁺ cells undergoing cell division require entry into the S phase before expressing IFN-γ *(84,86)*. It is important to note that chromatin remodeling can also occur rapidly, before entry into S phase. Thus, although changes in chromatin structure may be involved in regulating cytokine expression during cell division, several other mechanisms may also operate. One such possibility is the availability of appropriate transcription factors at specific stages of the cell cycle, which are required for the expression of IL-4 and IFN-γ. Whatever the process, if the cytokine phenotype is indeed fixed in a differentiated effector cell, this offers an attractive mechanism for rapid recall of cytokine production in response to antigenic restimulation.

Several studies have suggested that in the absence of selective pressure, cytokine expression is stochastic *(87)*. To examine allelic patterns of *IL-4* gene expression, Bix and Locksley analyzed the parental origin of *IL-4* transcripts in F1 mice by exploiting the existence of a polymorphism at the *IL-4* locus in the two parental strains *(87)*. The clones generated separated into those that expressed IL-4 biallelically or monoallelically and these states were maintained over time as an epigenetic heritable trait *(87)*. Riviere et al. derived CD4$^+$ cell lines from mice that had the human CD2 "knocked in" to the *IL-4* locus and found that a majority of the lines expressed IL-4 monoallelically *(88)*. The frequency of biallelic expression however increased with increasing strength of signal through the TCR *(88)*. The chromosomal location of *IL-4* is adjacent to two other Th2 cytokine genes *IL-5* and *IL-13*. It has been suggested that these genes may be regulated in a coordinate manner via a common enhancer or LCR *(78,83)*. It will be of interest to determine whether IL-5 and IL-13 are also regulated by the activation of a single allele.

The molecular mechanisms for such transcriptional regulation remain to be defined. Meanwhile, the physiological relevance of independent transcription of alleles is not evident. Aside from genes that are subject to dosage compensation, very few studies of single chromosomal expression exist. Thus, it is not clear whether the occurrence of monoallelic expression in cytokine genes is an important regulatory mechanism. It has been postulated that monoallelic activation may serve to control the levels of cytokines produced and that biallelic expression may serve as a marker of terminal differentiation to regulate the cessation of cytokine production *(87,88)*. It will be interesting to uncover whether stochastic regulation of cytokine gene expression and its proposed benefits, will constitute an exception rather than the rule.

4.1.3. Importance of Chromatin Remodeling of Cytokine Genes

Transcriptional regulation of cytokine gene expression by chromatin remodeling may provide a basis for regulation at the following levels:

1. *Accessibility:* Tissue-specific activators and repressors can recruit chromatin-modifying enzymes that alter the methylation state of DNA and/or the acetylation state of histones and confer specificity to the transcriptional process.
2. *Communication:* The long-range propagation of active chromatin domains or chromatin modifying activity between regulatory elements separated by long distances from the promoter may facilitate complex interactions.
3. *Epigenetic imprinting:* The chromatin remodeling activities and stability of multiple cooperative interactions may translate into an imprinting of a genetic locus leading to an epigenetic memory for maintenance of the differentiated state.

5. CONCLUSIONS

The identification of promoter elements and transcription factors over the past few years has greatly enhanced our understanding of cytokine gene transcription. Combinatorial networks of nonsubset-specific and tissue-restricted transcription factors harness associated proteins and cofactors in the context of chromatin structure to regulate the expression of cytokine genes. Transcriptional control is finely tuned at multiple levels to accommodate the stage and immunological context in which cytokines need to be activated during the course of an immune response. The development of naive T helper cells into Th1 and Th2 subsets has provided an excellent basis for studying transcriptional regulation within a biological context. We are now poised to apply these concepts to other cells of the immune system and to take advantage of the emerging paradigms and technical advances from the field of transcriptional regulation to investigate more detailed molecular processes. The incorporation of positive and negative signals from the T cell surface into complex signaling pathways leading to cytokine transcription in the nucleus is a dynamic process that offers many challenges for further experimentation.

REFERENCES

1. Mosmann, T. R., Cherwinski, H., Bond, M. W., Giedlin, M. A., and Coffman, R. L. (1986) Two types of murine helper T cell clone. I. Definition according to profiles of lymphokine activities and secreted proteins. *J. Immunol.* **136,** 2348–2357.
2. Paul, W. E. and Seder, R. A. (1994) Lymphocyte responses and cytokines. *Cell* **76,** 241–251.
3. Mosmann, T. R. and Sad, S. (1996) The expanding universe of T-cell subsets: Th1, Th2 and more. *Immunol. Today* **17,** 138–146.
4. Abbas, A. K., Murphy, K. M., and Sher, A. (1996) Functional diversity of helper T lymphocytes [Review]. *Nature* **383,** 787–793.
5. O'Garra, A. (1998) Cytokines induce the development of functionally heterogeneous T helper cell subsets. *Immunity* **8,** 275–283.
6. Constant, S. and Bottomly, K. (1997) Induction of Th1 and Th2 CD4+ T cell responses: the alternative approaches. *Annu. Rev. Immunol.* **15,** 297–322.
7. Carey, M. (1998) The enhanceosome and transcriptional synergy. *Cell* **92,** 5–8.
8. Fry, C. J. and Farnham, P. J. (1999) Context-dependent transcriptional regulation. *J. Biol. Chem.* **274,** 29,583–29,586.
9. Ernst, P. and Smale, S. T. (1995) Combinatorial regulation of transcription I: general aspects of transcriptional control. *Immunity* **2,** 311–319.
10. Umlauf, S. W., Beverly, B., Lantz, O., and Schwartz, R. H. (1995) Regulation of interleukin 2 gene expression by CD28 costimulation in mouse T-cell clones:

both nuclear and cytoplasmic RNAs are regulated with complex kinetics. *Mol. Cell. Biol.* **15,** 3197–3205.

11. Rothenberg, E. V. and Ward, S. B. (1996) A dynamic assembly of diverse transcription factors integrates activation and cell-type information for interleukin 2 gene regulation. *Proc. Natl. Acad. Sci. USA* **93,** 9358–9365.

12. Jain, J., Loh, C., and Rao, A. (1995) Transcriptional regulation of the IL-2 gene. *Curr. Biol.* **7,** 333–342.

13. Emmel, E. A., Verweij, C. L., Durand, D. B., Higgins, K. M., Lacy, E., and Crabtree, G. R. (1989) Cyclosporin A specifically inhibits function of nuclear proteins involved in T cell activation. *Science* **246,** 1617–1620.

14. Rooney, J., Sun, Y-L., Glimcher, L. H., and Hoey, T. (1995) Novel NFAT sites that mediate activation of the interleukin-2 promoter in response to T-cell receptor stimulation. *Mol. Cell. Biol.* **15,** 6299–6310.

15. Shapiro, V. S., Truitt, K. E., Imboden, J. B., and Weiss, A. (1997) CD28 mediates transcriptional upregulation of the interleukin-2 (IL-2) promoter through a composite element containing the CD28RE and NF-IL-2B AP-1 sites. *Mol. Cell. Biol.* **17,** 4051–4058.

16. Maggirwar, S. B., Harhaj, E. W., and Sun, S. C. (1997) Regulation of the interleukin-2 CD28-responsive element by NF-ATp and various NF-κB/Rel transcription factors. *Mol. Cell. Biol.* **17,** 2605–2614.

17. Shapiro, V. S., Mollenauer, M. N., and Weiss, A. (1998) Nuclear factor of activated T cells and AP-1 are insufficient for IL-2 promoter activation: requirement for CD28 up-regulation of RE/AP. *J. Immunol.* **161,** 6455–6458.

18. Himes, S. R., Coles, L. S., Reeves, R., and Shannon, M. F. (1996) High mobility group protein I(Y) is required for function and for c-Rel binding to CD28 response elements within the GM-CSF and IL-2 promoters. *Immunity* **5,** 479–489.

19. Ghosh, P., Tan, T. H., Rice, N. R., Sica, A., and Young, H. A. (1993) The interleukin 2 CD28-responsive complex contains at least three members of the NF κB family: c-Rel, p50, and p65. *Proc. Natl. Acad. Sci. USA* **90,** 1696–1700.

20. Siebenlist, U., Durand, D. B., Bressler, P., Holbrook, N. J., Norris, C. A., Kamoun, M., et al. (1986) Promoter region of interleukin-2 gene undergoes chromatin structure changes and confers inducibility on chloramphenicol acetyltransferase gene during activation of T cells. *Mol. Cell Biol.* **6,** 3042–3049.

21. Ward, S. B., Hernandez-Hoyos, G., Chen, F., Waterman, M., Reeves, R., and Rothenberg, E. V. (1998) Chromatin remodeling of the interleukin-2 gene: distinct alterations in the proximal versus distal enhancer regions. *Nucleic Acid Res.* **26,** 2923–2934.

22. Hollander, G. A., Zuklys, S., Morel, C., Mizoguchi, E., Mobisson, K., Simpson, S., et al. (1998) Monoallelic expression of the interleukin-2 locus. *Science* **279,** 2118–2121.

23. Naramura, M., Hu, R. J., and Gu, H. (1998) Mice with a fluorescent marker for interleukin 2 gene activation. *Immunity* **9,** 209–216.

24. Saparov, A., Wagner, F. H., Zheng, R., Oliver, J. R., Maeda, H., Hockett, R. D., and Weaver, C. T. (1999) Interleukin-2 expression by a subpopulation of primary T cells is linked to enhanced memory/effector function. *Immunity* **11,** 271–280.

25. Lederer, J. A., Perez, V. L., DesRoches, L., Kim, S. M., Abbas, A. K., and Lichtman, A. H. (1996) Cytokine transcriptional events during helper T cell subset differentiation. *J. Exp. Med.* **184,** 397–406.
26. Todd, M. D., Grusby, M. J., Lederer, J. A., Lacy, E., Lichtman, A. H., and Glimcher, L. H. (1993) Transcription of the interleukin 4 gene is regulated by multiple promoter elements. *J. Exp. Med.* **177,** 1663–1674.
27. Szabo, S. J., Gold, J. S., Murphy, T. L., and Murphy, K. M. (1993) Identification of *cis*-acting regulatory elements controlling interleukin-4 gene expression in T cells: roles for NF-Y and NF-ATc. *Mol. Cell. Biol.* **13,** 4793–4805.
28. Bruhn, K. W., Nelms, K., Boulay, J-L., Paul, W. E., and Lenardo, M. J. (1993) Molecular dissection of the mouse interleukin-4 promoter. *Proc. Natl. Acad. Sci. USA* **90,** 9707–9711.
29. Szabo, S. J., Glimcher, L. H., and Ho, I. C. (1997) Genes that regulate interleukin-4 expression in T cells. *Curr. Opin. Immunol.* **9,** 776–781.
30. Brown, M. A. and Hural, J. (1997) Functions of IL-4 and control of its expression. *Crit. Rev. Immunol.* **17,** 1–32.
31. Chuvpilo, S., Schomberg, C., Gerwig, R., Heinfling, A., Reeves, R., Grummt, F., and Serfling, E. (1993) Multiple closely-linked NFAT/octamer and HMG I (Y) binding sites are part of the interleukin-4 promoter. *Nuc. Acid Res.* **21,** 5694–5704.
32. Rooney, J. W., Hodge, M. R., McCaffrey, P. G., Rao, A., and Glimcher, L. H. (1994) A common factor regulates both Th1- and Th2-specific cytokine gene expression. *EMBO J.* **13,** 625–633.
33. Rooney, J. W., Hoey, T., and Glimcher, L. H. (1995) Coordinate and cooperative roles for NF-AT and AP-1 in the regulation of the murine IL-4 gene. *Immunity* **2,** 545–553.
34. Hodge, M. J., Rooney, J. W., and Glimcher, L. H. (1995) The proximal promoter of the IL-4 gene is composed of multiple essential regulatory sites which bind at least two distinct factors. *J. Immunol.* **154,** 6397–6405.
35. Hodge, M. R., Ranger, A. M., Charles de la Brousse, F., Hoey, T., Grusby, M. J., and Glimcher, L. H. (1996) Hyperproliferation and dysregulation of IL-4 expression in NF-ATp-deficient mice. *Immunity* **4,** 1–20.
36. Xanthoudakis, S., Viola, J. P., Shaw, K. T., Luo, C., Wallace, J. D., Bozza, P. T., et al. (1996) An enhanced immune response in mice lacking the transcription factor NFAT1. *Science* **272,** 892–895.
37. Kiani, A., Viola, J. P. B., Lichtman, A. H., and Rao, A. (1997) Down-regulation of IL-4 gene transcription and control of Th2 cell differentiation by a mechanism involving NFAT1. *Immunity* **7,** 849–860.
38. Ranger, A. M., Oukka, M., Rengarajan, J., and Glimcher, L. H. (1998) Inhibitory function of two NFAT family members in lymphoid homeostasis and Th2 development. *Immunity* **9,** 627–635.
39. Ranger, A. M., Hodge, M. R., Gravallese, E. M., Oukka, M., Davidson, L., Alt, F. W., et al. (1998) Delayed lymphoid repopulation with defects in IL-4-driven responses produced by inactivation of NFATc. *Immunity* **8,** 125–134.
40. Ho, I-C., Hodge, M. R., Rooney, J. W., and Glimcher, L. H. (1996) The proto-oncogene c-maf is responsible for tissue-specific expression of interleukin-4. *Cell* **85,** 973–983.

41. Hodge, M. R., Chun, H. J., Rengarajan, J., Alt, A., Lieberson, R., and Glimcher, L. H. (1996) NFAT-driven interleukin-4 transcription potentiated by NIP45. *Science* **274**, 1903–1905.

42. Kim, J., Ho, I. C., Grusby, M., and Glimcher, L. H. (1999) The transcription factor c-maf controls the production of IL-4 but not other Th2 cytokines. *Immunity* **10**, 745–751.

43. Ho, I-C., Lo, D., and Glimcher, L. H. (1998) C-maf promotes Th2 and attenuates Th1 differentiation by both IL-4 dependent and independent mechanisms. *J. Exp. Med.* **188**, 1859–1866.

44. Kubo, M., Ransom, J., Webb, D., Hashimoto, Y., Tada, T., and Nakayama, T. (1997) T-cell subset-specific expression of the IL-4 gene is regulated by a silencer element and STAT6. *EMBO J.* **16**, 4007–4020.

45. Ho, I. C., Vorhees, P., Marin, N., Oakley, B. K., Tsai, S. F., Orkin, S. H., and Leiden, J. M. (1991) Human GATA-3: a lineage-restricted transcription factor that regulates the expression of the T cell receptor alpha gene. *EMBO J.* **10**, 1187–1192.

46. Ting, C. N., Olson, M. C., Barton, K. P., and Leiden, J. M. (1996) Transcription factor GATA-3 is required for development of the T-cell lineage. *Nature* **384**, 474–478.

47. Hattori, N., Kawamoto, H., Fujimoto, S., Kuno, K., and Katsura, Y. (1996) Involvement of transcription factors TCF-1 and GATA-3 in the initiation of the earliest step of T cell development in the thymus. *J. Exp. Med.* **184**, 1137–1147.

48. Zheng, W-P. and Flavell, R. A. (1997) The transcription factor GATA-3 is necessary and sufficient for Th2 cytokine gene expression in CD4 T cells. *Cell* **89**, 587–596.

49. Zhang, D. H., Cohn, L., Ray, P., Bottomly, K., and Ray, A. (1997) Transcription factor GATA-3 is differentially expressed in murine Th1 and Th2 cells and controls Th2-specific expression of the interleukin-5 gene. *J. Biol. Chem.* **272**, 21,597–21,603.

50. Ranganath, S., Ouyang, W., Bhattarcharya, D., Sha, W. C., Grupe, A., Peltz, G., and Murphy, K. M. (1998) Cutting Edge: GATA-3-Dependent Enhancer Activity in IL-4 Gene Regulation. *J. Immunol.* **161**, 3822–3826.

51. Zhang, D. -H, Yang, L., Cohn, L., Parkyn, L., Homer, R., Ray, P., and Ray, A. (1999) Inhibition of allergic inflammation in a murine model of asthma by expression of a dominant-negative mutant of GATA-3. *Immunity* **11**, 473–482.

52. Zhang, D. H., Yang, L., and Ray, A. (1998) Cutting edge: differential responsiveness of the IL-5 and IL-4 genes to transcription factor GATA-3. *J. Immunol.* **161**, 3817–3821.

53. Ouyang, W., Ranganath, S. H., Weindel, K., Bhattacharya, D., Murphy, T. L., Sha, W. C., and Murphy, K. M. (1998) Inhibition of Th1 developmental mediated by GATA-3 through an IL-4 independent mechanism. *Immunity* **9**, 745–755.

54. Kaplan, M. H., Schindler, U., Smiley, S. T., and Grusby, M. J. (1996) Stat6 is required for mediating responses to IL-4 and for the development of Th2 cells. *Immunity* **4**, 313–319.

55. Shimoda, K., van Deursen, J., Sangster, M. Y., Sarawar, S. R., Carson, R. T., Tripp, R. A., et al. (1996) Lack of IL-4-induced Th2 response and IgE class switching in mice with disrupted Stat6 gene. *Nature* **380,** 630–633.

56. Takeda, K., Tanaka, T., Shi, W., Matsumoto, M., Minami, M., Kashiwamura, S., et al. (1996) Essential role of Stat6 in IL-4 signalling. *Nature* **380,** 627–630.

57. Kurata, H., Lee, H. J., O'Garra, A., and Arai, N. (1999) Ectopic Expression of Activated Stat6 Induces the Expression of Th2-Specific Cytokines and Transcription Factors in Developing Th1 Cells. *Immunity* **11,** 677–688.

58. Dent, A. L., Shaffer, A. L., Yu, X., Allman, D., and Staudt, L. M. (1997) Control of inflammation, cytokine expression, and germinal center formation by BCL-6. *Science* **276,** 589–592.

59. Dent, A. L., Hu-Li, J., Paul, W. E., and Staudt, L. M. (1998) T helper type 2 inflammatory disease in the absence of interleukin 4 and transcription factor STAT6. *Proc. Natl. Acad. Sci. USA* **95,** 13,823–13,828.

60. Ouyang, W., Lohning, M., Gao, Z., Assenmacher, M., Ranganath, S., Radbruch, A., and Murphy, K. M. (2000) Stat6-independent GATA-3 autoactivation directs IL-4-independent Th2 development and commitment. *Immunity* **12,** 27–37.

61. Hardy, K. J., Pererlin, B. M., Atchison, R. E., and Stobo, J. D. (1985) Regulation of expression of the human interferon γ gene. *Immunology* **82,** 8173–8177.

62. Hardy, K. J., Manger, B., Newton, M., and Stobo, J. D. (1987) Molecular events involved in regulating human interferon-γ gene expression during T cell activation. *J. of Immuno.* **138,** 2353–2358.

63. Young, H. A., Ghosh, P., Ye, J., Lederer, J., Lichtman, A., Gerard, J. R., et al. (1994) Differentiation of the T helper phenotypes by analysis of methylation state of the IFN-γ gene. *J. Immunol.* **153,** 3603–3610.

64. Penix, L., Weaver, W. M., Pang, Y., Young, H. A., and Wilson, C. B. (1993) Two essential regulatory elements in the human interferon γ promoter confer activation specific expression in T cells. *J. Exp. Med.* **178,** 1483–1496.

65. Penix, L. A., Sweetser, M. T., Weaver, W. M., Hoeffler, J. P., Kerppola, T. K., and Wilson, C. B. (1996) The proximal regulatory element of the interferon-γ promoter mediates selective expression in T cells. *J. Biol. Chem.* **271,** 31,964–31,972.

66. Sica, A., Dorman, L., Viggiano, V., Cippitelli, M., Ghosh, P., Rice, N., and Young, H. A. (1997) Interaction of NF-κB and NFAT with the interferon-γ promoter. *J. Biol. Chem.* **272,** 30,412–30,420.

67. Sweetser, M. T., Hoey, T., Sun, Y. L., Weaver, W. M., Price, G. A., and Wilson, C. B. (1998) The roles of nuclear factor of activated T cells and Ying-Yang 1 in activation-induced expression of the interferon-γ promoter in T cells. *J. Biol. Chem.* **273,** 34,775–34,783.

68. Campbell, P. M., Pimm, J., Ramassar, V., and Haloran, P. F. (1996) Identification of a calcium-inducible, cyclosporine sensitive element in the IFN-gamma promoter that is a potential NFAT binding site. *Transplantation* **61,** 933.

69. Ye, J., Cippitelli, M., Dorman, L., Ortaldo, J. R., and Young, H. A. (1996) The nuclear factor YY1 suppresses the human gamma interferon promoter through

two mechanisms: inhibition of AP1 binding and activation of a silencer element. *Mol. Cell. Biol.* **16,** 4744–4753.

70. Thierfelder, W. E., van Deursen, J. M., Yamamoto, K., Tripp, R. A., Sarawar, S. R., Carson, R. T., et al. (1996) Requirement for Stat4 in interleukin-12-mediated responses of natural killer and T cells. *Nature* **382,** 171–174.

71. Lohoff, M., Ferrick, D., Mittrucker, H. W., Duncan, G. S., Bischof, S., Rollinghoff, M., and Mak, T. W. (1997) Interferon regulatory factor-1 is required for a T helper 1 immune response in vivo. *Immunity* **6(6),** 681–689.

72. Kaplan, M. H., Sun, Y. L., Hoey, T., and Grusby, M. J. (1996) Impaired IL-12 responses and enhanced development of Th2 cells in Stat4-deficient mice. *Nature* **382,** 174–177.

73. Coccia, E. M., Passini, N., Battistini, A., Pini, C., Sinigaglia, F., and Rogge, L. (1999) Interleukin-12 induces expression of interferon regulatory factor-1 via signal transducer and activator of transcription-4 in human T helper type 1 cells. *J. Biol. Chem.* **274,** 6698.

74. Ouyang, W., Jacobson, N. G., Bhattacharya, D., Gorham, J. D., Fenoglio, D., Sha, W. C., et al. (1999) The Ets transcription factor ERM is Th1-specific and induced by IL-12 through a Stat4-dependent pathway. *Proc. Natl. Acad. Sci. USA* **96,** 3888–3893.

75. Rengarajan, J. R., Mittelstadt, P. R., Mages, H. W., Gerth, A. J., Kroczek, R. A., Ashwell, J. D., and Glimcher, L. H. (2000) Sequential involvement of NFAT and Egr transcription factors in FasL regulation. *Immunity* **12,** 293–300.

76. Szabo, S. J., Kim, S. T., Costa, G. L., Zhang, X., Fathman, C. G., and Glimcher, L. H. (2000) A novel transcription factor T-bet, directs Th1 lineage commitment. *Cell* **100,** 655–669.

77. Kadonaga, J. T. (1998) Eukaryotic transcription: an interlaced network of transcription factors and chromatin-modifying machines. *Cell* **92,** 307–313.

78. Agarwal, S. and Rao, A. (1998) Long-range transcriptional regulation of cytokine gene expression. *Curr. Opin. Immunol.* **10,** 345–352.

79. Agarwal, S., Viola, J. P. B., and Rao, A. (1999) Chromatin-based regulatory mechanisms governing cytokine gene transcription. *J. Allergy Clin. Immunol.* **103,** 990–999.

80. Reiner, S. L. and Seder, R. A. (1999) Dealing from the evolutionary pawnshop: how lymphocytes make decisions. *Immunity* **11,** 1–10.

81. Bucy, R. P., Panoskaltsis-Mortari, A., Huang, G. Q., Li, J., Karr, L., Ross, M., et al. (1994) Heterogeneity of single cell cytokine gene expression in clonal T cell populations. *J. Exp. Med.* **180,** 1251–1262.

82. Wenner, C. A., Szabo, S. J., and Murphy, K. M. (1997) Identification of IL-4 promoter elements conferring Th2-restricted expression during T helper cell subset development. *J. Immunol.* **158,** 765–773.

83. Agarwal, S. and Rao, A. (1998) Modulation of chromatin structure regulates cytokine gene expression during T cell differentiation. *Immunity* **9,** 765–775.

84. Bird, J. J., Brown, D. R., Mullen, A. C., Moskowitz, N. H., Mahowald, M. A., Sider, J. R., et al. (1998) Helper T cell differentiation is controlled by the cell cycle. *Immunity* **9,** 229–237.

85. Fitzpatrick, D. R., Shirley, K. M., and Kelso, A. (1999) Stable epigenetic inheritance of regional IFN-γ promoter demethylation in CD44^{high}CD8$^+$ T lymphocytes. *J. Immunol.* **162,** 5053–5057.
86. Richter, A., Lohning, M., and Radbruch, A. (1999) Instruction for cytokine expression in T helper lymphocytes in relation to proliferation and cell cycle progression. *J. Exp. Med.* **190,** 1439–1450.
87. Bix, M. and Locksley, R. M. (1998) Independent and epigenetic regulation of the interleukin-4 alleles in CD4+ T cells. *Science* **281,** 1352–1354.
88. Riviere, I., Sunshine, M. J., and Littman, D. R. (1998) Regulation of IL-4 expression by activation of individual alleles. *Immunity* **9,** 217–228.

2

Chromatin Remodeling and Transcriptional Regulation of Cytokine Gene Expression in T Cells

M. Frances Shannon and Adele F. Holloway

1. INTRODUCTION

The activation of T cells by antigen leads to the expression of a large number of cytokines that are important for the correct orchestration of an immune response. The specific array of cytokines produced depends on the antigen that is encountered and the environment of the T cell at the time of that encounter. These cytokines range from those required for T cell proliferation (e.g., interleukin-2 [IL-2]), activators of other cells of the immune system (e.g., IL-4 or granulocyte-macrophage colony-stimulating factor [GM-CSF]), to negative modulators of cell function (e.g., IL-10 or TGB-β). The aberrant expression of these cytokines can lead to immune related disease such as autoimmune disease or chronic inflammation and modulating the profile of cytokine expression or function has been long touted as a possible treatment for these diseases.

Cytokine expression is largely controlled at the level of gene transcription although there is significant evidence that mRNA stability as well as translational control also operate to govern the final level of protein produced. This chapter will focus entirely on the transcriptional control of cytokine gene expression. Cytokine genes are mostly maintained in a silent state until cells receive an appropriate activation signal. Then follows a transient burst of high level transcription followed by a return to baseline. This pattern of expression of gene transcription means that several control mechanisms have to play a role. First, the cytokine genes, while silent in resting T cells, are likely to be in a distinct chromatin configuration in the nucleus to those genes that are either permanently switched on or off in the cells. In other words, they may be "marked" in some way as genes that are silent but responsive to cell activation. The chromatin context of these inducible genes is currently an area of considerable interest. Second, they must be switched

From: *Cytokines and Autoimmune Diseases*
Edited by: V. K. Kuchroo, et al. © Humana Press Inc., Totowa, NJ

on in response to the correct set of environment signals, and this appears to be achieved by the assembly of a precise complex of transcription factors on promoter/enhancer regions. The requirement for a complex of transcription factors to switch on gene transcription means that the gene will not respond to signals that activate only one or two of the required transcription factors but will only respond when the correct array of factors is present. The third requirement, that the response be transient, may be a passive depletion of signaling or transcription factors or may require an active mechanism of repression but this is not yet well understood.

T cell activation is a complex process that depends on both activation of the T cell receptor (TCR) and so called costimulatory signals (reviewed in refs. *1,2*). While the TCR interacts with peptide MHC complexes on the surface of antigen-presenting cells (APCs), other cell surface molecules on APCs pair up with their counterparts on T cells to enhance the interaction of the APC with the T cells. The best-described costimulatory signal is the interaction of B7.1/B7.2 (CD80/CD86) on APCs with the CD28 receptor on T cells (reviewed in refs. *3,4*). CD28 signals serve to augment TCR signals and are thought to lower the threshold of TCR signal strength that is required for T cell activation. CD28 activation has been clearly shown to augment cytokine gene transcription in T cells to higher levels than that seen with TCR activation alone *(1–4)*. Blocking the interaction of B7 with CD28 alleviates the pathogenic response in many mouse models of autoimmunity and other immune-related diseases (reviewed in ref. *5*). The importance of this costimulatory pathway in regulating T cell activation has led to great interest in determining the mechanism of signal transduction by CD28 and the resultant mechanism of cytokine gene transcription.

While T cells produce a vast array of cytokines in response to activation, these cytokines can be divided into several groups depending on their time of production or their ultimate function (reviewed in refs. *6,7*). Activation of naive T cells leads first to the production of IL-2, GM-CSF, and IL-3 among others. These cytokines appear to have common patterns of activation although IL-2 and IL-3 are T cell specific, whereas GM-CSF can be produced by a variety of cells. The control of IL-2 production is a critical point in determining the outcome of the T cell response. If T cells are activated below a specific threshold and the IL-2 gene is not switched on, then the cells become anergic or unresponsive to further activation (reviewed in ref. *8*). On the other hand, too much IL-2 can lead to activation induced cell death *(8)*. Thus there is a critical range of IL-2 that must be produced to generate a productive immune response. Understanding the control of IL-2 gene transcription is crucial in understanding the mechanism of naive T cell activation. Other cytokines produced in this initial phase of T cell activation such as GM-CSF and IL-3, while not directly governing the T cell response can control the activation or production of other immune-related cells such as APCs.

Depending on the immune stimulus and the environment, the dividing helper T cells will mature in to either Th1 or Th2 effector cells (reviewed in refs. *6,7*). Th1 cells are associated with inflammatory reactions and delayed-type hypersensitivity and are characterized by the production of interferon-γ (IFNγ). These cells are thought to mediate many autoimmune diseases. On the other hand, cell mediated immunity and allergy are associated with Th2 type T cells, which produce an array of cytokines (IL-4, IL-5, IL-13, etc.), the prototype of which is IL-4. The differentiation of Th cells and their ability to produce different population of cytokines has been well-reviewed and will not be discussed in detail here. It should be noted, however, that the Th1/Th2 paradigm is best understood at a population level and that individual cells appear have a great plasticity to produce both Th1 and Th2 type cytokines *(9)*. Cytokines produced by the Th subtypes appear to have overlapping but distinct requirements governing their transcription and differ also from the cytokines activated immediately following naive T cell activation.

This chapter will focus on the more recent advances in understanding cytokine gene expression as well as those aspects such as CD28 activation that are possible therapeutic targets in autoimmune disease.

2. MECHANISMS OF TRANSCRIPTIONAL RESPONSE TO T CELL ACTIVATION

As described earlier, one step in the induction of cytokine gene transcription is the assembly of a transcription-factor complex on the promoter/enhancer regions of the gene that allows the recruitment of the basal-transcriptional machinery and hence activation of the RNA polymerase activity. T cell activation leads to either the production or nuclear localization of several families of transcription factors, the most important of which appear to be the NFAT, NF-κB, and AP-1 families (reviewed in refs. *10,11*). A detailed understanding of the role of individual members of these families is being obtained from gene-deletion studies in mice and this information has been recently reviewed *(11)*. These activation-dependent transcription factors bind to promoter/enhancer regions and together with constitutive factors and architectural proteins form the transcriptional-activation complex. There have been many detailed studies documenting the transcription factors and their binding sites that can play roles in activating cytokine genes such as IL-2, GM-CSF, IFN-γ, and IL-4 and these data have been extensively reviewed *(12–15)*. Several general principles have emerged from this work that are useful in terms of understanding the mechanisms of inducible cytokine gene expression.

For many of the T cell-expressed cytokine genes the proximal promoter region (i.e., the first 100–300 bp upstream from the start of transcription) is crowded with potential transcription factor-binding sites. Cooperation between the factors binding to many of these sites seems to be critical for promoter/enhancer activity. Many of the binding sites on these promoters are low-affinity sites for their cognate transcription factors and so do not have significant activity when tested in isolation. Furthermore, altering these low-affinity sites to high-affinity consensus sites not only leads to their ability to act alone but can disrupt the tissue-specific activity of the promoter. This has been well-demonstrated in the case of the IL-2 promoter and suggests that this cytokine promoter has been fine-tuned for both tissue specificity and induction in response to appropriate signals *(16,17)*. The need for cooperation between a number of transcription factors has been demonstrated in a number of ways. First, mutation of individual sites leads to a dramatic reduction in the activity of the promoter. This is illustrated by studies of the GM-CSF promoter where mutation of any of the known transcription factor-binding sites in the proximal promoter has a major effect on activity (reviewed in ref. *14*). Second, loss of a single factor can, in some cases, greatly reduce activity and this will be discussed in more detail later. Third, there is evidence from in vivo footprinting experiments that for the IL-2 promoter there is an all or nothing occupation of the promoter, implying cooperative promoter occupancy *(18)*. Finally, overexpression of transcription factors can lead to highly synergistic activation of promoter activity. This is illustrated by studies with the GM-CSF promoter where overexpression of Ets1, AP-1 (c-fos and c-jun), and NF-κB proteins (RelA and p50) showed highly synergistic activation in transient transfections in Jurkat T cells *(19)*.

Cooperation between transcription factors can be manifested in several ways. First, cooperative protein binding has been observed for some of the T cell transcription factors. A good example of this is the cooperative binding of NFAT and AP-1 proteins to many sites in the IL-2 and IL-4 promoters and the GM-CSF enhancer (reviewed in refs. *20,21*). For many of these sites, the individual factors bind very weakly but show strong cooperative binding. The precise positioning of the sites is essential for this cooperative binding and this leads to high levels of synergy at the level of function *(22)*. There are many other sites in cytokine genes that bind NFAT or AP-1 individually without any observation of cooperative binding or function, although it is not clear what the functional implications are.

   Cooperation may also be manifested at the level of function and not DNA binding. A very good example of this is the activity of the CD28 response region (CD28RR) of IL-2. Here adjacent NF-κB and AP-1 sites are required for activity but show no cooperative binding of their cognate transcription factors *(23)*. Cooperative activation in such cases may be related to the ability of the combination of factors, but not the individual factors, to recruit coactivators or components of the basal machinery. The function of the CD28RR will be discussed in detail in Subheading 3.

   Not just the presence of the correct set of proteins but the specific architecture of the complex appears to be important for optimal promoter activity. Altering the relative position of transcription factor-binding sites can have dramatic effects on transcription. This presumably disrupts the cooperative activities of the transcription factors either for DNA binding or recruitment of coactivators. The DNA structure can also alter transcription-factor interactions and the assembly of a functional complex. Architectural proteins that can alter DNA structure and also modulate transcription-factor binding have been implicated in cytokine expression. One such example is the HMGI(Y) family of architectural proteins that seem to play a major role in the activity of the IL-2 gene promoter *(24)*. These proteins are thought to be involved in the assembly of an active complex. Such an activation complex that forms on the IFN-β promoter in response to virus induction has been dubbed an enhanceosome (reviewed in ref. *25*). The formation of this enhanceosome allows the recruitment of coactivators such as CBP and also components of the basal machinery such as TFIIB to the promoter *(26,27)*. This recruitment appears to be the basis of enhanceosome activity. Such a complex structure may play an important role in allowing the promoter to respond only to the set of signals that result in the activation of the entire set of transcription factors required for enhanceosome assembly; for example, virus infection probably leads to the activation of an array of signal-transduction pathways that is interpreted at the IFN-β promoter by the assembly of the enhanceosome. The promoter is, thus, designed not to respond to the activation of only one of these signaling pathways. Similarly, T cell activation requires the precise interpretation of several cooperating signals to lead to the correct level and type of cytokine gene transcription. Given the examples described earlier of cooperative activation of cytokine promoters by different families of transcription factors, it is likely that enhanceosome-like complexes also form on many of the T cell cytokine promoters and dictate the response of the genes to T cell activation (*see* Fig. 1).

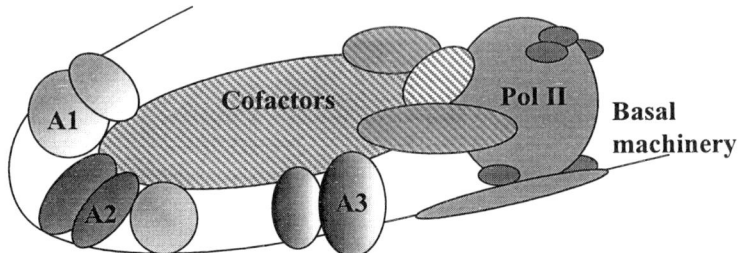

Fig. 1. A hypothetical model of the formation of an enhanceosome on a cytokine promoter, following T cell activation. Activated transcription factors (A1, A2, A3) bind to specific sequences on the DNA. This combination of factors serves as a recruitment "surface" for coactivators that may link the transcription factors to the basal transcriptional machinery represented by Pol II (RNA polymerase II) and associated factors. The cofactors may also possess chromatin-modifying activity as described in the text.

3. TRANSCRIPTIONAL RESPONSES TO COSTIMULATION IN T CELLS

The CD28 signal is clearly an important one in T cell activation as described earlier. It has been shown that inhibiting the interaction of CD28 with the B7 molecules has a significant impact on the pathology of experimental models of autoimmune disease. Therefore, a detailed understanding of the signal-transduction pathways that are activated by CD28 should provide many new targets for drugs to modify the immune response.

It has clearly been demonstrated that CD28 costimulation of T cells leads to an increase in transcription from the *IL-2* gene as well as many of the other cytokine genes expressed in T cells *(3,4)*. It is probably this increase in IL-2 expression and the subsequent T cell proliferation that is responsible for the ability of CD28 to overcome the anergic response that can be the result of TCR engagement in the absence of costimulation.

The mechanism of CD28 signal transduction is still a matter of debate but the end result appears to be an increase in the level or activity of some of the transcription factors that are known to activate cytokine gene transcription. The two best-described examples of transcription factor response to CD28 are the increased level of NF-κB family members and the increased activity of the AP-1 family (reviewed in refs. *3,4*). On the other hand, the NFAT family, which is also important in cytokine gene expression, does not appear to be affected. The ability of CD28 to increase the activity of AP-1 is most likely mediated by its ability to increase the activity of the JNK signal-transduction pathway *(28)*. JNK can, in turn, specifically phosphorylate c-jun to increase its DNA binding activity.

NF-κB proteins are located in the cytoplasm prior to activation in a complex with IκB inhibitory proteins. Upon cell activation, IκB proteins are phosphorylated by the IκB kinase complexes (IKKs), which targets them for degradation by the S26 proteosome pathway. The NF-κB proteins then translocate to the nucleus where they bind to their cognate recognition sites (reviewed in ref. *29*). CD28 activation appears to lead to both an increase in the level as well as a prolonged presence of certain NF-κB proteins in the nucleus. The level of RelA but in particular, c-Rel increases in response to CD28 *(30,31)*. Unlike, RelA there appears to be little c-Rel stored in the cytoplasm in resting cells. c-Rel appears in the nucleus at late times (>4 h) following activation and its presence is the result of increased expression from the c-Rel gene *(32)*. *c-Rel* gene transcription appears to be controlled at least in part by RelA or other NF-κB proteins and thus may be responding to the increase in these or other transcription factors following CD28 activation. A change in the degradation kinetics of IκB-β has been described in response to CD28 but there is also evidence for increased and sustained degradation of IκB-α *(33,34)*. There has been evidence presented recently that there may be crosstalk between the JNK and the NF-κB activation pathways. It has been shown that the JNK cascade can selectively activate the IKK-β but not the IKK-α pathway that leads to IκB phosphorylation and degradation *(35)*. The fact that the same pathways of AP-1 and NF-κB activation appear to be responsible for sensing the CD28 signal as the TCR signal supports the hypothesis that CD28 simply augments some of the TCR signals.

The region of the IL-2 promoter that is required for and most highly responsive to CD28 activation has been defined and studied in detail (*see* Fig. 2). Not surprisingly, it is a composite site for NF-κB and AP-1 transcription factors and will be referred to here as the CD28 responsive region (CD28RR). The CD28RR contains a nonclassical NF-κB binding site called the CD28RE (or CK-1) as well as an adjacent AP-1 binding site. There have been many studies of the proteins that bind to and mediate the activity of the CD28RR. There appears to be a general consensus that the binding of c-Rel to the CD28RE is important for its activity, although RelA has also been shown to play a role here *(23,31)*. The binding of c-Rel is highly dependent on the presence of the small nuclear architectural factor, HMGI(Y) *(31)*. HMGI(Y) binds to the A/T rich core of the site and although it promotes c-Rel binding, it appears to have little impact on the binding of RelA *(31)*. The basis for this difference is unknown. There have been several studies of the proteins that bind to and activate the AP-1 half of the CD28RR but the results

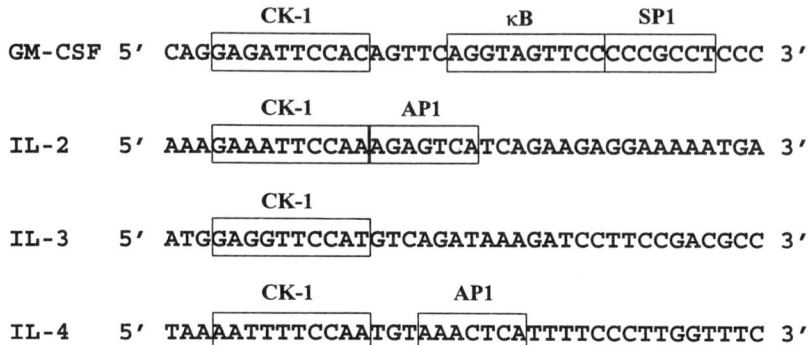

Fig. 2. Sequences of the CD28 response regions (CD28RRs) that have been identified in the promoters of IL-2, GM-CSF, IL-3, and IL-4. The sequences of the human genes are shown. The boxed areas of the sequence represent regions that are known transcription factor-binding sites. The names given to the boxes are those usually used in the literature. The CK-1 element is the conserved region across all the sequences.

are not consistent. It has been shown that combinations of RelA and c-jun as well as c-Rel and ATF-1/CREB2 could transactivate the CD28RR in transient transfection assays *(36,37)*. However, an analysis of the protein complexes binding to the CD28RR in Jurkat T cells or peripheral blood mononuclear cells (PBMCs) has revealed that c-Rel, c-jun, and c-fos are the dominant proteins present in the inducible complexes *(38)*. Neither of these sites functions well alone and there is a strong synergy in the context of the native promoter. The proteins that bind to these sites do not do so cooperatively, suggesting that the synergy is manifested at the level of recruitment of coactivators or the basal transcriptional machinery.

The GM-CSF and IL-3 promoters contain a highly related CD28RE/CK-1 to that found in the IL-2 gene *(see* Fig. 2). The IL-3 CD28RE-like region has not been well-studied, but the GM-CSF CD28RE/CK-1 has very similar properties to that of the IL-2 CD28RE, having a high affinity for the c-Rel transcription factor, binding HMGI(Y), and requiring adjacent sequences for activity *(31)*. However, the GM-CSF CD28RE is not flanked by an AP-1 binding site and requires an NF-κB/Sp-1 region located just downstream for its activity. This entire region is referred to as the CD28RR for GM-CSF. The NF-κB/SP-1 site of GM-CSF contains a classical NF-κB site that binds RelA/p50 heterodimers in response to TCR activation and does not appear to respond directly to CD28 at least in terms of DNA binding. The Sp1 site located immediately adjacent to the NF-κB site also appears to have a functional role in this region. Why two genes which appear to be coordinately regulated by CD28 have developed distinct modules for this response remains to be determined. Many NF-κB sites, or in particular multiple copies of NF-κB sites, can also respond weakly to CD28 signals, e.g., in the human immunodeficiency virus long terminal repeat (HIV LTR) *(39)*. There are also examples of NFAT/AP-1 composite sites that are responsive to CD28 *(40)*. This raises the question of whether there is a specific CD28 responsive element/region or whether any region containing an NF-κB or AP-1 site can respond to CD28. Given the hypothesis outlined earlier, that the role of CD28 may be simply to augment the TCR signal then the latter may in fact be true. On the other hand, the IL-2 gene in particular may have developed a specialized CD28RR that enables the promoter to sense the CD28 increase in TCR signal, in a very precise manner. Thus combining a low-affinity, specialized NF-κB site with a low-affinity AP-1 site may have generated an element that requires both cognate transcription factors to reach a specific functional threshold. This threshold would only be reached in the appropriate costimulatory environment. It is interesting to note that the G-CSF gene, which is not expressed in T cells, has utilized a highly related CD28RE-like sequence to regulate its response to TNF-α and IL-1 in fibroblasts *(41)*. Here the "CD28RE"/CK-1 operates in synergy with adjacent C/EBP binding sites. The IL-8 and I-CAM-1 promoters also respond with a similar combination of sites to inflammatory stimuli, raising the possibility of a CK-1/C/EBP module as a general mechanism of response to inflammatory stimuli *(42,43)*. Thus, a nonconsensus NF-κB site that cannot operate alone has been usurped by several different responses required for both innate and adaptive immunity.

The cytokines previously described are those that respond to initial T cell activation in naïve cells. It is important to ask if the effector cytokines produced by Th1 and Th2 cells are directly affected by CD28 activation signals. One could envisage a situation where CD28 is only necessary for the initial steps of naive T cell activation and once proliferation is established by the expression of IL-2 and its high-affinity receptor, the CD28 signal becomes redundant, being superseded by IL-2, IL-4, IL-12, or other cytokine-signaling events. Indeed, restimulation of memory T cells is generally thought to be independent of costimulation. There are no clearly defined CD28RR regions in any of the effector cytokine gene promoters. A recent report, however, showed that IL-4 did respond to CD28 activation in Jurkat T cells and that this was manifested at the level of promoter activity *(44)*. A region of the promoter known as P1 was identified as a CD28RR and was shown to bind c-Rel and AP-1 proteins (*see* Fig. 2) *(44)*. Compared to the level of CD28 response reported for the IL-2 CD28RR, the P1 region of IL-4 responded only weakly to the CD28 signal. Rooney et al. *(40)*, have also described the CD28 activation of an NFAT/AP-1 region in the IL-4 promoter as described earlier. There is no direct evidence on whether CD28 directly affects the activity of other Th2 cytokines such as IL-5, IL-13, or IFN-γ in Th1 cells and this area requires further investigation before any useful conclusion can be drawn. There is, however, experimental evidence that CD28 signaling is necessary for the development of the Th1/Th2 phenotypes in animal models. It has been shown that CD28 is necessary for the development of Th2-mediated, allergic airway responses in mice and that blocking B7.2:CD28 interactions reduced allergen-specific responses in T cells from atopic asthmatics *(45–47)*. The development of autoreactive effector cells in models of autoimmunity has also been shown to respond to CD28 blockade or absence (reviewed in ref. *5*). These effects, however, may not be direct and are consistent with the hypothesis that the major role of CD28 is in the initial production of IL-2 and the priming of T cells for proliferation and differentiation.

4. THE ROLE OF ARCHITECTURAL TRANSCRIPTION FACTORS IN CYTOKINE GENE TRANSCRIPTION

As discussed previously, the promoter/enhancer regions of cytokine genes assemble a complex array of transcription factors in a structure referred to as an enhanceosome. The architecture of this complex depends on DNA structure, protein:protein as well as protein:DNA interactions. The HMGI(Y) family of architectural transcription factors appear to play an important role in the assembly and stability of these complexes (reviewed in ref. *48*). The HMGI(Y) family consists of three members; HMGI, HMGY, and HMGI-C. HMGI and HMGY are the products of alternately spliced mRNAs from the same gene, whereas HMGI-C is the product of a separate gene. All three proteins are approx 100 amino acids in length and are highly related. Each protein contains three conserved DNA-binding domains known as A/T hooks. The DNA-binding domains recognize the minor groove structure of A/T stretches in DNA and can use each A/T hook to bind to adjacent A/T stretches on DNA. HMGI(Y) proteins have been shown to have many possible modes of action. They can alter DNA structure by modulating the natural bends on DNA. HMGI(Y) proteins have been well-documented to modulate the binding of many transcription factor families to DNA. HMGI(Y) has also been shown to interact directly with many transcription factors such as the ATF bZIP proteins. Thus, HMGI(Y) could have a major role in the assembly of enhanceosome complexes. In addition,

HMGI(Y) has been shown to bind to nucleosomes assembled on DNA in vitro and affect the rotational setting of the nucleosome. It has also been shown to antagonize the repressive effect of histone H1 on transcription in vitro. The highest level of HMGI(Y) proteins appears to be associated with actively dividing cells and abnormal levels have also been found in some tumors. The DNA-binding capacity of HMGI(Y) can be affected by phosphorylation of the protein by cdc2 kinase or caesin kinase II, thus leading to speculation about its role in the cell-cycle and signal transduction.

Recent studies have shown that HMGI(Y) may play a major role in the regulation of T cell cytokines. The IL-2 gene promoter is highly A/T rich and it was not surprising to find that HMGI(Y) had many binding sites across the first 300-bp region of the promoter *(24)*. The most important aspect of this was that the HMGI(Y) binding sites were all located within or close to known transcription factor-binding sites. Subsequent experiments showed that HMGI(Y) could modulate the binding of many of the transcription-factor families that are thought to play an important role in the activity of the IL-2 promoter *(24)*. This can be illustrated by an analysis of the effects of HMGI(Y) on the binding of factors to the IL-2 CD28RR *(24,31)*. The CD28RE/NF-κB binding site can bind c-Rel with high efficiency but only in the presence of HMGI(Y), whereas the binding of RelA to this site is much less dependent on HMGI(Y). The CD28RE of IL-2 or GM-CSF can also bind members of the NFAT family of transcription factors and HMGI(Y) either promotes or inhibits the binding of NFATp depending on the relative ratio of the proteins in the in vitro binding assays. Binding of AP-1 to the adjacent site in IL-2 (which does not have an A/T sequence) is also affected by HMGI(Y). The relevance of these in vitro binding studies is borne out by transfection studies in either T cell lines or primary T cells where depleting the level of HMGI(Y) by antisense expression greatly inhibits IL-2 promoter activity *(24)*. Of even greater significance is the fact that reducing HMGI(Y) levels leads to a decrease in the production of IL-2 from the endogenous gene, which in turn leads to reduced proliferation of the primary T cells *(24)*. On the other hand, overexpression of HMGI(Y) in Jurkat T cells or primary T cells leads to increased expression of IL-2 and thus increased proliferation in the primary cells. It has also been shown that the activity of the IL-2 receptor alpha promoter is dependent on HMGI(Y), leading to the conclusion that HMGI(Y) levels plays an important role in T cell proliferation *(49,50)*. Indeed, the levels of HMGI(Y) in Jurkat T cells are increased by stimulation with mitogenic signals *(24)*.

Other cytokines that are coexpressed with IL-2 such as GM-CSF and IL-3 also seem to be positively regulated by HMGI(Y). On the other hand, it has been shown that HMGI(Y) plays an inhibitory role in the regulation of IL-4 and this may be owing to the fact that HMGI(Y) can inhibit the binding of NFAT proteins to certain sites on the IL-4 promoter *(51)*. Intriguingly, IL-4 signaling has been shown to lead to phosphorylation of HMGI(Y) on casein kinase II consensus sites at the C-terminus *(52)*. This in turn leads to decreased DNA binding and may, in turn, reduce the inhibitory effect of HMGI(Y) on the binding of certain transcription factors such as NFAT to DNA. It is possible to speculate that the phosphorylation of HMGI(Y) by IL-4 is one mechanism by which IL-4 increases its own expression in Th2 type cells. Whether HMGI(Y) plays a distinct role in Th2 compared to Th1 cells has yet to be determined. Its positive transcription-activation role may be limited to the cytokine genes that are activated immediately following T cell activation becuase increases in HMGI(Y) levels are associated with proliferation.

Another family of architectural transcription factors that may play a role in the regulation of cytokine gene transcription are the Sry-like HMG box factors. This family of proteins is very distinct from the HMGI(Y) proteins discussed earlier. They are a large family of proteins including Sry, the many related Sox proteins, and TCF/LEF proteins and are related by the presence of a so-called HMG box that is required for DNA binding. These proteins can have major effects on DNA structure and generate large bends in DNA, thus affecting the structure of protein:DNA complexes and hence transcription (reviewed in ref. 53). TCF-1 and LEF-1 are highly related proteins that appear to play a major role in T cell differentiation *(53)*. Their role in differentiation parallels the role of other HMG-box proteins in development of other tissues. They have been shown to affect the transcription of genes such as those encoding CD4 and T cell receptor genes whose expression is important in the differentiation of the T cell repertoire in the thymus. Because the expression of some of the cytokines discussed in this chapter is restricted to T cells, it is possible that factors such as TCF/LEF are involved in their T cell-specific expression rather than inducible expression *per se*. A recent detailed accessibility mapping of a region 600 bp upstream of the IL-2 transcription start site has revealed a region between −350 and −600 that is constitutively accessible to DNase I cleavage in unstimulated as well as activated EL-4 T cells *(54)*. In contrast, the more proximal region between −1 and −350 is only accessible in activated cells. It is possible that the upstream region in some way marks the gene for expression in T cells, whereas the proximal region is required for inducible responses. The complexes that bind to a part of the upstream region have been shown to contain TCF/LEF, Oct proteins, and HMGI(Y) *(54)*. This raises the intriguing possibility that TCF/LEF may be involved in the T cell-specific expression of IL-2.

Such a "marking" phenomenon may occur during differentiation of T cells in the thymus. More investigation is, however, required to determine if this possibility is correct.

5. TRANSCRIPTIONAL REGULATION VIA CHROMATIN REMODELING AND MODIFICATION

Most of the information and models described previously comes from an analysis of cytokine promoter/enhancer regions in transient transfection assays in cell lines in culture. These experiments generally deal with short DNA fragments (hundreds of base pairs) linked to reporter genes and transfected into cells in large numbers (hundreds of copies per cell). The chromatin context of these plasmids has not been considered. Cellular genes are normally incorporated into chromatin and this forms an important level of regulatory control of gene transcription. In general, inactive genes are found in condensed chromatin, containing unmodified histones and densely methylated DNA, whereas acetylated histones and demethylated DNA characterize transcriptionally competent genes.

The structural unit of chromatin is the nucleosome, which is composed of 147 bp of DNA wrapped around a histone octamer (reviewed in ref. *55*). The histone proteins are composed of two domains: a central fold, which contributes to the histone core of the nucleosome and is constrained by the DNA; and a flexible amino terminal histone tail extending out of the core, which contains conserved residues that can be postranscriptionally modified by either acetylation or phosphorylation. The histones can be considered general gene repressors, and can regulate gene accessibility by at least two mechanisms. First, transcription factor-binding sites on DNA positioned within the nucleosome core may be inaccessible, preventing binding of transcription factors to these sites. A first step in "opening" silent loci may therefore involve remodeling of the chromatin so that promoter regions become accessible to transcription factors (reviewed in refs. *56,57*). Multi-subunit ATP-dependent remodeling complexes have been found in yeast (the yeast SWI/SNF complex and RSC complex), Drosophila (NURF, CHRAC, and ACF), and mammalian cells (BRG1 and hBRM-associated complexes), which are able to remodel chromatin by destabilizing the nucleosome or repositioning it on the DNA (reviewed in refs. *58–60*). Second, acetylation of the histone tails may also alter the nucleosomal structure. Acetylation of lysine residues neutrilizes positive charges, decreasing the affinity for DNA, thus altering the nucleosomal conformation and increasing accessibility of DNA elements to transcription factors. The histone tails are also proposed to contribute to the formation of higher order chromatin structures, possibly through contacts with adjacent nucleosomes. In vitro at least, acetylation of nucleosome arrays can disrupt higher-order chromatin structure, which may increase chromatin accessibility. Recently, a range of proteins have been found to contain histone acetyltransferase (HAT) activity including GCN5, p300/CBP, P/CAF, SRC-1, and TAFII250 or histone deacetylase activity (HDACs), including yeast RPD3 and human HDAC1 (reviewed in ref. *60*). Many of the proteins possessing HAT or HDAC activity are proteins that have previously been identified as having a role in transcription. For example several HATS are known transcriptional coactivators (for example, CBP/p300, ACTR, and SRC-1), whereas HDACs are often components of multiprotein complexes that contain proteins involved in transcriptional repression. Epigenetic modification of DNA by methylation is also a hallmark of silent genes, and it is becoming clear that the demethylation of CpG dinucleotides may be an important step in derepressing silent genes.

Chromatin structure may play a role in the regulation of cytokine gene expression, either in controlling the cell-type-specific expression of certain cytokines or in the induction of cytokine genes following T cell activation. Alterations in chromatin structure are frequently detected on the basis of changes in the accessibility to DNase I. DNase I sites have been mapped for a number of cytokine genes and changes in these sites observed in response to activation. For example, DNase I hypersensitivity mapping has identified inducible DNase I hypersensitive (DH) sites 3-kb upstream of the *GM-CSF* gene and 14-kb upstream of the *IL-3* gene *(61,62)*. The IL-3 DH site is inducible only in T cells, suggesting that this site plays a role in T cell-specific expression of IL-3. The GM-CSF DH site is inducible in all cell types expressing GM-CSF. Both of these inducible DH sites contain binding sites for activation-dependent transcription factors. The IL-3 site contains 4 NFAT sites, one of which overlaps with and cooperates with an Oct binding site. The GM-CSF site contains 3 NFAT binding sites linked to AP-1 sites. Similarly, chromatin remodeling of the *IL-2* gene has been detected upon T cell activation *(54)*. In vivo footprinting with DNaseI or restriction enzyme-accessibility studies have revealed inducible accessibility in the promoter region upon activation of T cells only. The fact that in all three genes these inducible hypersensitive sites only occur in cells expressing the cognate genes suggests a functional role for these regions. DNase I footprinting of a more distal region of the *IL-2* gene revealed constitutive DH sites between −300 and −600 in resting EL-4 T cells, but not non-T cells *(54)*. This region has been proposed to play a role in the T cell specificity of IL-2. Protein-DNA complexes containing the HMG proteins HMGI/Y and LEF-I were found to bind in this region. The presence of LEF-1 is particularly interesting because, LEF-1 is thought to be important in T cell development.

Comparison of the chromatin structure of the Th1 cytokine IFN-γ and the Th2 cytokine IL-4 in naive T cells and differentiated Th1 and Th2 cells revealed tissue-specific chromatin remodeling *(63)*. Terminally differentiated Th1 or Th2 cell clones showed marked differences in their chromatin configuration on the IL-4 and INF-γ loci as assessed by DNase I accessibilitiy. In Th2 clones, which express IL-4, the IL-4 locus was found to be accessible, whereas the IFN-γ locus displayed a closed configuration. The converse was true in Th1 clones. In agreement with this, naive T cells did not display accessible configurations of either gene, but upon differentiation to either Th1 or Th2 acquired IFN-γ or IL-4 accessible patterns, respectively. Therefore, the differentiation of T cells was associated with the remodeling of genes that confer the effector phenotype of the differentiated cells. In support of this, a second study has shown that three DH sites, occur in the intergenic region between IL-4 and IL-13 and although one of these sites appears in both Th1 and Th2 cells, as well as CD4$^+$ naive T cells, the other two sites appear exclusively in differentiated Th2 cells *(64)*.

These studies then demonstrate that chromatin is disrupted upon activation of T cells, and that the chromatin configuration of a cytokine locus may be involved in regulation of cell-type specificity. These chromatin-remodeling studies suggest that nucleosomes positioned across the cytokine genes in naive cells are remodeled upon activation (e.g., IL-2, GM-CSF, and IL-3) or Th-cell differentiation (e.g., IFN-γ and IL-4). There have been as yet no direct studies of nucleosome positioning on T cell cytokines. A recent study of the IL-12 p40 promoter in macrophages, however, presents a model that may be applicable to many inducible cytokine genes. High-resolution micrococcal-nuclease analysis showed that a positioned nucleosome spans the IL-12 p40 promoter, followed by a linker region and three nucleosomes positioned further upstream *(65)*. Upon activation of macrophages with lipopolysaccharide (LPS) or heat-killed Listeria monocytogenes (HKLM) the promoter positioned nucleosome was selectively remodeled, but the upstream nucleosomes remained in position. Although such studies have not been done in T cells, this study supports the notion that chromatin remodelling contributes to the rapid induction of cytokine genes, by increasing promoter accessibility. Other studies also support the idea that nucleosome remodeling is important in inducible gene transcription. For example, a link between T cell activation and chromatin remodeling has been indicated by studies showing that upon activation, the chromatin-remodeling Swi/Snf complex becomes stably associated with chromatin *(66)*. Similarly a link between chromatin modification and inducible gene expression has been shown by studies of the *IFN*-β gene in which the histones associated with the gene become hyperacetylated upon viral induction in HeLa cells *(67)*.

A link between CpG methylation of mammalian DNA and transcriptional silencing of genes has been proposed for many years, although the methods by which methylation represses transcription are not completely understood. Methylation of CpG dinucleotides may act directly to inhibit binding of transcription factors or the transcription machinery to DNA. Alternatively, methylation may influence the chromatin structure (reviewed in refs. *68–70*). There is now evidence that CpG methylation stimulates histone deacetylation, because complexes have been found that contain methyl-binding proteins and histone deactylases. The model suggested is that the methyl-binding protein MeCP2 recruits the corepressor mSin3A and the deacetylases HDAC1 and HDAC2 forming a repressor complex on methylated DNA that mediates histone deacetylation. Although control of cytokine gene transcription by methylation has not been widely studied, there is growing evidence that it is an important control mechanism in the generation and maintainence of Th1 and Th2 specific gene expression. Demethylation has been correlated with the activity of *IL-3, IL-4, IL-5,* and *IFN-γ* genes.

The most studied cytokine in this respect is INF-γ. The 108 base pair IFN-γ proximal promoter contains two important regulatory control elements, and the most proximal of these sites is able to reproduce the PMA/ionophore inducible, cyclosporin-sensitive expression of IFN-γ and also appears critical for the Th1-specific expression profile of IFN-γ *(71)*. A CpG dinucleotide within this element is methylated in naive T cells and Th2 clones, but becomes demethylated during Th1 differentiation. Methylation at this site correlates with the inability of naive T cells and Th2 clones to express IFN-γ *(72)*. A further study extended this finding, showing that thymocytes, neonatal T cells, and naive T cells are hypermethylated at this proximal site, whereas adult CD8[+] T cells and Th2 cells are hypomethylated *(73)*. This regulatory element has been shown to bind the transcription factors CREB, ATF-2, Jun, and electrophoretic mobility shift assay (EMSA) using oligonucleotides incorporating a methylated CpG dinucleotide at the critical position demonstrated reduced binding of all these factors, although the effect was more pronounced for CREB *(71)*. Although the above data was generated using methyl-sensitive restriction enzyme, bisulfite genomic sequencing of CpG dinucleotides across the IFN-γ promoter has confirmed the link between demethylation of the IFN-γ promoter and gene expression *(74)*. This study also showed that the ability of cells to produce IL-3 can similarly be linked to demethylation of the gene. CpG dinucleotides within the IL-3 promoter are mostly associated with transcription factor-binding sites, and therefore methylation may also affect transcription factor binding to this promoter. A further study has shown that in Th2 cells the IL-4 and IL-13 genes are demethylated. Although in naive T cells, the IL-4 and IL-13 genes are hypermethylated, the differentiation to Th2 cells is characterized by both chromatin remodeling and demethylation of the IL-4/IL-13 locus *(63)*. Therefore, the derepression of silent cytokine genes probably involves the coordinate demethylation and remodeling of the chromatin. This supports the model referred to earlier in which methylation and histone deacetylation are linked through the action of multiprotein complexes.

Recently a link between deregulation of cytokine gene transcription and gene methylation has been demonstrated in T cells. It is well-established that HIV or human T leukemia virus (HTLV) infection of T cells results in disregulated production of cytokines. Mikovits et al. *(75)* have shown that acute infection of T cells with HIV results in upregulation of DNA methyltransferase mRNA expression and activity. They established that this correlated with a general increase in genome methylation, but in particular it resulted in altered methylation of the IFN-γ gene in Th1 cells, via *de novo* methylation at the site that was shown in the aforementioned studies to be critical for transcriptional regulation of this gene. This correlated with decreased IFN-γ mRNA and protein expression.

Finally, it is well-established that differentiated effector Th cells respond far more rapidly and with much higher cytokine production than naive T cells. Although cytokine expression is only transient following initial stimulation, the cells can essentially remember this expression pattern, which is reflected later by the same and more rapid cytokine production following restimulation. This may well be explained in large part by the fact that the chromatin is remodeled and demethylated upon differentiation and that this state is then maintained stably. For example, analysis of the IFN-γ promoter through eight generations has shown that the methylation patterns, once established, can be faithfully inherited in the absence of stimuli *(74)*.

There is now also evidence appearing that links the differentiation of Th cells with the cell cycle. Bird et al. *(76)* have demonstrated that although IL-2 expression is independent of cell cycle, cells must enter S-phase of the first cell cycle after activation before they are able to express IFN-γ and must undergo at least three cell cycles before they express IL-4. Two further studies support this idea, demonstrating that, like IL-4 and IFN-γ, the expression of IL-3, IL-5, and IL-10 are also linked to the cell cycle *(77,78)*. DNA synthesis has long been proposed as an opportunity for remodeling of a gene from an inactive to an active state. DNA synthesis during S phase may then correlate with epigenetic modification of the DNA. Modifications such as acetylation or demethylation may occur following new DNA synthesis, which is carried through to the next cell generation. These studies speculate that one mechanism by which cytokine expression is repressed in naive T

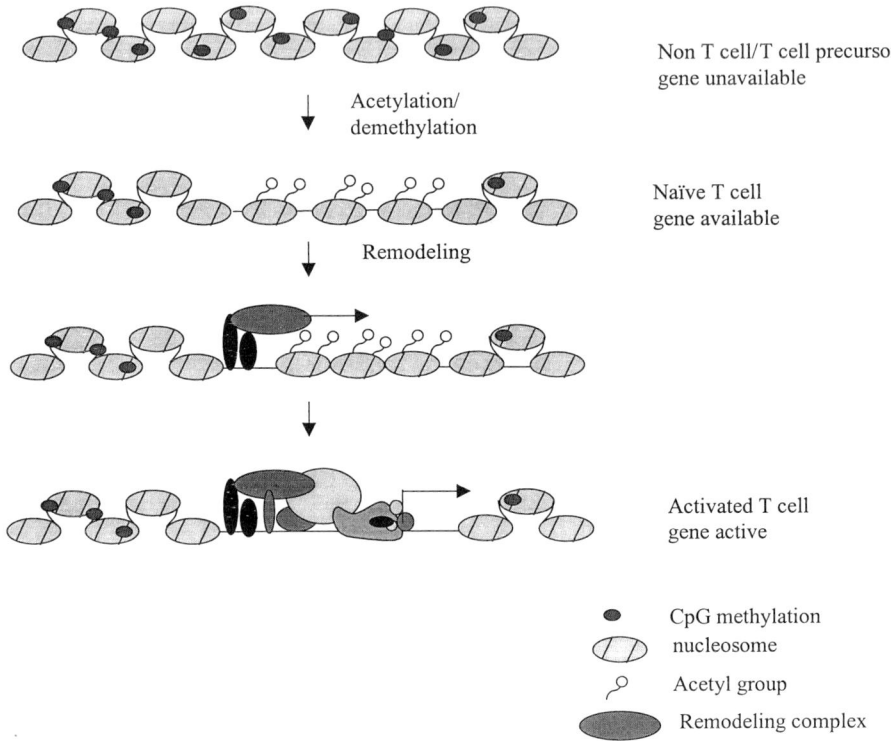

Non T cell/T cell precursor
gene unavailable

↓ Acetylation/
   demethylation

Naïve T cell
gene available

↓ Remodeling

Activated T cell
gene active

● CpG methylation
⬭ nucleosome
♀ Acetyl group
⬬ Remodeling complex

Fig. 3. A hypothetical model of the steps involved in the activation of a cytokine gene in T cells. In a non-T cell or precursor T cell, a cytokine gene may be in inactive chromatin characterized by unacetylated histones and DNA methylation at CpG dinucleotides. The development of a T cell may involve acetylation and/or demethylation of the genes that will respond to T cell activation generating an "available" chromatin configuration in a naive T cell. Similar modifications may occur for Th1 and Th2 expressed cytokines during Th-cell differentiation. Upon T cell activation, transcription factors bind to the promoter/enhancer regions of the gene, recruit chromatin remodeling complexes, and, in turn, allow the formation of an active enhanceosome.

cells is owing to methylation of the genes, and that progression through the cell cycle provides an opportunity for demethylation of these genes to occur.

It is clear that chromatin remodeling and modification is important in the regulation of cytokine genes. It has been shown that the inability of naive T cells to express certain cytokines may be owing to repressive chromatin effects. The differentiation to Th1 or Th2 subtypes involves chromatin remodeling and demethylation of, for example, the *IFN-γ* and *IL-4* genes, respectively, and once differentiated the open or active chromatin states are stably maintained and inherited, providing a cellular memory. Upon T cell activation, chromatin remodeling occurs, increasing promoter accessibility and allowing rapid induction of cytokine genes. A possible model for these events is described in Fig. 3.

6. CONCLUSION

We have previously described many of the important principles underlying inducible cytokine gene transcription in T cells. It is now necessary to integrate this information into a model that considers the chromatin context of the genes. It will be important to map precisely the nucleosome positions across the control regions of the cytokine genes and to monitor the changes that occur in response to activation. It will also be necessary to reproduce this chromatin structure in vitro in order to understand the molecular mechanisms that govern chromatin remodeling at the cytokine loci. Finally, transgenic-mouse models in which transcription can be analyzed in the context of chromatin in normal T cells will be important. Given the enormous recent development in regard to chromatin remodeling and its relationship to gene transcription, these goals should be achievable.

REFERENCES

1. Lanzavecchia, A., Iezzi, G., and Viola, A. (1999) From TCR engagement to T cell activation: a kinetic view of T cell behavior. *Cell* **96,** 1–4.
2. Sprent, J. (1999) Presidential address to the American Association of Immunologists. Stimulating naïve T cells. *J. Immunol.* **163,** 4629–4636.
3. Greenfield, E. A., Nguyen, K. A., and Kuchroo, V. K. (1998) CD28/B7 costimulation: a review. *Crit. Rev. Immunol.* **18,** 389–418.
4. Chambers, C. A. and Allison, J. P. (1999) Costimulatory regulation of T cell function. *Curr. Opin. Cell Biol.* **11,** 203–210.
5. Khoury, S., Sayegh, M. H., and Turka, L. A. (1999) Blocking costimulatory signals to induce transplantation tolerance and prevent autoimmune disease. *Intl. Rev. Immunol.* **18,** 185–199.
6. Abbas, A. K., Murphy, K. M., and Sherr, A. (1996) Functional diversity of helper T lymphocytes. *Nature* **383,** 787–793.
7. O'Garra, A. (1998) Cytokines induce the development of functionally heterogeneous T helper cell subsets. *Immunity* **8,** 275–283.
8. Lenardo, M., Chan, F. K-M., Hornung, F., McFarland, H., Siegel, R., Wang, J., et al. (1999) Mature T lymphocyte apoptosis-immune regulation in a dynamic and unpredictable antigenic environment. *Annu. Rev. Immunol.* **17,** 221–253.
9. Fitzpatrick, D. R. and Kelso, A. (1998) Independent regulation of cytokine genes in T cells: the paradox in the paradigm. *Transplantation* **65,** 1–5.
10. Glimcher, L. and Singh, H. (1999) Transcription factors in lymphocyte development-T and B cells get together. *Cell* **96,** 13–23.

11. Kuo, C. T. and Leiden, J. M. (1999) Transcriptional regulation of T lymphocyte development and function. *Annu. Rev. Immunol.* **17,** 149–187.
12. Avots, A., Escher, C., Muller-Deubert, S., Neumann, M., and Serfling, E. (1995) The interplay between lymphoid-specific and ubiquitous transcription factors controls the expression of the interleukin 2 gene in T lymphocytes. *Immunobiology* **193,** 254–258.
13. Jain, J., Loh, C., and Rao, A. (1995) Transcriptional regulation of the IL-2 gene. *Curr. Opin. Immunol.* **7,** 333–342.
14. Shannon, M. F., Coles, L. S., Vadas, M. A., and Cockerill, P. N. (1997) Signals for activation of the GM-CSF promoter and enhancer in T cells. *Crit. Rev. Immunol.* **17,** 301–323.
15. Brown, M. A. and Hural, J. (1997) Functions of IL-4 and control of its expression. *Crit. Rev. Immunol.* **17,** 1–32.
16. Briegel, K., Hentsch, B., Pfeuffer, I., and Serfling, E. (1991) One base pair change abolishes the T cell-restricted activity of a kB-like proto-enhancer element from the interleukin 2 promoter. *Nucleic Acids Res.* **19,** 5929–5936.
17. Hentsch, B., Mouzaki, A., Pfeuffer, I., Rungger, D., and Serfling, E. (1992) The weak, fine-tuned binding of ubiquitous transcription factors to the IL-2 enhancer contributes to its T cell-restricted activity. *Nucleic Acids Res.* **20,** 2657–2665.
18. Rothenberg, E. V. and Ward, S. B. (1996) A dynamic assembly of diverse transcription factors integrates activation and cell-type information for interleukin-2 gene regulation. *Proc. Natl. Acad. Sci. USA* **93,** 9358–9365.
19. Thomas, R. S., Tymms, M. J., McKinlay, L. H., Shannon, M. F., Seth, A., and Kola, I. (1997) ETS1, NF-kappaB and AP1 synergistically transactivate the human GM-CSF promoter. *Oncogene* **14,** 2845–2855.
20. Rao, A. (1994) NF-ATp: a transcription factor required for the co-ordinate induction of several cytokine genes. *Immunol. Today* **15,** 274–281.
21. Rao, A., Luo, C., and Hogan P. G. (1997) Transcription factors of the NFAT family: regulation and function. *Annu. Rev. Immunol.* **15,** 707–747.
22. Cockerill, P. N., Bert, A. G., Jenkins, F., Ryan, G. R., Shannon, M. F., and Vadas, M. A. (1995) Human granulocyte-macrophage colony-stimulating factor enhancer function is associated with cooperative interactions between AP-1 and NFATp/c. *Mol. Cell Biol.* **15,** 2071–2079.
23. Shapiro, V. S., Truitt, K. E., Imboden, J. B., and Weiss, A. (1997) CD28 mediates transcriptional upregulation of the interleukin-2 (IL-2) promoter through a composite element containing the CD28RE and NF-IL-2B AP-1 sites. *Mol. Cell Biol.* **17,** 4051–4058.
24. Himes, S. R., Reeves, R., Attema, J., Nissen, M., Li, Y., and Shannon, M. F. (2000) The role of high-mobility group I(Y) proteins in expression of IL-2 and T cell proliferation. *J. Immunol.* **164,** 3157–3168.
25. Carey, M. (1998) The enhanceosome and transcriptional synergy. *Cell* **92,** 5–8.
26. Merika, M., Williams, A. J., Chen, G., Collins, T., and Thanos, D. (1998) Recruitment of CBP/p300 by the IFNβ enhanceosome is required for synergistic activation of transcription. *Mol. Cell* **1,** 277–287.

27. Kim, T. K., Kim, T. H., and Maniatis, T. (1998) Efficient recruitment of TFIIB and CBP-RNA polymerase II holoenzyme by an interferon-β enhanceosome in vitro. *Proc. Natl. Acad. Sci. USA* **95,** 12,191–12,196.

28. Su, B., Jacinto, E., Hibi, M., Kallunki, T., Karin, M., and Ben-Neriah, Y. (1994) JNK is involved in signal integration during costimulation of T lymphocytes. *Cell* **77,** 727–736.

29. Baldwin, A. S. (1996) The NF-κB and IκB proteins: new discoveries and insights. *Annu. Rev. Immunol.* **14,** 649–683.

30. Bryan, R. G., Li, Y., Lai, J. H., Van, M., Rice, N. R., Rich, R. R., et al. (1994) Effect of CD28 signal transduction on c-Rel in human peripheral blood T cells. *Mol. Cell Biol.* **14,** 7933–7942.

31. Himes, S. R., Coles, L. S., Reeves, R., and Shannon, M. F. (1996) High mobility group protein I(Y) is required for function and for c-Rel binding to CD28 response elements within the GM-CSF and IL-2 promoters. *Immunity* **5,** 479–489.

32. Grumont, R. J., Richardson, I. B., Gaff, C., and Gerondakis, S. (1993) Rel/NF-κB nuclear complexes that bind κB sites in the murine c-rel promoter are required for constitutive c-rel transcription in B-cells. *Cell Growth Differ.* **4,** 731–743.

33. Lai, J.-H. and Tan, T.-H. (1994) CD28 signaling causes a sustained down-regulation of IκBα which can be prevented by the immunosuppressant rapamycin. *J. Biol. Chem.* **269,** 30,077–30,080.

34. Harhaj, E. W., Maggirwar, S. B., Good, L., and Sun, S.-C. (1996) CD28 mediates a potent costimulatory signal for rapid degradation of IκBβ which is associated with accelerated activation of various NF-κB/Rel heterodimers. *Mol. Cell Biol.* **16,** 6736–6743.

35. Kempiak, S. J., Hiura, T. S., and Nel, A. E. (1999) The Jun kinase cascade is responsible for activating the CD28 response element of the IL-2 promoter; proof of cross-talk with the IκB kinase cascade. *J. Immunol.* **162,** 3176–3187.

36. Butscher, W. G., Powers, C., Olive, M., Vinson, C., and Gardner, K. (1998) Coordinate transactivation of the interleukin-2 CD28 response element by c-Rel and ATF-1/CREB2. *J. Biol. Chem.* **273,** 552–560.

37. Parra, E., McGuire, K., Hedlund, G., and Dohlsten, M. (1998) Overexpression of p65 and c-Jun substitutes for B7-1 costimulation by targeting the CD28RE within the IL-2 promoter. *J. Immunol.* **160,** 5374–5381.

38. McGuire, K. and Iacobelli, M. (1997) Involvement of Rel, Fos, and Jun proteins in binding activity to the IL-2 promoter CD28 response element/AP-1 sequence in human T cells. *J. Immunol.* **159,** 1319–1327.

39. Civil, A., Rensink, I., Aarden, L. A., and Verweij, C. L. (1999) Functional disparity of distinct CD28 response elements toward mitogenic responses. *J. Biol. Chem.* **274,** 34,369–34,374.

40. Rooney, J. W., Sun, Y. L., Glimcher, L. H., and Hoey, T. (1995) Novel NFAT sites that mediate activation of the interleukin-2 promoter in response to T cell receptor stimulation. *Mol. Cell Biol.* **15,** 6299–6310.

41. Dunn, S. M., Coles, L. S., Lang, R. K., Gerondakis, S., Vadas, M. A., and Shannon, M. F. (1994) Requirement for nuclear factor (NF)-kappa B p65 and NF-interleukin-6 binding elements in the tumor necrosis factor response region of the granulocyte colony-stimulating factor promoter. *Blood* **83,** 2469–2479.

42. Kunsch, C., Lang, R. K., Rosen, C. A., and Shannon, M. F. (1994) Synergistic transcriptional activation of the IL-8 gene by NF-κB p65 (RelA) and NF-IL-6. *J. Immunol.* **153,** 153–164.

43. Catron, K. M., Brickwood, J. R., Shang, C., Li, Y., Shannon, M. F., and Parks, T. P. (1998) Cooperative binding and synergistic activation by RelA and C/EBPβ on the intercellular adhesion mclecule-1 promoter. *Cell Growth Differ.* **9,** 949–959.

44. Li-Weber, M., Giasi, M., and Krammer, P. H. (1998) Involvement of Jun and Rel proteins in up-regulation of interleukin-4 gene activity by the T cell accessory molecule CD28. *J. Biol. Chem.* **273,** 32,460–32,466.

45. Keane-Myers, A., Gause, W. C., Linsley, P. S., Chen, S.-J., and Wills-Karp, M. (1997) B7-CD28/CTLA-4 costimulatory pathways are required for the development of T helper cell 2-mediated allergic airway responses to inhaled antigens. *J. Immunol.* **158,** 2042–2049.

46. Tsuyuki, S., Tsuyuki, J., Einsle, K., Kopf, M., and Coyle, A. J. (1997) Costimulation through B7-2 (CD86) is required for the induction of a lung mucosal T helper cell 2 (TH2) immune response and altered airway responsiveness. *J. Exp. Med.* **185,** 1671–1679.

47. Larché, M., Till, S. J., Haselden, B. M., North, J., Barkans, J., Corrigan, C. J., et al. (1998) Costimulation through CD86 is involved in airway antigen-presenting cell and T cell responses to allergen in atopic asthmatics. *J. Immunol.* **161,** 6375–6382.

48. Bustin, M. and Reeves, R. (1996) High-mobility-group chromosomal proteins: architectural components that facilitate chromatin function. *Prog. Nucleic Acid Res. Mol. Biol.* **54,** 35–100.

49. John, S., Reeves, R. B., Lin, J.-X., Child, R., Leiden, J. M., Thompson, C. B., and Leonard, W. J. (1995) Regulation of cell type-specific interleukin-2 receptor α-chain gene expression: potential role of physical interactions between Elf-1, HMG-I(Y), and NF-κB family proteins. *Mol. Cell Biol.* **15,** 1786–1796.

50. John, S., Robbins, C. M., and Leonard, W. J. (1996) An IL-2 response element in the human IL-2 receptor α chain promoter is a composite element that binds Stat5, Elf-1, HMG-I(Y) and a GATA family protein. *EMBO J.* **15,** 5627–5635.

51. Klein-Hessling, S., Schneider, G., Heinfling, A., Chuvpilo, S., and Serfling, E. (1996) HMG I(Y) interferes with the DNA binding of NF-AT factors and the induction of the interleukin 4 promoter in T cells. *Proc. Natl. Acad. Sci. USA* **93,** 15,311–15,316.

52. Wang, D.-Z., Ray, P., and Boothby, M. (1995) Interleukin 4-inducible phosphorylation of HMG-I(Y) is inhibited by rapamycin. *J. Biol. Chem.* **270,** 22,924–22,932.

53. Schilham, M. W. and Clevers, H. (1998) HMG box containing transcription factors in lymphocyte differentiation. *Semin. Immunol.* **10,** 127–132.

54. Ward, S. B., Hernandez-Hoyos, G., Chen, F., Waterman, M., Reeves, R., and Rothenberg, E. V. (1998) Chromatin remodeling of the interleukin-2 gene: distinct alterations in the proximal versus distal enhancer regions. *Nucleic Acids Res.* **26,** 2923–2934.

55. Kornberg, R. D. and Lorch, Y. (1999) Twenty-five years of the nucleosome, fundamental particle of the eukaryote chromosome. *Cell* **98,** 285–294.
56. Struhl, K. (1998) Histone acetylation and transcriptional regulatory mechanisms. *Genes Develop.* **12,** 599–606.
57. Kadonaga, J. T. (1998) Eukaryotic transcription: an interlaced network of transcription factors and chromatin-modifying machines. *Cell* **92,** 307–313.
58. Varga-Weisz, P. D. and Becker, P. B. (1998) Chromatin-remodeling factors: machines that regulate? *Curr. Opin. Cell Biol.* **10,** 346–353.
59. Gusthin, D. and Wolffe, A. P. (1999) Transcriptional control: Swltched-on mobility. *Curr. Biol.* **9,** R742–R746.
60. Björklund, S., Almouzni, G., Davidson, I., Nightingale, K. P., and Weiss, K. (1999) Global transcription regulators of eukaryotes. *Cell* **96,** 759–767.
61. Cockerill, P. N., Shannon, M. F., Bert, A. G., Ryan, G. R., and Vadas, M. A. (1993) The granulocyte-macrophage colony-stimulating factor/interleukin 3 locus is regulated by an inducible cyclosporin A-sensitive enhancer. *Proc. Natl. Acad. Sci. USA* **90,** 2466–2470.
62. Duncliffe, K. N., Bert, A. G., Vadas, M. A., and Cockerill, P. N. (1997) A T cell-specific enhancer in the interleukin-3 locus is activated cooperatively by Oct and NFAT elements within a DNase I-hypersensitive site. *Immunity* **6,** 175–185.
63. Agarwal, S. and Rao, A. (1998) Modulation of chromatin structure regulates cytokine gene expression during T cell differentiation. *Immunity* **9,** 765–775.
64. Takemoto, N., Koyano-Nakagawa, N., Yokota, T., Arai, N., Miyatake, S., and Arai, K. (1998) T_h2-specific DNase I-hypersensitive sites in the murine IL-13 and IL-4 intergenic region. *Intl. Immunol.* **10,** 1981–1985.
65. Weinmann, A. S., Plevy, S. E., and Smale, S. T. (1999) Rapid and selective remodeling of a positioned nucleosome during the induction of IL-12 p40 transcription. *Immunity* **11,** 665–695.
66. Zhao, K., Wang, W., Rando, O. J., Xue, Y., Swiderek, K., Kuo, A., and Crabtree, G. R. (1998) Rapid and phosphoinositol-dependent binding of the SWI/SNF-like BAF complex to chromatin after T lymphocyte receptor signaling. *Cell* **95,** 625–636.
67. Parekh, B. S. and Maniatis, T. (1999) Virus infection leads to localized hyperacetylation of histones H3 and H4 at the IFN-β promoter. *Mol. Cell* **3,** 125–129.
68. Jones, P. L. and Wolffe, A. P. (1999) Relationships between chromatin organization and DNA methylation in determining gene expression. *Semin. Cancer Biol.* **9,** 339–347.
69. Razin, A. (1998) CpG methylation, chromatin structure and gene silencing-a three-way connection. *EMBO J.* **17,** 4905–4908.
70. Bird, A. P. and Wolffe, A. P. (1999) Methylation-induced repression-belts, braces, and chromatin. *Cell* **99,** 451–454.
71. Penix, L. A., Sweetser, M. T., Weaver, W. M., Hoeffler, J. P., Kerppola, T. K., and Wilson, C. B. (1996) The proximal regulatory element of the interferon-γ promoter mediates selective expression in T cells. *J. Biol. Chem.* **271,** 31,964–31,972.

72. Young, H. A., Ghosh, P., Ye, J., Lederer, J., Lichtman, A., Gerard, J. R., et al. (1994) Differentiation of the T helper phenotypes by analysis of the methylation state of the IFN-γ gene. *J. Immunol.* **153,** 3603–3610.

73. Melvin, A. J., McGurn, M. E., Bort, S. J., Gibson, C., and Lewis, D. B. (1995) Hypomethylation of the interferon-γ gene correlates with its expression by primary T-lineage cells. *Eur. J. Immunol.* **25,** 426–430.

74. Fitzpatrick, D. R., Shirley, K. M., McDonald, L. E., Bielefeldt-Ohmann, H., Kay, G. F., and Kelso, A. (1998) Distinct methylation of the interferon γ (IFN-γ) and interleukin 3 (IL-3) genes in newly activated primary CD8+ T lymphocytes: regional IFN-γ promoter demethylation and mRNA expression are heritable in CD44^{high} CD8+ T cells. *J. Exp. Med.* **188,** 103–117.

75. Mikovits, J. A., Young, H. A., Vertino, P., Issa, J.-P. J., Pitha, P. A., Turcoski-Corrales, S., et al. (1998) Infection with human immunodeficiency virus type 1 upregulates DNA methyltransferase, resulting in de novo methylation of the gamma interferon (IFN-γ) promoter and subsequent downregulation of IFN-γ production. *Mol. Cell Biol.* **18,** 5166–5177.

76. Bird, J. J., Brown, D. R., Mullen, A. C., Moskowitz, N. H., Mahowald, M. A., Sider, J. R., et al. (1998) Helper T cell differentiation is controlled by the cell cycle. *Immunity* **9,** 229–237.

77. Gett, A. V. and Hodgkin, P. D. (1998) Cell division regulates the T cell cytokine repertoire, revealing a mechanism underlying immune class regulation. *Proc. Natl. Acad. Sci. USA* **95,** 9488–9493.

78. Richter, A., Löhning, M., and Radbruch, A. (1999) Instruction for cytokine expression in T helper lymphocytes in relation to proliferation and cell cycle progression. *J. Exp. Med.* **190,** 1439–1450.

3

Variant Ligands, Altered T Cell Receptor Signaling, Hierarchical Response Thresholds, and CD4$^+$ Effector Responses

Yasushi Itoh and Ronald N. Germain

1. INTRODUCTION

T-lymphocytes expressing $\alpha\beta$ receptors for antigen (T cell receptors [TCR]) play a central role in adaptive immune responses. The mature T cell repertoire is produced by selection in the thymus of precursor T cells bearing clonally distributed TCR, based on the nature of signals generated by receptor interaction with ligands comprised of self-peptides bound to major histocompatibility complex (MHC) class I or class II molecules *(1)*. In the periphery, the mature CD4$^+$ and CD8$^+$ T cells develop effector activity in response to the combination of intracellular signals generated by TCR recognition of ligands composed of foreign peptide bound to the same set of MHC molecules (p/MHC) and by binding of other surface receptors to cell-associated counterreceptors or cytokines. T cells show a complex array of activation-related responses following such ligand recognition and the initiation of TCR signaling, including but not limited to proliferation, production of a diverse set of cytokines, expression of new surface proteins, cytotoxicity, and altered migratory behavior. For CD8$^+$ T cells recognizing p/MHC class I ligands, most studies have been largely confined to measurements of cell killing or production of a limited set of cytokines, most notably interferon-γ (IFN-γ). A much wider range of responses has been characterized for CD4$^+$ T cells. Particular attention has been paid in the past decade to the notion of polarized CD4$^+$ T cell phenotypes, typically referred to as Th1 and Th2. Th1 cells produce several characteristic cytokines, including IL-2, IFN-γ, tumor necrocis factor-β (TNF-β), and FasL, whereas Th2 cells typically produce IL-4, IL-5, IL-9, IL-10, and IL-13, although the bulk of published reports focus on analysis of Th1 and Th2 defined by the signature cytokines IFN-γ and IL-4, respectively *(2)*.

From: *Cytokines and Autoimmune Diseases*
Edited by: V. K. Kuchroo, et al. © Humana Press Inc., Totowa, NJ

Many factors in addition to those directly involving the TCR have been shown to influence Th1 vs Th2 differentiation, including cytokines such as IL-12, IFN-γ, or IL-4 *(3,4)*, costimulation by CD80 and CD86 via CD28 *(5–7)*, the physical form of the antigen *(8)*, signals arising from pattern recognition receptors interacting with microbial components *(9,10)*, and the route of antigen administration *(11,12)*. Despite the importance of nonantigen specific factors in controlling CD4$^+$ T cell differentiation, however, an important question in this area of research remains how the nature (quantity/quality) of TCR signaling in response to either self-ligands (autoantigens) or foreign ligands influences Th polarization. This brief chapter will focus on what is currently known about how the extent and nature of signaling via the TCR in response to alternations in ligand quality participate in regulating the effector properties of T cells. These findings will be related to the quantitative issues discussed in depth in the preceding chapter.

2. VARIANT TCR LIGANDS AND FUNCTIONAL PARTIAL ACTIVATION OR ANTAGONISM

2.1. The Occupancy Model of T Cell Activation

For many years, it was generally assumed that antigens (more specifically, peptides) that did not activate T cells as measured by proliferation, cytokine release, or cell killing were not antigenic. In the case of a failure to prime T cells in the intact animal, this lack of antigenicity was attributed to a failure of effective presentation by available MHC molecules (that is, the analyzed peptides were unable to bind to available MHC molecules and create a TCR ligand) rather than to holes in the repertoire (the absence of T cells able to respond to those peptide/MHC molecule combinations that could be formed) *(13–15)*. In the case of already primed T cells, peptides that could bind to the relevant MHC molecule but not elicit one of these commonly measured responses were considered to produce ligands unable to interact with the TCR of the T cells in question, at least to the degree necessary for effective intracellular signal generation *(16)*. The basis for this view was the notion that all occupancy events involving the TCR were equivalent in their signaling outcomes and hence, their effect on the T cell. If p/MHC complexes were created at sufficient density, but the T cell did not produce IL-2 or proliferate, then the simple view was that the TCR had such a low affinity for the complexes that no substantial occupancy occurred, no signals were generated, and hence, no responses ensued.

2.2. Partial Agonists

Two sets of data obtained in the early 1990s involving the biological effects of sequence analogs of known stimulatory peptides changed this view of TCR signaling and T cell responses. The first observation involved a study of mouse Th2 cells *(17)*. The Th2 cells in question responded to an antigenic peptide derived from hemoglobin when bound to the MHC class II I-E^k molecule by proliferating and secreting IL-4. Presentation to these T cells by the same I-E^k molecules of a variant peptide antigen that had a single amino acid substitution resulted instead in secretion of nearly the same amount of IL-4, but no measurable proliferation. It was proposed that the small change in ligand structure resulting from the amino acid substitution in the hemoglobin sequence modified affinity of the p/MHC ligand for the TCR, resulting in a change in intracellular signaling that affected the proliferative responses differently from transcription of the IL-4 gene.

One complicating feature of this study was the ability of IL-1, which is not a T cell product, to rescue the proliferative response. Production of IL-1 by antigen-presenting cells (APC) can be modified by ligation of their MHC class II molecules *(18,19)*. Thus, an alternative interpretation of these data was that the change in affinity of the TCR for the variant peptide/I-E^k ligand altered signals received by the APC via class II engagement by the TCR, limiting IL-1 production and hence, IL-4 dependent induction of proliferation that can require IL-1 *(20,21)*. If this were the case in the hemoglobin model, then altered TCR signaling might not account for the differential responses to the original and altered ligands. This caveat aside, ligands with the characteristics of the variant hemoglobin/I-E^k combination that elicit only a subset of biological responses have been referred to as "partial agonists" and the existence of such ligands has now been reported in many other experimental systems (reviewed in refs. *22–24*).

It is important to note the distinction between "partial agonists" and "weak agonists." The latter can induce all the responses that can be elicited by strong agonists in the same relative proportion, whereas the former fail to induce one or more responses that the T cell is potentially able to make, or induces them with a substantial alteration in their relative proportions at any given ligand concentration *(25)* (Fig. 1). This distinction is of significance in considering whether such variant ligands merely induce less signaling or alter the nature of the signals transmitted through the TCR in what is operationally a qualitatively distinct manner. Another issue of some confusion is the difference between a primary defect in TCR-induced responsiveness and a secondary effect of the limited TCR-dependent response. In the hemoglobin model, it was reported that anergy (defined as defective IL-2 production in response to an otherwise stimulatory ligand/APC combination by T cells previously exposed to antigen) resulted directly from altered signaling experienced during partial agonist pretreatment *(26,27)*. However, other studies suggest that this is a secondary consequence of the failure of the

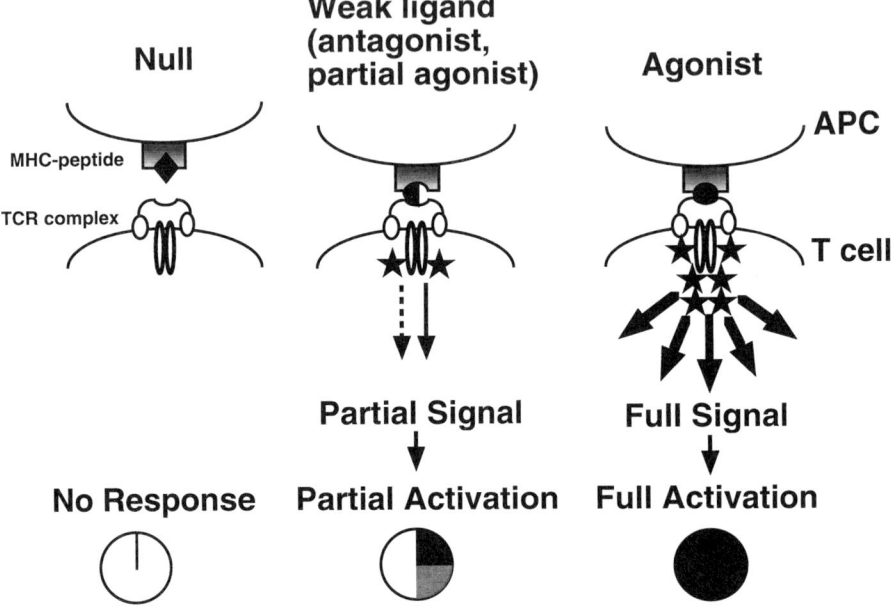

Fig. 1. Types of T cell receptor ligands. Agonist ligands induce full phosphorylation (stars) of ITAMs within the TCR complex followed by elicitation of the entire set of effector responses. Partial agonists induce incomplete phosphorylation of TCR ζ-chain ITAMs and induce a limited subset of effector responses. Antagonists also induce partial ζ phosphorylation and inhibit the responses to simultaneously offered agonist ligand.

cells to produce IL-2, rather than a direct intracellular disturbance resulting from altered TCR signaling itself *(28)* (Fig. 1).

2.3. Antagonists

The second novel category of TCR ligands was discovered in studies of variant peptides like those used in the Evavold experiment with Th2, but in which both a stimulatory peptide and a variant peptide were bound to the same APC membrane. The variant p/MHC ligands in question did not evoke any measurable T cell responses when presented by themselves, which would conventionally define them as nonantigenic or nonagonist in nature. However, these nonstimulatory ligands were not "null" in terms of effects on the TCR, because when copresented they inhibited the response to a stimulatory ligand, i.e., they acted as antagonists. In the first report on this phenomenon, human T cell proliferation and IL-2 responses were inhibited by p/MHC ligands formed using peptides that were single amino acid variants of the antigenic peptide, but these responses were not inhibited by unrelated peptides even if they bound to MHC molecules on the same cell surface *(29)*. In combination with the fact that the stimulatory peptides were allowed to form complexes with MHC molecules before addition of the inhibitory variant peptide, these data argued strongly against the possibility that the nonstimulatory peptide simply competed with the stimulatory peptide for binding to MHC presenting molecules.

In the second independent description of TCR antagonism, a mouse T cell clone responsive to pigeon cytochrome *c* peptide bound to wild-type I-E^k MHC class II molecules or to a mutant form of I-E^k in the absence of cytochrome peptide was studied *(30)*. The response to the mutant MHC class II molecule was inhibited rather than augmented by addition of pigeon cytochrome *c* and as in the human clone results, unrelated peptides that bound to I-E^k, or even cytochrome peptides altered in the major epitopic contact residue that bound equally well to I-E^k, failed to cause such inhibition. This again argued in favor of a TCR-mediated negative effect and not interference with stimulatory ligand formation. This study also provided several other additional insights into the activity of altered ligands for the TCR. In this case, the peptide was not changed (it remained wild-type pigeon cytochrome *c* in sequence), but the ligand formed was altered because of the mutation in the MHC molecule. This emphasizes that it is the complete p/MHC ligand that is relevant and points out that the term "altered peptide ligand" applies only to a subset of all possible "variant TCR ligands" with distinct functional properties (partial agonist, antagonist). Perhaps of greater significance, tests involving a hybridoma expressing the identical TCR showed an IL-3 but not IL-2 response to the combination of mutant MHC class II plus cytochrome peptide, rather than antagonism. This made clear the capacity of this ligand to engage and apparently signal actively through the TCR, implying that the inhibitory function of antagonists was not likely to lie solely with the ability to compete for TCR engagement with agonist ligand without generating any signals, as was originally proposed *(31)*. The contribution of active signaling by TCR antagonists to their inhibitory function has been recently confirmed in two different studies *(32,33)*, although some contribution of passive TCR competition cannot be ruled out at present *(34,35)*. A final new point made in this study was that increased costimulation through the CD28 pathway could not overcome the action of the antagonist, in contrast to the IL-1 data in the Th2/hemoglobin model, implying that the defect truly resided within the T cell and not the APC. A third early study then extended these observations to mouse CD8$^+$ T cells *(36)*. Both partial agonists and antagonists were identified for cytotoxic T cells specific for the ovalbumin peptide SIINFEKL bound to the MHC class

I molecule H-2K^b, helping to generalize the concept of pharmacologically distinct TCR ligand subclasses beyond the CD4$^+$ subset.

3. VARIANT LIGANDS AND ALTERED TCR SIGNALING

3.1. Effects of Variant Ligand Recognition on ζ Chain and ZAP-70 Phosphorylation

The recognition that TCR ligands existed with partial agonist and antagonist properties raised the question of whether the distinct functional characteristics of these ligands arose owing to differences in the nature of intracellular signals generated upon their binding to the TCR. The data in the cytochrome system in particular suggested that this might be the case *(30)*. The earliest known biochemical events induced by TCR ligation involve activation/recruitment of src family kinases, particularly Lck, and the tyrosine phosphorylation of specific residues in the intracellular domains of the CD3 (γ, δ, and ε) and TCR ζ chains physically associated with TCR αβ on the cell surface *(37)*. These tyrosine residues are located within a unique consensus amino acid sequence called immune receptor tyrosine-based activation motif (ITAM = YxxL [..6–8 residues..] YxxL) (38). Each of the CD3 subunits has one ITAM, whereas the TCR ζ chain has three ITAMs in each of the subunits that comprised this disulfide-bonded dimeric protein. Early studies of ζ phosphorylation showed that all six tyrosines on each chain could be modified in response to strong ligation of the TCR *(39,40)*. This raised the possibility that only some and not other of these sites might undergo effective modification when the TCR was engaged with a less effective ligand. Because the mobility of the TCR ζ chain in sodium dodecyl sulfate-polyacrylamide gel electrophoresis (SDS-PAGE) depends on the extent of its phosphorylation, analysis of phospho-ζ chains by SDS-PAGE and blotting with anti-phosphotyrosine antibodies seemed a reasonable approach to testing whether variant TCR ligands affected the earliest stages of intracellular signal generation. Such studies in both the hemoglobin and cytochrome models showed congruent data, revealing the generation of similar proportions of two isoforms of phosphorylated ζ chain monomers migrating with apparent molecular masses of 23 and 21 kD (p23 and p21) when strong stimulatory ligands were used, and an excess of p21 with little p23 ζ when either partial agonist or even nonstimulatory antagonists were employed *(27,41)*. Strikingly, using lower amounts of the strong ligands did not result in the p21 ζ dominant pattern seen with partial agonists or antagonists, indicating that the difference between agonists and antagonists was not simply the result of less TCR occupancy.

These two early studies reached different conclusions about whether or not ZAP-70 kinase was recruited to the partially phosphorylated ζ chains, with the data in the hemoglobin system taken to indicate a lack of such recruitment and the results in the cytochrome model indicating binding but not tyrosine phosphorylation nor activation of ZAP-70. More recent results have confirmed that in the hemoglobin model *(42)*, as in the cytochrome *(41)* and other systems analyzed more recently using both mouse and human lymphocytes *(33,43–46)*, ZAP-70 is bound to the partially phosphorylated ζ chains, but it typically remains nonphosphorylated and inactive. This is in contrast to the ZAP-70 bound to the ITAMs present in TCR complexes stimulated with agonist ligands, in which case the ZAP-70 becomes tyrosine phosphorylated and acquires kinase activity.

These same later studies have confirmed and extended the initial observations of differential ζ chain phosphorylation as well using mouse and also human CD4+ cells (in the latter case, nonreduced conditions are frequently employed, producing dimeric ζ with apparent mobilities of p32 = p21 monomer, and p38 = p23 monomer). Furthermore, similar results are seen using CD8+ cells *(47)*. Analysis with phosphopeptide specific antibodies confirmed, as expected from the earlier two-dimensional gel analysis, that p23 corresponds to ζ chains with all six tyrosines phosphorylated *(42)*. Unexpectedly, however, this same analysis indicated that p21 ζ is actually a mixture of several phosphorylated species, and most significantly, that the ITAMs in these p21 ζ isoforms are singly phosphorylated, that is, rather than having one or two ITAMs each dually phosphorylated, p21 ζ consists of chains initially having only one of two tyrosines in up to three ITAMs modified. Because of the effect of dual ZAP-70 SH2 domain engagement of phosphotyrosines within an ITAM on the structure of this kinase, its modification by src kinases, and its catalytic activity *(48–50)*, these data provide a possible explanation for how ZAP-70 can be recruited to partially phosphorylated ζ chains within a TCR complex and fail to be efficiently phosphorylated and activated.

3.2. Relationship Between the Kinetics of TCR:Ligand Interactions and Altered Signaling

Although a full molecular explanation for the altered phosphorylation patterns seen with partial agonists and antagonists has not been achieved, several important advances have been made in this area in the past several years. Measurements of the kinetics and affinity of soluble TCR for various soluble forms of p/MHC combinations using surface plasmon resonance *(51–54)* have indicated a general correlation between affinity and more specifically, TCR-ligand dissociation-rate, partial agonist/antagonists functional properties, and altered signaling *(53–58)*. These findings indicate that the life-time of engagement between the TCR and its ligand plays a crucial role in establishing the altered intracellular events that are ultimately translated into distinct biological outcomes. How the dissociation rate leads to incomplete ζ chain phosphorylation is not yet resolved. One model proposes that initiation of signaling involves sequestration of Lck-associated TCR away from CD45 *(59,60)*; once ligand binding is terminated, CD45 would gain access to the activated receptor complex and interrupt signaling by dephosphorylating Lck at the activating tyrosine 394 and by removing phosphates from ζ *(61,62)*. Very recent data indicate that the initial burst of kinase function produces tyrosine phosphorylated SHP-1 phosphatase *(63)* that then binds to Lck. Activation of this bound SHP-1 by other phospho-proteins within the activated TCR complex could the result in dephosphorylation of Lck, ZAP-70, and possibly ζ, resulting in a similar picture of bound inactive ZAP-70 and partially phosphorylated ζ *(24*; Stefanova et al., submitted). Unexpectedly, it was recently discovered that inhibition of such SHP-1 recruitment can be mediated by ERK-1 modification of Lck and that stimulatory ligands produce a more rapid rise in ERK-1 activity that inhibits TCR desensitization by this phosphatase *(24*; Stefanova et al., submitted). Thus, the very early limitation of signal duration by CD45 action on TCR disengaged from weakly binding ligands may be translated into inefficient downstream signaling for ERK activity, further depressing effective TCR signals owing to the unopposed action of a second phosphatase, SHP-1.

3.3. Coreceptor Function and Altered Signaling in Response to Variant TCR Ligands

The stability of TCR-ligand interaction depends not only on the intrinsic affinity of these interacting proteins, but also the additional avidity contributed by coassociation of the CD4 or CD8 coreceptors. These coreceptors are also bound to Lck, which contributes to the development of intracellular signals through tyrosine phosphorylation of various substrates *(64,65)*. Thus, it is not surprising that the effective recruitment of CD4 or CD8 plays an important role in the generation of fully phosphorylated TCR-associated chains, and that interference with coreceptor function through use of blocking antibodies or the use of mutant MHC molecules unable to bind these coreceptors *(66–68)* interferes with full activation, as analyzed by the state of phosphorylation of TCR ζ and ZAP-70. One attractive model is that the rapidity of TCR-ligand dissociation determines in large measure whether CD4 or CD8 has time to enter into a trimeric association with the TCR-ligand pair or not, based on the rate of diffusion of the respective complexes in the membrane. Rapidly dissociating TCR-ligand complexes would not have a high likelihood of remaining intact during the time it takes for a coreceptor to come

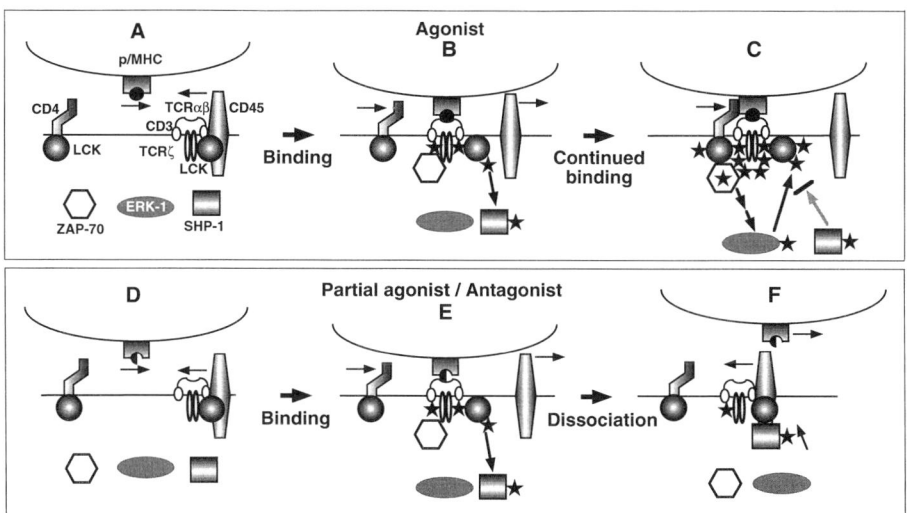

Fig. 2. Model for the origin of altered TCR signaling by partial agonists/antagonists. When TCR encounter agonist ligands on an APC membrane (upper panel **A**), receptor-associated kinase (?Lck) is activated and begins to phosphorylate tyrosines in ITAMs in proteins such as TCR ζ as well as on SHP-1 (**B**). Because the agonist-MHC:TCR interaction is relatively stable, i.e., the half-life of agonist-MHC:TCR contact is long enough (B→C), CD4-Lck can be recruited to the agonist:TCR pair (**C**). By both preventing ligand dissociation and also providing an additional source of kinase, this leads to further phosphorylation of ITAMs and ZAP-70 recruitment/ activation, followed by the subsequent modification of adapter proteins such as LAT and translation of the TCR-ligand interaction into a cascade of second messenger activities. Among these in ERK-1, which modifies the Lck and prevents recruitment of phosphorylated SHP-1, helping to extend the duration of signaling and fostering proper synapse formation. In contrast, when partial agonists/antagonists engage TCR (lower panel **D**), the initial events are similar, involving initiation of ITAM phosphorylation along with phosphorylation of SHP-1 (**E**). Dissociation of ligand prior to coreceptor recruitment interferes with activation of ZAP-70 even when bound to the partially phosphorylated ITAMs of TCR-associated chains (E→F), which in turn prevents efficient production of downstream messengers such as activate ERK-1 (**F**). This leaves the TCR complex susceptible to binding and activation of SHP-1, which in turn inactivates Lck and aborts the signaling process.

into close association. This would prevent such ligands from enhancing their time of association with the TCR through the action of the coreceptor, accentuating the difference in lifetime of the two types of complexes *(68,69)*. These considerations of coreceptor action may be of significance in understanding the contributions of CD4 to T cell functional polarization, as discussed later (Fig. 2).

4. MEMBRANE PROTEIN DYNAMICS AND T CELL ACTIVATION

Analyses involving sequential or real-time analysis of the distribution of proteins in the interface between a T cell and an antigen-bearing APC have revealed a remarkably precise organization of various receptors and their ligands on the two cell membranes. Rather than a random clustering, zones in which the concentration of certain molecules is substantially increased or diminished regularly form with a particular pattern. When T cells recognize agonist antigens on the APC, ICAM-1 molecules (LFA-1 is the counterreceptor on the T cells) cluster in the central area of T cell-APC contact and p/MHC complexes that are engaged by the TCR on the opposing cell membrane surround the ICAM-1 zone at a very early time-point (30 s after engagement). By 10 min, MHC-peptide complexes move to center of the contact area and ICAM-1 is now concentrated in a surrounding ring *(70,71)*. Protein kinase C (PKC)-θ is also included in the center of contact area *(70)*. This organized structure is called the SMAC (supramolecular activation complex) or immunological synapse. The efficiency of this cluster formation and the final density of TCR in the cluster is determined by the affinity of the offered ligand for the TCR, in other words, weak ligands like partial agonists or antagonists do not concentrate TCR on the central contact area *(71)* (Fig. 3).

A key point is understanding the significance of the cluster. As clearly pointed out by Grakoui et al. *(71)*, the apparent function of this structure is to provide for the sustained signaling over many hours that is necessary for the gene activation involved in effector-cell differentiation and function. The synapse is only fully formed well after the initial burst of high-level tyrosine phosphorylation or rise in intracellular Ca^{++} characteristic of effective TCR signal transduction, which occurs in less than a minute or two *(24,38,72)*. Thus, the correlation between synapse organization and ligand quality reflects the requirement for effective TCR signaling to actively form the synapse, not the need for synapse formation to achieve an agonist quality of proximal TCR signaling. Seen in this way, one can consider three time scales involved in TCR signaling: a "micro" scale involving the very rapid (less than a second to a few seconds) association/dissociation of individual receptors and p/MHC that determine the level of initial downstream second messenger production. This in turn influences the balance of the negative (SHP-1) and positive (ERK-1) feedback pathways that control the duration and quality of the early phosphorylation response (1 to 20–40 min) *(24)*. This "meso" scale signaling in turn contributes to the efficiency of synapse formation (Délon et al., unpublished observations), which then dictates the time scale over which chronic, presumably low intensity signaling occurs

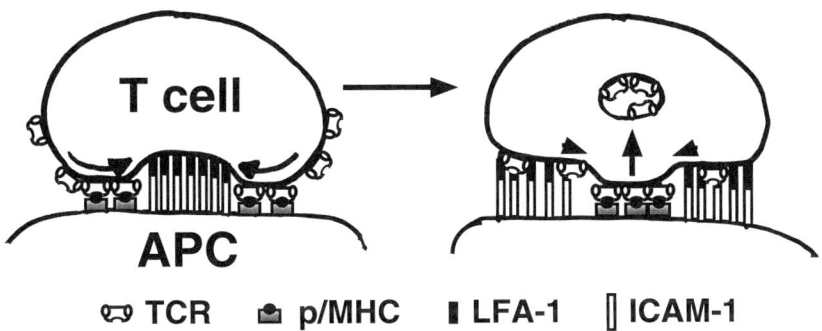

Fig. 3. Immunological synapse formation. When a migrating T cell encounters an APC bearing specific antigens, it stops its movement and adheres to APC using high-affinity LFA-1 binding *(144)*. At this point LFA-1:ICAM-1 complexes are located in the center of the contact area surrounded by TCR-ligand complexes. Soon thereafter, TCR-ligand complexes gather into the center of the T cell:APC attachment zone and LFA-1:ICAM-1 complexes are excluded from the center, forming a ring around the concentrated TCR-ligand pairs. This patch keeps the local density of TCRs high, perhaps allowing ligand rebinding to augment effective occupancy *(145)*. Fully activated TCR complexes are internalized (downmodulated) and degraded, replaced by new TCR from outside the synaptic zone. This permits serial engagement of multiple TCRs by the same pool of ligands, amplifying the effective signal intensity *(79,80)*.

(30 min—several hours). The magnitude and duration of early signaling events may determine the number of responding cells that reach the threshold necessarily for stable synapse formation and any functional response *(73)*, whereas the duration of these late signaling events may determine which gene products are produced *(74)*.

The synapse is not a static structure. Rather, TCR and possibly coreceptors appear to enter and exit the central zone over time, with TCR complexes being targeted for endocytic uptake and degradation, resulting in net TCR and CD4 or CD8 downmodulation *(75–78)*. This sequential binding of TCR by a fixed pool of p/MHC ligands has been termed serial engagement *(79,80)* (Fig. 3). The resulting TCR downmodulation is well correlated with the quality and quantity of the ligands recognized *(44,79–82)* because TCR downregulation is antigen dose-dependent and strong agonists induce more effective modulation, consistent with a requirement for full phosphorylation to induce internalization of receptors *(44,80,83,84)*. This process may amplify the effect of small number of ligands by allowing signals to be generated from a greater number of TCR. The partial phosphorylation events characteristic of antagonists are not adequate to modulate TCR expression, although the kinase activation leading to these partial phosphorylation events does induce SHP-1 phosphatase recruitment and inhibition of TCR function upon engagement of agonist ligands *(24,33)* and correlates with inhibitory activity *(85)*.

5. RESPONSE THRESHOLDS, RESPONSE HIERARCHY, AND EFFECTOR POLARIZATION

5.1. Intraclonal Heterogeneity in CD4⁺ Cytokine Responses

In trying to relate these emerging concepts of pharmacologically distinct ligand classes and patterns of TCR signaling to effector polarization and function of T cells, it is important to also consider another key idea to emerge from studies over the past few years. Early analyses of T cell responses made the simplifying assumption that once "triggered," a T cell would play out a fixed-response program, that is, produce the entire set of effector functions of which it is capable. The major debate was whether the magnitude (not the quality) of the response of each cell differed with the strength of stimulus (analog response), or whether variations in response within cell populations reflected only a difference in the number of cells passing the triggering threshold (digital response). It now appears that both can occur, with a rise in the number of responding cells *(73,86)* and in the amount of cytokine made per cell also scaling to some extent with signal intensity *(87,88)*. However, these studies did not address the question of whether the quality or set of effector functions elicited from a cell was unchanging over a dose-response of stimulation. CD4⁺ T cells in particular have many effector functions. Th1 cells make IL-2, IFN-γ, and TNF-β as soluble factors and upregulate FasL and CD40L to interact with other cells. Th2 cells make IL-4, IL-5, IL-9, IL-13, and help B cell responses *(2)*. The advent of single-cell analysis using either *in situ* hybridization or more commonly, intracellular cytokine staining, has now made it clear that individual Th1 or Th2 cells do not make all of these cytokines simultaneously *(87–95)*. Some of this heterogeneity comes from individual cells gaining competence to transcribe one but not another cytokine gene *(96–99)*, but even among cells that are potentially able to transcribe multiple cytokine genes, whether a product is made can vary with the extent of TCR signaling, all others things being equal.

5.2. Hierarchical Organization of Individual Effector Response Thresholds

We and other groups have formulated these series of observations into a "hierarchical" model of T cell effector functions, which proposes that each effector function has a different triggering threshold (Fig. 4). For example,

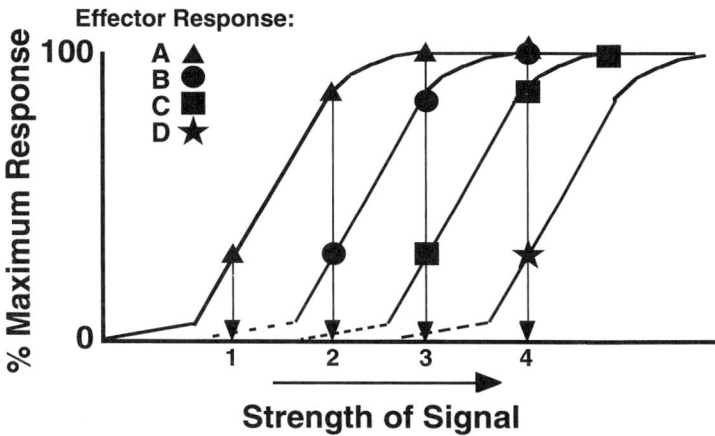

Fig. 4. Hierarchical response threshold model. (**A**), (**B**), (**C**), and (**D**) are different effector responses. They have different signal-intensity thresholds that must be reached for their elicitation. With a very weak signal (1), only response (A) is produced. (B) needs a stronger signal than A and so an appreciable response is not seen until signal strength 2 is reached. (C) is less easily elicited than (B) and requires signal strength 3, whereas (D) requires signal strength 4. This gives rise to very different ratios of effector products at distinct points in the dose-response curve and can account for very distinct biological behaviors of the T cell immune system at low and high antigen density.

with CD8$^+$ CTL cytolytic activity is seen at very low densities of p/MHC ligand *(100)*, but cytokine production of the same T cells needs much greater levels of ligand than cytotoxicity *(47,101)*. This may reflect the difference between a transcription-independent and transcript-dependent response, such that formation of a synapse resulting in prolonged signaling is not necessary for killing by granule release, but is required for maintaining the proper set of activated transcription factors for synthesis of cytokine mRNA. A hierarchy of T cell effector responses has also been seen with CD4$^+$ T cells. Typically, IFN-γ production is observed at a lower concentration of antigen than that of IL-2 *(88,101–104)*. Using Th0 cells, IL-4 production is often obtained at a lower ligand density than IFN-γ *(44,105)*. Because of such differences in the triggering thresholds for distinct effector functions, responses induced by a low concentration of agonist ligand often look phenotypically like the responses to partial agonists *(44)*. This may arise because the cells primarily respond to the number of fully signaling TCR complexes, which may be similar with both ligands types when each is used at a suitable concentration. In this manner, quantitative variations in receptor triggering can be translated to qualitative difference in immune responses owing to the distinct mix of cytokines produced at different points in a dose-response curve (Fig. 4).

The hierarchical nature of cytokine response thresholds is likely to play a major role in dictating the functional responses of populations of CD4$^+$ T cells. Because achieving the magnitude and/or duration of signaling necessary to exceed a particular response threshold in turn depends strongly on not just the quantity, but also the quality of the ligand, it is thus not surprising that these parameters have been found to have a strong impact on the quality of immune responses. Regulation of Th polarization by antigen dose has been repeatedly documented in experiments analyzing the induction of Th1 or Th2 cells from naive T cells. IL-4 production is seen using T cells from TCR transgenic mice primed in vitro with a low concentration of peptide. On the other hand, IFN-γ production is seen with cells primed at a relatively high concentration of antigen *(106,107)*. The initial interpretation of these data involved a simple version of the hierarchy model, in which the threshold for eliciting IL-4 was lower than that for IFN-γ, hence a low density of ligand promoted Th2 development, which is self-reinforcing *(2)*. High concentrations of ligand presumably allowed the cells to reach the threshold necessary for IFN-γ production, which is reinforced by a combination of positive and negative regulatory effects of this cytokine when it is at adequate concentrations *(108,109)*. Similar data were obtained using partial agonist ligands *(110)*, which favored Th2 development just as seen at low agonist ligand density, arguing again that limited signaling is adequate for Th2 but not Th1 differentiation owing to threshold differences (Fig. 5).

It was thus unexpected that limiting dilution studies in a transgenic model did not show a bias in IL-4 vs IFN-γ producing cells when either ligand density or ligand quality was varied *(111)*. Rather, the requirement for a high dose of antigen for Th1 polarization was explained by effects of the cytokines themselves acting *in trans* on populations of cells. At low antigen concentrations or with partial agonist ligands, too little IFN-γ was produced to outweigh the self-amplifying effects of IL-4 on its own production, hence the predominance of Th2 polarization. As ligand density/efficacy increased, a greater absolute amount of IFN-γ was generated that eventually reached a sufficient concentration to override the effect of IL-4 and move the population in the Th1 direction. These data emphasize the complexity of the final response patterns of T cell populations and the indirect relationship between altered ligand function and these outcomes. At the same time, it is probable that populations effects such as these are relevant during the generation of in vivo immune responses, a view consistent with the tendency of partial agonist ligands to promote Th2 polarization in in vivo model systems *(103,112)*.

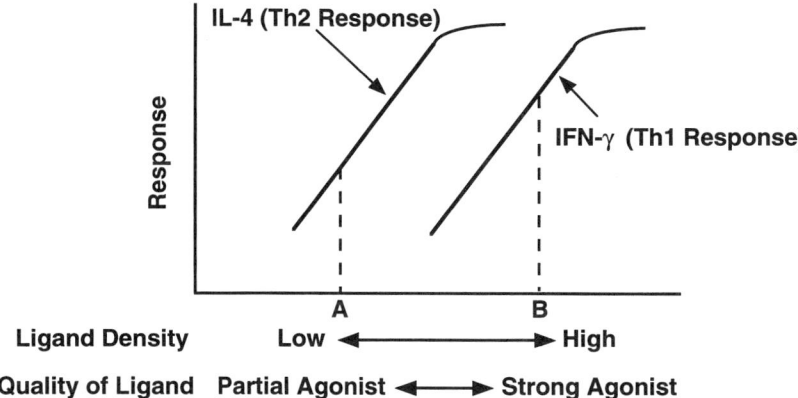

Fig. 5. Hierarchical order of Th1 and Th2 responses. During the induction of effector Th cells from naive T cells, a low quantity and/or low affinity of ligand for the TCR preferentially elicits IL-4 and polarization to the Th2 phenotype (**A**). In contrast, high concentrations of antigen or agonists with high affinity induce Th1 responses (**B**), presumably because as IL-4 production plateaus, increasing IFN-γ production can override the IL-4 drive to Th2 and produce Th1 polarization.

They also support a key importance of the hierarchical model when considered on the cell-population level with respect to the relative levels of polarizing cytokines made during an early phase of an immune response at various ligand densities or with varying quality of ligand-TCR relationship.

6. CALCIUM SIGNALS AND TRANSCRIPTION-FACTOR ACTIVATION

Whether affecting an individual cell's response by operating in a quantitative manner with respect to the hierarchy of triggering thresholds, affecting the response by changing the pattern of intracellular signaling in a qualitative manner, or influencing population behavior by modifying the overall strength of response among individual cells, it is clear that changing the quality of a TCR ligand influences the biology of the responding system. How the altered proximal signaling and the downstream effects on synapse formation and signal duration that result from TCR binding to variant ligands operates at a molecular level remains to be deciphered, but several clues have emerged and some models can be proposed. The obvious place to seek connections is in the downstream signaling pathways that connect the proximal phosphorylation events described earlier to the activation of transcription factors that regulate gene expression.

One second messenger whose pattern and extent of modification has been well-studied in T cells is intracellular Ca^{++}, which is both released from intracellular stores via the action of IP_3 and admitted into the cell through the action of Ca^{++} channels *(113,114)*. Using microscopic methods to trace single cells and indicators to detect cytosolic calcium, calcium responses have been characterized according to the frequency of responding cells, the onset of responses, the frequency of oscillations and the shape of peak (full, reduced, partial, and transient signals) *(23,115,116)*. Full agonists induced a singular rapid increase or a transient and small sinusoidal peak with a sustained level of calcium elevation lasting for more than 10 min. This sustained rise in Ca^{++} correlates with induction of proliferation *(117)*. Partial agonists, in contrast, induce only a transient elevation of intracellular calcium levels, with a rapid return to resting levels, whereas no initial peak and only a series of oscillations (3–5 times/min) are seen with antagonists.

These different patterns of intracellular Ca^{++} modulation in cells exposed to ligands of distinct quality are likely to have major influence on gene activity. A study using B cells showed a clear relationship between calcium signaling patterns and activation of transcription factors *(118)*. Activation of NF-κB and JNK (c-Jun N-terminal kinase)-1 required a large transient calcium increase, whereas NF-ATp/c (NF-AT 1/2) were translocated to the nucleus in the face of only a low sustained calcium rise. Therefore, stimulation of a low calcium rise can lead to NF-ATp/c translocation without accompany activation of NF-κB or JNK1, with obvious implications for activation of genes with differential dependence on these two sets of transcription factors. The frequency of oscillations in cytosolic calcium concentration, as well as the peak or mean levels of Ca^{++} rise, have been documented to control gene expression in T cells *(119,120)*. NF-AT, NF-κB, and Oct/OAP activities are dependent on intracellular calcium concentration and reach plateau activation at a high mean intracellular Ca^{++} concentration. Oscillation of $[Ca^{++}]_i$, however, has different effects on these factors depending on the frequency of the changes. NF-κB activation can be sustained with an oscillation period as long as 1800 s, in contrast to NF-AT and Oct/OAP, whose activity vanishes at a period longer than 400 s. Based on these observations and the measurements of Ca^{++} changes induced by ligands of different quality, it appears that full agonist ligands capable of inducing sustained high-amplitude calcium influx would likely activate NF-AT, NF-kB, and Oct/OAP, whereas partial agonists and antagonists producing a low-amplitude response with but high-frequency oscillations might preferentially activate the NF-κB pathway. Such differential activation of key transcription factors presumably plays a major role in the capacity of variant ligands to elicit only some of the full range of potential effector responses from a given T cell.

7. VARIANT LIGANDS AND THE DEVELOPMENT OF TH1/ TH2 EFFECTOR PHENOTYPES: RELATING SIGNALING TO FUNCTION

7.1. Variant Ligands and Polarization of Naive T Cells

Altered ligands can have dramatic effects on the differentiation of naive T cells *(121)*. In several model systems in which the original p/MHC combination typical induces a strong Th1 type response (collagen IV *[112]* or proteolipid protein (PLP) *[103]*), altered peptides produce ligands favoring Th2 generation, as evidenced by production of IL-4 and/or IL-10. In the study with collagen, the wild-type collagen peptide had a different affinity for MHC molecules compared to the variant peptides tested; whether this feature of the peptides, or different binding of the smaller number of ligands generated to the available TCR, contributed to this effect has not been resolved. PLP antigen induces experimental autoimmune encephalomyelitis (EAE) owing to generation of Th1-type autoreactive T cells in response to wild type PLP antigen *(122)*. Immunization with an altered PLP peptide induces not only IFN-γ production but also IL-4 and IL-10 production that appears to modulate the pathology induced by a Th1 response to the wild-type PLP *(123)*. Similarly, T cells expressing the same transgenic TCR differentiate into Th1 or Th2 cells with strong agonists or weak ligands, respectively *(110)*. In the context of the data presented in preceding sections, it is likely that these variant ligands produce only incomplete signals whose effect on transcription factor activity favors IL-4 secretion without production of an amount of IFN-γ sufficient to overcome the feedback amplification of the former cytokine, leading to a dominant Th2 response (Fig. 5).

7.2. Altered TCR Signaling to Agonist Ligands in Polarized Th2 Cells

Using a TCR transgenic system, biochemical signals induced by agonists and altered ligands were analyzed in already polarized Th1 and Th2 cells *(124)*. Partial phosphorylation pattern of the ζ chain was seen when T cells encountering altered ligands during a first stimulation and developing into Th2 cells were restimulated with an agonist ligand that could elicit a full phosphorylation pattern with naive or Th1 cells bearing the same TCR. Other reports also suggest that TCR signaling in established Th2 cells more closely resembles the partial agonist pattern described for Th1 and Tc1 cells in many systems, including little or no detectable TCR-associated protein phosphorylation and limited activation/phosphorylation of Fyn, Lck, ZAP-70, PLC-γ 1, or Lnk *(124–126)*. In addition, Th2 cells without Lck activity still have an ability to make Th2 cytokines *(126,127)*, suggesting that Lck is not the primary src family kinase mediating even the limited signaling seen in such cells. In a like manner, calcium elevations in Th2 cells are transient and of lower amplitude than those seen with Th1 cells with the same TCR and using the same ligand *(23,124,128)*. Thus, not only does an initial partial pattern of signaling favor generation of Th2 cells, but these Th2 cells then show signaling of this constrained type even when exposed to what for their TCR would be considered a full agonist ligand, one that with Th1 cells bearing identical TCR elicits full phosphorylation and downstream second-messenger production.

Although it is perhaps simple to imagine why weak signals might favor Th2 generation, if IL-4 can be produced with less robust signaling than can IFN-γ, it is more surprising that once differentiated, Th2 should need to continue to signal in this manner even when exposed to a ligand with (relatively) high affinity for the TCR. This raises two questions: First, what changes in coupling of the TCR to the signaling apparatus result in a different translation of the same affinity of ligand binding in Th2 cells as compared to naive cells or Th1 cells, and second, why is this important to the proper functioning of Th2 cells? With respect to the first issue, recent data from this laboratory suggest that one possible difference between Th1 and Th2 may be in the level of CD4 expression, with the level being lower in Th2 (Itoh, Y., et al., in preparation). This would fit with our previous proposal that the rate of recruitment of CD4 to engaged TCR complexes, which is determined by the surface density of CD4, sets a threshold for effective signal generation *(68)* (Fig. 2). In terms of the second issue, one possible rationale is based on the hierarchical threshold model (Fig. 5). If IFN-γ requires more robust signaling that IL-4 for production, then constraining the extent of signaling in Th2 helps enforce the selective production of Th2 cytokines, IL-4 in particular. In Th1 cells, extensive signaling would be necessary to evoke IFN-γ and signal transduction would need to be optimal. Although such strong signaling would exceed the theoretic threshold for IL-4 production, the changes in transcription-factor activity in Th1 cells prevents IL-4 gene activation even when a high level of TCR signaling occurs, avoiding inappropriate Th2 cytokine production. Thus, Th1 and Th2 may use somewhat different mechanisms to maintain their polarized production of cytokines.

This model is not without its flaws. In particular, it does not explain several observations suggesting that Th2 development requires more potent signaling that production of Th1. Using CD4 deficient mice or APC with mutant

MHC class II molecules unable to engage CD4, it was observed that Th2 differentiation was severely impaired though Th1 responses were normal *(129,130)*. Further, dominant-negative Lck transgenic mice develop very weak Th2 responses *(131)* and the Ras/MAPK pathway is required for Th2 differentiation *(132)*. These data seem to imply that differentiation and polarization for Th2 cells need better/greater signals than for Th1 in contrast to the findings of preferential Th2 generation using low concentrations of agonist or partial agonist ligands *(106,107,111,124)*. It is not obvious at the present time how to reconcile these two sets of apparently divergent observations.

8. CONCLUSION

8.1. Self-Ligands as Partial Agonists

Given the crucial role of specific cytokines in the pathology of autoimmune diseases, it is clear that the effects of variant TCR ligands on Th polarization and effector function is of significance both for understanding disease and potentially also for use in treatment. One issue that has not been raised here is whether the self-ligands that are involved in autoimmunity fall into the agonist or partial agonist categories in any predictable manner. In a study of human T cell TCR signaling using variant p/MHC combinations, it was found that the pattern of ζ phosphorylation seen using the nominal "agonist" antigen for myelin basic protein (MBP)-specific T cells was suboptimal in terms of the p32/p38 phospho-ζ ratio, and that the proportion of p38 ζ increased when a variant ligand selected based on enhanced functional potency (superagonist) was identified and tested *(44)*. These data have been interpreted to imply that the MBP specific T cell clones analyzed see this self-antigen as a partial agonist, rather than a fully potent agonist *(24)*. Trimming of the repertoire in the thymus and periphery by various tolerance-inducing mechanisms that primarily affect the highest affinity T cells in the repertoire can account for this finding and would be consistent with the general notion that most self-specific T cells eluding these tolerance mechanisms see their ligands with less than an optimal affinity.

Nevertheless, these cells are clearly capable of effector responses to such ligands. One way in which this can occur relates to the widely held "mimicry" model of autoimmunity *(133)*. Pathogen-derived peptides might resemble the "superagonist" peptides identified for the human MBP specific clones by artificial means *(134)*. In the context of signals from the innate immune responses to the pathogen itself, such effective TCR signaling can generate polarized effector memory cells. Some evidence exists to suggest that such primed cells are more sensitive to ligand than their naive precursors *(135–138)*, in which case a partial agonist ligand that might not activate the corresponding naive cell or that would induce a nonpathogenic set of effector responses might now have the capacity to elicit damaging cytokines from these primed cells. This is an issue deserving of additional investigation.

8.2. Variant Ligands in Disease Prophylaxis and Therapy

On the therapeutic side, variant ligands have been used successfully in prophylaxis (but less so for therapy) *(139)* of autoimmune disease models in animals, especially experimental allergic encephalomyelitis *(123)*. The mechanism of disease prevention has not been fully determined, but some data suggest that induction of Th2 cells that suppress Th1 pathogenic cell priming in *trans* is a key factor in the efficacy of such treatments *(123,140–142)*. Other models include the induction of anergy in the potentially pathogenic precursor T cells *(26)*, or even deletion through selective induction of cell death pathways without effector cytokine generation *(143)*.

These latter therapeutic considerations apply primarily to disease based on Th1-induced pathology. Antibody-mediated autoimmunity, especially if the Ig isotypes involved are those dependent on Th2 cytokine for switching, would presumably have a distinct relationship to variant ligand function. One could imagine that the altered signaling by a low level of a self-ligand seen as a partial agonist would induce polarization of cells to the Th2 phenotype, and that such cells under the right circumstances could support pathogenic autoantibody production. In this case, the use of variant ligands for therapy is questionable, as they would either augment the production of the disease-causing antibodies, or if used as "superagonists" to try to generate Th1 counterregulatory cells, result in a different form of immune damage.

Considerations such as these imply that expanding our knowledge of how variant TCR ligands induce intracellular signals, how such altered signals control T cell behavior, and how T cells responding to variant ligands contribute to and modify autoimmune disease is an area of research with specific importance in relating cytokines to immune pathology. Knowledge of the intracellular pathways that are affected by variant TCR signaling may also provide helpful clues in designing pharmacologic agents to modify cytokine production for patient benefit, beyond its relevance to our basic understanding of the biology of T cells.

REFERECES

1. Robey, E., and Fowlkes, B. J. (1994) Selective events in T cell development. *Annu. Rev. Immunol.* **12**, 675–705.
2. Seder, R. A., and Paul, W. E. (1994) Acquisition of lymphokine-producing phenotype by CD4+ T cells. *Annu. Rev. Immunol.* **12**, 635–673.

3. Swain, S. L., Weinberg, A. D., English, M., and Huston, G. (1990) IL-4 directs the development of Th2-like helper effectors. *J. Immunnol.* **145**, 3796–3806.
4. Le Gros, G., Ben-Sasson, S. Z., Seder, R., Finkelman, F. D., and Paul, W. E. (1990) Generation of interleukin 4 (IL-4)-producing cells in vivo and in vitro: IL-2 and IL-4 are required for in vitro generation of IL-4-producing cells. *J. Exp. Med.* **172**, 921–929.
5. Kuchroo, V. K., Das, M. P., Brown, J. A., Ranger, A. M., Zamvil, S. S., Sobel, R. A., et al. (1995) B7-1 and B7-2 costimulatory molecules activate differentially the Th1/Th2 develpomental pathways: application to autoimmune disease therapy. *Cell* **80**, 707–718.
6. Freeman, G. J., Boussiotis, V. A., Anumanthan, A., Bernstein, G. M., Ke, X.-Y., Rennert, P. D., et al. (1995) B7-1 and B7-2 do not deliver indentical costimulatory signals, since B7-2 but not B7-1 preferentially costimulates the initial production of IL-4. *Immunity* **2**, 523–532.
7. Lenschow, D. J., Herold, K. C., Rhee, L., Patel, B., Koons, A., Qin, H.-Y., Fuchs, E., et al. (1996) CD28/B7 regulation of Th1 and Th2 subsets in the development of autoimmune diabetes. *Immunity* **5**, 285–293.
8. Degermann, S., Pria, E., and Adorini, L. (1996) Soluble protein but not peptide administration diverts the immune response of a clonal CD4$^+$ T cell population to the T helper 2 cell pathway. *J. Immunol.* **157**, 3260–3269.
9. Bretsher, P. A., Wei, G., Menon, J. N., and Bielefeldt-Ohmann, H. (1992) Establishment of stable, cell-mediated immunity that makes "susceptible" mice resistant to Leishmania major. *Science* **257**, 539–542.
10. Bancroft, A. J., Else, K. J., and Grencis, R. K. (1994) Low-level infection with Trichuris muris significantly affects the polarization of the CD4 response. *Eur. J. Immunol.* **24**, 3113–3118.
11. Chen, Y., Kuchroo, V. K., Inobe, J., Hafler, D. A., and Weiner, H. L. (1994) Regulatory T cell clones induced by oral tolerance: suppression of autoimmune encephalomyelitis. *Science* **265**, 1237–1240.
12. Guery, J.-C., Galbiati, F., Smiroldo, S., and Adorini, L. (1996) Selective development of T helper (Th)2 cells induced by continuous administration of low dose soluble proteins to normal and β2-microglobulin-deficient BALB/c mice. *J. Exp. Med.* **183**, 485–497.
13. Rosenthal, A. S. (1978) Determinant selection and macrophage function in genetic control of the immune response. *Immunol. Rev.* **40**, 136–152.
14. Ogasawara, K., Maloy, W. L., and Schwartz, R. H. (1987) Failure to find holes in the T cell repertoire. *Nature* **325**, 450-452.
15. Schaeffer, E. B., Sette, A., Johnson, D. L., Bekoff, M. C., Smith, J. A., Grey, H. M., and Buus, S. (1989) Relative contribution of "determinant selection" and "holes in the T cell repertoire" to T cell responses. *Proc. Natl. Acad. Sci. USA* **86**, 4649–4653.
16. Ashwell, J. D., Fox, B. S., and Schwartz, R. H. (1986) Functional analysis of the interaction of the antigen-specific T cell receptor with its ligands. *J. Immunol.* **136**, 757–768.
17. Evavold, B. D. and Allen, P. M. (1991) Separation of IL-4 production from Th cell proliferation by an altered T cell receptor ligand. *Science* **252**, 1308–1310.

18. Gilman, S. C., Rosenberg, J. S., and Feldman, J. D. (1983) Inhibition of interleukin synthesis and T cell proliferation by a monoclonal anti-Ia antibody. *J. Immunol.* **130**, 1236–1240.

19. Palacios, R. (1985) Monoclonal antibodies against human Ia antigens stimulate monocytes to secrete interleukin 1. *Proc. Natl. Acad. Sci. USA* **82**, 6652–6656.

20. Lichtman, A. H., Chin, J., Schmidt, J. A., and Abbas, A. K. (1988) Role of interleukin 1 in the activation of T lymphocytes. *Proc. Natl. Acad. Sci. USA* **85**, 9699–9703.

21. Janeway, C. J., Rojo, J., Saizawa, K., Dianzani, U., Portoles, P., Tite, J., Haque, S., and Jones, B. (1989), Selective induction of growth factor production and growth factor receptor expression by different signals to a single T cell. *Eur. J. Immunol.* **19**, 2061–2067.

22. Jameson, S. C. and Bevan, M. J. (1995) T cell receptor antagonists and partial agonists. *Immunity* **2**, 1–11.

23. Sloan-Lancaster, J., Steinberg, T. H., and Allen, P. M. (1997) Selective loss of the calcium ion signaling pathway in T cells maturing toward a T helper 2 phenotype. *J. Immunol.* **159**, 1160–1168.

24. Germain, R. N. and Stefanova, I. (1999) The dynamics of T cell receptor signaling: complex orchestration and the key roles of tempo and cooperation. *Annu. Rev. Immunol.* **17**, 467–522.

25. Madrenas, J. and Germain, R. N. (1996) Variant TCR ligands: new insights into the molecular basis of antigen-dependent signal transduction and T cell activation. *Sem. Immunol.* **8**, 83–101.

26. Sloan-Lancaster, J., Evavold, B. D., and Allen, P. M. (1993) Induction of T cell anergy by altered T cell-receptor ligand on live antigen-presenting cells. *Nature* **363**, 156–159.

27. Sloan-Lancaster, J., Shaw, A. S., Rothbard, J. B., and Allen, P. M. (1994) Partial T cell signaling: altered phospho-ζ and lack of ZAP70 recruitment in APL-induced T cell anergy. *Cell* **79**, 913–922.

28. Madrenas, J., Schwartz, R. H., and Germain, R. N. (1996) Interleukin 2 production, not the pattern of early T cell antigen receptor-dependent tyrosine phosphorylation, controls anergy induction by both agonists and partial agonists. *Proc. Natl. Acad. Sci. USA* **93**, 9736–9741.

29. De Magistris, M. T., Alexander, J., Coggeshall, M., Altman, A., Gaeta, F. C. A., Grey, H. M., and Sette, A. (1992) Antigen analog-major histocompatibility complexes act as antagonists of the T cell receptor. *Cell* **68**, 625–634.

30. Racioppi, L., Ronchese, F., Matis, L. A., and Germain, R. N. (1993) Peptide-major histocompatibility complex class II complexes with mixed agonist/ antagonist properties provide evidence for ligand-related differences in T cell receptor-dependent intracellular signaling. *J. Exp. Med.* **177**, 1047–1060.

31. Ruppert, J., Alexander, J., Snoke, K., Coggeshall, M., Herbert, E., McKenzie, D., et al. (1993) Effect of T cell receptor antagonism on interaction between T cells and antigen-presenting cells and on T cell signaling events. *Proc. Natl. Acad. Sci. USA* **90**, 2671–2675.

32. Robertson, J. M. and Evavold, B. D. (1999) Cutting edge: dueling TCRs: peptide antagonism of CD4+ T cells with dual antigen specificities. *J. Immunol.* **163**, 1750–1754.

33. Dittel, B. N., Stefanova, I., Germain, R. N., and Janeway, C. A., Jr. (1999) Cross-antagonism of a T cell clone expressing two distinct T cell receptors. *Immunity* **11**, 289–298.

34. Stotz, S. H., Bolliger, L., Carbone, F. R., and Palmer, E. (1999) T cell receptor (TCR) antagonism without a negative signal: evidence from T cell hybridomas expressing two independent TCRs. *J. Exp. Med.* **189**, 253–264.

35. Daniels, M. A., Schober, S. L., Hogquist, K. A., and Jameson, S. C. (1999) Cutting Edge: A test of the dominant negative signal model for TCR antagonism. *J. Immunol.* **162**, 3761–3764.

36. Jameson, S. C., Carbone, F. R., and Bevan, M. J. (1993) Clone-specific T cell receptor antagonists of major histocompatibility complex class I-restricted cytotoxic T cells. *J. Exp. Med.* **177**, 541–1550.

37. Weiss, A. (1993) T cell antigen receptor signal transduction: a tale of tails and cytoplasmic protein-tyrosine kinases. *Cell* **73**, 209–212.

38. Weiss, A. and Littman, D. R. (1994) Signal transduction by lymphocyte antigen receptors. *Cell* **76**, 263–274.

39. Samelson, L. E., Patel, M. D., Weissman, A. M., Harford, J. B., and Klausner, R. D. (1986) Antigen activation of murine T cells induces tyrosine phosphorylation of a polypeptide associated with the T cell antigen receptor. *Cell* **46**, 1083–1090.

40. Klausner, R. D., O'Shea, J. J., Luong, H., Ross, P., Bluestone, J. A., and Samelson, L. E. (1987) T cell receptor tyrosine phosphorylation. Variable coupling for different activating ligands. *J. Biol. Chem.* **262**, 12,654–12,659.

41. Madrenas, J., Wange, R. L., Wang, J. L., Isakov, N., Samelson, L. E., and Germain, R. N. (1995) ζ phosphorylation without ZAP-70 activation induced by TCR antagonists or partial agonists. *Science* **267**, 515–518.

42. Kersh, E. N., Shaw, A. S., and Allen, M. A. (1998) Fidelity of T cell activation through multistep T cell receptor ζ phosphorylation. *Science* **281**, 572–575.

43. La Face, D. M., Couture, C., Anderson, K., Shih, G., Alexander, J., Sette, A., et al. (1997) Differential T cell signaling induced by antagonist peptide-MHC complexes and the associated phenotypic responses. *J. Immunol.* **158**, 2057–2064.

44. Hemmer, B., Stefanova, I., Vergelli, M., Germain, R. N., and Martin, R. (1998) Relationships among TCR ligand potency, thresholds for effector function elicitation, and the quality of early signaling events in human T cells. *J. Immunol.* **160**, 5807–5814.

45. Smyth, L. A., Williams, O., Huby, R. D., Norton, T., Acuto, O., Ley, S. C., and Kioussis, D. (1998) Altered peptide ligands induce quantitatively but not qualitatively different intracellular signals in primary thymocytes. *Proc. Natl. Acad. Sci. USA* **98**, 8193–8198.

46. Lucas, B., Stefanova, I., Yasutomo, K., Dautigny, N., and Germain, R. N. (1999) Divergent changes in the sensitivity of maturing T cells to structurally related ligands underlies formation of a useful T cell repertoire. *Immunity* **10**, 367–376.

47. Reis e Sousa, C., Levine, E. H., and Germain, R. N. (1996) Partial signaling by CD8⁺ T cells in response to antagonist ligands. *J. Exp. Med.* **184**, 149–157.

48. Hatada, M. H., Lu, X., Laird, E. R., Green, J., Morgenstern, J. P., Lou, M., Marr, C. S., et al. (1995) Molecular basis for interaction of the protein tyrosine kinase ZAP-70 with the T cell receptor. *Nature* **377**, 32–38.

49. LoGrasso, P. V., Hawkins, J., Frank, L. J., Wisniewski, D., and Marcy, A. (1996) Mechanism of activation for Zap-70 catalytic activity. *Proc. Natl. Acad. Sci. USA* **93**, 12,165–12,170.

50. Magistrelli, G., Bosotti, R., Valsasina, B., Visco, C., Perego, R., Toma, S., et al. (1999) Role of the Src homology 2 domains and interdomain regions in ZAP-70 phosphorylation and enzymatic activity. *Eur. J. Biochem.* **266**, 1166–1173.

51. Matsui, K., Boniface, J. J., Steffner, P., Reay, P. A., and Davis, M. M. (1994) Kinetics of T cell receptor binding to peptide/I-E^k complexes: correlation of the dissociation rate with T cell responsiveness. *Proc. Natl. Acad. Sci. USA* **91**, 12,862–12,866.

52. Corr, M., Slanetz, A. E., Boyd, L. F., Jelonek, M. T., Khilko, S., al-Ramadi, B. K., et al. (1994) T cell receptor-MHC class I peptide interactions: affinity, kinetics, and specificity. *Science* **265**, 946–949.

53. Alam, S. M., Travers, P. J., Wung, J. L., Nasholds, W., Redpath, S., Jameson, S. C., and Gascoigne, N. R. J. (1996) T cell-receptor affinity and thymocyte positive selection. *Nature* **381**, 616–620.

54. Lyons, D. S., Lieberman, S. A., Hampl, J., Boniface, J. J., Chien, Y.-h., Berg, L. J., and Davis, M. M. (1996) A TCR binds to antagonist ligands with lower affinities and faster dissociation rates than to agonists. *Immunity* **5**, 53–61.

55. Kessler, B. M., Bassanini, P., Cerottini, J. C., and Luescher, I. F. (1997) Effects of epitope modification on T cell receptor-ligand binding and antigen recognition by seven H-2K^d-restricted cytotoxic T lymphocyte clones specific for a photoreactive peptide derivative. *J. Exp. Med.* **185**, 629–640.

56. Crawford, F., Kozono, H., White, J., Marrack, P., and Kappler, J. (1998) Detection of antigen-specific T cells with multivalent soluble class II MHC covalent peptide complexes. *Immunity* **8**, 675–682.

57. Kersh, G. J., Kersh, E. N., Fremont, D. H., and Allen, P. M. (1998) High- and low-potency ligands with similar affinities for the TCR: the importance of kinetics in TCR signaling. *Immunity* **9**, 817–826.

58. Williams, C. B., Engle, D. L., Kersh, G. J., White, J. M., and Allen, P. M. (1999) A kinetics threshold between negative and positive selection based on the longevity of the T cell receptor-ligand complex. *J. Exp. Med.* **189**, 1531–1544.

59. Davis, S. J. and van der Merwe, P. A. (1996) The structure and ligand interactions of CD2: implications for T cell function. *Immunol. Today* **17**, 177–187.

60. Leitenberg, D., Boutin, Y., Lu, D. D., and Bottomly, K. (1999) Biochemical association of CD45 with the T cell receptor complex: regulation by CD45 isoform and during T cell activation. *Immunity* **10**, 701–711.

61. Volarevic, S., Niklinska, B. B., Burns, C. M., Yamada, H., June, C. H., Dumont, F. J., and Ashwell, J. D. (1992) The CD45 tyrosine phosphatase regulates phosphotyrosine homeostasis and its loss reveals a novel pattern of late T cell receptor-induced Ca^{2+} oscillations. *J. Exp. Med.* **176**, 835–844.

62. D'Oro, U. and Ashwell, J. D. (1999) Cutting Edge: The CD45 tyrosine phosphatase is an inhibitor of Lck activity in thymocytes. *J. Immunol.* **162**, 1879–1883.

63. Lorenz, U., Ravichandran, K. S., Pei, D., Walsh, C. T., Burakoff, S. J., and Neel, B. G. (1994), Lck-dependent tyrosyl phosphorylation of the phosphotyrosine phosphatase SH-PTP1 in murine T cells. *Mol. Cell. Biol.* **14**, 1824–1834.

64. Glaichenhaus, N., Shastri, N., Littman, D. R., and Turner, J. M. (1991) Requirement for association of p56lck with CD4 in antigen-specific signal transduction in T cells. *Cell* **64**, 511–520.

65. Ravichandran, K. S., Collins, T. L., and Burakoff, S. J. (1996) CD4 and signal transduction. *Curr. Top. Microbiol. Immunol.* **205**, 47–62.

66. Konig, R., Huang, L. -Y., and Germain, R. N. (1992) MHC class II interaction with CD4 mediated by a region analogous to the MHC class I binding site for CD8. *Nature* **356**, 796–798.

67. Luescher, I. F., Vivier, E., Layer, A., Mahiou, J., Godeau, F., Malissen, B., and Romero, P. (1995) CD8 modulation of T cell antigen receptor-ligand interactions on living cytotoxic T lymphocytes. *Nature* **373**, 353–356.

68. Madrenas, J., Chau, L. A., Smith, J., Bluestone, J. A., and Germain, R. N. (1997) The efficiency of CD4 recruitment to ligand-engaged TCR controls the agonist/partial agonist properties of peptide-MHC molecule ligands. *J. Exp. Med.* **185**, 219–229.

69. Hampl, J., Chien, Y. H., and Davis, M. M. (1997) CD4 augments the response of a T cell to agonist but not to antagonist ligands. *Immunity* **7**, 379–385.

70. Monks, C. R. F., Freiberg, B. A., Kupfer, H., Sciaky, N., and Kupfer, A. (1998) Three-dimentional segregation of supramolecular activation clusters in T cells. *Nature* **395**, 82–86.

71. Grakoui, A., Bromley, S. K., Sumen, C., Davis, M. M., Shaw, A. S., Allen, P. M., and L., D. M. (1999) The immunological synapse: a molecular machine controlling T cell activation. *Science* **285**, 221–227.

72. June, C. H., Fletcher, M. C., Ledbetter, J. A., and Samelson, L. E. (1990) Increases in tyrosine phosphorylation are detectable before phospholipase C activation after T cell receptor stimulation. *J. Immunol.* **144**, 1591–1599.

73. Fiering, S., Northrop, J. P., Nolan, G. P., Mattila, P. S., Crabtree, G. R., and Herzenberg, L. A. (1990) Single cell assay of a transcription factor reveals a threshold in transcription activated by signals emanating from the T cell antigen receptor. *Genes Dev.* **4**, 1823–1834.

74. Iezzi, G., Karjalainen, K., and Lanzavecchia, A. (1998) The duration of antigenic stimulation determines the fate of naive and effector T cells. *Immunity* **8**, 89–95.

75. Boyer, C., Auphan, N., Gabert, J., Blanc, D., Malissen, B., and Schmitt-Verhulst, A. M. (1989) Comparison of phosphorylation and internalization of the antigen receptor/CD3 complex, CD8, and class I MHC-encoded proteins on T cells. Role of intracytoplasmic domains analyzed with hybrid CD8/class I molecules. *J. Immunol.* **143**, 1905–1914.

76. Minami, Y., Samelson, L. E., and Klausner, R. D. (1987) Internalization and cycling of the T cell antigen receptor. *J. Biol. Chem.* **262**, 13,342–13,347.

77. Krangel, M. S. (1987) Endocytosis and recycling of the T3-T cell receptor complex: the role of T3 phosphorylation. *J. Exp. Med.* **165**, 1141–1159.

78. Thuillier, L., Pérignon, J.-L., Selz, F., Griscelli, C., and Fischer, A. (1991) Opposing effects of protein tyrosine kinase inhibitors on the monoclonal antibody induced internalization of CD3 and CD4 antigens. *Eur. J. Immunol.* **21**, 2641–2643.

79. Valitutti, S., Muller, S., Cella, M., Padovan, E., and Lanzavecchia, A. (1995) Serial triggering of many T cell receptors by a few peptide-MHC complexes. *Nature* **375**, 148–151.

80. Itoh, Y., Hemmer, B., Martin, R., and Germain, R. N. (1999) Serial TCR engagement and down-modulation by peptide:MHC molecule ligands: relationship to the quality of individual TCR signaling events. *J. Immunol.* **162,** 2073–2080.

81. Schodin, B. A., Tsomides, T. J., and Kranz, D. M. (1996) Correlation between the number of T cell receptors required for T cell activation and TCR-ligand affinity. *Immunity* **5**, 137–146.

82. Bachmann, M. F., Oxenius, A., Speiser, D. E., Mariathasan, S., Hengartner, H., Zinkernagel, R. M., and Ohashi, P. S. (1997) Peptide-induced T cell receptor down-regulation on naive T cells predicts agonist/partial agonist properties and strictly correlates with T cell activation. *Eur. J. Immunol.* **27**, 2195–2203.

83. Dietrich, J., Hou, X., Wegener, A.-M. K., and Geisler, C. (1994) CD3γ contains a phosphoserine dependent di-leucine motif involved in down-regulation of the T cell receptor. *EMBO J.* **13**, 2156–2166.

84. Luton, F., Buferne, M., Davoust, J., Schmitt-Verhulst, A.-M., and Boyer, C. (1994) Evidence for protein tyrosine kinase involvement in ligand-induced TCR/CD3 internalization and surface redistribution. *J. Immunol.* **153**, 63–72.

85. Kersh, B. E., Kersh, G. J., and Allen, P. M. (1999) Partially phosphorylated T cell receptor zeta molecules can inhibit T cell activation. *J. Exp. Med.* **190**, 1627–1636.

86. Karttunen, J. and Shastri, N. (1991) Measurement of ligand-induced activation in single viable T cells using the lacZ reporter gene. *Proc. Natl. Acad. Sci. USA* **88**, 3972–3976.

87. Bucy, R. P., Panoskaltsis-Mortani, A., Huang, G.-Q., Li, J., Karr, L., Ross, M., Russell, J. H., Murphy, K. M., and Weaver, C. T. (1994) Heterogeneity of single-cell cytokine gene expression in clonal T cell populations. *J. Exp. Med.* **180**, 1251–1262.

88. Itoh, Y. and Germain, R. N. (1997) Single cell analysis reveals regulated hierarchical T cell antigen receptor signaling thresholds and intraclonal heterogeneity for individual cytokine responses of CD4+ T cells. *J. Exp. Med.* **186**, 757–766.

89. Street, N. E., Schumacher, J. H., Fong, T. A. T., Bass, H., Fiorentino, D. F., Leverah, J. A., and Mosmann, T. R. (1990) Heterogeneity of mouse helper T cells: evidence from bulk cultures and limiting dilution cloning for precursors of Th1 and Th2 cells. *J. Immunol.* **14,** 1629–1639.

90. Assenmacher, M., Schmitz, J., and Radbruch, A. (1994) Flow cytometric determination of cytokines in activated murine T helper lymphocytes: expression of interleukin-10 in interferon-γ and in interleukin-4-expressing cells. *Eur. J. Immunol.* **24**, 1097–1101.

91. Jung, T., Schauer, U., Rieger, C., Wagner, K., Einsle, K., Neumann, C., and Heusser, C. (1995) Interleukin-4 and interleukin-5 are rarely coexpressed by human T cells. *Eur. J. Immunol.* **25**, 2413–2416.

92. Bucy, R. P., Karr, L., Huang, G. Q., Li, J., Carter, D., Honjo, K., et al. (1995) Single cell analysis of cytokine gene coexpression during CD4⁺ T cell phenotype development. *Proc. Natl. Acad. Sci. USA* **92**, 7565–7569.

93. Kelso, A. (1995) Th1 and Th2 subsets: paradigms lost? *Immunol. Today* **16**, 374–379.

94. Openshaw, P., Murphy, E. E., hosken, N. A., Maino, V., Davis, K., Murphy, K., and O'Garra, A. (1995) Heterogeneity of intracellular cytokine synthesis at the single-cell level in polarized T helper 1 and T helper 2 population. *J. Exp. Med.* **182**, 1357–1367.

95. Kelso, A., Groves, P., Ramm, L., and Doyle, A. G. (1999) Single-cell analysis by RT-PCR reveals differential expression of multiple type 1 and 2 cytokine genes among cells within polarized CD4⁺ T cell populations. *Intl. Immunol.* **11**, 617–621.

96. Agarwal, S. and Rao, A. (1998) Long-range transcriptional regulation of cytokine gene expression. *Curr. Opin. Immunol.* **10**, 345–352.

97. Bix, M. and Locksley, R. M. (1998) Independent and epigenetic regulation of the interleukin-4 alleles in CD4⁺ T cells. *Science* **281**, 1352–1354.

98. Bix, M., Wang, Z. E., Thiel, B., Schork, N. J., and Locksley, R. M. (1998) Genetic regulation of commitment to interleukin 4 production by a CD4(+) T cell-intrinsic mechanism. *J. Exp. Med.* **188**, 2289–2299.

99. Riviere, I., Sunshine, M. J., and Littman, D. R. (1998) Regulation of IL-4 expression by activation of individual alleles. *Immunity* **9**, 217–228.

100. Sykulev, Y., Joo, M., Vturina, I., Tsomides, T. J., and Eisen, H. N. (1996) Evidence that a single peptide-MHC complex on a target cell can elicit a cytolytic T cell response. *Immunity* **4**, 565–571.

101. Valitutti, S., Muller, S., Dessing, M., and Lanzavecchia, A. (1996) Different responses are elicited in cytotoxic T lymphocytes by different levels of T cell receptor occupancy. *J. Exp. Med.* **183**, 1917–21.

102. Viola, A. and Lanzavecchia, A. (1996) T cell activation determined by T cell receptor number and tunable thresholds. *Science* **273**, 104–106.

103. Nicholson, L. B., Waldner, H., Carrizosa, A. M., Sette, A., Collins, M., and Kuchroo, V. K. (1998) Heteroclitic proliferative responses and changes in cytokine profile induced by altered peptides: Implications for autoimmunity. *Proc. Natl. Acad. Sci. USA* **95**, 264–269.

104. Waldrop, S. L., Davis, K. A., Maino, V. C., and Picker, L. J. (1998) Normal human CD4⁺ memory T cells display broad heterogeneity in their activation threshold for cytokine synthesis. *J. Immunol.* **161**, 5284–5295.

105. Windhagen, A., Scholz, C., Hollsberg, P., Fukaura, H., Sette, A., and Hafler, D. A. (1995) Modulation of cytokine patterns of human autoreactive T cell clones by a single amino acid substitution of their peptide ligand. *Immunity* **2**, 373–380.

106. Hosken, N. A., Shibuya, K., Heath, A. W., Murphy, K. M., and O'Garra, A. (1995) The effect of antigen dose on CD4⁺ T helper cell phenotype developement in a T cell receptor-αβ transgenic model. *J. Exp. Med.* **182**, 1579–1584.

107. Constant, S., Pfeiffer, C., Woodard, A., Pasqualini, T., and Bottomly, K. (1995) Extent of T cell receptor ligation can determine the functional differentiation of naive CD4+ T cells. *J. Exp. Med.* **182**, 1591–1596.

108. Murphy, K. M., Ouyang, W., Szabo, S. J., Jacobson, N. G., Guler, M. L., Gorham, J. D., et al. (1999) T helper differentiation proceeds through Stat1-dependent, Stat4- dependent and Stat4-independent phases. *Curr. Top. Microbiol. Immunol.* **238**, 13-26.

109. Wenner, C. A., Guler, M. L., Macatonia, S. E., O'Garra, A., and Murphy, K. M. (1996) Roles of IFN-gamma and IFN-alpha in IL-12-induced T helper cell-1 development. *J. Immunol.* **156**, 1442–1447.

110. Tao, X., Grant, C., Constant, S., and Bottomly, K. (1997) Induction of IL-4-producing CD4+ T cells by antigenic peptides altered for TCR binding. *J. Immunol.* **158**, 4237–4244.

111. Grakoui, A., Donermeyer, D. L., Kanagawa, O., Murphy, K. M., and Allen, P. M. (1999) TCR-independent pathways mediate the effects of antigen does and altered peptide ligands on Th cell polarization. *J. Immunol.* **162**, 1923–1930.

112. Pfeiffer, C., Stein, J., Southwood, S., Ketelaar, H., Sette, A., and Bottomly, K. (1995) Altered peptide ligands can control CD4 T lymphocyte differenciation in vivo. *J. Exp. Med.* **181**, 1569–1574.

113. Lewis, R. S. and Calahan, M. D. (1995) Potassium and calcium channels in lymphocytes. *Annu. Rev. Immunol.* **13**, 623–653.

114. Parekh, A. B., Fleig, A., and Penner, R. (1997) The store-operated calcium current I(CRAC): nonlinear activation by InsP3 and dissociation from calcium release. *Cell* **89**, 973–980.

115. Wulfing, C., Rabinowitz, J. D., Beeson, C., Sjaastad, M. D., McConnell, H. M., and Davis, M. M. (1997) Kinetics and extent of T cell activation as measured with the calcium signal. *J. Exp. Med.* **185**, 1815–1825.

116. Chen, Y.-Z., Lai, Z.-F., Nishi, K., and Nishimura, Y. (1998) Modulation of calcium responses by altered peptide ligands in a human T cell clone. *Eur. J. Immunol.* **28**, 3929–3939.

117. Rabinowitz, J. D., Beeson, C., Wulfing, C., Tate, K., Allen, P. M., Davis, M. M., and McConnell, H. M. (1996) Altered T cell receptor ligands trigger a subset of early T cell signals. *Immunity* **5**, 125–135.

118. Dolmetsch, R. E., Lewis, R. S., Goodnow, C. C., and Healy, J. I. (1997) Differential activation of transcription factors induced by Ca^{2+} response amplitude and duration. *Nature* **386**, 855–858.

119. Dolmetsch, R. E., Xu, K., and Lewis, R. S. (1998) Calcium oscillations increase the efficiency and specificity of gene expression. *Nature* **392**, 933–936.

120. Li, W.-h., Llopis, J., Whitney, M., Zlokarnik, G., and Tsien, R. Y. (1998) Cell-permeant caged InsP3 ester shows that Ca^{2+} spike frequency can optimize gene expression. *Nature* **392**, 936–941.

121. Nakamura, T., Kamogawa, Y., Bottomly, K., and Flavell, R. A. (1997) Polarization of IL-4- and IFN-γ-producing CD4+ T cells following activation of naive CD4+ T cells. *J. Immunol.* **158**, 1085–1094.

122. Miller, S. D., and Karpus, W. J. (1994) The immunopahogenesis and regulation of T cell-mediated demyelinating diseases. *Immunol. Today* **15**, 356–361.

123. Nicholson, L. B., Greer, J. M., Sobel, R. A., Lees, M. B., and Kuchroo, V. K. (1995) An altered peptide ligand mediates immune deviation and prevents autoimmune encephalomyelitis. *Immunity* **3**, 397–405.

124. Boutin, Y., Leitenberg, D., Tao, X., and Bottomly, K. (1997) Distinct biochemical signals characterize agonist- and altered peptide ligand-induced differentiation of naive CD4$^+$ T cells into Th1 and Th2 subsets. *J. Immunol.* **159**, 5802–5809.

125. Tamura, T., Nakano, H., Nagase, H., Morokata, T., Igarashi, O., Oshimi, Y., et al. (1995) Early activation signal transduction pathways of Th1 and Th2 cell clones stimulated with anti-CD3. *J. Immunol.* **155**, 4692–4701.

126. al-Ramadi, B. K., Nakamura, T., Leitenberg, D., and Bothwell, A. L. M. (1996) Deficient expression of p56lck in Th2 cells leads to partial TCR signaling and a dysregulation in lympholkine mRNA levels. *J. Immunol.* **157**, 4751–4761.

127. Faith, A., Akdis, C. A., Akdis, M., Simon, H.-U., and Blaser, K. (1997) Defective TCR stimulation in anegized type 2 T helper cells correlated with abroagted p56lck and ZAP-70 tyrosine kinase activities. *J. Immunol.* **159**, 53–60.

128. Gajewski, T. F., Schell, S. R., and Fitch, F. W. (1990) Evidence implicating utilization of different T cell receptor-associated signaling pathways by TH1 and TH2 clones. *J. Immunol.* **144**, 4110–4120.

129. Fowell, D. J., Magram, J., Turck, C. W., Killeen, N., and Locksley, R. M. (1997) Impaired Th2 subset development in the absence of CD4. *Immunity* **6**, 559–569.

130. Leitenberg, D., Boutin, Y., Constant, S., and Bottomly, K. (1998) CD4 regulation of TCR signaling and T cell differentiation following stimulation with peptides of different affinities for the TCR. *J. Immunol.* **161**, 1194–1203.

131. Yamashita, M., Hashimoto, K., Kimura, M., Kubo, M., Tada, T., and Nakayama, T. (1998) Requirement for p56lck tyrosine kinase activation in Th subset differentiation. *Intl. Immunol.* **10**, 577–591.

132. Yamashita, M., Kimura, M., Kubo, M., Shimizu, C., Tada, T., Perlmutter, R. M., and Nakayama, T. (1999) T cell antigen receptor-mediated activation of the Ras/mitogen-activated protein kinase pathway controls interleukin 4 receptor function and type-2 helper T cell differentiation. *Proc. Natl. Acad. Sci. USA* **96**, 1024–1029.

133. Wucherpfennig, K. W. and Strominger, J. L. (1995) Molecular mimicry in T cell-mediated autoimmunity, viral peptides activate human T cell clones specific for myelin basic protein. *Cell* **80**, 695–705.

134. Hemmer, B., Vergelli, M., Pinilla, C., Houghten, R., and Martin, R. (1998) Probing degeneracy in T cell recognition using peptide combinatorial libraries. *Immunol. Today* **19**, 163–168.

135. Ericsson, P. O., Orchansky, P. L., Carlow, D. A., and Teh, H. S. (1996) Differential activation of phospholipase C-gamma 1 and mitogen-activated protein kinase in naive and antigen-primed CD4 T cells by the peptide/MHC ligand. *J. Immunol.* **156**, 2045–2053.

136. Pihlgren, M., Dubois, P. M., Tomkowiak, M., Sjogren, T., and Marvel, J. (1996) Resting memory CD8$^+$ T cells are hyperreactive to antigenic challenge in vitro. *J. Exp. Med.* **184**, 2141–2151.

137. Curtsinger, J. M., Lins, D. C., and Mescher, M. F. (1998) CD8$^+$ memory T cells (CD44^{high}, Ly-6C$^+$) are more sensitive than naive cells to (CD44^{low}, Ly-6C$^-$) to TCR/CD8 signaling in response to antigen. *J. Immunol.* **160**, 3236–3243.

138. Bachmann, M. F., Gallimore, A., Linkert, S., Cerundolo, V., Lanzavecchia, A., Kopf, M., and Viola, A. (1999) Developmental regulation of Lck targeting to the CD8 coreceptor controls signaling in naive and memory T cells. *J. Exp. Med.* **189**, 1521–1530.

139. Anderton, S. M., Kissler, S., Lamont, A. G., and Wraith, D. C. (1999) Therapeutic potential of TCR antagonists is determined by their ability to modulate a diverse repertoire of autoreactive T cells. *Eur. J. Immunol.* **29**, 1850–1857.

140. Khoury, S. J., Hancock, W. W., and Weiner, H. L. (1992) Oral tolerance to myelin basic protein and natural recovery from experimental autoimmune encephalomyelitis are associated with downregulation of inflammatory cytokines and differential upregulation of transforming growth factor B, interleukin 4, and prostaglandin E expression in the brain. *J. Exp. Med.* **176**, 1355–1364.

141. Myers, L. K., Tang, B., Rosloniec, E. F., Stuart, J. M., Chiang, T. M., and Kang, A. H. (1998) Characterization of a peptide analog of a determinant of type II collagen that suppresses collagen-induced arthritis. *J. Immunol.* **161**, 3589–3595.

142. Ruiz, P. J., Garren, H., Hirschberg, D. L., Langer-Gould, A. M., Levite, M., Karpuj, M. V., et al. (1999) Microbial epitopes act as altered peptide ligands to prevent experimental autoimmune encephalomyelitis. *J. Exp. Med.* **189**, 1275–1284.

143. Combadiere, B., Reis e Sousa, C., Germain, R. N., and Lenardo, M. J. (1998) Selective induction of apoptosis in mature T lymphocytes by variant T cell receptor ligands. *J. Exp. Med.* **187**, 349–355.

144. Dustin, M. L., Bromley, S. K., Kan, Z., Peterson, D. A., and Unanue, E. R. (1997) Antigen receptor engagement delivers a stop signal to migrating T lymphocytes. *Proc. Natl. Acad. Sci.USA* **94**, 3909–3913.

145. Germain, R. N. (1997) T cell signaling, the importance of receptor clustering. *Curr. Biol.* **7**, R640–644.

4

The Role of Costimulation in T Cell Differentiation

Janet E. Buhlmann and Arlene H. Sharpe

1. WHAT IS COSTIMULATION?

The last 15 years has seen great advances in our understanding of the events necessary for the activation of T cells. From this work, what has come to be accepted as the "two-signal hypothesis of T cell activation" has evolved. This hypothesis was adapted from studies orginally done by Bretscher and Cohn investigating the activation of B cells *(1)*. According to this hypothesis, the first required activation signal for T cells is received after recognition of specific peptide antigens complexed to class I or class II major histocompatibility molecules (MHC) by the T cells receptor (TCR). If this is the only signal received by the T cells a state of unresponsiveness or anergy may be induced *(2)*. The second signal, which can prevent the induction of anergy, comes from an antigen-nonspecific receptor, the costimulatory molecule. This costimulatory signal can have multiple effects on the responding T cells including enhanced proliferation, cytokine production, T cell-effector differentiation and survival *(3)*. Although there are many receptor-ligand pairs that have been implicated in costimulation, this chapter will focus on two major pathways, the B7-CD28/CTLA-4 pathway and the CD40-CD154 pathway, and their effects on T helper (Th) differentiation. These pathways utilize important regulatory molecules that affect both the T cell and the antigen presenting cell (APC). The B7-CD28/CTLA-4 pathway provides critical costimulatory signals directly to T cells via members of the CD28 family. In contrast, the CD40-CD154 pathway has a more indirect affect on Th differentiation by altering the functional capacity of the APC via CD40.

From: *Cytokines and Autoimmune Diseases*
Edited by: V. K. Kuchroo, et al. © Humana Press Inc., Totowa, NJ

2. T CELL COSTIMULATORY PLAYERS: RECEPTORS , LIGANDS AND THEIR EFFECTS ON TH DIFFERENTIATION

2.1. T Cell Costimulatory Receptors: CD28, CTLA-4, and ICOS

The CD28 and CTLA-4 receptors share many features: both are members of the Ig superfamily, are expressed on T cells, and interact with the B7-1 and B7-2 ligands. Although there is ~30% conservation at the amino acid level, including the MYPPPY sequence essential for B7 binding, these receptors also have distinct properties. CD28 and CTLA-4 have distinct expression kinetics. CD28 is constitutively expressed on the surface of naive T cells, whereas CTLA-4 is upregulated following T cell activation, with peak expression ~48–72 h after activation *(4,5)*. The subcellular distributions also differ: Although CTLA-4 is expressed on the surface of activated T cells, the majority of CTLA-4 remains intracellular within endocytic compartments, whereas CD28 is on the cell surface.

Another difference is the distinct roles that CD28 and CTLA-4 have in regulating T cell responses. The CD28 costimulatory receptor transmits a signal that synergizes with the TCR signal to promote T cell activation. Studies using CD28 deficient mice and CD28 blockade have revealed that CD28 signaling has multiple functional consequences. CD28 costimulation results in sustained T cell proliferation, stimulation of anti-apoptotic molecules (bcl-xl), increased expression of cell cycle proteins, upregulation of CD154 expression, the stimulation of multiple cytokine production, and regulation of cytokine receptors, which will be discussed in greater detail later within this chapter. In addition, CD28 signaling regulates the threshold for T cell activation: CD28 costimulation significantly decreases the degree of TCR engagement needed for effective T cell activation *(6)*.

While the costimulatory function of CD28 is well established, the function of CTLA-4 has been more controversial. Some studies have suggested that CTLA-4 functions similarly to CD28 as a positive costimulator, but the majority of the data support a role for CTLA-4 as a negative regulator of T cell activation. The lymphoproliferative disease with massive lymphadenopathy, splenomegaly, and multi-organ lymphocytic infiltrates that develops in mice lacking CTLA-4 provides compelling evidence of a critical role for CTLA-4 in downregulating T cell activation and regulating lymphocyte homeostasis *(7–9)*. As will be discussed later, antibodies to CTLA-4 administered in vivo exacerbate autoimmune diseases.

The newly discovered CD28 homolog, ICOS (inducible costimulatory molecule), is a T cell costimulatory molecule, first reported on activated human T cells *(10)*. Whereas CD28 is constitutively expressed, ICOS is not detectable on unstimulated human peripheral blood $CD4^+$ or $CD8^+$ T cells, but is induced upon TCR engagement. The mouse homolog of ICOS also has been identified recently with expression detected on activated T cells and resting memory cells *(11)*.

2.2. T Cell Costimulatory Receptor Ligands: B7-1, B7-2, B7h/B7RP-1, and B7-H1

Until recently, B7-1 and B7-2 were the only members of the B7 family. B7-1 was the first molecule identified on B cells that could bind CD28 and provide costimulation *(12)*. Later studies identified a second molecule, B7-2, which could also bind CD28 and CTLA-4 *(13,14)*. Although B7-1 and B7-2 share approx 25% amino acid identity *(15)*, there are many differences between these molecules.

The kinetics of B7-1 and B7-2 expression are distinct: B7-2 is constitutively expressed at low levels on dendritic cells, macrophages, and B cells and is rapidly upregulated on APCs in response to many stimuli, including cytokines, activation signals, and infection (reviewed in ref. *16*) *(15,17)*. Significantly, B7-1 expression is upregulated later than B7-2. This distinct temporal expression pattern has suggested that B7-2 may be important for the initiation of responses whereas B7-1 may regulate or amplify responses. Indeed, as discussed later, studies using B7 antagonists and B7$^{-/-}$ mice indicate that this is true in many situations. MHC class II molecules and CD40 crosslinking upregulate both B7-1 and B7-2. Cytokines also regulate B7-1 and B7-2 expression, which will be discussed in depth later within this chapter. Additionally, B7-1 and B7-2 are expressed on T cells, but the functional role of these molecules on T cells is not clear. The B7-1 and B7-2 costimulators have dual specificity for CD28 and CTLA-4. CTLA-4 is the high-affinity receptor for both B7 costimulators, but the fine specificities of B7-1 and B7-2 interactions with CTLA-4 are distinct. B7-1 has a slower "off" rate than B7-2 from both CD28 and CTLA-4 *(18)*, which may account for distinct functional roles of these molecules in different types of in vivo immune responses.

B7h, a newly isolated member of the B7 family, was identified while screening genes which were tumor necrosis factor-α (TNF-α) inducible and RelA-dependent *(19)*. B7h is a surface protein, with homology to B7-1 and B7-2, which is expressed on splenocytes, purified B cells, and within the lung, thymus, lymph nodes, and spleen. Inducible expression can be seen on 3T3 cells and embryonic fibroblasts after treatment with TNF-α. Treatment of mice with LPS, which stimulates TNF-α production, elicits increased B7h mRNA expression in the testes, kidneys, and the peritoneum. Recent work by two groups has discovered that B7h is the counter-receptor for ICOS *(11,20)*. Studies done by Yoshinaga et al. also identified B7h, however, they termed the protein B7RP-1 *(11)*. Using ICOS-Ig to visualize expression, B7RP-1 (B7h) was detected on B cells and macrophages but B7RP-1/B7h was not identified on dendritc cells (DC) derived from cultured PBMCs. Further expression analysis awaits the generation of antibodies directed against B7h/B7RP-1.

Yet another family member, termed B7-H1 *(21)*, is constitutively expressed on human monocytes and is upregulated on the majority of activated monocytes. B7-H1 also is found on activated T cells and B cells. This fourth member of the B7 family is reported to bind an undefined receptor as studies with all three known counter-receptors, CD28, CTLA-4, and ICOS, did not demonstrate binding. However, B7-H1 interactions share some similarities with the reported effects of ICOS stimulation. Ligation of B7-H1 costimulated T cell responses and produced high levels of interleukin-10 (IL-10), which was dependent upon the presence of IL-2.

2.3. B7-CD28 Costimulatory Family in Th Cell Differentiation

Following initial activation, CD4$^+$ T cells (Th) differentiate into two subpopulations that produce distinct patterns of cytokines *(22)*. Th1 differentation results in production of IL-2 and/or interferon-γ (IFN-γ) and TNF-α, which elicit delayed type hypersensitivity (DTH) responses and activate macrophages. Th2 differentiation results in production of IL-4, IL-5, IL-10, and IL-13, and are especially important for IgE production, eosinophilic inflammation, and also may suppress cell mediated immunity. These two Th cell populations cross regulate each other because their respective cytokines act antagonistically. IL-4 and IFN-γ show reciprocal inhibition *(23)*. The differentiation of CD4 Th cells into Th1 or Th2 subsets has profound effects on the outcome of autoimmune diseases, infectious diseases, and graft rejection. CD4$^+$ T cell differentiation is influenced by three key factors: antigen dose, cytokine milieu at the time of T cell priming, and costimulation.

2.4. Role of B7-1 vs B7-2

The roles for B7-1 and B7-2 in Th differentiation have been an area of intense investigation. In vitro and in vivo studies using MAbs against B7-1 and B7-2 and in vitro studies with B7-1 or B7-2 transfected Chinese hamster ovary (CHO) cells indicated that B7-1 and B7-2 may be distinct in their capacity to induce T cell differentiation. Early studies suggested that B7-1 directed Th1 responses, whereas B7-2 directed Th2 responses. However, this has not been seen in all systems.

Initial studies done with B7 transfectants demonstrated that B7-1 and B7-2 costimulation induced comparable levels of IL-2 and IFN-γ production along with IL-2R subunit expression. However, B7-2 was able to induce higher levels of IL-4 than was seen with B7-1 costimulation, especially from naive T cells *(24)*. Repetitive stimulation with B7-2 resulted in modest levels of IL-2 and IL-4, whereas B7-1 induced high levels of IL-2 and low levels of IL-4. Together, these results suggested that B7-1 and B7-2 may have specific roles in Th differentiation. However, subsequent studies found B7-1 and B7-2 could have similar effects when used to costimulate T cells and argued against distinct roles for B7-1 and B7-2 in controlling Th differentiation *(25,26)*. Adding to the controversy were studies in which antibodies to either B7-1 or B7-2 were added to an in vitro culture during the primary stimulation of naive TCR transgenic T cells with specific peptide (27). Cells were harvested and then restimulated to determine how the responding T cells differentiated. Anti-B7-2 during the primary resulted in decreased IL-4 after restimulation without a similar decrease in IL-2 and IFN-γ. However, anti-B7-1 during the primary caused an increase in IL-4 and a decrease in both IL-2 and IFN-γ. Again, these results suggested that B7-1 engagement supports Th1 differentiation, whereas B7-2 favors Th2 development.

Later studies done by Schweitzer et al. evaluated the contributions of individual B7 molecules during the priming and differentiation of naive T cells by using APCs deficient for either B7-1 or B7-2 during primary stimulation of TCR transgenic T cells *(28)*. Similar to the studies of Ranger et al., B7-deficient APC presented specific peptide during the primary stimulation after which T cells were restimulated with wild-type APC. These studies indicated: (1) B7-1 and B7-2 both contribute to Th1 and Th2 cytokine production, with a greater role for B7-2 than B7-1 and (2) IL-4 production is more sensitive to a decrease in the level of B7 costimulation than is IFN-γ. Thus, these studies concluded that B7-1 and B7-2 costimulation provide similar signals to T cells and that apparent differences result from quantitative (temporal and/or spatial) differences in expression of these molecules.

Although in vitro studies suggest overlapping roles for B7-1 and B7-2 costimulation in Th differentiation, several in vivo studies suggest that B7s can have differential effects. Using a mouse model of experimental allergic encephalomyelitis (EAE), a Th1-mediated autoimmune disease, Kuchroo et al. found that anti-B7-1 treatment prevented disease and resulted in a predominantly Th2 response. Conversely, anti-B7-2 antibody exacerbated disease suggesting that engagement of B7-1 by CD28 or CTLA-4 leads to the development of Th1 cells *(29)*, whereas B7-2 engagement leads to Th2 differentiation. Additional studies using the Th2 biased model of leishmaniasis, found that treatment with anti-B7-2 antibodies was able to downregulate the deleterious Th2 response in susceptible mice and allow clearance of infection *(30)*. Another autoimmune model that showed differential effects of B7-1 and B7-2 is the development of diabetes in nonobese mice (NOD) *(31)*. Lenschow and coworkers found distinct effects of anti-B7-1 and anti-B7-2, which depended upon when the antibodies were administered. If antibodies were given early (prior to the onset of insulitis), anti-B7-2 inhibited diabetes but not insulitis, whereas anti-B7-1 or the two antibodies together exacerbated disease. Neither anti-B7 antibody affected diabetes if given late (once insulitis had developed). A later study by these investigators showed that NOD-backcrossed CD28 deficient mice or NOD mice expressing a CTLA-4Ig gene systemically had more frequent or rapid diabetes than littermate controls. This difference was attributed to reduced IL-4 production and Th2 differentiation. Likewise, administration of anti-CD28 antibodies into NOD mice beginning at 2 wk of age prevented diabetes and insulitis, which could be reversed by coinjection of anti-IL-4 antibody *(32)*. These in vivo studies suggest that B7-1 and B7-2 may in fact have differential functions and highlight the complex nature of interactions that occur within an immune response that may not be reproduced in vitro. Some of the differences may involve the level and kinetics of antigen exposure, strength of stimulus, and costimulatory molecule expression that is distinct to the in vivo microenvironment.

Another potential means by which B7 may regulate cytokine production is through B7 expressed on T cells. Although the role of B7 on T cells is not well understood, a recent study indicates that B7-1 on T cells may regulate the production of IL-4 *(33)*. In vitro studies using TCR transgenic T cells cocultured with peptide and wild-type APC found that B7-1 deficient (B7-1$^{-/-}$) T cells produced more IL-4 and less IFN-γ than wild-type T cells under the same conditions. These results suggest that B7-1 on T cells plays a role in regulating IL-4 production. In addition, IL-4 affected the expression of B7-1 on wild-type T cells. Wild-type cells cultured in the presence of IL-4 express less B7-1 whereas neutralization of IL-4 leads to enhanced B7-1 expression. The function of B7-1 on T cells seems to oppose the function of B7s on APCs: B7-1 on T cells downregulates cytokine production whereas B7-1 on APCs enhances cytokine production. Further studies to elucidate the function of B7-1 on T cells are needed, however, the initial work suggests that B7-1 may have an important role in the fine tuning of Th differentiation during an immune response. During the course of an immune response, under Th1 biased conditions, B7-1 expression on T cells would be high, thus downregulating IL-4 production helping to drive further Th1 differentiation. Conversely, under Th2 conditions, B7-1 expression on T cells would be low, enhancing IL-4 production and Th2 deviation. A functional role for B7-1 on T cells in regulating Th differentiation has potential implications for autoimmune diseases. For example, because B7-1 expression on

T cells is markedly upregulated in EAE and multiple sclerosis (MS) patients, B7-1 on T cells may have a role in regulating the pathogenicity of self-reactive T cells *(34–36)*. Additionally, administration of intact anti-B7-1 antibodies and anti-B7-1 Fab fragments in a relapsing EAE model have opposing effects. It is possible that these opposing outcomes may reflect the effects of B7-1 crosslinking vs B7-1 blockade on the T cell.

2.5. Role of B7-CD28 Interactions

In addition to providing proliferative and survival signals to T cells *(37,38)*, CD28 has a critical role in regulating cytokine production. Early studies investigating the effects of crosslinking CD28 on activated T cells found CD28 profoundly enhanced IL-2 production. In addition to IL-2, increases in TNF-α, lymphotoxin, IFN-γ, IL-4, IL-5, IL-6, IL-13, and granulocyte-macrophage colony stimulating factor (GM-CSF) were detected *(15,39–41)*. In synergy with CD28 costimulation, IL-1 augments IL-6 production and IL-4 responsiveness *(40,42)*. Another synergistic interaction occurs between IL-12 and CD28. IL-12 in combination with CD28 costimulation enhances IFN-γ and IL-10 production along with a slight inhibition of IL-4 and IL-5 production *(43)*. The effects on cytokine production result from both increased gene transcription as well as increased mRNA stability of cytokine transcripts *(44,45)*. Another property of CD28 costimulation is to lower the threshold of TCR engagement necessary for a functional response to be generated *(6)*. In a study using altered peptide ligands, Ding and Shevach demonstrated that a weak agonist peptide was unable to induce any measure of T cell activation. However, when the peptide was augmented with CD28 costimulation T cells produced both IL-2 and IL-3 *(46)*.

CD28 also has a critical role regulating Th differentiation. In the absence of CD28 costimulation, the differentiation of naive T cells is skewed toward a Th1 response owing to impaired IL-4 production *(47)*. CD28 deficient TCR transgenic T cells were not capable of producing IL-4 after antigenic stimulation, however, IL-4 could be recovered if rIL-4 was present during stimulation. Studies done by Schweitzer et al. using B7-1/B7-2-deficient APCs demonstrated that IL-4 was severely compromised in the absence of B7-mediated signals, even after restimulation with wild-type APCs *(48)*. Production of IL-4 could be restored either by CD28 crosslinking or addition of rIL-4 to the in vitro cultures. Whereas a lack of CD28 stimulation inhibits IL-4 production, increasing amounts of CD28 costimulation promotes Th2 differentiation by enhancing IL-4 and IL-5 production *(47)*. Taken together, these studies suggest that CD28 provides signals critical for IL-4 production and thus Th2 differentiation. However, there are situations where IL-4 production does not have such a strong dependence on CD28 costimulation. For example, repeated immunization of mice expressing a CTLA-4-Ig transgene that blocks the B7:CD28 interaction resulted in detectable IL-4 production following in vitro restimulation *(49)*. In addition, when CD28$^{-/-}$ BALB/c mice were infected with *Leishmania major*, which causes a progressive Th2-mediated disease in wild-type BALB/c mice, the CD28$^{-/-}$ mice were susceptible to disease. Cytokine analysis showed that although IL-4 production was reduced following in vitro restimulation, ELISA enzyme linked immunosorbant assay (ELISPOT) analysis directly ex vivo revealed that wild-type and CD28$^{-/-}$ mice had the same number of IL-4-producing cells *(50)*.

Other cytokines seem to have variable dependence upon CD28 costimulation. For example, TCR transgenic CD4$^+$ T cells from CD28$^{-/-}$ mice were able to produce IL-2 at high concentrations of antigenic peptide, although high levels of IL-2 production, and sustained proliferation, appeared to be CD28-dependent *(49)*. These results were consistent with other studies that had demonstrated a quantitative effect of B7-mediated costimulation on a T cell clone *(6)*. Additionally, studies with B7-deficient APC found that, with high-dose peptide stimulation, IL-2 production was detectable but severely inhibited compared to wild-type APC *(48)*. Upon restimulation with wild-type APCs, IL-2 production was still decreased after priming in the absence of CD28 stimulation. Together these data suggest that while CD28 stimulation is important for maximal sustained production of IL-2, the need for CD28 costimulation can be overcome by strong stimulation through TCR engagement.

Studies of the role of B7 costimulation on IFN-γ production by CD4$^+$ T cells have yielded conflicting results. Early studies using T cell clones reported that IFN-γ production is only partially dependent on costimulation *(51)*. Parallel results were found with TCR transgenic cells by some investigators, who found that primary or secondary stimulation elicited IFN-γ that was relatively B7-independent *(52)*. In contrast, a different study using TCR transgenic T cells found that production of IFN-γ following priming in the absence of B7 costimulation was ablated *(41)*. Like IL-4 production, IFN-γ production was dependent on the presence of IL-2 during priming. Because IL-2 production was absent without costimulation under the conditions used, IFN-γ production was also ablated. Studies using CD28$^{-/-}$ TCR transgenic T cells indicated that whereas IFN-γ production was reduced in the absence of CD28 expression, crosslinking CD28 on wild-type T cells did not significantly influence the ability to produce IFN-γ upon subsequent stimulation *(47)*. In studies using B7-deficient APCs, with intentionally high levels of peptide stimulation where IL-2 production was detectable during priming, naive TCR transgenic T cells primed with B7-1/B7-2$^{-/-}$ APCs were able to produce near wild type levels of IFN-γ upon restimulation with wild-type APCs *(48)*. Likewise, T cells primed with wild type APCs, which were capable of producing high levels of IFN-γ, continued to produce high levels of IFN-γ upon restimulation with B7-1/B7-2$^{-/-}$ APCs.

Taken together, the data indicate that B7-CD28-mediated costimulation mainly affects IL-4 and IL-2 production by naive T cells. From this work, some general rules describing direct and downstream effects of B7-CD28 costimulation on cytokine production by CD4$^+$ cells have emerged. First, there is the distinct hierarchy in costimulation-dependence of cytokines produced by naive vs primed T cells. For naive T cells, the dependence on B7-CD28 decreases from IL-4 > IL-2 > IFN-γ; for previously activated T cells, IL-2 > IL-4 = IFN-γ. The costimulation dependence of IL-2 is relatively great for both naive and previously activated T cells, whereas that of IFN-γ is relatively small for both naive and previously activated T cells. The main difference in B7 dependence between naive and previously activated T cells is for IL-4 production, which is highly B7 dependent in naive T cells and relatively independent in previously activated T cells. Second, there is interdependence in the production of certain cytokines. During T cell differentiation, the Th2-promoting effects of IL-4 dominate over Th1-promoting effects of IL-12 *(53)*. Thus, during the development of an immune response, the amount of B7-CD28 costimulation can play a pivotal role in determining the level of IL-4 production, which then drives Th1 vs Th2 differentiation. However, once differentiation is achieved, there seems to be little dependence upon costimulation to maintain the response.

2.6. Role of B7-CTLA-4 Interactions

Whereas B7-CD28 interacts to promote T cell activation, B7-CTLA-4 interactions inhibit or downregulate T cell activation. CTLA-4 blockade in vitro increases T cell proliferation and cytokine production. However, CTLA-4 engagement inhibits proliferation and cytokine secretion, most notably decreasing IL-2 production *(54,55)*. Additionally, studies utilizing T cells lacking CTLA-4 indicate that CTLA-4 regulates Th-cell differentiation. The short lifespan of CTLA-4$^{-/-}$ mice, death within 3-4 wk of birth, and the extensive in vivo activation of T cells has made the study of naive CTLA-4$^{-/-}$ T cells difficult. This problem has resulted in the generation of several mouse strains that enable isolation of unactivated T cells that are CTLA-4 deficient. One strategy was to cross TCR transgenes onto the CTLA-4$^{-/-}$ background to decrease the frequency of spontaneous activation in vivo. The second approach was to generate a triple knockout (TKO) mouse by breeding the CTLA-4$^{-/-}$ mice with B7-1/B7-2$^{-/-}$ mice, which prevented in vivo activation of normal T cells. In studies using TCR transgenic CTLA-4$^{-/-}$ cells or T cells from TKO mice, T cells without CTLA-4 demonstrated skewing toward Th2 differentiation by secreting large quantities of IL-4, IL-5, and IL-10 *(56,57)*. Paralleling the in vitro studies, injection of TKO mice with anti-CD28 antibodies lead to Th2 differentiation in vivo. CD4$^+$ T cells from TKO mice produced high levels of IL-4 *(56)*. A similar result was seen when anti-CTLA-4 antibodies were used to inhibit staphylococcal enterotoxin B (SEB)-induced T cell responses in vivo *(58)*. Additionally, a role for CTLA-4 in regulating TGF-β production has been described recently *(59)*, suggesting another means by which CTLA-4 may influence T cell differentiation and self-reactive T cells.

2.7. Potential Role of the Newest Family Members: ICOS and B7-H1

Like CD28, ICOS has positive costimulatory activity, enhancing proliferation and cytokine production (IL-4, IL-5, IFN-γ, and GM-CSF) *(10)*. However, it has several properties that are distinct from CD28 and make it particularly intriguing. In contrast to CD28, ICOS is rapidly induced after T cell activation and does not stimulate IL-2 production, but superinduces IL-10 production. Murine studies investigating the effects of ICOS engagement showed enhanced proliferation and increased secretion of IFN-γ with no effect on IL-2 production, but IL-10 was not tested *(11)*. Similar to ICOS stimulation, ligation of B7-H1 costimulated T cell responses and produced high levels of IL-10, which was dependent upon the presence of IL-2. The function of B7RP-1/B7h-ICOS and B7-H1 interactions on Th differentiation is currently an active area of reseach. Given the inducible expression of B7h/B7-RP1 and B7H-1 receptors on activated T cells, these pathways may influence T cell function and differentiation. Because of the effects of B7h/B7-RP1 and B7-H1 on IL-10 secretion, these new receptor/ligand pairs may be another important regulatory control in the development of immune responses and may play a role in the development of autoimmunity.

3. APC COSTIMULATORY PLAYERS: RECEPTORS, LIGANDS, AND THEIR EFFECTS ON TH DIFFERENTIATION

3.1. APC Costimulatory Receptor: CD40

Another costimulatory pathway that may function independently or synergize with the B7-CD28 pathway is the CD40-CD154 pathway. This pathway has a key role in regulating lymphocyte activation with more profound direct effects on the antigen presenting cell which, in turn, affects T cell differentiation. Although early studies demonstrated a critical role of the CD40-CD154 pathway in B cell biology, more recent studies have shown that this pathway is important for both cell-mediated and humoral immune responses. CD40, a member of the tumor necrosis factor receptor (TNF-R) family is expressed on a wide variety of cell types. CD40 is constitutively expressed on B cells from very early in development, and is upregulated slightly on B cells upon activation with polyclonal activators or cytokines *(60)*. Additionally, CD40 is expressed on monocytes *(61)*, dendritic cells (DC) *(62)*, microglia *(63)*, follicular dendritic cells, hematopoetic progenitors (CD34$^+$), fibroblasts *(64)*, thymic epithelial cells *(65)*, endothelial cells *(66,67)*, keratinocytes *(68)*, and human vascular smooth muscle cells *(69)*.

3.2. Ligand: CD154 (gp39, CD40L)

CD154, the ligand for CD40, is a TNF family member that is expressed on mature activated CD4$^+$ T cells, some CD8$^+$ T cells, monocytes/macrophages, natural killer (NK) cells, human mast cells, basophils, eosinophils, platelets (as reviewed in ref. *64)*, germinal center B cells *(70)*, vascular endothelial cells, and smooth-muscle cells *(69)*. The expression of CD154 is highly regulated; CD154 is rapidly induced on CD4$^+$ T cells, a subset of CD8$^+$ T cells and is found expressed on Th0, Th1, and Th2 cells *(71)*. In vitro CD154 expression is induced within 4–6 h after activation, peaks by 24 h, and then decreases. In vivo injection of antigen leads to a somewhat slower kinetics of expression, with maximal frequency of CD154$^+$ T cells by 3–4 d after T-dependent antigen administration.

3.3. Role of the CD40-CD154 Pathway

Initially, studies on CD40 function focused on B cell activation and antibody production. Hyper-IgM syndrome demonstrates the critical role of CD40 signaling in B cell function. Hyper-IgM syndrome in humans or mice results from mutations in or the loss of either CD40 or it's cognate ligand, CD154 *(72)*. Loss of the CD40-CD154 pathway function causes defects in germinal center formation, isotype switching, and B cell memory development *(60)*. Recent work also has demonstrated that CD40 stimulation leads to enhanced cytokine production by a variety of cell types. When B cells are stimulated via engagement of both surface IgM and CD40, there is enhanced production of IL-1β, IL-6, IL-10, GM-CSF, and TNF-α *(73,74)*. However, CD40 stimulation alone can enhance B cell production of IL-10. Addition of IL-4 during CD40 stimulation can have differential effects on B cell cytokine production. IL-4 plus anti-CD40 enhances the production of IL-6 *(75,76)* whereas, IL-10 production is inhibited *(77)*. Although murine B cells have not been shown to secrete IL-12, human B cells have been shown to produce IL-12 in response to CD40 stimulation *(76)*. IL-12 production can be enhanced further by the addition of IFN-γ, however, IL-4 severely inhibits IL-12 and IL-10 completely abrogates IL-12 production in response to CD40 engagement. Late during B cell activation, IL-2, and IL-13 mRNA can be detected after stimulation first with anti-CD40 and then PMA plus ionomycin *(78)*.

CD40 is also an important signaling molecule for many other cell types. CD40 signals to DC increase secretion of IL-1α, IL-1β, IL-6, IL-8, IL-10, IL-12, IL-15, TNF-α, and MIP-1α *(79–82)*. The cytokine profile produced by DC after CD40 stimulation also can be modulated if cytokines are present during stimulation. Peripheral blood mononuclear cells (PBMCs) can be cultured in the presence of GM-CSF and IL-4 to generate DC. When IFN-β is added to the DC differentiation culture, IL-12 production is selectively inhibited after CD40 engagement with no alterations seen in IL-8 or TNF-α production *(83)* while IL-6 can be augmented *(84)*. Similar to B cells, addition of IL-4 impairs DC IL-12 secretion, IL-10 dramatically inhibits IL-12 production and the cytokines together have additive effects *(80,81)*. In contrast to the effects on IL-12, IL-10 synergizes with CD40 to upregulate IL-8 and TNF-α production *(85)*. Although IL-12 can be produced by DC, it also modulates the production of other cytokines. DCs produce IFN-γ in response to IL-12, which can be enhanced by the addition of IL-4 *(86)*.

Monocytes, macrophages, and microglia cells are related to the myeloid lineage of DCs. Thus, it is not surprising that CD40 engagement on these cells leads to production of a similar profile of cytokines. CD40 signals stimulate monocytes/macrophages to produce IL-1, IL-6, IL-8, IL-10, IL-12, TNF-α, and MIP-1α *(79,87–89)*. Addition of GM-CSF, IL-3, or IFN-γ to monocytes stimulated with CD40 enhances the production of IL-6, IL-8, and TNF-α *(61)*. Microglia cells produce TNF-α and IL-12, which is IFN-γ-dependent, in response to CD40 ligation *(90,91)*. Like other APC populations, IL-10 as well as TGFβ1 can inhibit CD40 induced TNF-α production by microglia cells *(92)*.

Even some nonprofessional APCs produce cytokines in response to CD40 stimulation. Engagement of CD40 on human vascular smooth muscle cells induces the expression of proinflammatory cytokines *(69)*. Additionally, CD40 ligation of keratinocytes leads to IL-8 production *(68)*. Finally, CD40 stimulation of thymic epithelial cells in the presence of IFN-γ and IL-1 induces GM-CSF secretion *(65)*. In summary, CD40 critically regulates the expression of proinflammatory cytokines by many APCs, which then influences the Th1-Th2 differentiation of responding T cells.

3.4. A Direct Role of CD154 on T Cells

Although the work regarding direct signaling into T cells via CD154 has been limited, some studies suggest that CD154 modulates T cell cytokine production. In a system utilizing antibodies to CD3, CD28, and CD154 for

T cell stimulation in the absence of APCs, low doses of anti-CD3 plus anti-CD28 produced very low levels of IL-4. Addition of anti-CD154 greatly enhanced the production of IL-4, however, IL-4 synthesis was inhibited with maximal CD3 stimulation *(93)*. Another study that implicated direct signaling into T cells via CD154 demonstrated that CD154 engagement in the presence of CD3 or phytohemagglutinin (PHA) stimulation augmented production of a number of cytokines including IL-2, IFN-γ TNF-α, IL-4, IL-5, and IL-10 *(94,95)*. Addition of IL-12 to cultures caused even greater production of IFN-γ. Although these studies do not implicate CD154 as a modulator of Th differentiation, they suggest that this molecule may have a more general role in enhancing T cell cytokine production.

4. CYTOKINE REGULATION OF COSTIMULATORY MOLECULE EXPRESSION

4.1. Regulation of Costimulatory Ligands: B7 Family and CD154

Costimulatory molecules provide signals that are critical for the proper development of an immune reponse. One key determinant of costimulation is the proper regulated expression of both costimulatory receptors and ligands. Owing to the importance of costimulation, it is possible that aberrant expression of costimulatory molecules can result in inappropriate immune responses. In fact, altered expression of costimulatory molecules has been seen in many autoimmune disorders *(96–99)*. Often the expression of costimulatory molecules is controlled by stimulatory signals to the responding cell, whether a T cell or an APC. However, another key regulatory determinant is the effect of cytokines on the expression of costimulatory molecules.

Multiple cytokines can have distinct effects on the expression of B7 molecules depending upon the type of cell along with the activation status of the cells *(see* Table 1). For B cells, initial studies demonstrated that IL-4 could dramatically upregulate B7-1 and B7-2 expression *(100,101)*. Additionally, Valle et al. showed that IL-2 could also enhance B7 expression on activated B cells. In a study investigating the T cell-dependent induction of B7-1 on B cells, Ranheim and Kipps demonstrated that TNF-α and TNF-β also augmented the expression of B7-1 on B cells *(102)*. TNF-α mediated B7-1 expression was dependent on CD120 (p75 TNFRβ) and could be inhibited by antibodies to TNF-α. IL-10 was also found to have differential effects on B7-1 depending upon the stimulation conditions. In combination with CD40 stimulation, IL-10 enhanced B7-1 expression, however, IL-10 was able to inhibit B7-1 expression induced by crosslinking of CD120.

DC also exhibit a complex pattern of cytokine-regulated B7 expression, which is dependent on the source of DC analyzed. Both IFN-γ and IL-10 can

Table 1
Cytokine Regulation of B7-1 and B7-2 Expression

Cell type/cytokine	B7-1	B7-2	Refs.
B cells			
IL-4	↑	↑	*(100,101)*
IL-2	↑	↑	*(101)*
TNF-α, TNF-α	↑	NR	*(102)*
α-TNFR + IL-10	↓	NR	
α-CD40 + IL-10	↑	NR	
Dendritic cells			
Langerhans cells			
IL-10	↓	NC	*(103)*
IFN-γ	↓	NC	
GM-CSF + IFN-γ	↑	NR	
GM-CSF + IL-10	↓	NR	
Blood-derived DC			
IL-10	NC	↓	*(104)*
Dermal DC			
IL-10	NC	↓	*(105)*
α-GM-CSF	NC	↓	
Monocytes			
GM-CSF	NC or ↑	↑	*(105–107)*
IFN-γ	↑	↑	*(106,107)*
IL-10	↑	↓	*(107)*
IL-4, TNF-α	NC	↓	
Macrophages			
IFN-γ	↓	↑	*(108)*
IFN-γ + IL-10	↓	↓	
Microglia			
GM-CSF	↑	↑	*(109)*
GM-CSF + IL-4	NC	↓	
GM-CSF + IL-11	NC	↓	
GM-CSF + TGF-β	NC	↓	
GM-CSF + NGF	NC	↓	
IFN-γ	NC	↑	
IFN-γ + IL-10	NC	↓	

NC, no change; NR, not reported. Upward arrows indicate there was an increased B7 expression as a result of the listed treatment and downward arrows indicate that B7 expression decreased from this treatment.

inhibit B7-1 expression on Langerhans cells (LC) without affecting the expression of B7-2 *(103)*. GM-CSF can partially restore B7-1 expression in the presence of IFN-γ but not IL-10. In contrast to LC, blood-derived DC downregulate B7-2 but not B7-1 in response to IL-10 *(104)*. Like blood DC, dermal DC downregulate only B7-2 in response to IL-10 *(105)*. Additionally, treatment with anti-GM-CSF caused the downregulation of B7-2 only on dermal DC.

Similar to DC, monocytes demonstrate preferential upregulation of B7-2 in response to GM-CSF *(105)*, however, in some studies, both B7-1 and B7-2 are upregulated in response to either GM-CSF or IFN-γ *(106,107)*. IL-10 was shown to downregulate B7-2 expression on monocytes, while slightly enhancing B7-1 *(107)*. Selective B7-2 downregulation on monocytes can also be mediated by IL-4 or TNF-α *(107)*. Macrophages selectively downregulate B7-1 while upregulating B7-2 in response to IFN-γ. Addition of IL-10 and IFN-γ will lead to decreased expression of both B7-1 and B7-2 (as reviewed in ref. *108*). Similar to monocytes, GM-CSF will upregulate both B7s on microglia, while IFN-γ will selectively enhance B7-2 expression (109). Similar to macrophages, addition of IL-10 will inhibit IFN-γ-mediated microglial expression. GM-CSF induced upregulation of B7-2 also can be inhibited by the addition of IL-4, TGF-β, IL-11, or nerve growth factor (NGF) while B7-1 upregulation is unaffected. Finally, although not generally considered a professional APC, fibroblasts that constitutively express B7-1 upregulate B7-1 in response to IFN-γ and TNF-α stimulation *(110)*.

Although B7h/B7RP-1 has only recently been identified, initial studies have indicated that TNF-α induces B7h/B7RP-1 mRNA expression on fibroblasts *(19)*. IFN-γ or IL-1α alone was unable to induce B7h/B7RP-1 mRNA expression, but addition of TNF-α, alone or in combination with IFN-γ or IL-1α, dramatically upregulated B7h/B7RP-1 mRNA in cultured fibroblasts. Additionally, in vivo administration of lipopolysaccharide (LPS), a potent stimulus for TNF-α production, led to increased B7h/B7RP-1 mRNA expression in several nonlymphoid tissues including the testes, kidneys, and peritoneum with modest downregulation in the spleen. Much work still needs to be done to elucidate the expression pattern of B7h/B7RP-1 and to determine what are the key regulators of B7h/B7RP-1 expression. Unlike B7h/B7RP-1, no information is currently available regarding the cytokine regulation of B7-H1 expression, however, future studies will undoubtedly investigate this question.

In addition to modulating B7 expression, some cytokines alter the expression of CD154, which triggers signals through CD40. In studies using murine Th clones as well as purified CD4 T cells, Roy et al. found that IFN-γ

was a potent inhibitor of CD154 expression for either CD4$^+$ T cells or both
Th1 and Th2 clones *(71)*. Additionally, the authors found that TGF-β inhibited CD154 expression on Th2 clones. Studies examining CD154 expression in human T cells also found IFN-γ to be inhibitory while IL-4 was able
to upregulate CD154 mRNA *(111)*. In contrast to the effects of IFN-γ, IL-12
has been shown to upregulate CD154, both at the mRNA and protein level,
on human peripheral-blood T cells *(112)*. Optimal induction was seen in the
presence of multiple stimuli including IL-2, IL-12, and B7/CD28
costimulation. Additionally, Hirohata et al. found that IL-12 along with anti-
CD3 upregulated CD154 expression on human T cells *(113)*. However, this
in study the presence of either IL-4 or IL-10 during anti-CD3 stimulation
decreased surface levels of CD154, but IFN-γ had no effect. Recently,
CD154 has been identified on human macrophages, vascular endothelial
cells, and smooth-muscle cells. Stimulation with IL-1β, TNF-α, or IFN-γ
increased both surface expression and synthesis of CD154 on all three cell
types *(69)*.

4.2. Regulation of Costimulatory Receptors: CD28 Family and CD40

Despite the critical role of CD28 and CTLA-4 in costimulating cytokine
production there appears to be little information on the regulation of these
receptors by cytokines. Shindo et al. have demonstrated that CD28 expression is downregulated in response to IL-2 and this is dependent on expression of the IL-2Rβ subunit *(114)*. IL-2 also has been shown to enhance
expression of CTLA-4 on anti-CD3-stimulated T cells *(115)*. CTLA-4 was
modestly enhanced by the addition of IL-4, IL-6, IL-7, or IL-12. Another
study suggests that IL-12 may enhance CTLA-4 expression, while IL-10
downregulates CTLA-4. Patients infected with *Mycobacterium tuberculosis*
have depressed CTLA-4 expression on PBMCs *(116)*. Treatment of these
cells with either anti-IL-10 or exogenous IL-12 upregulated expression of
CTLA-4, suggesting that IL-10 inhibits CTLA-4, whereas IL12 enhances
expression. How IL-12 modulates CTLA-4 expression was not addressed
and may result from either direct effects of IL-12 or indirect effects via regulation of other cytokines, such as IFN-γ. At this point, studies have yet to
investigate the effects of cytokines on the expression of ICOS; however,
future studies will likely address this question.

Similar to the regulation of B7s, CD28, CTLA-4, and CD154, cytokines
differentially regulate the expression of CD40 on various cells types. When
CD40 was initially identified, IFN-γ was shown to increase CD40 mRNA in
both B cells and epithelial neoplasms *(117)*. Since then, IL-4 alone has been
shown to upregulate CD40 expression on human B cells. When combined
with stimulation through surface IgM, either IL-2 or IL-4 can augment

expression *(118)*. Monocytes have been shown to upregulate CD40 expression of both mRNA and surface protein in response to GM-CSF, IL-3, or IFN-γ *(61,88)*. CD40 on microglia has a complicated regulatory pattern. GM-CSF or IFN-γ alone will enhance the expression of CD40 *(109,119)*. However, TGFβ can repress IFN-γ inducible expression *(119)* and IL-4, TGFβ1, or NGF can repress GM-CSF inducible CD40 expression *(109)*. For thymic epithelial cells, CD40 expression is augmented by IL-1α, TNF-α, and IFN-γ but not by IL-4 *(65)*. Although keratinocytes and endothelial cells are not considered professional APCs, they also show cytokine regulated expression of CD40. Keratinocytes demonstrate upregulated expression after exposure to IFN-γ but not TNF-α or IL-1β *(68)* whereas endothelial cells show augmented expression after treatment with TNF-α, IL-1, IFN-β, and IFN-γ *(67)*. Additionally, the interferons show synergistic enhancement when combined with either TNF-α or IL-1. Thus, while these receptor-ligand interactions serve to regulate cytokine expression, cytokines act as part of a feedback loop to either limit or sustain signals that will alter costimulatory molecule expression, ultimately determining the duration of cytokine production.

5. REGULATION OF COSTIMULATORY MOLECULES AND CYTOKINE RECEPTORS BY COSTIMULATION

One of the most important aspects of CD40-CD154 function is its functional relationship with the B7-CD28 costimulatory pathway. As stated earlier, CD40 stimulation leads to upregulation of B7-1 and B7-2, which greatly enhances the costimulatory capacity of B cells, macrophages, and DC *(79,120–122)*. Although CD154 can be upregulated in the absence of costimulation *(122–124)*, B7-CD28 interactions can lead to upregulation of CD154 *(124,125)*. One in vivo study using the injection of anti-CD28 saw a dramatic increase in the number of peripheral B cells *(126)*. The authors found that the B cell expansion was owing to the upregulation of CD154 after CD28 engagement. There is an important synergy between the CD40-CD154 and B7-CD28 pathways to initiate and amplify T cell-dependent immune responses. Although the effects of ICOS signaling are not yet fully understood, stimulation via ICOS also results in upregulation of CD154 *(10)*. This could be yet another level of control that is critical to the careful balance between protective immunity and autoimmunity. The biological significance of this synergy has been demonstrated in a variety of studies showing the synergistic ability of CD154 and B7 antagonists in vivo to block autoimmune diseases, graft rejection, and antibody production in murine model systems *(127,128)*. Elegant studies have shown that the injection of

B7-1 expressing B cells into CD154-deficient mice can restore Th1 responses in a model of autoimmunity *(129)*. Thus, the B7-CD28 and CD40-CD154 pathways are inter-related and synergistic.

Cytokines must bind their cognate receptor on the cell surface to mediate their biological effects. This is yet another level where costimulation can modulate cytokine responses. Studies by Armitage et al. demonstrate that CD154 ligation leads to increased CD25 expression on human T cells *(94)*. Additionally, studies have shown that CD28 ligation can lead to the upregulation of the IL-2R *(130,131)*. More recent studies have indicated that CD28 costimulation also enhances IL-12R expression *(132)*. In addition to the direct effects of CD28 signaling, IL-2 and IL-12, which are produced in response to CD28 engagement, enhance IL-12R β subunit expression *(133)*. Thus, B7-CD28 interactions play an important regulatory role in the expression of the IL-12 β receptor subunit, which is a key determinant of IL-12 responsiveness and Th1 lineage commitment. In contrast to the effects of CD28, CTLA-4 has been shown to downregulate both the IL-2R *(54,134)* and the IL-12R *(133)*, further emphasizing the opposing roles that CD28 and CTLA-4 have during an immune response.

6. ROLE OF COSTIMULATION IN AUTOIMMUNITY

6.1. Manipulation of the B7-CD28/CTLA-4 and CD40-CD154 Pathways in Animal Models of Autoimmunity

The identification of the B7-CD28/CTLA-4 and CD40-CD154 pathways as key immunoregulatory pathways has prompted investigation of the roles of these pathways in the pathogenesis of autoimmune diseases and their therapeutic potential for controlling autoimmune diseases. Numerous studies have indicated that these pathways have key roles in both the initiation and effector phases of autoimmune diseases. The roles of the receptors and ligands in these pathways have been probed using monoclonal antibodies (MAbs) that recognize these receptors or ligands, chimeric fusion proteins, and mice deficient in receptors or ligands. Each of these approaches has its advantages and disadvantages. For example, studies using antibodies may be misleading owing to artifacts resulting from crosslinking events, Fc-receptor-mediated effects, or incomplete penetration. In studies using knockout mice, developmental effects (e.g., affecting TCR repertoire or activation threshold) need to be considered in the interpretation of results.

6.2. Blockade or Elimination of B7 Costimulation

Manipulation of the B7-CD28/CTLA-4 costimulatory pathway can prevent the initiation of an autoimmune disease, as well as suppress an ongoing autoimmune process. Initial studies of the role of the B7-CD28/CTLA-4 pathway used CTLA-4Ig, a chimeric fusion protein of the extracellular domain of CTLA-4 fused to an Ig tail that binds to both B7 molecules, to block the natural interaction of B7s with both CD28 and CTLA-4 receptors. Studies in the NOD model of diabetes demonstrated that CTLA-4Ig treatment early (at 2–3 wk of age) for 2 wk markedly reduced the incidence of diabetes *(31)*. NOD mice treated with CTLA-4Ig after the onset of insulitis also had a reduced incidence of diabetes. Likewise, in the systemic lupus erythematosus (SLE)-like disease model using New Zealand black/New Zealand white mice, administration of CTLA-4Ig blocked autoantibody production and prolonged the survival of lupus-prone mice *(135)*. Beneficial effects of CTLA-4Ig were still seen in this lupus model even if treatment was started after the development of advanced clinical signs of disease. CTLA-4Ig also prevented Collagen-induced arthritis (CIA) *(136)*. Similarly, in the murine model for MS of EAE, CTLA-4Ig treatment protected against EAE induced by either active immunization or adoptive transfer. This profound inhibition of the clinical and histological manifestations of EAE continued after CTLA-4Ig treatment was ended *(137–141)*. However, CTLA-4Ig treatment after the priming of encephalitogenic T cells has had limited or no effects in many cases. Administration of CTLA-4Ig following the adoptive transfer of encephalitogenic T cells delayed disease onset or reduced severity of disease in some murine studies, but did not ameliorate EAE in other studies. One potential explanation for the inability of CTLA-4Ig treatment to inhibit EAE after induction of the disease is that the CTLA-4Ig does not efficiently enter the central nervous system (CNS) to block the B7:CD28 interactions at the site of effector T cell activation. Recent studies indicate that this is the case. Local CNS delivery of CTLA-4Ig using a nonreplicating adenoviral vector was able to ameliorate ongoing EAE, while systemic administration of CTLA-4Ig had a minimal effect on disease *(142)*.

Certain CTLA-4Ig treatment protocols exacerbated rather than ameliorated disease. The timing of CTLA-4Ig administration appears to influence the outcome of disease. These results may reflect the complex interactions among receptors and ligands in this pathway and the opposing effects on the outcome of an immune response may depend on whether positive or negative signaling through this pathway is disrupted. The mechanism by which CTLA-4Ig exerts its protective effects is not clear and is an active area of investigation. Splenocytes derived from CTLA-4Ig-treated mice proliferated in response to PLP in vitro, indicating that EAE prevention was not owing to tolerance to antigen.

The role of B7 costimulation also has been examined in murine models of autoimmunity using mice lacking both B7-1and B7-2 (B7-1/B7-2$^{-/-}$ mice) and anti-B7-1 plus anti-B7-2 MAb treatment *(143,144)*. Webb and coworkers found that anti-B7-1 or anti-B7-2 alone could not inhibit CIA but combined administration effectively blocked CIA, even if treatment was delayed until after onset of clinical disease *(145)*. The importance of the B7:CD28 costimulatory pathway was examined during the initiation of the autoimmune response in EAE, by directly immunizing C57BL/6 B7-1/B7-2-deficient mice with the myelin oligodendrocyte glycoprotein (MOG) epitope 35-55. Mice lacking both B7-1 and B7-2 were highly resistant to EAE induction. T cells in the B7-1/B7-2$^{-/-}$ mice were primed to MOG 35-55, although their proliferative responses were impaired. Resistance to EAE was not owing to a lack of induction of Th1 cytokines, because T cells from B7-1/B7-2$^{-/-}$ mice produced more IFN-γ, as compared to T cells from wild-type mice. The role of B7 costimulation during the effector phase of the EAE was examined by adoptively transferring wild-type MOG 35-55 activated T cell lines into B7-1/B7-2$^{-/-}$ vs wild-type mice *(143)*. EAE was markedly reduced in B7-1/B7-2$^{-/-}$ recipients following adoptive transfer of MOG-specific wild-type T cells, demonstrating that B7 costimulatory molecules have a critical role in the effector phase of EAE. Thus, B7 costimulators have key roles in both the initial activation and/or expansion of MOG-reactive T cells in the periphery and in their activation within the target organ.

Although B7-1/B7-2$^{-/-}$ mice are highly resistant to the development of clinical EAE, they do develop some inflammatory foci, but these lesions are limited almost exclusively to the meninges *(143)*. These histological findings suggest previously unappreciated roles for B7-mediated costimulation in the target organ: B7 costimulation may be needed: (1) to stimulate the production of chemokines and adhesion molecules that enable T cell entry into the CNS parenchyma and/or prevent trafficking of activated T cells out of the CNS parenchyma; (2) to stimulate the production of growth and survival factors that sustain activation of T cells that enter the CNS parenchyma; and/or (3) to enable activated T cells in the CNS parenchyma to recruit other lymphocytes and leukocytes to the CNS. Further studies are needed to distinguish among these possibilities.

6.3. Comparison of the Roles of B7-1 and B7-2

Many in vivo studies investigating the roles of B7-1 vs B7-2 costimulation in the expansion of T cells and the induction of Th1 vs Th2 cytokines have suggested that B7-1 and B7-2 are fairly comparable. At times B7-2 plays a more dominant costimulatory role, primarily because it is the costimulatory molecule present during initial T cell priming. However, there is a considerable amount of data that indicate that B7-1 and B7-2 costimulation may have different roles in the initiation or regulation of autoimmune diseases.

Although these studies clearly show a key role for B7 costimulation in the initiation and/or progression of Th1-mediated autoimmune diseases, the individual roles of B7-1 and B7-2 have not been clear.

B7-1 and B7-2 expression during autoimmune diseases has been examined, because manipulation of this pathway to block an immune response must take into account B7 expression patterns. For example, in EAE, there is selective upregulation of B7-1 in the spleen and CNS in actively induced or adoptively transferred EAE. Similar observations have been made in MS correlating preferential B7-1 expression with disease activity. Immunohistochemical staining of MS plaques and inflammatory stroke lesions from the same brains demonstrated that while B7-2 expression was found in both types of lesions, B7-1 was uniquely associated with the MS plaques *(146–148)*. Interestingly, after treatment with IFNβ-1b, one of the three FDA-approved treatments for the relapsing-remitting form of MS, the frequency of B7-1 expressing B cells decreased, while the number of B7-2$^+$ B cells remained unchanged. These findings suggest that distinct kinetics of B7-1 and B7-2 expression at different locations could lead to distinct roles for these costimulators in different diseases and immune settings.

Studies addressing the individual role of B7-1 and B7-2 in the induction and effector phases of autoimmune diseases using anti-B7 MAbs have yielded conflicting and confusing results. In the NOD mouse diabetes model, early treatment with anti-B7-2 (like CTLA-4Ig treatment) prevented clinical disease, whereas later treatment had no effect on the incidence of overt diabetes. However, both anti-B7-1 administration and a combination of anti-B7-1 plus anti-B7-2 led to accelerated and more severe diabetes. In contrast, treatment of mice with anti-B7-1 MAb in vivo during the induction of EAE protected mice from disease, whereas anti-B7-2 MAb exacerbated disease severity. The effectiveness of the anti-B7-1 MAb required continuous therapy for 30 d postimmunization *(149,150)*. Administration of anti-B7-1 MAbs in vivo at the time of immunization did not inhibit the induction of antigen-specific T cells, but did alter the cytokine profile of the responding cells and resulted in predominant generation of Th2 clones whose transfer prevented EAE induction and abrogated established disease. Treatment with anti-B7-2 MAb was correlated with skewing towards a Th1 phenotype. Consistent with these observations, administration of noncrosslinking anti-B7-1 Fab fragments, but not anti-B7-2 MAbs, after the first clinical remission of EAE significantly decreased the incidence of relapses in these mice *(151)*. There was a reduction in the number of T cells generated that react with a second epitope, suggesting that anti-B7-1 MAb treatment prevents epitope spreading. In a follow-up study, the authors demonstrated that APCs isolated from the spinal cords of mice with acute EAE preferentially utilized B7-1 costimulation, as anti-B7-1 MAb but not anti-B7-2 MAb significantly inhibited T cell activation when these cells were used as a source of APCs *(152)*. Together, these results support separate functional roles for B7-1 and B7-2 during EAE induction and progression.

However, the interpretation of these data are complicated because the efficacy of MAb therapy will depend on the effectiveness of the blockade based on the type or the dose of MAb used and may be influenced by the potential signaling capacity of the MAbs. The latter is perhaps best exemplified by the observation that treatment of SJL mice with intact anti-B7-1 MAbs during EAE disease remission results in accelerated relapses, pathology, and epitope spreading. Because T cells are the major cell type expressing B7-1 and B7-2 in the CNS during acute, relapsing, and chronic EAE, the potential effects of MAbs signaling into the T cell need to be considered in interpreting the results of experiments using anti-B7 MAbs. As discussed earlier, a role for B7-1 on T cells in limiting IL-4 production has been described recently *(33)*. It may be that B7-1 on T cells inhibits IL-4 production by these T cells, and promotes autopathogenic T cell responses Thus, anti-B7-1 Fab fragments may protect against EAE by enhancing IL-4 production and protective Th2 responses.

More recently, studies have used mice lacking either B7-1 or B7-2 as another means to examine the individual roles of these B7 costimulators in autoimmune disease. Although studies with anti-B7 MAbs have demonstrated a primary role for B7-1 costimulation in the pathogenesis of EAE using SJL/PLP 139-151 model of EAE, studies with mice lacking either B7-1 or B7-2 alone have found that B7-1 and B7-2 have overlapping roles in PLP-induced EAE, and that B7-1 did not have a preferential role in the pathogenesis of PLP-induced EAE. The induction of EAE also has been examined in NOD mice lacking expression of B7-1 or B7-2. Disease severity was significantly more reduced in B7-2$^{-/-}$ NOD mice than in B7-1, and absent in CD28$^{-/-}$ NOD mice as compared with wild type NOD animals. It should be noted that neither anti-B7-1 nor anti-B7-2 MAb inhibited EAE in NOD mice, but together these anti-B7 MAbs delayed NOD onset and severity, and anti-B7-1 MAb treatment of B7-2$^{-/-}$ mice further reduced disease severity. Differences in efficacy of MAb blockade in different tissues, especially the periphery lymphoid organs vs the CNS, may explain the differences between the use of anti-B7 MAbs and costimulator deficient mice. Because the timing and level of B7-1 expression are unchanged in B7-2$^{-/-}$ mice and likewise, B7-2 expression is unaffected in B7-1$^{-/-}$ mice, the difference in conclusions drawn from the two systems is not likely to be attributable to alterations of B7 expression in B7-1- or B7-2-deficient mice. The relative importance of B7-1 and B7-2 may differ between MOG-induced

EAE in C57BL/6 mice and PLP (proteolipid protein) or MBP (myelin basic protein) induced EAE in SJL mice or NOD mice. Differences in myelin antigens and/or genetic background may influence the respective roles of B7-1 and B7-2 in the induction of EAE. Additionally, there may be differences in the T cell repertoires between different strains of mice. Background, non-MHC-linked genes that differ among inbred strains of mice may also influence the avidity of interactions between T cells and APCs. Induction and level of B7-1 and B7-2 expression may differ on various genetic backgrounds. As will be discussed later, genetic analyses have identified chromosomal regions containing the CD28/CTLA-4 and B7-1/B7-2 loci as important for the development of EAE. Such differences in the B7-CD28/CTLA-4 costimulatory pathway on different genetic backgrounds may contribute to the relative role of B7-1 vs B7-2 or CD28 in the pathogenesis of EAE and human autoimmune diseases.

How may differences in B7-1 and B7-2 costimulation in autoimmune diseases be explained? At least two factors may play critical roles in determining the relative effects of B7-1 vs B7-2 costimulation on the activation of T cells: the strength of signal delivered through the TCR and the activation and/or differentiation state of the T cell during activation. One study has found that human CD4 T cell clones responded to B7-1 and B7-2 costimulation equivalently when activated with their cognate ligand, MBP p85-99 *(153)*. However, when a weak agonist peptide with lower affinity for the TCR was used to activate the T cell clones, B7-1 costimulation clearly provided a more potent costimulatory signal than did B7-2. A similar quantitative difference between B7-1 and B7-2 costimulation was observed when B7-1 or B7-2 cell transfectants were used to stimulate naive CD8 TCR-transgenic T cells *(154)*. However, the responses of primed CD8 TCR-transgenic T cells to costimulation by B7-1 and B7-2 were quantitatively similar.

6.4. Effects of CD28 Manipulation

Recent studies have more specifically assessed the role of CD28 in EAE using anti-CD28 Fabs and CD28$^{-/-}$ mice. Anti-CD28 Fab administered either during priming or later, before disease onset, significantly ameliorated EAE and suppressed TNF-α production by lymph node cells. CD28 blockade during the first disease episode attenuated established EAE and treated mice did not undergo subsequent relapses, suggesting that short-term CD28 blockade may provide a means to ameliorate an established autoimmune response. Whereas MBP TCR^{+} RAG$^{-/-}$ mice spontaneously develop EAE, MBP TCR^{+} RAG$^{-/-}$ CD28$^{-/-}$ mice do not develop EAE, indicating a critical role for CD28 costimulation. MBP TCR^{+} RAG$^{-/-}$ CD28$^{-/-}$ T cells proliferate and produce IL-2 in response to MBP peptide, demonstrating that these T cells are not anergized. The proliferation of encephalitogenic T cells depended on the concentration of MBP peptide, as did the development of MBP-induced EAE in CD28$^{-/-}$ PL/J mice. CD28$^{-/-}$ NOD mice were completely resistant to the induction of EAE with PLP 56-70 *(144)*. CD28$^{-/-}$ C57BL/6 mice do not develop MOG-induced EAE, but develop meningeal inflammation. Taken together, these studies suggest that CD28 is required to lower the threshold for effective TCR activation of autoaggressive CD4^{+} T cells, which trigger the autoimmune response in EAE.

The role of CD28 also has been examined in the NOD diabetes model. NOD mice lacking CD28 exhibited more rapid and increased incidence of diabetes, as compared to littermate controls *(155)*. Exacerbated diabetes was attributed to reduced IL-4 production and Th2 cell functions. Administration of intact anti-CD28 MAb (presumably acting as an agonist) into wild-type NOD mice beginning at 2 wk of age inhibited insulitis and diabetes *(32)* and these striking effects could be reversed by coinjection of anti-CD28 and anti-IL-4 MAb. In contrast, when anti-CD28 was given later, it had no significant effect on diabetes. These studies point to a role for CD28 costimulation early in this autoimmune disease, but it is not yet clear whether CD28 exerts its effects prior to the onset of insulitis and/or following the development of insulitis.

6.5. Effects of CTLA-4 Manipulation

In contrast to CD28, CTLA-4 inhibits T cell activation. The phenotype of the CTLA-4$^{-/-}$ mouse suggested a key role for CTLA-4 in inducing and/or maintaining peripheral tolerance and provided impetus for studying the role of CTLA-4 in autoimmunity and peripheral tolerance. A number of studies have examined whether signaling via CTLA-4 on self antigen-specific T cells is critical for downregulating activated self-reactive T cells. For example, anti-CTLA-4 antibodies can promote expansion of antigen-specific T cells in vivo and exacerbate autoimmune T cell responses. CTLA-4 appears to have an important role in downregulating T cell responses throughout the course of EAE *(156–158)*. Addition of anti-CTLA-4 MAb to in vitro restimulation cultures of primed PLP 139-151-specific T cells potentiated the capacity of these cells to transfer EAE. Anti-CTLA-4 treatment also exacerbated EAE when administered following adoptive transfer of primed T cells. When given at the peak of disease, anti-CTLA-4 blunted disease remission and worsened relapses. Additionally, anti-CTLA-4 led to greater incidence and severity of relapses when administered during the first disease remission. These effects were correlated with elevated production of IFN-γ, TNF-α, and IL-2 *(156–158)*. Similarly, anti-CTLA-4 MAb injection greatly accelerated the onset of diabetes in a TCR transgenic model of diabetes and enhanced its penetrance, but only when given before the onset of insulitis *(159)*. This was not owing to global activation of T lymphocytes, but reflected a markedly more aggressive T cell infiltrate in the pancreatic islets. When administered after the onset of insulitis, anti-CTLA-4 had no detectable effect on the development of diabetes. Thus, CTLA-4 appears to have a key role in the initiation of diabetes. Recent studies also support an important role for B7-CTLA-4 interactions during the induction of anergy. Adoptive transfer of TCR transgenic T cells and administration of anti-CTLA-4 MAbs to mice given antigen by a tolerizing regimen resulted in the development of antigen-reactive T cells and cytokine production, suggesting that tolerance induction may require productive B7-CTLA-4 interactions *(160)*. Whether CTLA-4 signals can be manipulated to induce/ sustain tolerance to self-antigens is an area of active investigation.

6.6. CD40 Blockade

CIA was one of the first model systems in which disruption of costimulatory interactions was shown to have therapeutic value. Durie et al. found that disruption of CD40-CD154 interactions prevented the onset of CIA *(161)*. Treatment of NOD mice with anti-CD154 also prevented insulitis and diabetes if antibody was administered at 3–4 wk of age *(162)*. Cytokine analysis of treated mice revealed a decrease in IL-2 and IFN-γ production without an increase in IL-4. However, if anti-CD154 treatment was started later than 9 wk of age, insulitis and diabetes developed, suggesting a limited period of time when CD40-CD154 are required.

Like the B7/CD28 pathway, the role of CD40-CD154 interactions also has been evaluated in EAE. Initial studies focused on the expression of CD40 and CD154 within the brain of MS patients. Activated T cells expressing CD154 were found in MS brains but not control brains *(97)*. Additionally, these T cells were colocalized with CD40 positive monocytes and microglia cells in active lesions. Gerritse et al. also treated mice with an antibody to CD154, which disrupted the interaction with CD40. Treatment with anti-CD154 either at the time of induction or after initial onset resulted in dramatic disease reduction. Work done by Samoilova et al. demonstrated that anti-CD154 treatment did not cause anergy or deletion of autoreactive T cells, but instead caused a Th2 skewing *(163)*. IFN-γ was markedly suppressed while IL-4 was elevated in anti-CD154 treated mice. However, another study suggests that inhibition of Th1 responses and not Th2 skewing may mediate the beneficial effects of CD40-CD154 blockade. In a model of relapsing EAE, anti-CD154 administration at either the peak of disease or during remission did not affect T cell proliferation, IL-2, IL-4, IL-5, or IL-10 production *(164)*. However, IFN-γ production was dramatically decreased along with peptide specific delayed-type hypersensitivity responses and generation of encephalitogenic effector cells. Adding support to the importance of CD40 for Th1 differentiation in EAE is a study indicating that the protective effects of anti-CD154 blockade can be overcome by coadministration of IL-12 *(165)*.

Similar protective effects were seen with CD40 blockade *(166,167)* and long-term disease inhibition was generated after combined treatment blocking both CD40 and CD28 pathways *(168)* in lupus models. Several studies have investigated the expression of costimulatory molecules in SLE patients and have found elevated levels of CD154 *(169,170)* and dysregulated expression of B7-1 and B7-2 *(171)*.

In summary, many studies indicate the CD40-CD154 and B7-CD28 pathways have a key role in the pathogenesis of autoimmunity and that blockade of these costimulatory interactions has therapeutic potential during the initiation and/or progression of autoimmune disease. B7-CTLA-4 interactions, in contrast play a critical role in preventing the activation of self-reactive T cells and blockade of B7-CTLA-4 interactions can exacerbate autoimmunity. However, the need for B7-CD28 costimulation differs among naive, recently activated, and memory T cells, but CD28 and CTLA-4 appear to have opposing effects on T cells with various activation histories. CD28 lowers the threshold for effective TCR activation, and may enhance lower avidity interactions during autoreactive T cell responses. In contrast, CTLA-4 may increase the threshold for T cell activation and thereby prevent undesired activation by low-strength TCR signals, which may be needed for survival of naive and memory T cells and protect against autoimmune responses.

6.7. Genetics of Autoimmune Disease and Costimulation

Mutations in genes encoding critical immunoregulatory molecules can lead to immunodeficiency or lymphoproliferative syndromes in mice and humans. The importance of the B7-CD28/CTLA-4 pathway for T cell activation, tolerance, and autoimmunity has suggested that dysregulated expression or mutations in the genes encoding ligands and/or receptors could play a significant role in the pathogenesis of human disease. Rodent models for the major human autoimmune diseases are under intense genetic analysis. Genome-wide linkage studies have indicated that in each model, multiple genetic loci are involved. Candidate genes are being identified. Strikingly, in a number of animal models of autoimmune diseases including diabetes, lupus, autoimmune ovarian dysgenesis, and EAE models, there is a linkage to a genetic interval on chromosome 1 that encompasses the CD28/CTLA-4 locus. The significance of this linkage is further highlighted by reports that in human type I diabetes, there is linkage in a syntenic region containing the CD28/CTLA-4 locus *(172,173)*. There are numerous reports of polymorphisms in the CTLA-4 gene in autoimmune diseases including type I diabetes, Grave's disease, Addison's Disease, and MS *(174)*. Further studies are needed to determine if the etiological mutation is within or in close proximity to the CTLA-4 gene and whether these polymorphisms lead to altered expression of genes or altered protein function. The locus encompassing B7-1 and B7-2 also has been identified as an important susceptibility locus. For example, in a genetic analysis of susceptibility to EAE , two of seven loci showing evidence of significant linkage mapped to mouse chromosome 16 ($p < 0.05$), but the two loci with strongest linkage to EAE mapped to other chromosomes *(175)*. Autoimmune ovarian dysgenesis maps to a single major immunoregulatory locus on mouse chromosome 16, but further studies are needed to determine its proximity to the B7 locus on chromosome 16.

7. CONCLUSION

Although there are many factors that regulate the differentiation and response of a naive T cell, one critical interaction is that of costimulatory molecules. Engagement of CD28 on T cells provides key secondary activation signals that can prevent the induction of anergy, upregulate additional costimulatory molecules and cytokine receptors, and promote T cell survival. These same signals enhance the production of cytokines by increasing both transcription and mRNA stability, which can influence T cell differentiation. In contrast to the effects of CD28, CTLA-4 functions to downregulate T cell responses by limiting proliferation and downregulating cytokine receptors. Additionally, recent studies indicate that CTLA-4 has an important role in regulating the differentiation of Th cells because in the absence of CTLA-4, T cells are skewed toward Th2 production. CTLA-4 also may stimulate TGF-β production. Engagement of CD40 on APC parallels the effects of CD28 on T cells. CD40 functions to activate the APC to express B7-1 and B-2, along with upregulating cytokine production and promoting survival. The cytokines produced by the APC act as part of a critical regulatory loop that controls the differentiation of naive T cells. Cytokines can regulate the expression of both costimulatory receptors and ligands. The dramatic effects of disruption of the B7-CD28/CTLA-4 and CD40-CD154 pathways in a number of models of autoimmunity demonstrate the critical role of these pathways in the pathogenesis of autoimmunity. Therefore, these pathways represent important therapeutic targets for controlling human autoimmune diseases. Further studies are needed to learn how to most effectively manipulate these pathways to control autoimmune disease.

REFERENCES

1. Bretscher, P. and Cohn, M. (1970) A theory of self-nonself discrimination. *Science* **169,** 1042–1049.
2. Jenkins, M. K., Pardoll, D. M., Mizuguchi, J., Quill, H., and Schwartz, R. H. (1987) T cell unresponsiveness in vivo and in vitro: fine specificity of induction and molecular characterization of the unresponsive state. *Immunol. Rev.* **95,** 113–135.
3. Bluestone, J. A., Khattri, R., and van Seventer, G. A. (1999) *Accessory Molecules.* Lippincott-Raven, Philadelphia. pp. 449–478.
4. Walunas, T. L., Lenschow, D. J., Bakker, C. Y., Linsley, P. S., Freeman, G. J., Green, J. M., et al. (1994) CTLA-4 can function as a negative regulator of T cell activation. *Immunity* **1,** 405–413.
5. Linsley, P. S., Greene, J. L., Tan, P., Bradshaw, J., Ledbetter, J. A., Anasetti, C., et al. (1992) Coexpression and functional cooperation of CTLA-4 and CD28 on activated T lymphocytes. *J. Exp. Med.* **176,** 1595–1604.
6. Viola, A. and Lanzavecchia, A. (1996) T cell activation determined by T cell receptor number and tunable thresholds. *Science* **273,** 104–106.
7. Tivol, E., Borriello, F., Schweitzer, A., Lynch, W., Bluestone, J., and Sharpe. A. (1995) Loss of CTLA-4 leads to massive lymphoproliferation and fatal multiorgan destruction, revealing a critical negative regulatory role of CTLA-4. *Immunity* **3,** 541–547.
8. Waterhouse, P., Penninger, J., Timms, E., Wakeham, A., Shahinian, A., Lee, K., et al. (1995) Lymphoproliferative disorders with early lethality in mice deficient in CTLA-4. *Science* **270,** 985–988.
9. Chambers, C. A., Cado, D., Truong, T., and Allison, J. P. (1997) Thymocyte development is normal in CTLA-4-deficient mice. *Proc Natl Acad Sci USA* **94,** 9296–9301.
10. Hutloff, A., Dittrich, A. M., Beier, K. C., Eljaschewitsch, Kraft, R., Anagnostopoulos, I., and Kroczek, R. A. (1999) ICOS is an inducible T cell costimulator structurally and functionally related to CD28. *Nature* 397, 263–266.
11. Yoshinaga, S. K., W. J. S., Khare, S. D., Sarmiento, U., Guo, J., Horan, T., et al. (1999) T cell co-stimulation through B7RP-1 and ICOS. *Nature* **402,** 827–832.
12. Linsley, P. S., Clark, E. A., and Ledbetter, J. A. (1990) T cell antigen CD28 mediates adhesion with B cells by interacting with activation antigen B7/BB-1. *Proc. Natl. Acad. Sci. USA* **87,** 5031–5035.
13. Azuma, M., Ito, D., Yagita, H., Okumura, K., Phillips, J. H., Lanier, L. L., and Somoza, C. (1993) B70 antigen is a second ligand for CTLA-4 and CD28. *Nature* **366,** 76–79.
14. Freeman, G. J., Gribben, J. G., Boussiotis, V. A., Ng, J. W., Restivo, V., Lombard, L., et al. (1993) Cloning of B7-2: a CTLA4 counter-receptor that costimulates human T cell proliferation. *Science* **262,** 909–911.
15. June, C. H., Bluestone, J. A., Nadler, L. M., and Thompson, C. B. (1994) The B7 and CD28 receptor families. *Immunol. Today* **15,** 321–331.
16. Tivol, E. A., Schweitzer, A. N., and Sharpe, A. H. (1996) Costimulation and autoimmunity. *Curr. Opin. Immunol.* **8,** 822–830.

17. Boussiotis, V. A., Gribben, J. G., Freeman, G. J., and Nadler, L. M. (1994) Blockade of the CD28 costimulatory pathway: a means to induce tolerance. *Curr. Opin. Immunol.* **6,** 797–807

18. Linsley, P. S., Greene, J. L., Brady, W., Bayorath, J., Ledbetter, J. A., and Peach, R. (1994) Human B7-1 (CD80) and B7-2 (CD86) bind with similar avidities but distinct kinetics to CD28 and CTLA4 receptors. *Immunity* **1,** 793–801.

19. Swallow, M., Wallin, J., and Sha, W. (1999) B7h, a novel costimulatory homolog of B7. 1 and B7. 2, is induced by TNFα. *Immunity* **11,** 423–432.

20. Ling, V., Wu, P. W., Finnerty, H. F., Bean, K. M., Spaulding, V., Fouser, L. A., et al. (2000) Identification of GL50, a novel B7-like protein which functionally binds to ICOS receptor. *J. Immunol.* **164,** 1653–1657.

21. Dong, H., Zhu, G., Tamada, K., and Chen, L. (1999) B7-H1, a third member of the B7 family, co-stimulates T cell proliferation and interleukin-10 secretion. *Nat. Med.* **5,** 1365–1369.

22. Mosmann, T. R. and Sad, S. (1996) The expanding universe of T cell subsets: Th1, Th2 and more [see comments]. *Immunol. Today* **17,** 138–146.

23. Paul, W. (1991) Interleukin 4: a prototypic immunoregulatory lymphokine. *Blood* **77,** 1859.

24. Freeman, G. J., Boussiotis, V. A., Anumanthan, A., Bernstein, G. M., Ke, K.-Y., Rennert, P. D., et al. (1995) B7-1 and B7-2 do not deliver identical costimulatory signals, since B7-2 but not B7-1 preferentially costimulates the initial production of IL-4. *Immunity* **2,** 523–532.

25. Levine, B. L., Ueda, Y., Craighead, N., Huang, M. L., and June, C. H. (1995) CD28 ligands CD80 (B7-1) and CD86 (B7-2) induce long-term autocrine growth of CD4+ T cells and induce similar patterns of cytokine secretion in vitro. *Intl. Immunol.* **7,** 891–904.

26. Natesan, M., Razi-Wolf, Z., and Reiser, H. (1996) Costimulation of IL-4 production by murine B7-1 and B7-2 molecules. *J. Immunol.* **156,** 2783–2791.

27. Ranger, A. M., Prabhu Das, M., Kuchroo, V. K., and Glimcher, L. H. (1996) B7-2 (CD86) is essential for the development of IL-4-producing T cells. *Intl. Immunol.* **8,** 1549–1560.

28. Schweitzer, A. N., Borriello, F., Wong, R. C., Abbas, A. K., and Sharpe, A. H. (1997) Role of costimulators in T cell differentiation: studies using antigen-presenting cells lacking expression of CD80 or CD86. *J. Immunol.* **158,** 2713–2722.

29. Kuchroo, V., Prabhu Das, M., Brown, J. A., Ranger, A. M., Zamvil, S. S., Sobel, R. A., et al. (1995) B7-1 and B7-2 costimulatory molecules differentially activate the Th1/Th2 developmental pathways: application to autoimmune disease therapy. *Cell* **80,** 707–716.

30. Brown, J. A., Titus, R. G., Nabavi, N., and Glimcher, L. H. (1996) Blockade of CD86 ameliorates Leishmania major infection by down-regulating the Th2 response. *J. Infect. Dis.* **174,** 1303–1308.

31. Lenschow, D. J., Ho, S. C., Sattar, H., Rhee, L., Gray, G., Nabavi, N., et al. (1995) Differential effects of anti-B7-1 and anti-B7-2 monoclonal antibody treatment on the development of diabetes in the nonobese diabetic mouse. *J. Exp. Med.* **181,** 1145–1155.

32. Arreaza, G. A., Cameron, M. J., Jaramillo, A., Gill, B. M., Hardy, D., Laupland, K. B., et al. (1997) Neonatal activation of CD28 signaling overcomes T cell anergy and prevents autoimmune diabetes by an IL-4-dependent mechanism. *J. Clin. Invest.* **100,** 2243–2253.

33. Schweitzer, A. N. and Sharpe, A. H. (2000) Mutual regulation between B7-1 (CD80) expressed on T cells and IL-4. *J. Immunol.* **163,** 4819–4825.

34. Windhagen, A., Newcombe, J., Dangond, F., Strand, C., Woodroofe, M. N., Cuzner, M. L., et al. (1995) Expression of costimulatory molecules B7-1 (CD80), B7-2 (CD86), and interleukin 12 cytokine in multiple sclerosis lesions. *J. Exp. Med.* **182,** 1985–1996.

35. Mena, E. and Rohowsky-Kochan, C. (1999) Expression of costimulatory molecules on peripheral blood mononuclear cells in multiple sclerosis. *Acta Neurol. Scand.* **100,** 92–96.

36. De Simone, R., Giampaolo, A., Giometto, B., Gallo, P., Levi, G., Peschle, C., et al. (1995) The costimulatory molecule B7 is expressed on human microglia in culture and in multiple sclerosis acute lesions. *J. Neuropathol. Exp. Neurol.* **54,** 175–187.

37. Lucas, P. J., Negishi, I., Nakayama, K., Fields, L. E., and Loh, D. Y. (1995) Naive CD28-deficient T cells can initiate but not sustain an in vitro antigen-specific Immune response. *J. Immunol.* **154,** 5757–5768.

38. Hsueh, Y. P., Liang, H. E., Ng, S. Y., and Lai, M. Z. (1997) CD28-costimulation activates cyclic AMP-responsive element-binding protein in T lymphocytes. *J. Immunol.* **158,** 85–93.

39. Thompson, C. B., Lindsten, T., Ledbetter, J. A., Kunkel, S. L., Young, H. A., Emerson, S. G., et al. (1989) CD28 activation pathway regulates the production of multiple T cell- derived lymphokines/cytokines. *Proc. Natl. Acad. Sci. USA* **86,** 1333–1337.

40. Lorre, K., Kasran, A., Van Vaeck, F., de Boer, M., and Ceuppens, J. L. (1994) Interleukin-1 and B7/CD28 interaction regulate interleukin-6 production by human T cells. *Clin. Immunol. Immunopathol.* **70,** 81–90.

41. Seder, R. A., Germain, R. N., Linsley, P. S., and Paul, W. E. (1994) CD28-mediated costimulation of interleukin 2 (IL-2) production plays a critical role in T cell priming for IL-4 and interferon gamma production. *J. Exp. Med.* **179,** 299–304.

42. Ward, S. G. (1996) CD28: a signalling perspective. *Biochem. J.* **318,** 361–377.

43. Peng, X., Kasran, A., and Ceuppens, J. L. (1997) Interleukin 12 and B7/CD28 interaction synergistically upregulate interleukin 10 production by human T cells. *Cytokine* 9, 499–506.

44. Fraser, J. D., Irving, B. A., Crabtree, G. R., and Weiss, A. (1991) Regulation of interleukin-2 gene enhancer activity by the T cell accessory molecule CD28. *Science* **251,** 313–316.

45. Lindsten, T., June, C. H., Ledbetter, J. A., Stella, G., and Thompson, C. B. (1989) Regulation of lymphokine messenger RNA stability by a surface-mediated T cell activation pathway. *Science* **244,** 339–343.

46. Ding, L. and Shevach, E. M. (1998) Differential effects of CD28 engagement and IL-12 on T cell activation by altered peptide ligands. *J. Immunol.* **161,** 6614–6621.

47. Rulifson, I. C., Sperling, A. I., Fields, P. E., Fitch, F. W., and Bluestone, J. A. (1997) CD28 costimulation promotes the production of Th2 cytokines. *J. Immunol.* **158,** 658–665.

48. Schweitzer, A. N. and Sharpe, A. H. (1998) Studies using antigen-presenting cells lacking expression of both B7-1 (CD80) and B7-2 (CD86) show distinct requirements for B7 molecules during priming versus restimulation of Th2 but not Th1 cytokine production. *J. Immunol.* **161,** 2762–2771.

49. Ronchese, F., Hausmann, B., Hubele, S., and Lane, P. (1994) Mice transgenic for a soluble form of murine CTLA4 show enhanced expansion of antigen-specific CD4+ T cells and defective antibody production in vivo. *J. Exp. Med.* **179,** 809–817.

50. Brown, D. R., Green, J. M., Moskowitz, N. H., Davis, M., Thompson, C. B., and Reiner, S. L. (1996) Limited role of CD28-mediated signals in T helper subset differentiation. *J. Exp. Med.* **184,** 803–810.

51. Jenkins, M. K., Chen, C. A., Jung, G., Mueller, D. L., and Schwartz, R. H. (1990) Inhibition of antigen-specific proliferation of type 1 murine T cell clones after stimulation with immobilized anti-CD3 monoclonal antibody. *J. Immunol.* **144,** 16–22.

52. McKnight, A. J., Perez, V. L., Shea, C. M., Gray, G. S., and Abbas, A. K. (1994) Costimulator dependence of lymphokine secretion by naive and activated CD4$^+$ T lymphocytes from TCR transgenic mice. *J. Immunol.* **152,** 5220–5225.

53. Perez, V. L., Lederer, J. A., Lichtman, A. H., and Abbas, A. K. (1995) Stability of Th1 and Th2 populations. *Intl. Immunol.* **7,** 869–875.

54. Walunas, T. L., Bakker, C. Y., and Bluestone, J. A. (1996) CTLA-4 ligation blocks CD28-dependent T cell activation. *J. Exp. Med.* **183,** 2541–2550.

55. Krummel, M. and Allison, J. (1995) CD28 and CTLA4 have opposing effects on the response of T cells to stimulation. *J. Exp. Med.* **182,** 459–466.

56. Oosterwegel, M. A., Mandelbrot, D. A., Boyd, S. D., Lorsbach, R. B., Jarrett, D. Y., Abbas, A. K., and Sharpe, A. H. (1999) The role of CTLA-4 in regulating Th2 differentiation. *J. Immunol.* **163,** 2634–2639.

57. Khattri, R., Auger, J. A., Griffin, M. D., Sharpe, A. H., and Bluestone, J. A. (1999) Lymphoproliferative disorder in CTLA-4 knockout mice is characterized by CD28-regulated activation of Th2 responses. *J. Immunol.* **162,** 5784–5791.

58. Walunas, T. L. and Bluestone, J. A. (1998) CTLA-4 regulates tolerance induction and T cell differentiation in vivo. *J. Immunol.* **160,** 3855–3860.

59. Chen, W., Jin, W., and Wahl, S. M. (1998) Engagement of cytotoxic T lymphocyte-associated antigen 4 (CTLA-4) induces transforming growth factor beta (TGF-beta) production by murine CD4(+) T cells. *J. Exp. Med.* **188,** 1849–1857.

60. Van Kooten, C. and Banchereau, J. (1996) CD40-CD40 ligand: a multifunctional receptor-ligand pair. *Adv. Immunol.* **61,** 1–77.

61. Alderson, M. R., Armitage, R. J., Tough, T. W., Strockbine, L., Fanslow, W. C., and Spriggs, M. K. (1993) CD40 expression by human monocytes: regulation by cytokines and activation of monocytes by the ligand for CD40. *J. Exp. Med.* **178,** 669–674.

62. Banchereau, J., Dubois, B., Fayette, J., Burdin, N., Briere, F., Miossec, P., et al. (1995) Functional CD40 antigen on B cells, dendritic cells and fibroblasts. *Adv. Exp. Med. Biol.* **378,** 79–83.

63. Havenith, C. E., Askew, D., and Walker,W. S. (1998) Mouse resident microglia: isolation and characterization of immunoregulatory properties with naive CD4+ and CD8+ T cells. *Glia* **22,** 348–359.

64. Vogel, L. A. and Noelle, R. J. (1998) CD40 and its crucial role as a member of the TNFR family. *Semin. Immunol.* **10,** 435–442.

65. Galy, A. H. and Spits, H. (1992) CD40 is functionally expressed on human thymic epithelial cells. *J. Immunol.* **149,** 775–782.

66. Hollenbaugh, D., Ochs, H. D., Noelle, R. J., Ledbetter, J. A., and Aruffo, A. (1994) The role of CD40 and its ligand in the regulation of the immune response. *Immunol. Rev.* **138,** 23–37.

67. Karmann, K., Hughes, C. C., Schechner, J., Fanslow, W. C., and Pober, J. S. (1995) CD40 on human endothelial cells: inducibility by cytokines and functional regulation of adhesion molecule expression. *Proc. Natl. Acad. Sci. USA* **92,** 4342–4346.

68. Denfeld, R. W., Hollenbaugh, D., Fehrenbach, A., Weiss, J. M., von Leoprechting, A., Mai, B., et al. (1996) CD40 is functionally expressed on human keratinocytes. *Eur. J. Immunol.* **26,** 2329–2334.

69. Mach, F., Schonbeck, U., Sukhova, G. K., Bourcier, T., Bonnefoy, J. Y., Pober, J. S., and Libby, P. (1997) Functional CD40 ligand is expressed on human vascular endothelial cells, smooth muscle cells, and macrophages: implications for CD40-CD40 ligand signaling in atherosclerosis. *Proc. Natl. Acad. Sci. USA* **94,** 1931–1936.

70. Grammer, A. C., McFarland, R. D., Heaney, J., Darnell, B. F., and Lipsky, P. E. (1999) Expression, regulation, and function of B cell-expressed CD154 in germinal centers. *J. Immunol.* **163,** 4150–4159.

71. Roy, M., Waldschmidt, T., Aruffo, A., Ledbetter, J. A., and Noelle, R. J. (1993) The regulation of the expression of gp39, the CD40 ligand, on normal and cloned CD4+ T cells. *J. Immunol.* **151,** 2497–2510.

72. Ramesh, N., Morio, T., Fuleihan, R., Worm, M., Horner, A., Tsitsikov, E., et al. (1995) CD40-CD40 ligand (CD40L) interactions and X-linked hyperIgM syndrome (HIGMX-1). *Clin. Immunol. Immunopathol.* 76, S208–213.

73. Burdin, N., Van Kooten, C., Galibert, L., Abrams, J. S., Wijdenes, J., Banchereau, J., et al. (1995) Endogenous IL-6 and IL-10 contribute to the differentiation of CD40- activated human B lymphocytes. *J. Immunol.* **154,** 2533–2544.

74. Skok, J., Poudrier, J., and Gray, D. (1999) Dendritic cell-derived IL-12 promotes B cell induction of Th2 differentiation: a feedback regulation of Th1 development. *J. Immunol.* **163,** 4284–4291.

75. Jeppson, J. D., Patel, H. R., Sakata, N., Domenico, J., Terada, N., and Gelfand, E. W. (1998) Requirement for dual signals by anti-CD40 and IL-4 for the induction of nuclear factor-kappa B, IL-6, and IgE in human B lymphocytes. *J. Immunol.* **161,** 1738–1742.

76. Schultze, J. L., Michalak, S., Lowne, J., Wong, A., Gilleece, M. H., Gribben, J. G., and Nadler, L. M. (1999) Human non-germinal center B cell interleukin (IL)-12 production is primarily regulated by T cell signals CD40 ligand, interferon gamma, and IL-10: role of B cells in the maintenance of T cell responses. *J. Exp. Med.* **189,** 1–12.

77. Burdin, N., Rousset, F., and Banchereau, J. (1997) B-cell-derived IL-10: production and function. *Methods* 11, 98–111.
78. Kindler, V., Matthes, T., Jeannin, P., and Zubler, R. H. (1995) Interleukin-2 secretion by human B lymphocytes occurs as a late event and requires additional stimulation after CD40 cross-linking. *Eur. J. Immunol.* **25,** 1239–1243.
79. Caux, C., Massacrier, C., Vanbervliet, B., Dubois, B., Van Kooten, C., Durand, I., and Banchereau, J. (1994) Activation of human dendritic cells through CD40 cross-linking. *J. Exp. Med.* **180,** 1263–1272.
80. Kelsall, B. L., Stuber, E., Neurath, M., and Strober, W. (1996) Interleukin-12 production by dendritic cells. The role of CD40-CD40L interactions in Th1 T cell responses. *Ann. NY Acad. Sci.* **795,** 116–126.
81. Koch, F., Stanzl, U., Jennewein, P., Janke, K., Heufler, C., Kampgen, E., et al. (1996) High level IL-12 production by murine dendritic cells: upregulation via MHC class II and CD40 molecules and downregulation by IL-4 and IL-10. *J. Exp. Med.* **184,** 741–746.
82. Kuniyoshi, J. S., Kuniyoshi, C. J., Lim, A. M., Wang, F. Y., Bade, E. R., Lau, R., et al. (1999) Dendritic cell secretion of IL-15 is induced by recombinant huCD40LT and augments the stimulation of antigen-specific cytolytic T cells. *Cell Immunol.* **193,** 48–58.
83. Bartholome, E. J., Willems, F., Crusiaux, A., Thielemans, K., Schandene, L., and Goldman, M. (1999) IFN-beta interferes with the differentiation of dendritic cells from peripheral blood mononuclear cells: selective inhibition of CD40- dependent interleukin-12 secretion. *J. Interferon Cytokine Res.* **19,** 471–478.
84. McRae, B. L., Beilfuss, B. A., and Seventer, G. A. (2000) IFN-beta differentially regulates CD40-induced cytokine secretion by human dendritic cells. *J. Immunol.* **164,** 23–28.
85. Buelens, C., Verhasselt, V., De Groote, D., Thielemans, K., Goldman, M., and Willems, F. (1997) Human dendritic cell responses to lipopolysaccharide and CD40 ligation are differentially regulated by interleukin-10. *Eur. J. Immunol.* **27,** 1848–1852.
86. Fukao, T., Matsuda, S., and Koyasu, S. (2000) Synergistic effects of IL-4 and IL-18 on IL-12-dependent IFN-gamma production by dendritic cells. *J. Immunol.* **164,** 64–71.
87. Wagner, D. H., Jr., Stout, R. D., and Suttles, J. (1994) Role of the CD40-CD40 ligand interaction in CD4+ T cell contact- dependent activation of monocyte interleukin-1 synthesis. *Eur. J. Immunol.* **24,** 3148–3154.
88. Kiener, P. A., Moran-Davis, P., Rankin, B. M., Wahl, A. F., Aruffo, A., and Hollenbaugh, D. (1995) Stimulation of CD40 with purified soluble gp39 induces proinflammatory responses in human monocytes. *J. Immunol.* **155,** 4917–4925.
89. Kato, T., Yamane, H., and Nariuchi, H. (1997) Differential effects of LPS and CD40 ligand stimulations on the induction of IL-12 production by dendritic cells and macrophages. *Cell Immunol.* **181,** 59–67.
90. Tan, J., Town, T., Paris, D., Placzek, A., Parker, T., Crawford, F., et al. (1999) Activation of microglial cells by the CD40 pathway: relevance to multiple sclerosis. *J. Neuroimmunol.* **97,** 77–85.

91. Aloisi, F., Penna, G., Polazzi, E., Minghetti, L., and Adorini, L. (1999) CD40-CD154 interaction and IFN-gamma are required for IL-12 but not prostaglandin E2 secretion by microglia during antigen presentation to Th1 cells. *J. Immunol.* **162,** 1384–1391.

92. Tan, J., Town, T., Saxe, M., Paris, D., Wu, Y., and Mullan, M. (1999) Ligation of microglial CD40 Results in p44/42 mitogen-activated protein kinase-dependent TNF-alpha production that is opposed by TGF-beta1 and IL-10. *J. Immunol.* **163,** 6614–6621.

93. Blotta, M. H., Marshall, J. D., DeKruyff, R. H., and Umetsu, D. T. (1996) Cross-linking of the CD40 ligand on human CD4+ T lymphocytes generates a costimulatory signal that up-regulates IL-4 synthesis. *J. Immunol.* **156,** 3133–3140.

94. Armitage, R. J., Tough, T. W., Macduff, B. M., Fanslow, W. C., Spriggs, M. K., Ramsdell, F., et al. (1993) CD40 ligand is a T cell growth factor. *Eur. J. Immunol.* **23,** 2326–2331.

95. Peng, X., Kasran, A., Warmerdam, P. A., de Boer, M., and Ceuppens, J. L. (1996) Accessory signaling by CD40 for T cell activation: induction of Th1 and Th2 cytokines and synergy with interleukin-12 for interferon-gamma production. *Eur. J. Immunol.* **26,** 1621–1627.

96. Balashov, K. E., Smith, D. R., Khoury, S. J., Hafler, D. A., and Weiner, H. L. (1997) Increased interleukin 12 production in progressive multiple sclerosis: induction by activated CD4+ T cells via CD40 ligand. *Proc. Natl. Acad. Sci. USA* **94,** 599–603.

97. Gerritse, K., Laman, J. D., Noelle, R. J., Aruffo, A., Ledbetter, J. A., Boersma, W. J., et al. (1996) CD40-CD40 ligand interactions in experimental allergic encephalomyelitis and multiple sclerosis. *Proc. Natl. Acad. Sci. USA* **93,** 2499–2504.

98. Miller, S., Vanderlugt, C., Lenschow, D., Pope, J., Karandikar, N., Canto, M. D., and Bluestone, J. (1995) Blockade of CD28-B7-1 interaction prevents epitope spreading and clinical relapses of murine EAE. *Immunity* **3,** 739–745.

99. Issazadeh, S., Navikas, V., Schaub, M., Sayegh, M., and Khoury, S. (1998) Kinetics of expression of costimulatory molecules and their ligands in murine relapsing experimental autoimmune encephalomyelitis in vivo. *J. Immunol.* **161,** 1104–1112.

100. Stack, R. M., Lenschow, D. J., Gray, G. S., Bluestone, J. A., and Fitch, F. W. (1994) IL-4 treatment of small splenic B cells induces costimulatory molecules B7-1 and B7-2. *J. Immunol.* **152,** 5723–5733.

101. Valle, A., Aubry, J. P., Durand, I., and Banchereau, J. (1991) IL-4 and IL-2 upregulate the expression of antigen B7, the B cell counterstructure to T cell CD28: an amplification mechanism for T-B cell interactions. *Intl. Immunol.* **3,** 229–235.

102. Ranheim, E. A. and Kipps, T. J. (1995) Tumor necrosis factor-alpha facilitates induction of CD80 (B7-1) and CD54 on human B cells by activated T cells: complex regulation by IL-4, IL-10, and CD40L. *Cell Immunol.* **161,** 226–235.

103. Ozawa, H., Aiba, Nakagawa, S., and Tagami, H. (1996) Interferon-gamma and interleukin-10 inhibit antigen presentation by Langerhans cells for T helper type 1 cells by suppressing their CD80 (B7-1) expression. *Eur. J. Immunol.* **26,** 648–652.

104. Buelens, C., Willems, F., Delvaux, A., Pierard, G., Delville, J. P., Velu, T., and Goldman, M. (1995) Interleukin-10 differentially regulates B7-1 (CD80) and B7-2 (CD86) expression on human peripheral blood dendritic cells. *Eur. J. Immunol.* **25**, 2668–2672.

105. Mitra, R. S., Judge, T. A., Nestle, F. O., Turka L. A., and Nickoloff, B. J. (1995) Psoriatic skin-derived dendritic cell function is inhibited by exogenous IL-10. Differential modulation of B7-1 (CD80) and B7-2 (CD86) expression. *J. Immunol.* **154**, 2668–2677.

106. Barcy, S., Wettendorff, M., Leo, O., Urbain, J., Kruger, M., Ceuppens, J. L., et al. (1995) FcR cross-linking on monocytes results in impaired T cell stimulatory capacity. *Intl. Immunol.* **7**, 179–189.

107. Creery, W. D., Diaz-Mitoma, F., Filion, L., and Kumar, A. (1996) Differential modulation of B7-1 and B7-2 isoform expression on human monocytes by cytokines which influence the development of T helper cell phenotype. *Eur. J. Immunol.* **26**, 1273–1277.

108. Lenschow, D. J., Walunas, T. L., and Bluestone, J. A. (1996) CD28/B7 system of T cell costimulation. *Ann. Rev. Immunol.* **14**, 233–258.

109. Wei, R. and Jonakait, G. M. (1999) Neurotrophins and the anti-inflammatory agents interleukin-4 (IL-4), IL- 10, IL-11 and transforming growth factor-beta1 (TGF-beta1) down- regulate T cell costimulatory molecules B7 and CD40 on cultured rat microglia. *J. Neuroimmunol.* **95**, 8–18.

110. Pechhold, K., Patterson, N. B., Craighead, N., Lee, K. P., June, C. H., and Harlan, D. M. (1997) Inflammatory cytokines IFN-gamma plus TNF-alpha induce regulated expression of CD80 (B7-1) but not CD86 (B7-2) on murine fibroblasts. *J. Immunol.* **158**, 4921–4929.

111. Gauchat, J. F., Aubry, J. P., Mazzei, G., Life, P., Jomotte, T., Elson, G., et al. (1993) Human CD40-ligand: molecular cloning, cellular distribution and regulation of expression by factors controlling IgE production. *FEBS Lett.* **315**, 259–266.

112. Peng, X., Remacle, J. E., Kasran, A., Huylebroeck, D., and Ceuppens, J. L. (1998) IL-12 up-regulates CD40 ligand (CD154) expression on human T cells. *J. Immunol.* **160**, 1166–1172.

113. Hirohata, S. (1999) Human Th1 responses driven by IL-12 are associated with enhanced expression of CD40 ligand. *Clin. Exp. Immunol.* **115**, 78–85.

114. Shindo, T., Sugie, K. Nakamura,, K., Tagaya, Y., Maeda, M., Uchiyama, T., et al. (1990) Down-regulation of KOLT-2 antigen (CD28) by interleukin 2; role of IL-2R (p70). *Immunology* **71**, 63–69.

115. Alegre, M. L., Noel, P. J., Eisfelder, B. J., Chuang, E.,. Clark, M. R, Reiner, S. L., and Thompson, C. B. (1996) Regulation of surface and intracellular expression of CTLA4 on mouse T cells. *J. Immunol.* **157**, 4762–4770.

116. Gong, J. H., Zhang, M., Modlin, R. L., Linsley, P. S., Iyer, D., Lin, Y., et al. (1996) Interleukin-10 downregulates Mycobacterium tuberculosis-induced Th1 responses and CTLA-4 expression. *Infect. Immun.* **64**, 913–918.

117. Stamenkovic, I., Clark, E. A., and Seed, B. (1989) A B-lymphocyte activation molecule related to the nerve growth factor receptor and induced by cytokines in carcinomas. *EMBO J.* **8**, 1403–1410.

118. Bjorck, P., Axelsson, B., and Paulie, S. (1991) Expression of CD40 and CD43 during activation of human B lymphocytes. *Scand. J. Immunol.* **33,** 211–218.
119. Nguyen, V. T., Walker, W. S., and Benveniste, E. N. (1998) Post-transcriptional inhibition of CD40 gene expression in microglia by transforming growth factor-beta. *Eur. J. Immunol.* **28,** 2537–2548.
120. Ranheim, E. A. and Kipps, T. J. (1993) Activated T cells induce expression of B7/BB1 on normal or leukemic B cells through a CD40-dependent signal. *J. Exp. Med.* **177,** 925–935.
121. Yellin, M. J., Sinning, J., Covey, L. R., Sherman, W., Lee, J. J., Glickman-Nir, E., et al. (1994) T lymphocyte T cell-B cell-activating molecule/CD40-L molecules induce normal B cells or chronic lymphocytic leukemia B cells to express CD80 (B7/BB-1) and enhance their costimulatory activity. *J. Immunol.* **153,** 666–674.
122. Roy, M., Aruffo, A., Ledbetter, J., Linsley, P., Kehry, M., and Noelle, R. (1995) Studies on the interdependence of gp39 and B7 expression and function during antigen-specific immune responses. *Eur. J. Immunol.* **25,** 596–603.
123. Jaiswal, A. I., Dubey, C., Swain, S. L., and Croft, M. (1996) Regulation of CD40 ligand expression on naive CD4 T cells: a role for TCR but not co-stimulatory signals. *Intl. Immunol.* **8,** 275–285.
124. Ding, L., Green, J. M., Thompson, C. B., and Shevach, E. M. (1995) B7/CD28-dependent and -independent induction of CD40 ligand expression. *J. Immunol.* **155,** 5124–5132.
125. de Boer, M., Kasran, A., Kwekkeboom, J., Walter, H., Vandenberghe, P., and Ceuppens, J. L. (1993) Ligation of B7 with CD28/CTLA-4 on T cells results in CD40 ligand expression, interleukin-4 secretion and efficient help for antibody production by B cells. *Eur. J. Immunol.* **23,** 3120–3125.
126. Yin, D., Zhang, L., Wang, R., Radvanyi, L., Haudenschild, C., Fang, Q., et al. (1999) Ligation of CD28 in vivo induces CD40 ligand expression and promotes B cell survival. *J. Immunol.* **163,** 4328–4334.
127. Schaub, M., Issazadeh, S., Stadlbauer, T. H., Peach, R., Sayegh, M. H., and Khoury, S. J. (1999) Costimulatory signal blockade in murine relapsing experimental autoimmune encephalomyelitis. *J. Neuroimmunol.* **96,** 158–166.
128. Larsen, C. P., Elwood, E. T., Alexander, D. Z., Ritchie, S. C., Hendrix, R., Tucker-Burden, C., et al. (1996) Long-term acceptance of skin and cardiac allografts after blocking CD40 and CD28 pathways. *Nature* **381,** 434–438.
129. Grewal, I. S., Foellmer, H. G., Grewal, K. D., Xu, J., Hardardottir, F., Baron, J. L., et al. (1996). Requirement for CD40 ligand in costimulation induction, T cell activation, and experimental allergic encephalomyelitis. *Science* **273,** 1864–1867.
130. Cerdan, C., Martin, Y., Courcoul, M., Mawas, C., Birg, F., and Olive, D. (1995) CD28 costimulation regulates long-term expression of the three genes (alpha, beta, gamma) encoding the high-affinity IL2 receptor. *Res. Immunol.* **146,** 164–168.
131. Cerdan, C., Martin, Y., Courcoul, M., Mawas, C., Birg, F., and Olive, D. (1995) CD28 costimulation up-regulates long-term IL-2R beta expression in human T cells through combined transcriptional and post-transcriptional regulation. *J. Immunol.* **154,** 1007–1013.

132. Wu, C., Warrier, R. R., Wang, X., Presky, D. H., and Gately, M. K. (1997) Regulation of interleukin-12 receptor beta1 chain expression and interleukin-12 binding by human peripheral blood mononuclear cells. *Eur. J. Immunol.* **27,** 147–154.
133. Chang, J. T., Segal, B. M., and Shevach, E. M. (2000) Role of costimulation in the induction of the IL-12/IL-12 receptor pathway and the development of autoimmunity. *J. Immunol.* **164,** 100–106.
134. Bluestone, J. A. (1997) Is CTLA-4 a master switch for peripheral T cell tolerance? *J. Immunol.* **158,** 1989–1993.
135. Finck, B., Linsley, P., and Wofsy, D. (1994) Treatment of murine lupus with CTLA4Ig. *Science* **265,** 1225–1227.
136. Knoerzer, D. B., Karr, R. W., Schwartz, B. D., and Mengle-Gaw, L. J. (1995) Collagen-induced arthritis in the BB rat. Prevention of disease by treatment with CTLA-4-Ig. *J. Clin. Invest.* **96,** 987–993.
137. Cross, A. H., Girard, T. J., Giacoletto, K. S., Evans, R. J., Keeling, R. M., Lin, R. F., Trotter, J. L., and Karr, R. W. (1995) Long-term inhibition of murine experimental autoimmune encephalomyelitis using CTLA-4-Fc supports a key role for CD28 costimulation [see comments]. *J. Clin. Invest.* **95,** 2783–2789.
138. Khoury, S., Akalin, E., Chandraker, A., Turka, L., Linsely, P., Sayegh, M., and Hancock, W. (1995) CD28-B7 costimulatory blockade by CTLA4Ig prevents actively induced experimental autoimmune encephalomyelitis and inhibits Th1 but spares Th2 cytokines in the central nervous system. *J. Immunol.* **155,** 4521–4524.
139. Perrin, P. J., Scott, D., Quigley, L., Albert, P. S., Feder, O., Gray, G. S., et al. (1995) Role of B7/CD28 CTLA-4 in the induction of chronic relapsing experimental allergic encephalomyelitis. *J. Immunol.* **154,** 1481–1490.
140. Arima, T., Rehman, A., Hickey, W. F., and Flye, M. W. (1996) Inhibition by CTLA4Ig of experimental allergic encephalomyelitis. *J. Immunol.* **156,** 4916–4924.
141. Gallon, L., Chandraker, A., Issazadeh, S., Peach, R., Linsley, P. S., Turka, L. A., et al. (1997) Differential effects of B7-1 blockade in the rat experimental autoimmune encephalomyelitis model. *J. Immunol.* **159,** 4212–4216.
142. Croxford, J. L., O'Neill, J. K., Ali, R. R., Browne, K., Byrnes, A. P., Dallman, M. J., et al. (1998) Local gene therapy with CTLA4-immunoglobulin fusion protein in experimental allergic encephalomyelitis. *Eur. J. Immunol.* **28,** 3904–3916.
143. Chang, T. C., Jabs, C., Sobel, R. A., Kuchroo, V. K., and Sharpe, A. H. (1999) Studies in B7-deficient mice reveal a critical role for B7 costimulation in both the initiation and effector phases of. *J. Exp. Med.* **190,** 733–740.
144. Girvin, A. M., Dal Canto, M. C., Rhee, L., Salomon, B., Sharpe, A., Bluestone, J. A., et al. (2000) A critical role for B7/CD28 costimulation in experimental autoimmune encephalomyelitis: a comparative study using costimulatory molecule- deficient mice and monoclonal antibody blockade. *J. Immunol.* **164,** 136–143.
145. Webb, L. M., Walmsley, M. J., and Feldmann, M. (1996) Prevention and amelioration of collagen-induced arthritis by blockade of the CD28 co-stimulatory pathway: requirement for both B7-1 and B7-2. *Eur. J. Immunol.* **26,** 2320–2328.

146. Windhagen, A., Newcombe, J., Dangond, F., Strand, C., Woodroofe, M., Cuzner, M., et al. (1995) Expression of costimulatory molecules B7-1 (CD80), B7-2 (CD86), and interleukin 12 in multiple sclerosis lesions. *J. Exp. Med.* **182,** 1985–1996.

147. Williams, K. C., Ulvestad, E., and Hickey, W. F. (1994) Immunology of multiple sclerosis. *Clin. Neurosci.* **2,** 229–245.

148. Genc, K., Dona, D. L., and Reder, A. T. (1997) Increased CD80(+) B cells in active multiple sclerosis and reversal by interferon beta-1b therapy. *J. Clin. Invest.* **99,** 2664–2671.

149. Kuchroo, V. K., Das, M. P., Brown, J. A., Ranger, A. M., Zamvil, S. S., Sobel, R. A., et al. (1995) B7-1 and B7-2 costimulatory molecules activate differentially the Th1/Th2 developmental pathways: application to autoimmune disease therapy. *Cell* **80,** 707–718.

150. Racke, M., Scott, D., Quigley, L., Gray, G., Abe, R., June, C., et al. (1995) Distinct roles of B7-1 (CD-80) and B7-2 (CD-86) in the initiation of Experimental Allergic Encephalomyelitis. *J. Clin. Invest.* **96,** 2195–2203.

151. Vanderlugt, C. L., Karandikar, N. J., Lenschow, D. J., Dal Canto, M. C., Bluestone, J. A., and Miller, S. D. (1997) Treatment with intact anti-B7-1 mAb during disease remission enhances epitope spreading and exacerbates relapses in R-EAE. *J. Neuroimmunol.* **79,** 113–118.

152. Karandikar, N. J., Vanderlugt, C. L., Eagar, T., Tan, L., Bluestone, J. A., and Miller, S. D. (1998) Tissue-specific up-regulation of B7-1 expression and function during the course of murine relapsing experimental autoimmune encephalomyelitis. *J. Immunol.* **161,** 192–199.

153. Anderson, D. E., Ausubel, L. J., Krieger, J., Hollsberg, P., Freeman, G. J., and Hafler, D. A. (1997) Weak peptide agonists reveal functional differences in B7-1 and B7-2 costimulation of human T cell clones. *J. Immunol.* **159,** 1669–1675.

154. Fields, P. E., Finch, R. J., Gray, G. S., Zollner, R., Thomas, J. L., Sturmhoefel, K., et al. (1998) B7. 1 is a quantitatively stronger costimulus than B7. 2 in the activation of naive CD8+ TCR-transgenic T cells. *J. Immunol.* **161,** 5268–5275.

155. Lenschow, D., Herold, K., Ree, L., Patel, B., Koons, A., Singh, B., et al. (1996) CD28/B7 regualtion of Th1 and Th2 subsets in the development of autoimmune diabetes. *Immunity* **5,** 285–293.

156. Perrin, P. J., Maldonado, J. H., Davis, T. A., June, C. H., and Racke, M. K. (1996) CTLA-4 blockade enhances clinical disease and cytokine production during experimental allergic encephalomyelitis. *J. Immunol.* **157,** 1333–1336.

157. Karandikar, N., Vanderlugt, C., Walnus, T., Miller, S., and Bluestone, J. (1996) CTLA-4-a negative regulator of autoimmune disease. *J. Exp. Med.* **184,** 783–788.

158. Hurwitz, A. A., Sullivan, T. J., Krummel, M. F., Sobel, R. A., and Allison, J. P. (1997) Specific blockade of CTLA-4/B7 interactions results in exacerbated clinical and histologic disease in an actively-induced model of experimental allergic encephalomyelitis. *J. Neuroimmunol.* **73,** 57–62.

159. Luhder, F., Hoglund, P., Allison, J. P., Benoist, C., and Mathis, D. (1998) Cytotoxic T lymphocyte-associated antigen 4 (CTLA-4) regulates the unfolding of autoimmune diabetes. *J. Exp. Med.* **187,** 427–432.

160. Perez, V., Vanparijis, L., Biuckians, A., Zheng, X., Strom, T., and Abbas, A. (1997) Induction of peripheral T cell tolerance in vivo requires CTLA-4 engagement. *Immunity* **6,** 411–417.

161. Durie, F. H., Fava, R. A., Foy, T. M., Aruffo, A., Ledbetter, J. A., and Noelle, R. J. (1993) Prevention of Collagen-Induced Arthritis with an Antibody to gp39, the Ligand for CD40. *Science* **261,** 1328–1330.

162. Balasa, B., Krahl, T., Patstone, G., Lee, J., Tisch, R., McDevitt, H. O., et al. (1997) CD40 ligand-CD40 interactions are necessary for the initiation of insulitis and diabetes in nonobese diabetic mice. *J. Immunol.* **159,** 4620–4627.

163. Samoilova, E. B., Horton, J. L., Zhang, H., and Chen, Y. (1997) CD40L blockade prevents autoimmune encephalomyelitis and hampers TH1 but not TH2 pathway of T cell differentiation. *J. Mol. Med.* **75,** 603–608.

164. Howard, L. M., Miga, A. J., Vanderlugt, C. L., Dal Canto, M. C., Laman, J. D., Noelle, R. J., et al. (1999) Mechanisms of immunotherapeutic intervention by anti-CD40L (CD154) antibody in an animal model of multiple sclerosis. *J. Clin. Invest.* **103,** 281–290.

165. Constantinescu, C. S., Hilliard, B., Wysocka, M., Ventura, E. S., Bhopale, M. K., Trinchieri, G., and Rostami, A. M. (1999) IL-12 reverses the suppressive effect of the CD40 ligand blockade on experimental autoimmune encephalomyelitis (EAE). *J. Neurol. Sci.* **171,** 60–64.

166. Mohan, C., Shi, Y., Laman, J. D., and Datta, S. K. (1995) Interaction between CD40 and its ligand gp39 in the development of murine lupus nephritis. *J. Immunol.* **154,** 1470–1480.

167. Early, G. S., Zhao, W., and Burns, C. M. (1996) Anti-CD40 ligand antibody treatment prevents the development of lupus- like nephritis in a subset of New Zealand black x New Zealand white mice. Response correlates with the absence of an anti-antibody response. *J. Immunol.* **157,** 3159–3164.

168. Daikh, D. I., Finck, B. K., Linsley, P. S., Hollenbaugh, D., and Wofsy, D. (1997) Long-term inhibition of murine lupus by brief simultaneous blockade of the B7/CD28 and CD40/gp39 costimulation pathways. *J. Immunol.* **159,** 3104–3108.

169. Koshy, M., Berger, D., and Crow, M. K. (1996) Increased expression of CD40 ligand on systemic lupus erythematosus lymphocytes. *J. Clin. Invest.* **98,** 826–837.

170. Devi, B. S., Van Noordin, S., Krausz, T., and Davies, K. A. (1998) Peripheral blood lymphocytes in SLE—hyperexpression of CD154 on T and B lymphocytes and increased number of double negative T cells. *J. Autoimmun.* **11,** 471–475.

171. Takasaki, Y., Abe, K., Tokano, Y., and Hashimoto, H. (1999) The expression of LFA-1, ICAM-1, CD80 and CD86 molecules in lupus patients: implication for immunotherapy. *Intern. Med.* **38,** 175–177.

172. Nistico, L., Buzzetti, R., Pritchard, L. E., Van der Auwera, B., Giovannini, C., Bosi, E., et al. (1996) The CTLA-4 gene region of chromosome 2q33 is linked to, and associated with, type 1 diabetes. Belgian Diabetes Registry. *Human Mol. Genet.* **5,** 1075–1080.

173. Donner, H., Braun, J., Seidl, C., Rau, H., Finke, R., Ventz, M., et al. (1997) Codon 17 polymorphism of the cytotoxic T lymphocyte antigen 4 gene in Hashimoto's thyroiditis and Addison's disease. *J. Clin. Endocrinol. Metab.* **82,** 4130–4132.
174. Harbo, H. F., Celius, E. G., Vartdal, F., and Spurkland, A. (1999) CTLA4 promoter and exon 1 dimorphisms in multiple sclerosis. *Tissue Antigens* **53,** 106–110.
175. Encinas, J. A., Lees, M. B., Sobel, R. A., Symonowicz, C., Greer, J. M., Shovlin, C. L., et al. (1996) Genetic analysis of susceptibility to experimental autoimmune encephalomyelitis in a cross between SJL/J and B10. S mice. *J. Immunol.* **157,** 2186–2192.

5

CD1d-Restricted NK T Cells and Autoimmunity

Mark Exley and S. Brian Wilson

1. INTRODUCTION

Autoimmune diseases are disorders of complex etiology, involving environmental triggers interacting with a polygenic susceptibility background. Genetic studies demonstrate that a combinatorial admixture of susceptibility and protective genes influences development of disease *(1)*. Longitudinal studies on twins or large cohorts of at-risk individuals indicate that many high-risk subjects do not develop overt disease *(2,3)*. In fact, once the nefarious event initiating these disorders occurs, the subsequent autoimmune diseases are typically characterized by a chronic smoldering inflammation. This is in marked contrast to the tempo of most host-immune responses to infectious agents. Although epigenetic events may explain incomplete penetrance of genetic risk, it is less clear why autoreactive T cells and antibodies are often detectable in the circulation of at-risk relatives as well as in healthy human leukocyte antigen (HLA)-matched controls that never go on to develop disease *(4)*. The same is true in animal models of autoimmunity, where a significant fraction of the animals in a homogeneous colony remain disease-free despite prominent evidence of autorecognition *(5–7)*. These observations suggest that the presence of autoreactive T cells and antibodies are not sufficient to confer disease but that additional immune abnormalities must occur to result in disease.

The definition of a spectrum of Th phenotypes, with extremes of T helper 1 (Th1) and Th2 subsets of CD4$^+$ T cells has provided a framework to explain the cellular basis for the diversity of T and B cell responses seen in normal immune responses and autoimmunity *(8)*. For example, Type 1 diabetes is T cell-mediated disorder with a strong and requisite Th1 bias *(9–11)*. Th1 cells are biased toward secretion of interferon-γ (IFN-γ), tumor necrosis factor-β (TNF-β), and interleukin-2 (IL-2) and promote inflammatory cellular

From: *Cytokines and Autoimmune Diseases*
Edited by: V. K. Kuchroo, et al. © Humana Press Inc., Totowa, NJ

immune responses *(12,13)*. Th2 cells are biased toward secretion of IL-4, IL-5, IL-6, IL-10, and IL-13, induce strong humoral immunity dominated by distinct antibody isotypes, and reciprocally inhibit Th1 responses. The cellular mechanisms integrating the drive to Th1 or Th2 effector-cell differentiation are poorly understood.

Over the past 10 years, several studies identified a unique family of CD1d-reactive T cells with many of the functional characteristics expected of a regulatory cell important for integrating Th-balance and peripheral tolerance *(14)*. The original subset of CD1d-reactive T cells were historically called natural killer (NK) T cells because they were found to express cell surface markers for both αβTCR+ T cells and NK cells *(15)*. Although the role of CD1d-reactive T cells in the immune system is not yet fully understood, it is now clear that their dysfunction correlates with the pathogenesis of T cell-mediated autoimmune diseases *(16–20)*. This chapter will discuss mechanisms of CD1d-reactive T cell function and the relationship of this lineage to the development of disease.

2. CELL SURFACE PHENOTYPE AND TISSUE DISTRIBUTION OF CD1d-RESTRICTED T CELLS

2.1. CD1d-Restricted T Cell Receptor Repertoire

CD1d-restricted T cells are a family of T cells originally identified through the convergence of many lines of investigation associating canonical T cell receptor (TCR) rearrangements with a regulatory function. Taniguchi and associates reported the first hint of this function. When these investigators sequenced the TCRs of several hybridoma clones made from KLH-specific suppressor cells, the presence of an invariant TCR-α chain (TCRAV14) was noted *(21)*. The sequence detected had a TCR-α chain rearrangement where AV14-AJ281 recombination occurred in the germline configuration. This means that there were no N/P additions found at the V-J junction, whereas random additions are a characteristic feature of most TCR rearrangements. The same workers went on to demonstrate that the invariant rearrangement was present at a relatively high frequency, 0.5–1% in the thymus and spleen, respectively. In later work, the thymus was noted to have a similar population of mature thymocytes that did not express CD4 or CD8, i.e., double-negative (DN) T cells. The invariant Vα14Jα281+ population was found to preferentially express TCR Vβ8 chains and the NK marker CD161 *(14,22)*. The TCR β chains pairing with the invariant Vα14Jα281 α chains were, in decreasing order of frequency, Vβ8.2, Vαβ7, Vβ8.3, Vβ2, and Vβ8.1.

In a seminal series of experiments, Bendelac and coworkers noted that thymic and other CD4$^+$, CD161$^+$ T cells were able to secrete burst amounts of IL-4, as well as IFN-γ in response to mitogen stimulation in vivo without requiring prior IL-4 priming *(15,23,24)*. This is in marked contrast to the majority of naive peripheral T cells, which require IL-4 priming to acquire the capacity to secrete this cytokine. The capacity of unprimed IL-4 secretion made NK T cells a candidate source for early IL-4 required for the initiation of Th2 responses. Furthermore, unlike most CD4$^+$ and CD8$^+$ $\alpha\beta$TCR$^+$ T cells, which recognize major histocompatibility complex (MHC) class II and class I proteins, respectively, invariant Vα14Jα281 and other NK T cells are restricted by the nonpolymorphic MHC Class Ib molecule, CD1d. The development of these T cells was subsequently definitively shown to be dependent on expression of CD1d by the observation that they did not develop in mice with targeted gene disruptions of the CD1 locus *(25,26)*.

In parallel studies, it was noted that humans had a strikingly homologous Vα24JαQ invariant rearrangement whose frequency was also enriched in the CD4/CD8 DN compartment *(27)*. The murine and human α-chain sequences are highly conserved. Through the coding region of the CDR3 loop, the two TCR α-chains share 90% amino acid identity and the two amino acids that differ are conservative substitutions *(28)*. Consistent with the hypothesis of conserved function suggested by the high degree of sequence homology, murine CD1d-restricted NK T cell clones are cross-restricted with human CD1d and human Vα24JαQ clones can recognize murine CD1d *(29)*. The Vα24JαQ TCR also pairs with a restricted set of TCR β chains, with Vβ11 (the human homolog of Vβ8), Vβ13, Vβ8, Vβ9, and Vβ6 found in decreasing order of prevalence *(30,31)*.

The invariant TCR α-chain was for many years considered a hallmark feature of NK T cells. For human Vα24JαQ$^+$ T cells the requirement for an invariant rearrangement is not absolute. Both asp and thr were found as naturally occuring functional substitutions for the ser residue encoded as the terminal amino acid of AV24 exon *(32)*. Subsequent experiments done in mice defined other noninvariant clones and hybridomas, both with and without the CD161 marker, that are restricted by CD1d *(33–36)*. Despite the use of other noninvariant Vα chains in these murine clones, Vβ8 was still the preferential TCR β-chain partner *(33)*. Both human and murine peripheral NK T cells were reported to have a nominal three to five amino acid motif in the CDR3 loop of the TCR β chain *(33,37)*. In contrast, most of the CD1d-restricted T cells in the bone marrow of mice are not invariant, and they seem to preferentially use Vβ2 TCR chains *(38)*. While in human bone marrow, invariant Vα24JαQ T cells are detectable, a much larger set of random rearrangements is found *(39)*. In summary, the cross-species conservation of CD1d function and the significant homology of invariant TCR sequences strongly suggests that a restricted set of antigens/ligands is presented by CD1d *(40,41)*.

2.2. Surface Phenotype of CD1d-Restricted T Cells

Several cell-surface proteins or combinations of markers have been used to define the CD1d-restricted T cell population. To date, no single set of markers definitively identifies this subset of T cells. For example, the combination of Vα24 with Vβ11 is markedly enriched for CD1d reactive T cells in humans *(30)*. However, the use of this TCR pair to define CD1d-restricted T cells would exclude from analysis the large family of CD1d-restricted T cells that use other TCR α and/or β chains such as the bone-marrow population, and would include irrelevant Vα24[+] Vβ11[+] T cells using other J elements. Moreover, reports of function based solely on surface phenotyping should be interpreted with caution. Total NK T cell frequency can expand or remain stable while the invariant T cells are specifically lost during the development of disease *(19,42,43)*. In addition, many CD1a-c restricted lines and clones from human donors are CD161[+] *(40,44,45)*. For these and other reasons, it is best to functionally define "these" cells as CD1d-restricted, as opposed to the more general term of NK T cell.

Other than the TCR, the *sine qua non* of cell-surface proteins originally used to identify NK T cells was CD161 *(15)*. Prior to its CD designation, this protein was known as NKR-P1A in humans, the only known human homolog to the murine NKR-P1A-C proteins. In the mouse, the NK 1.1 allele refers to a form of the NKR-P1C protein recognized by monoclonal antibody (MAb) PK136 *(46)*. This allele is expressed in C57BL, FVB/N, NZB, and SJL strains of mice.

CD161 is a C-type lectin encoded in the NK locus. This protein is also expressed by NK cells and up to 10% of T cells. In the mouse, many T cells expressing CD161 do not recognize CD1d, as significant populations of CD161[+] T cells remain after targeted deletion of the CD1 locus, whereas there is no residual CD1d reactivity in these knockout mice *(25,26,35,41)*. Moreover, there are substantial numbers of CD1d-restricted T cells that are CD161[-]. The cognate ligand for CD161 on APC and the function of this protein remain to be defined. Murine NK T cells apparently secreted IFN-γ directly in response to ligation of CD161 by MAbs *(47)*. CD161 functions as a coactivator for CD1d recognition by human invariant clones and ligation of this molecule alone does not activate IFN-γ secretion *(48)*. An explanation for the discrepancy may be species-specific association of CD161 with lck. Rodent CD161 constitutively associates with lck whereas the human does not *(48,49)*.

In rodents, other surface markers have been identified on CD1d-restricted T cells, which vary according to the strain used. In thymic NK T cells from C57Bl/6 mice, ratios of 3:2 CD4$^+$ to CD4$^-$, and 4:1 NK lectins Ly49C$^+$ and Ly49A$^+$, respectively were found *(14)*. The cells are also Thy1^{hi}, CD5^{hi}, CD44^{hi}, CD45RB^{hi}, CD161^{int} (NK1.1), CD122^{int}(IL2Rb), CD69^{int}, CD16^{lo}, HAS$^-$, and CD62L$^-$ *(14)*. In the NOD mouse, a murine model for Type 1 diabetes, NK T cells were enriched for by sorting TCR$^+$, CD4/CD8$^-$ (DN) thymocytes, or CD3$^+$, CD112$^+$, Ly49A$^+$ cells from spleen *(16,17)*. Rats also have a subset of αβTCR$^+$ cells that express CD161 *(50)*. Unlike the mouse, this group of cells is largely CD8$^+$. In addition, many of these cells express RT6, and it this subset that is present in markedly reduced frequency in the diabetes-prone BB rat *(50,51)*.

The surface phenotyping of CD1d-restricted T cells in humans has been done using invariant CD1d-restricted clones *(19,45,52)*. Individual donors vary considerably in the frequency CD4$^+$ to CD4$^-$ CD1d-restricted T cells. Human clones derived from peripheral blood have all been CD69$^+$, CD161^{var}, CD94^{var}, CD16$^-$, CD57$^-$, and CD158$^-$ (Ig-domain NK cell killer inhibitory receptors, KIRs) *(19,32,45)*. The CD8 molecule appears to have activation-dependent expression with upregulation of only the CD8αα isoform after stimulation *(19,32)*. There is some uncertainty about CD56 expression *(53)*. Ex vivo, at least some invariant clones expressed CD56 that may be lost in culture *(54,55)*. Another large set of clones derived from peripheral blood of multiple donors were all CD56$^-$, suggesting the possibility of donor variability or differential regulation of cell-surface markers in vivo compared to in vitro *(19,32,45)*. Vα24JαQ lines and clones derived from liver biopsies variably expressed CD56$^+$ *(53)*. The CD56 marker was associated with enhanced cytolytic activity. Recently we have developed a MAb, 6B11, specific for the invariant CDR3 loop of the AV24AJ18 rearrangement. In the peripheral blood of healthy donors, the cell population that was both Vb11$^+$ and 6B11$^+$ were found to be 60–70% CD161$^+$, 20–30% CD56$^+$, 60–80% CD8αα$^+$, 20–60% CD4$^+$, and <5% CD158$^+$. In contrast, the bone marrow contains a high percentage of CD161+ CD1d-restricted T cells, which do not use the invariant Vα24JαQ TCR α chain *(39)*. Therefore, CD1d-restricted T cells includes invariant "NK T cells" and other more heterogeneous and ill-defined populations.

2.3. Tissue Distribution of CD1d-Restricted T Cells

CD1d-restricted T cells can be detected in most sites where T cells are found, but show preferential enrichment in certain tissues. They account for 10–30% of liver and bone-marrow T cells, 10–20% of mature thymocytes, and 0.5–1% of splenocytes *(14,56)*. In the gut, the lamina propia appears to be enriched for these cells, whereas they are excluded from the intra-epithelial lymphocyte (IEL) fraction *(57)*. The frequency of CD1d-restricted T cells in peripheral lymph nodes is quite variable. It is unclear at this time whether there is specific tissue recruitment during an inflammatory response. Conversely, there is only minimal published data on total NK T cell frequency indicating specific loss at sites of autoimmune destruction. We have found that the invariant $V\alpha14J\alpha281$ population is specifically lost from the Islets of NOD (diabetes-prone) during the transition to the destructive phase of insulitis.

In general, the tissue distribution of invariant CD1d-restricted cells appears to parallel antigen-presenting cells (APC) expressing CD1d, but comprehensive histologic analysis of the cellular architecture in different species is lacking. A limited number of histologic studies in the mouse suggest that CD1d-restricted T cells segregate to areas of immunologic interest *(58)*. In the MHC class II null mouse, where NK T cells make up 30% of CD4$^+$ T cells (notably not all NK T cells were CD1d-reactive), they were found clustered in B cell follicles and in the marginal zone of the spleen *(59–61)*. Moreover, during the development of anterior-chamber immune deviation (ACAID), which requires CD1d-reactive T cells, TCR$^+$, CD161$^+$ T cells were found in apposition to the F4/80$^+$ APC *(62)*. These clusters were located in marginal zone of the spleen and not in B cell follicles. The data suggests that these cells segregate to areas of intense sampling of antigen and apoptotic cells (e.g., thymus and gut) by APCs.

3. CD1d RECOGNITION AND LIPID LIGAND RECOGNITION

3.1. CD1 Expression

Five nonpolymorphic genes on chromosome 1 encode the human CD1 family. The intron-exon structures are similar to those for MHC class I genes from the MHC locus on chromosome 6. The encoded proteins have homology to both MHC class I and Class II proteins. Of the five genes, only CD1 a-d have been shown to be expressed as proteins. Calabi and Milstein designated the CD1a-c genes as group I, and CD1d (and e) as group II on the basis of sequence homology *(63)*. Rats and mice appear to have lost the group I genes and mice have a duplication of the CD1d locus giving the *CD1D1* and *CD1D2* genes *(14,40)*. In the C57/BL6 background there is a nonsense mutation in the *CD1D2* coding sequence that ablates expression. This point mutation is not present in BALB/c, AKR, NOD, or 129 strains of mice *(14)*. The group I proteins, CD1a-c, appear to function by sampling various intracellular compartments for presenting microbial glycolipid antigens to cytotoxic T lymphocyte (CTL) *(40,64,65)*. Current evidence suggests that CD1d-based activation primarily subserves an immunoregulatory function, although this axis may also be involved in the presentation of lipid antigens after infection by malarial or trypanasomal parasites *(66)*.

Many predictions based on sequence- and antigen-recognition studies were verified with the solution of the crystal structure of murine CD1d. CD1d forms a complex with β2 microglobulin and the overall architecture of the protein is strikingly similar to MHC Class I, although the nature of the antigen-binding groove is quite distinct *(67)*. The groove is narrower, deeper, and is very hydrophobic. In addition, both ends of the antigen-binding groove appear to be roofed over leaving a smaller central opening to two large hydrophobic "pockets," termed A' and F', respectively. Although the exact structure of the antigen could not be determined, the electron-density pattern of bound ligand was that of an unbranched chain. This structure is incompatible with the presence of a peptide. Confirmation that CD1d presents lipid was verified by: (1) the identification of α-galactosylceramide (α-GalCer) purified from marine sponges as a potent agonist for both murine Vα14Jα281 and human Vα24JαQ invariant T cells *(68–70)*; (2) elution of glycophosphatidylinositol from purified CD1d1 (which was not an activating ligand) *(71)*; and (3) direct demonstration that CD1d binds promiscuously to the lipid portion of the antigen *(72)*. This binding occurs in a fashion analogous to the presentation of lipids by the CD1a-c molecules *(40,64,65)* with the exquisite specificity of T cell recognition dictated by the polar head groups.

It has been shown that CD1d proteins are widely expressed on cells of hematopoetic origin in both humans and mice, although in humans its expression appears to be more tightly regulated. In the mouse CD1d expression is particularly strong on marginal-zone B cells and CD8αα+ dendritic cell (DC) populations *(58,73)*. The function of CD1d on marginal-zone B cells is unclear because it is not required for their development. In contrast, CD1d on the surface of DC may be of particular importance. DC appear to be necessary for the functional activation of invariant NK T cells in vivo by the administration of α-GalCer *(74–76)*.

In the peripheral blood of humans, CD1d is found at low levels on B cells and monocytes, but was not found on resting T cells *(40,77)*. Conversely, activated T cells can express low levels of CD1d. It does not appear that human T cells or B cells expressing CD1d are able to activate Vα24JαQ+ T cells, while in the mouse CD1d-restricted hybridomas clearly have a spectrum of APC preferences *(34,78)*. Monocytes promptly lose CD1d on culture in vitro but regain expression when differentiated into myeloid DC) by culturing with granulocyte-macrophage colony stimulating factor (GM-CSF) and IL-4 plus various maturation agents *(79–81)*. Immunohistochemical analysis confirmed that this molecule was preferentially expressed on DC in the paracortical T cell zones of the lymph node in vivo *(81)*. In lymph node biopsies demonstrating granulomatous inflammatory response, striking CD1d staining was also found on epithelioid histiocytes in both caseating granulomas of *Mycobacterium tuberculosis* infections and nonmycobacterial granulomas. Whereas in the mouse, the major form of CD1d found in the mouse is complexed with β2-microglobulin, structural variants lacking this association and of unclear function are expressed on human thymocytes and enterocytes *(77,82)*. Thus, the parallel patterns of CD1d expression by APC and CD1d-restricted T cell localization suggests that their regulatory function is effected by interaction with these APC, resulting in the subsequent functional activation of CD1d-restricted T cells.

3.2. Specificity of Lipid Antigen-Recognition by CD1d-Restricted T Cells

The identity and spectrum of endogenous lipid antigens recognized by CD1d-restricted T cells remains largely unknown. Inroads into the identification of the endogenous ligands have recently been made by the development of in vitro CD1d antigen-presentation systems. This approach was used to purify phosphatidylinositol from RMAS cell extracts and demonstrate that this was the cell-derived antigen for a single hybridoma expressing an invariant Vα14Jα281 TCR *(83)*. Additional unidentified lipids appear to be capable of activating other invariant as well as noninvariant hybridomas *(34,83)*. Murine CD1d-restricted hybridomas were also shown to have differential preference for APC reactivity *(78)*. Discriminatory recognition of APC did not appear to correlate with the presence of invariant TCR Vα chain *(34)*. Further analysis of CD1d restriction demonstrated that intracellular trafficking of the CD1d molecule appeared to dictate recognition. Invariant Vα14[+] hybridomas were strongly biased towards recognition of wild-type CD1d. The noninvariant hybridomas were activated with equivalent efficiency by wild-type CD1d, or a truncated molecule lacking the cytoplasmic tail that encodes an endosomal trafficking signal *(34)*. Activation by α-GalCer also appears to be relatively specific for invariant Vα14[+] and Vα24[+] cells *(39,68,84)*. Moreover, agents that interfere with endosome acidification abrogated recognition of this ligand by invariant NK T cells *(68)*. In contrast, most noninvariant NK T cells are relatively indifferent to the addition of α-GalCer.

Direct binding studies demonstrate that CD1d acts as a lipid sink without strict restriction on the di-acyl chain length for presentation *(72)*. Thereby sampling a variety of lipids available in APC in much the same way as MHC Class II proteins functions with peptides. However, CD1d-restricted T cells are exquisitely sensitive to structural variations in the glyscosyl head and are selectively activated only by those stereoisomers of the appropriate conformation *(68,70,84)*. Thus, the data suggests that the nature of the APC and subcellular source of the antigen regulate activation of CD1d-restricted T cells.

4. FUNCTION OF CD1D-RESTRICTED T CELLS

The early studies demonstrating that CD1d-restricted T cells were capable of burst secretion of IL-4 in an unprimed fashion made this family of T cells a primary candidate for initiating Th2 immune responses. The large body of data collected since this observation suggests a more complex role for these cells. CD1d-restricted T cells have been shown to be critical for tumor surveillance, control of viral infections, initiation of antigen-specific tolerance, maintenance of the gravid state, and in the control of autoimmune disorders *(16,19,62,85–87)*. Data from these various model systems will be discussed in order to help build an integrated model for the regulatory function of CD1d-restricted T cells.

4.1. Regulation of T Cell Th Phenotype

CD1d-restricted T cells were thought to effect a Th2 bias of immune responses through their capacity to secrete IL-4, but the direct cellular targets for their immunomodulatory function(s) have remained enigmatic. The early observation of burst IL-4 secretion initiating a Th2 response was in part supported by the generation of a $V\alpha14J\alpha281$ transgenic mouse *(23)*. In this animal, $CD4^+$ T cells exhibited a 10- to 100-fold increase in the capacity to secrete IL-4 on stimulation and had elevated levels of IgE. However, mice lacking $\beta2$-microglobulin as well as those whose CD1d locus was ablated by gene targeting retained the capacity to generate antigen-specific Th2 responses at both the cellular and antibody level *(25,26,88)*. An absolute requirement for IL-4 priming of Th2 responses by CD1d-restricted T cell population was also called into question when it was found that these T cells can support Th2 differentiation in an IL-4 receptor-deficient mouse *(89)*. In addition, CD1d-restricted T cells were the source of T cell help and IFN-γ required for functional $CD8^+$ CTL activation in murine leshmania infection *(90)*. Moreover, administration of α-GalCer to pregnant mice resulted in abortion, which was dependent on IFN-γ and perforin and not IL-4 *(86)*. Clearly, the context in which the activation of CD1d-restricted T cells occurs can have major and disparate effects on the function of these cells.

To investigate the consequences of TCR activation in human invariant T cells, clones were examined by transcriptional profiling using high-density oligonucleotide arrays. Significantly, this family of T cells was capable of

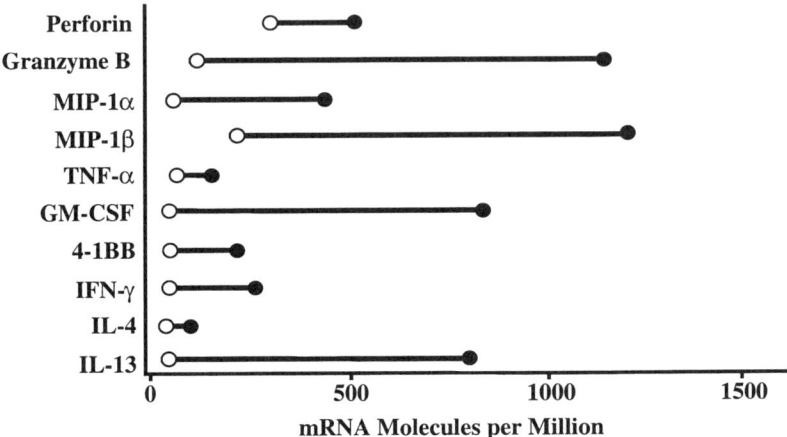

Fig. 1. Transcriptional induction of genes for cytokines and cytolytic enzymes in activated human Vα24JαQ T cells. Vα24JαQ T cell clones were activated with soluble anti-CD3 or IgG1 control, and specific mRNA levels were quantitated on a DNA microarray genechip (Affymetrix, San Jose, CA). The values for the number of copies of specific mRNA per million after treatment with IgG1 control are represented by open circles, and their corresponding copy numbers after activation with anti-CD3 treatment by closed circles.

expressing an unusually broad panel of cytokine, chemokines, and costimulatory proteins (Fig. 1). Activation of Vα24JαQ T cell clones resulted in transcriptional upregulation and secretion of cytokines important for the recruitment and differentiation of myeloid dendritic cells (DC1) including IL-4, GM-CSF, TNF-α, CD40L, and 4-1BB *(91)*. Peripheral-blood monocytes cultured in the presence of IL-4 and GM-CSF differentiated into DC1 DC and expressed CD1d *(81)*. Moreover, Vα24JαQ T cell clones efficiently lysed these cultured DC in a CD1d-restricted fashion. Because human DC1 DC are integral to the genesis of Th1 immune responses, their susceptibility to lysis by Vα24JαQ T cells may be part of a negative-feedback loop in cell-mediated immune responses (Fig. 2).

4.2. Tumor Surveillance

Several studies demonstrated that Vα14Jα281 T cells play a critical role in tumor surveillance and in control of metastasis. In the Jα281 knockout mice, which are incapable of generating the Vα14Jα281 TCR-α chain, these cells were shown to be required for IL-12-mediated rejection of tumors *(85)*. Vα14Jα281 T cells were shown to have NK-like activity, and be necessary and sufficient for the control of metastases of several types of sarcomas and carcinomas *(85,92)*. This function was markedly augmented by the addition

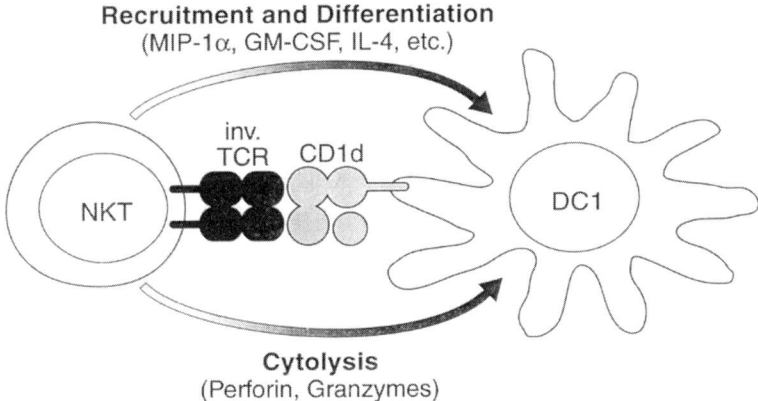

Fig. 2. A model demonstrating the interaction of CD1d-restricted T cells with myeloid dendritic cells (DC). Activation of invariant Vα24JαQ T cells results in the secretion of cytokines and chemokines important for myeloid DC recruitment and activation. In addition, important cell surface costimulatory molecules are also expressed. During myeloid DC maturation, CD1d is upregulated and activates CD1d-restricted T cells. In addition to the secretion of cytokines and chemokines, activated Vα24JαQ T cells upregulate perforin, granzyme B, and Granulysin. The CD1d-dependent secretion of these molecules then results in the lysis of myeloid DC.

of α-GalCer, and the immunopotentiating effect was the result of direct interaction with DCand necessitated the secretion of IL-12 by DC *(74–76)*. Importantly, Vα14Jα281 T cells were also required for endogenous IL-12-mediated protection from spontaneous tumors initiated by chemical carcinogens *(92)*. In another model, C57/Bl6 mice were protected from challenge with melanomas if they had first been vaccinated with an irradiated nonviable melanoma genetically engineered to secrete GM-CSF *(93)*. This protection was completely abrogated in the CD1d knock out mouse *(94)*. Furthermore, this loss of protection was demonstrated to be in part the result of a failure to functionally mature the myeloid DC lineage in the knockout mice.

Human patients with melanoma, like Type 1 diabetics, had fewer circulating CD161⁺ Vα24JαQ⁺ T cells *(95)*. These findings have been verified in patients with prostate cancer (Exley, M., unpublished results). Furthermore, and in complete contrast to the patients with Type 1 diabetes, the residual population of CD161⁺ Vα24JαQ⁺ T cells in the cancer patients had a striking Th2 polarization. This Th2 polarization was lost on recovery from disease as this profile was not found in prostate-cancer patients in remission (Exley, M., unpublished results).

There is also compelling evidence that tumor immunity and some forms of autoimmunity are closely related. The development of genetic and biochemical methods for the identification of tumor antigens has revealed that normal differentiation proteins, much like autoantigens, can serve as targets for T lymphocyte and antibody responses in patients with autoimmune disorders or cancer *(96–99)*. The most convincing example of immune surveilance as important for containing or rejecting tumors occurs in malignant melanoma *(93)*. Vaccination and adoptive T cell immunotherapies have induced both tumor destruction and the death of normal melanocytes in both murine models and in clinical trials of melanoma therapy. These connections between tumor immunity and autoimmunity suggest that common mechanisms may underly the development of both responses.

4.3. Autoimmunity

Several lines of evidence clearly show that dysfunction and/or diminished frequency of CD1d-restricted T cells correlates with the development of autoimmunity in both rodents and humans *(19,16,42,100)*. In several murine models of autoimmunity, Vα14Jα281$^+$ T cells were shown to be present in diminished numbers and to decrease in frequency prior to the onset of disease *(16,43,101)*. Autoimmunity in these rodents was temporally accelerated by depletion of CD161$^+$ T cells and delayed by generating mice transgenic for the Vα14Jα281 TCR *(43,87,102)*. Although the selective loss of CD1d-restricted T cells has been associated with several autoimmune disorders, qualitative changes in function of these cells are likely to be more important. The SJL mouse, a mouse strain highly susceptible to experimental allergic encephalomyelitis, has in addition to a decreased number of NK T cells, a striking functional defect in these cells on activation *(100)*. In this mouse there is a mutation in the promoter for CD161 resulting in diminished expression of this protein *(14)*. Whether this defect in expression relates to the noted functional defect and the development of disease has not yet been determined. Notably, the loss of invariant Vα24JαQ T cells is also an immunologic hallmark of multiple sclerosis (MS) *(20)*.

The nonobese diabetic mouse (NOD) and the diabetes-prone BB rat are also severely deficient in CD1d-restricted T cells, and the quantitative defects are associated with a reduced ability to secrete IL-4, IL-10, and IFN-γ in response to stimulation *(16,50,103)*. Development of diabetes in both these rodent models was prevented by adoptive transfer of CD1d-restricted T cells *(16,50)*. In the NOD mouse, the protective effect of adoptive transfer was dependent on IL-4 and IL-10 *(104)*. The concomitant administration of anti-IL-4 or anti-IL-10 cytokine-specific antibodies ablated the protective effect of the adoptively transferred Vα14Jα281 T cells. As indicated by experiments using anti-cytokine antibodies or transgenic overexpression of the Vα14Jα281 TCR α chain, protection was not dependent just on increased numbers of CD1d-restricted T cells. A direct demonstration of the importance of function was demonstrated by the generation of NOD mice with markedly elevated frequencies of CD1d-restricted T cells resulting from the transgenic overexpression of the Vα14Jα281 TCR α chain *(87)*. Despite the resultant large population of CD1d-restricted T cells, these transgenic mice were only partially protected from developing diabetes. Maximal protection was specifically associated with lines of transgenic mice whose CD1d-restricted T cells had the highest levels of cytokine production after activation. CD1d-restricted T cells lines derived from the spleens of NOD mice were also found to be markedly defective in cytokine secretion after activation. In fact, this family of cells responded particularly poorly to IL-12 coactivation of IFN-γ secretion *(17)*. In subsequent cell transfer experiments, protection from diabetes was associated with IL-12 treated lines which demonstrated an enhanced ability to secrete IFN-γ relative to IL-4. The apparent contradictory observations between the anti-IL-4 MAb treatment in vivo and the IL-12-matured transfer experiments is likely owing to different tissue sources of donor lines *(16,17,104)*, and that α-GalCer activation requires IL-12 and autocrine IL-4 in vivo *(105)*. Treatment of NOD mice with α-GalCer protects them from the subsequent development of diabetes (Wilson, S. B., unpublished results) Administration of the lipid results in the specific recruitment of Vα14Jα281 T cells to the Islets of Langerhans. Perhaps more importantly, α-GalCer administration specifically alters DC subsets in the pancreatic lymph nodes draining this organ. Treatment with α-GalCer results in a specific loss of CD11c$^+$ CD8α$^+$ DCs and accumulation of CD11c$^+$ CD8α$^-$ DCs. The CD11c$^+$ CD8α$^+$ subset of DCs are thought to be a major source of IL-12 and promote Th1-biased responses and CD11c$^+$ CD8α$^-$ DCs transfer protection from diabetes *(73,106–108)*. In the spontaneously diabetic NOD mouse, and in TCR transgenic models of diabetes, activation of insulitis occurs first through DC recruitment to the pancreatic Islets and lymph nodes (LNs) *(109–112)*. Therefore, changes in the CD1d-restricted T cell/DC axis is associated with the development of diabetes in the NOD mouse.

Defective function is also seen in CD1d-restricted T cells cloned from human patients with type 1 diabetes *(19)*. We recently demonstrated that in a set of monozygotic twins discordant for insulin-dependet diabetes mellitus (IDDM), invariant Vα24JαQ$^+$ T cells were found to be present at significantly higher frequencies in the nonprogressing sibling as compared to their diabetic twin *(19)*. Reduced circulating and tissue-specific frequencies of Vα24JαQ$^+$ T cells have also been seen in rheumatoid arthritis (RA),

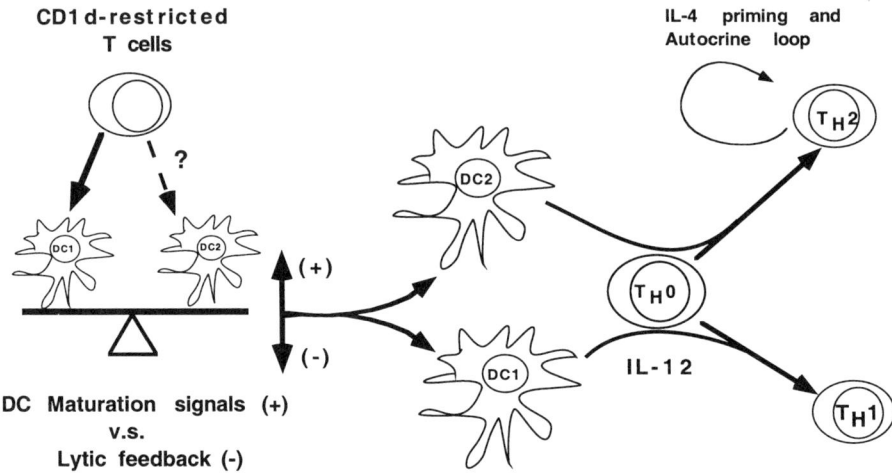

Fig. 3. Activation of CD1d-restricted T cells regulates immune responses by changing the balance of dendritic cell (DC) subsets. Because human myeloid-derived DC (DC1) and lymphoid-derived DC (DC2) regulate CD4⁺ Th cell responses, the specific lysis of DC1 cells by Vα24JαQ T cells suggests that their immunomodulatory function is not limited to Th2 bias induced by IL-4 secretion. When cocultured with T cells, DC1 cells secreted high levels of IL-12 and induced T cells with a Th1 phenotype. Coculture of T cells with DC2 cells induced a marked Th2 response. Thus, the specific lysis of myeloid dendritic (DC1) cells by Vα24JαQ T cells may serve as a negative feedback mechanism for limiting Th1 T cell responses. Although there is strong evidence in the mouse that different DC subsets reciprocally regulate T cell phenotypes, there is no data available on the direct interaction between murine invariant Vα14Jα281 T cells.

systemic sclerosis, and MS *(20,40,42)*. Moreover, Vα24JαQ⁺ T cell clones from autoimmune diabetics exhibited an extreme Th1 bias, secreting only IFN-γ while those from IDDM nonprogressors and normals secreted both IL-4 and IFN-γ *(19)*. When examined by DNA microarrays, activation of Vα24JαQ T cell clones demonstrated markedly discordant expression patterns for gene families representing cytokine/chemokines, anti-apoptotic genes, Ca²⁺ signaling molecules, and Th-specific transcription factors *(91)*. Therefore, the clones derived from diabetic patients were dysfunctional with regards to the expression of cytokine and costimulatory molecules important for regulating the immune deviation for which CD1d-restricted T cells are responsible. In addition, DC function has been noted to be defective in individuals at high risk for the development of type 1 diabetes and in patients with the disease *(113)*. The parallels in quantitative and qualitative dysfunction of CD1d-restricted T cells seen between the rodent models and human type 1 diabetes are therefore striking.

5. SUMMARY

CD1d-restricted T cells are important regulators of several different immune responses. Appropriate or inappropriate activation of this family of T cells has a profound impact on the course of the subsequent immune response. Although the spectrum of CD1d-restricted T cell populations and the functional consequences of CD1d expression on various APC remains to be defined, a critical two-way interaction of these T cells with DC subsets provides a unifying hypothesis for many of their reported functions (Fig. 3).

REFERENCES

1. Becker, K. G. (1999) Comparative genetics of type 1 diabetes and autoimmune disease: common loci, commmon pathways. *Diabetes* **48,** 1353–1358.
2. Verge, C. F., Gianani, R., Liping, Y., Pietropaolo, M., Smith, T., Jackson, R. A., et al. (1995) Late progression to diabetes and evidence for chronic b-cell autoimmunity in identical twins of patients with type I diabetes. *Diabetes* **44,** 1176–1179.
3. Verge, C. F., Gianani, R., Kawasaki, E., Yu, L., Pietropaolo, M., Jackson, R. A., et al. (1996) Prediction of type I diabetes in first-degree relatives using a combination of insulin, GAD, and ICA512bdc/IA-2 autoantibodies. *Diabetes* **45,** 926–933.
4. Roep, B. O. (1996) T cell responses to autoantigens in IDDM. The search for the holy grail. *Diabetes* **45,** 1147–1156.
5. Wicker, L. S., Todd, J. A., and Peterson, L. B. (1995) Genetic control of autoimmune diabetes in the NOD mouse. *Ann. Rev. Immunol.* **13,** 179–200.
6. Wherret, D. K., Singer, S. M., and McDevitt, H. O. (1997) Reduction in diabetes incidence in an I-A^{g7} transgenic nonobese diabetic mouse line. *Diabetes* **46,** 1970–1974.
7. Delovitch, T. L. and Singh, B. (1997) The nonobese diabetic mouse as a model of autoimmune diabetes: immune dysregulation gets the NOD. *Immunity* **7,** 727–738.
8. Abbas, A. K., Murphy, K. M., and Sher, A. (1996) Functional diversity of helper T lymphocytes. *Nature* **383,** 787–793.
9. Berman, M. A., Sandborg, C. I., Wang, Z., Imfeld, K. L., Zaldivar, F. J., Dadufalza, V., et al. (1996) Decreased IL-4 production in new onset type 1 insulin-dependent diabetes mellitus. *J. Immunol.* **157,** 4690–4696.
10. Serreze, D. V. and Leiter, E. H. (1994) Genetic and pathogenic basis of autoimmune diabetes in NOD mice. *Curr. Opin. Immunol.* **6,** 900–906.
11. Mueller, R., Krahl, T., and Sarvetnick, N. (1996) Pancreatic expression of interleukin-4 abrogates insulitis and autoimmune diabetes in nonobese diabetic (NOD) mice. *J. Exp. Med.* **184,** 1093–1099.
12. Cetkovic-Cvrlje, M., Gerling, I. C., Muir, A., Atkinson, M. A., Elliot, J. F., and Leiter, E. H. (1997) Retardation or acceleration of diabetes in NOD/Lt

mice mediated by intrathymic administration fo candidate β-cell antigens. *Diabetes* **46,** 1975–1982.

13. Bradley, L. M., Asensio, V. C., Schioetz, L. K., Harbertson, J., Krahl, T., Patstone, G., et al. (1999) Islet-specific Th1, but not Th2, cells secrete multiple chemokines and promote rapid induction of autoimmune diabetes. *J. Immunol.* **162,** 2511–2520.

14. Bendelac, A., Rivera, M. N., Park, H.-S., and Roark J. H. (1997) Mouse CD1-specific NK1 T cells: development, specificity, and function. *Ann. Rev. Immunol.* **15,** 535–562.

15. Bendelac, A., Lantz, O., Quimby, M. E., Yewdell, J. W., Bennink, J. R., and Brutkiewicz, R. R. (1995) CD1 recognition by mouse NK1+ T lymphocytes. *Science* **268,** 863–865.

16. Baxter, A. G., Kinder, S. J., Hammond, K. J. L., Scollay, R., and Godfrey, D. I. (1997) Association between αβTCR+CD4-CD8- T cell defiency and IDDM in NOD/Lt mice. *Diabetes* **46,** 572–582.

17. Falcone, M., Yeung, B., Tucker, L., Rodriguez, E., and Sarvetnick, N. (1999) A defect in interleukin 12-induced activation and interferon gamma secretion of peripheral natural killer T cells in nonobese diabetic mice suggests new pathogenic mechanisms for insulin-dependent diabetes mellitus. *J. Exp. Med.* **190,** 963–972.

18. Falcone, M. and Sarvetnick, N. (1999) Cytokines that regulate autoimmune responses. *Curr. Opin. Immunol.* **11,** 670–676.

19. Wilson, S. B., Kent, S. C., Patton, K. T., Orban, T., Jackson, R. A., Exley, M., et al. (1998) Extreme Th 1 bias of invariant Va24JaQ T cells in type 1 diabetes. *Nature* **391,** 177–181.

20. Illes, Z., Kondo, T., Newcombe, J., Oka, N., Tabira, T., and Yamamura, T. (2000) Differential expression of NK T cell Valpha24JalphaQ invariant TCR chains in the lesions of multiple sclerosis and chronic inflammatory demyelinating polyneuropathy. *J. Immunol.* **164,** 4375–4381.

21. Koseki, H., Imai, K., Ichikawa, T., Hayata, I., and Taniguchi, M. (1989) Predominant use of a particular alpha-chain in suppressor T cell hybridomas specific for keyhole limpet hemocyanin. *Intl. Immunol.* **1,** 557–564.

22. Ohteki, T. and MacDonald, H. R. (1996) Stringent V beta requirement for the development of NK1. 1+ T cell receptor-alpha/beta+ cells in mouse liver. J. Exp. Med. 183, 1277–1282.

23. Bendelac, A., Hunziker, R. D., and Lantz, O. (1996) Increased interleukin 4 and immunogloulin E production in transgenic mice overexpressing NK1 T cells. *J. Exp. Med.* **184,** 1285–1293.

24. Lantz, O. and Bendelac, A. (1994) An invariant T cell receptor alpha chain is used by a unique subset of major histocompatibility complex class I-specific CD4+ and CD4-8- T cells in mice and humans. *J. Exp. Med.* **180,** 1097–1106.

25. Mendiratta, S. K., Martin, W. D., Hong, S., Boesteanu, A., Joyce, S., and Van Kaer, L. (1997) *CD1d1* mutant mice are deficient in natural T cells that promptly produce IL-4. *Immunity* **6,** 469–477.

26. Smiley, S. T., Kaplan, M. H., and Grusby, M. J. (1997) Immunoglobulin E production in the absence of interleukin-4-secreting CD1-dependent cells. *Science* **275,** 977–979.
27. Porcelli, S., Yockey, C. E., Brenner, M. B., and Balk, S. P. (1993) Analysis of T cell antigen receptor (TCR) expression by human peripheral blood CD4-8-α/β T cells demonstrates preferential use of several Vβ genes and an invariant TCRα chain. *J. Exp. Med.* **178,** 1–16.
28. Bendelac, A. (1995) CD1: presenting unusual antigens to unusual T lymphocytes. *Science* **269,** 185,186.
29. Brossay, L. and Kronenberg, M. (1999) Highly conserved antigen-presenting function of CD1d molecules. *Immunogenetics* **50,** 146–151.
30. Dellabona, P., Padovan, E., Casorati, G., Brockhaus, M., and Lanzavecchia, A. (1994) An invariant Vα24-JαQ/Vb11 T cell receptor is expressed in all individuals by clonally expanded CD4-8- T cells. *J. Exp. Med.* **180,** 1171–1176.
31. Keino, H., Matsumoto, I., Okada, S., Kurokawa, M., Kato, T., Tokuhisa, T., et al. (1999) A single cell analysis of TCR AV24AJ18+ DN T cells. *Microbiol. Immunol.* **43,** 577–584.
32. Kent, S. C., Hafler, D. A., Strominger, J. L., and Wilson, S. B. (1999) Noncanonical Valpha24JalphaQ T cells with conservative alpha chain CDR3 region amino acid substitutions are restricted by CD1d. *Human Immunol.* **60,** 1080–1089.
33. Behar, S. M., Podrebarac, T. A., Roy, C. J., Wang, C. R., and Brenner, M. B. (1999) Diverse TCRs recognize murine CD1. *J. Immunol.* **162,** 161–167.
34. Chiu, Y. H., Jayawardena, J., Weiss, A., Lee, D., Park, S. H., Dautry-Varsat, A., and Bendelac, A. (1999) Distinct subsets of CD1d-restricted T cells recognize self-antigens loaded in different cellular compartments. *J. Exp. Med.* **189,** 103–110.
35. Hammond, K. J., Pelikan, S. B., Crowe, N. Y., Randle-Barrett, E., Nakayama, T., Taniguchi, M., et al. (1999) NKT cells are phenotypically and functionally diverse. *Eur. J. Immunol.* **29,** 3768–3781.
36. Eberl, G., Lees, R., Smiley, S. T., Taniguchi, M., Grusby, M. J., and MacDonald, H. R. (1999) Tissue-specific segregation of CD1d-dependent and CD1d-independent NK T cells. *J. Immunol.* **162,** 6410–6419.
37. Kawano, T., Tanaka, Y., Shimizu, E., Kaneko, Y., Kamata, N., Sato, H., et al. (1999) A novel recognition motif of human NKT antigen receptor for a glycolipid ligand. *Intl. Immunol.* **11,** 881–887.
38. Zeng, D., Lewis, D., Dejbakhsh-Jones, S., Lan, F., Garcia-Ojeda, M., Sibley, R., et al. (1999) Bone marrow NK1. 1(-) and NK1. 1(+) T cells reciprocally regulate acute graft versus host disease. *J. Exp. Med.* **189,** 1073–1081.
39. Exley, M., Tahir, S., Cheng, O., Shaulov, A. Joyce, R. Avigan, D., et al. Polyclonal human bone marrow-derived Th2-like non-invariant CD1d-reactive Tcells target lymphoid cells and suppress mixed lymphocyte responses, in press.
40. Porcelli, S. A. and Modlin, R. L. (1999) The CD1 system: antigen-presenting molecules for T cell recognition of lipids and glycolipids. *Ann. Rev. Immunol.* **17,** 297–329.

41. Hong, S., Scherer, D. C., Singh, N., Mendiratta, S. K., Serizawa, I., Koezuka, Y., and Van Kaer, L. (1999) Lipid antigen presentation in the immune system: lessons learned from CD1d knockout mice. *Immunol. Rev.* **169,** 31–44.

42. Sumida, T., Sakamoto, A., Murata, H., Makino, Y., Takahashi, H., Yoshida, S., et al. (1995) Selective reduction of T cells bearing invariant Vα24JαQ antigen receptor in patients with systemic sclerosis. *J. Exp. Med.* **182,** 1163–1168.

43. Mieza, M. A., Itoh, T., Cui, J. Q., Makino, Y., Kawano, T., Tsuchida, K., et al. (1996) Selective reduction of Vα14+ NK T cells associated with disease development in autoimmune-prone mice. *J. Immunol.* **156,** 4035–4040.

44. Beckman, E. M., Porcelli, S. A., Morita, C. T., Behar, S. M., Furlong, S. T., and Brenner, M. B. (1994) Recognition of a lipid antigen by CD1-restricted alpha beta+ T cells [see comments]. *Nature* **372,** 691–694.

45. Exley, M., Garcia, J., Balk, S. P., and Porcelli, S. (1997) Requirements for CD1d Recognition by Human Invariant Va24+ CD4-CD8- T Cells. *J. Exp. Med.* **186,** 1–11.

46. Yokoyama, W. M. and Seaman, W. E. (1993) The Ly-49 and NKR-P1 gene families encoding lectin-like receptors on natural killer cells: the NK gene complex. *Ann. Rev. Immunol.* **11,** 613–635.

47. Arase, H., Arase, N., and Saito, T. (1996) Interferon γ production by natural killer (NK) cells and NK1. 1+ T cells upon NKR-P1 cross-linking. *J. Exp. Med.* **183,** 2391–2396.

48. Exley, M., Porcelli, S., Furman, M., Garcia, J., and Balk, S. (1998) CD161 (NKR-P1A) costimulation of CD1d-dependent activation of human T cells expressing invariant V alpha 24 J alpha Q T cell receptor alpha chains. *J. Exp. Med.* **188,** 867–876.

49. Campbell, K. S. and Giorda, R. (1997) The cytoplasmic domain of rat NKR-P1 receptor interacts with the N- terminal domain of p56(lck) via cysteine residues. *Eur. J. Immunol.* **27,** 72–77.

50. Iwakoshi, N. N., Greiner, D. L., Rossini, A. A., and Mordes, J. P. (1999) Diabetes prone BB rats are severely deficient in natural killer T cells. *Autoimmunity* **31,** 1–14.

51. Greiner, D. L., Mordes, J. P., Handler, E. S., Angelillo, M., Nakamura, N., and Rossini, A. A. (1987) Depletion of RT6. 1+ T lymphocytes induces diabetes in resistant biobreeding/Worcester (BB/W) rats. *J. Exp. Med.* **166,** 461–475.

52. Dellabona, P., Casorati, G., Friedli, B., Angman, L., Sallusto, F., Tunnacliffe, A., et al. (1993) In vivo persistence of expanded clones specific for bacterial antigens within the human T cell receptor α/b CD4-8- subset. *J. Exp. Med.* **177,** 1763–1771.

53. Norris, S., Doherty, D. G., Collins, C., McEntee, G., Traynor, O., Hegarty, J. E., et al. (1999) Natural T cells in the human liver: cytotoxic lymphocytes with dual T cell and natural killer cell phenotype and function are phenotypically heterogenous and include Valpha24-JalphaQ and gammadelta T cell receptor bearing cells. *Human Immunol.* **60,** 20–31.

54. Prussin, C. and Foster, B. (1997) TCR V alpha 24 and V beta 11 coexpression defines a human NK1 T cell analog containing a unique Th0 subpopulation. *J. Immunol.* **159,** 5862–5870.

55. Nuti, S., Rosa, D., Valiante, N. M., Saletti, G., Caratozzolo, M., Dellabona, P., et al. (1998) Dynamics of intra-hepatic lymphocytes in chronic hepatitis C: enrichment for Valpha 24+ T cells and rapid elimination of effector cells by apoptis. *Eur. J. Immunol.* **28,** 3448–3455.

56. Masuda, K., Makino, Y., Cui, J., Ito, T., Tokuhisa, T., Takahama, Y., Koseki, H., et al. (1997) Phenotypes and invariant αβ TCR expression of peripheral Vα14+ NK T cells. *J. Immunol.* **158,** 2076–2082.

57. Ohteki, T. and MacDonald, H. R. (1994) Major histocompatibility complex class I related molecules control the development of CD4+8- and CD4-8- subsets of natural killer 1. 1+ T cell receptor-alpha/beta+ cells in the liver of mice. *J. Exp. Med.* **180,** 699–704.

58. Roark, J. H., Park, S. H., Jayawardena, J., Kavita, U., S. M., and Bendelac, A. (1998) CD1. 1 expression by mouse antigen-presenting cells and maginal zone B cells. *J. Immunol.* **160,** 3121–3127.

59. Cardell, S., Tangri, S., Chan, S., Kronenberg, M., Benoist, C., and Mathis, D. (1995) CD1-restricted CD4+ T cells in major histocompatibility complex class II-deficient mice. *J. Exp. Med.* **182,** 993–1004.

60. Amano, M., Baumgarth, N., Dick, M. D., Brossay, L., Kronenberg, M., Herzenberg, L. A., and Strober, S. (1998) CD1 expression defines subsets of follicular and marginal zone B cells in the spleen: beta 2-microglobulin-dependent and independent forms. *J. Immunol.* **161,** 1710–1717.

61. Brossay, L., Jullien, D., Cardell, S., Sydora, B. C., Burdin, N., Modlin, R. L., et al. (1997) Mouse CD1 is mainly expressed on hemopoietic-derived cells. *J. Immunol.* **159,** 1216–1224.

62. Sonoda, K. H., Exley, M., Snapper, S., Balk, S. P., and Stein-Streilein, J. (1999) CD1-reactive natural killer T cells are required for development of systemic tolerance through an immune-privileged site [see comments]. *J. Exp. Med.* **190,** 1215–1226.

63. Calabi, F., Jarvis, J. M., Martin, L., and Milstein, C. (1989) Two classes of CD1 genes. *Eur. J. Immunol.* **19,** 285–292.

64. Moody, D. B., Besra, G. S., Wilson, I. A., and Porcelli, S. A. (1999) The molecular basis of CD1-mediated presentation of lipid antigens. *Immunol. Rev.* **172,** 285–296.

65. Moody, D. B., Reinhold, B. B., Guy, M. R., Beckman, E. M., Frederique, D. E., Furlong, S. T., et al. (1997) Structural requirements for glycolipid antigen recognition by CD1b- restricted T cells. *Science* **278,** 283–286.

66. Schofield, L., McConville, M. J., Hansen, D., Campbell, A. S., Fraser-Reid, B., Grusby, M. J., and Tachado, S. D. (1999) CD1d-restricted immunoglobulin G formation to GPI-anchored antigens mediated by NKT cells. *Science* **283,** 225–229.

67. Zeng, Z.-H., Castano, A. R., Segelke, B. W., Stura, E. A., Peterson, P. A., and Wilson, I. A. (1997) Crystal structure of mouse CD1:an MHC-like fold with a large hydrophobic binding groove. *Science* **277,** 339–345.

68. Kawano, T., Cui, J., Koezuka, Y., Toura, I., Kaneko, Y., Motoki, K., et al. (1997) CD1d-restricted and TCR-mediated activation of valpha14 NKT cells by glycoceramides. *Science* **278,** 1626–1629.

69. Brossay, L., Chioda, M., Burdin, N., Koezuka, Y., Casorati, G., Dellabona, P., and Kronenberg, M. (1998) CD1d-mediated recognition of an alpha-galactosylceramide by natural killer T cells is highly conserved through mammalian evolution. *J. Exp. Med.* **188,** 1521–1528.

70. Spada, F. M., Koezuka, Y., and Porcelli, S. A. (1998) CD1d-restricted recognition of synthetic glycolipid antigens by human natural killer T cells. *J. Exp. Med.* **188,** 1529–1534.

71. Joyce, S., Woods, A. S., Yewdell, J. W., Bennink, J. R., De Silva, A. D., Boesteanu, A., et al. (1998) Natural ligand of mouse CD1d1: cellular glycosylphosphatidylinositol. *Science* **279,** 1541–1544.

72. Naidenko, O. V., Maher, J. K., Ernst, W. A., Sakai, T., Modllin, R. L., and Kronenberg, M. (1999) Binding and Antigen Presentation of Ceramide-containing glycolipids by Soluble Mouse and Human CD1d Molecules. *J. Exp. Med.* **190,** 1069–1079.

73. Pulendran, B., Lingappa, J., Kennedy, M. K., Smith, J., Teepe, M., Rudensky, A., et al. (1997) Developmental pathways of dendritic cells in vivo: distinct function, phenotype, and localization of dendritic cell subsets in FLT3 ligand-treated mice. *J. Immunol.* **159,** 2222–2231.

74. Kitamura, H., Iwanabe, K., Yahata, T., Nishimura, S.-i., Ohta, A., Ohmi, Y., et al. (1999) The natural killer (NKT) cell ligand alpha-galactosylceramide demonstrates its immunopotentiating effect by inducing interleukin (IL)-12 production by dendritic cells and IL-12 receptor expression on NKT cells. *J. Exp. Med.* **189,** 1121–1127.

75. Toura, I., Kawano, T., Akutsu, Y., Nakayama, T., Ochiai, T., and Taniguchi, M. (1999) Cutting edge: inhibition of experimental tumor metastasis by dendritic cells pulsed with alpha-galactosylceramide. *J. Immunol.* **163,** 2387–2391.

76. Tomura, M., Yu, W.-G., Ahn, H.-J., Yamashita, M., Yang, Y.-F., Ono, S., et al. (1999) A Novel Function of Valpha14+CD4+NKT Cells: Stimulation of IL-12 Production by Antigen-Presenting Cells in the Innate Immune System. *J. Immunol.* **163,** 93–101.

77. Exley, M., Garcia, J., Wilson, S. B., Spada, F., Gerdes, D., Tahir, S. M., et al. (2000) CD1d structure and regulation on human thymocytes, peripheral blood T cells,B cells and monocytes. *Immunology* **100,** 37–47.

78. Park, S. H., Roark, J. H., and Bendelac, A. (1998) Tissue-specific recognition of mouse CD1 molecules. *J. Immunol.* **160,** 3128–3134.

79. Nicol, A., Nieda, M., Koezuka, Y., Porcelli, S., Suzuki, K., Tadokoro, K., et al. (2000) Dendritic cells are targets for human invariant Valpha24+ natural killer T cell cytotoxic activity: an important immune regulatory function. *Exp. Hematol.* **28,** 276–282.

80. Takahashi, T., Nieda, M., Koezuka, Y., Nicol, A., Porcelli, S. A., Ishikawa, Y., et al. (2000) Analysis of human valpha24+ CD4+ NKT cells activated by alpha- glycosylceramide-pulsed monocyte-derived dendritic cells [in process citation]. *J. Immunol.* **164,** 4458–4464.

81. Yang, O., Racke, F. R., Nguyen, P. T., Gausling, R., Severino, M., Horton, H. F., et al. (2000) CD1d on myeloid dendritici cells timulates cytokine

secretion from and cytolytic activity of Va24JaQ T cells: a feedback mechanism for immune regulation. *J. Immunol.* **165,** 3239–3246.

82. Kim, H. S., Garcia, J., Exley, M., Johnson, K. W., Balk, S. P., and Blumberg, R. S. (1999) Biochemical characterization of CD1d expression in the absence of beta2- microglobulin. *J. Biol. Chem.* **274,** 9289–9295.

83. Gumperz, J. E., Roy, C., Makowska, A., Lum, D., Sugita, M., Podrebarac, T., et al. (2000) Murine CD1d-restricted T cell recognition of cellular lipids. *Immunity* **12,** 211–221.

84. Brossay, L., Naidenko, O., Burdin, N., Matsuda, J., Sakai, T., and Kronenberg, M. (1998) Structural requirements for galactosylceramide recognition by CD1- restricted NK T cells. *J. Immunol.* **161,** 5124–5128.

85. Cui, J., Shin, T., Kawano, T., Sato, H., Kondo, E., Toura, I., et al. (1997) Requirement for Vα14 NKT cells in IL-12-mediated rejection of tumors. *Science* **278,** 1623–1626.

86. Ito, K., Karasawa, M., Kawano, T., Akasaka, T., Koseki, H., Akutsu, Y., et al. (2000) Involvement of decidual Valpha14 NKT cells in abortion. *Proc Natl Acad Sci USA* **97,** 740–744.

87. Lehuen, A., Lantz, O., Beaudoin, L., Laloux, V., Carnaud, C., Bendelac, A., et al. (1998) Overexpression of natural killer T cells protects Valpha14-Jalpha281 transgenic nonobese diabetic mice against diabetes. *J. Exp. Med.* **188,** 1831–1839.

88. Brown, D. R., Fowell, D. J., Corry, D. B., Wynn, T. A., Moskowitz, N. H., Cheever, A. W., et al. (1996) Beta 2-microglobulin-dependent NK1. 1+ T cells are not essential for T helper cell 2 immune responses. *J. Exp. Med.* **184,** 1295–1304.

89. Noben-Trauth, N., Shultz, L. D., Brombacher, F., Urban, J. F., Jr., Gu, H., and Paul, W. E. (1997) An interleukin 4 (IL-4)-independent pathway for CD4+ T cell IL-4 production is revealed in IL-4 receptor-deficient mice. *Proc. Natl. Acad. Sci. USA* **94,** 10,838–10,843.

90. Wakil, A. E., Wang, Z. E., Ryan, J. C., Fowell, D. J., and Locksley, R. M. (1998) Interferon gamma derived from CD4(+) T cells is sufficient to mediate T helper cell type 1 development. *J. Exp. Med.* **188,** 1651–1656.

91. Wilson, S. B., Kent, S. C., Horton, H. F., Hill, A. A., Bollyky, P. L., Hafler, D. A., et al. (2000) Multiple differences in gene expression in regulatory Valpha24JalphaQ T cells from identical twins discordant for type I diabetes. *Proc. Natl. Acad. Sci. USA* **97,** 7411–7416.

92. Smyth, M. J., Thia, K. Y. T., Street, S. E. A., Cretney, E., Trapani, J. A., Taniguchi, M., et al. (2000) Differential tumor surveillance by natural killer (NK) and NKT cells. *J. Exp. Med.* **191,** 661–668.

93. Soiffer, R., Lynch, T., Mihm, M., Jung, K., Rhuda, C., Schmollinger, J. C., et al. (1998) Vaccination with irradiated autologous melanoma cells engineered to secrete human granulocyte-macrophage colony-stimulating factor generates potent antitumor immunity in patients with metastatic melanoma. *Proc. Natl. Acad. Sci. USA* **95,** 13,141–13,146.

94. Gillesen, S., Santambrogio, L., Naumov, Y., Lee, F. S., Wong, M.-L., Luster, A. D., et al. CD1d-restricted T cells regulate dendritic cell function and anti-tumor immunity in a GM-CSF-dependent fashion. *J. Exp. Med.*, submitted.

95. Kawano, T., Nakayama, T., Kamada, N., Kaneko, Y., Harada, M., Ogura, N., et al. (1999) Antitumor cytotoxicity mediated by ligand-activated human V alpha24 NKT cells. *Cancer Res.* **59,** 5102–5105.

96. Tamada, K., Shimozaki, K., Chapoval, A. I., Zhu, G., Sica, G., Flies, D., et al. (2000) Modulation of T cell-mediated immunity in tumor and graft-ver-sus-host disease models through the LIGHT co-stimulatory pathway. *Nat. Med.* **6,** 283–289.

97. Ludewig, B., Ochsenbein, A. F., Odermatt, B., Paulin, D., Hengartner, H., and Zinkernagel, R. M. (2000) Immunotherapy with dendritic cells directed against tumor antigens shared with normal host cells results in severe autoimmune disease. *J. Exp. Med.* **191,** 795–804.

98. Castelli, C., Rivoltini, L., Andreola, G., Carrabba, M., Renkvist, N., and Parmiani, G. (2000) T cell recognition of melanoma-associated antigens. *J. Cell. Physiol.* **182,** 323–331.

99. Pittet, M. J., Valmori, D., Dunbar, P. R., Speiser, D. E., Lienard, D., Lejeune, F., et al. (1999) High frequencies of naive Melan-A/MART-1-specific CD8(+) T cells in a large proportion of human histocompatibility leukocyte antigen (HLA)-A2 individuals. *J. Exp. Med.* **190,** 705–715.

100. Yoshimoto, T., Bendelac, A., Hu-Li, J., and Paul, W. E. (1995) Defective IgE production by SJL mice is linked to the absence of CD4+, NK1. 1+ T cells that promptly produce interleukin 4. *Proc. Natl. Acad. Sci. USA* **92,** 11,931–11,934.

101. Gombert, J. M., Herbelin, A., Tancrede-Bohin, E., Dy, M., Carnaud, C., and Bach, J. F. (1996) Early quantitative and functional deficiency of NK1+-like thymocytes in the NOD mouse. *Eur. J. Immunol.* **26,** 2989–2998.

102. Takeda, K. and Dennert, G. (1993) The development of autoimmunity in C57BL/6 *lpr* mice correlates with the disappearance of natural killer type 1-positive cells: evidence for their suppressive action on bone marrow stem cell proliferation, B cell immunoglobulin secretion, and autoimmune symptoms. *J. Exp. Med.* **177,** 155–164.

103. Wonigeit, K., Dinkel, A., Fangmann, J., and Thude, H. (1997) Expression of the ectoenzyme RT6 is not restricted to resting peripheral T cells and is differently regulated in normal peripheral T cells, intestinal IEL, and NK cells. *Adv. Exp. Med. Biol.* **419,** 229–240.

104. Hammond, K. I. L., Poulton, L. D., Palmisano, L. J., Silveira, P. A., Godfrey, D. I., and Baxter, A. G. (1998) alpha/beta-T cell receptor (TCR)+CD4-CD8-(NKT) thymocytes prevent insulin-dependent diabetes mellitus in nonobese diabetic (NOD)/Lt mice by the influence of interleukin (IL)-4 and/or IL-10. *J. Exp. Med.* 187, 1047–1056.

105. Kaneko, B. Y., Harada, M., Kawano, T., Yamashita, M., Shibata, Y., Gejyo, F., Nakayama, T., et al. (2000) Augmentation of Valpha14 NKT cell-mediated cytotoxicity by interleukin 4 in an autocrine mechanism resulting in the development of concanavalin A-induced hepatitis. *J. Exp. Med.* **191,** 105–114.

106. Reis e Sousa, C., Yap, G., Schulz, O., Rogers, N., Schito, M., Aliberti, J., et al. (1999) Paralysis of dendritic cell IL-12 production by microbial products prevents infection-induced immunopathology. *Immunity* **11,** 637–647.
107. Pulendran, B., Smith, J. L., Caspary, G., Brasel, K., Pettit, D., Maraskovsky, E., et al. (1999) Distinct dendritic cell subsets differentially regulate the class of immune response in vivo. *Proc. Natl. Acad. Sci. USA* **96,** 1036–1041.
108. Feili-Hariri, M., Dong, X., Alber, S. M., Watkins, S. C., Salter, R. D., and Morel, P. A. (1999) Immunotherapy of NOD mice with bone marrow-derived dendritic cells. *Diabetes* **48,** 2300–2308.
109. Jansen, A., Homo-Delarche, F., Hooijkaas, H., Leenen, P. J., Dardenne, M., and Drexhage, H. A. (1994) Immunohistochemical characterization of monocytes-macrophages and dendritic cells involved in the initiation of the insulitis and beta-cell destruction in NOD mice. *Diabetes* **43,** 667–675.
110. Ludewig, B., Odermatt, B., Ochsenbein, A. F., Zinkernagel, R. M., and Hengartner, H. (1999) Role of dendritic cells in the induction and maintenance of autoimmune diseases. *Immunol. Rev.* **169,** 45–54.
111. Ludewig, B., Odermatt, B., Landmann, S., Hengartner, H., and Zinkernagel, R. M. (1998) Dendritic cells induce autoimmune diabetes and maintain disease via de novo formation of local lymphoid tissue. *J. Exp. Med.* **188,** 1493–1501.
112. Hoglund, P., Mintern, J., Waltzinger, C., Heath, W., Benoist, C., and Mathis, D. (1999) Initiation of autoimmune diabetes by developmentally regulated presentation of islet cell antigens in the pancreatic lymph nodes. *J. Exp. Med.* **189,** 331–339.
113. Takahashi, K., Honeyman, M. C., and Harrison, L. C. (1998) Impaired yield, phenotype, and function of monocyte-derived dendritic cells in humans at risk for insulin-dependent diabetes. *J. Immunol.* **161,** 2629–2635.

6

Role of T Cell Death and Cytokines in Autoimmunity

Luk Van Parijs and Abul K. Abbas

1. INTRODUCTION: CELL DEATH IN THE IMMUNE SYSTEM

The immune system is effective at fighting a vast diversity of microbes and eliminating toxic substances. In contrast to most other organ systems, the total number of immune cells can increase by a factor of two or more in a few days following an infection. This increase is often attributable to a 1000- to 50,000-fold expansion of the lymphocytes specific for the antigens of the microbe. At the same time, the immune system continuously generates new lymphocytes, each specific for a different antigen, in the hope that one or more of these will prove useful against future infections. In the face of this massive production of cells, the immune system has developed mechanisms to eliminate lymphocytes, so that it can maintain an optimal size and a balanced representation of cells. These mechanisms rely on an event called programmed cell death, or apoptosis.

The immune system also faces the challenge of preventing lymphocytes that express receptors specific for self-antigens from becoming activated and causing autoimmunity. Many of these harmful cells are eliminated by apoptotic cell death, either as they mature in the bone marrow or thymus, or when they respond to autoantigens in the body.

To balance the opposing needs of the immune system to eliminate harmful and excess cells while maintaining and amplifying protective ones, apoptosis has to be tightly regulated. As we shall discuss in this chapter, many of the signals that control lymphocyte cell death are regulated by cytokines. These soluble proteins provide a mechanism whereby useful cells can be identified and protected from apoptosis, while those that are defective or that respond to self-antigens can be targeted for elimination. As a consequence, defects in cytokine production or their signaling pathways are

From: *Cytokines and Autoimmune Diseases*
Edited by: V. K. Kuchroo, et al. © Humana Press Inc., Totowa, NJ

frequently associated with defects in cell death, and often have pathologic consequences.

2. MOLECULAR BASIS OF PROGRAMMED CELL DEATH

Lymphocytes and other cells can die as a result of a number of insults, including infection with microbes, trauma, and exposure to toxic substances. In many cases, these insults disrupt cellular metabolism or the integrity of the plasma membrane to an extent that they cause the cell to take up water and swell, and, ultimately, burst, spilling the cellular contents into the extracellular milieu. This disorganized, unprogrammed, and pathologic form of cell death is known as necrosis (*see* Table 1).

Cells also die in a more orderly manner by apoptosis (*see* Table 1). This form of death is characterized by several morphological phases. After apoptosis has been initiated, a cell releases contacts with its neighbors and starts to shrink by condensing its nucleus and cytoplasm. At the same time the plasma membrane starts to involute, and, ultimately, the whole cell breaks down into smaller apoptotic bodies. During this process, the nuclear envelope and nucleolus dissolve, and the cell condenses its chromatin, which is then cleaved into characteristic fragments of about 180 bp by specific endonucleases. The cell signals that it is undergoing apoptosis by allowing certain phospholipids, such as phosphatidyl serine, to flip from the cytoplasmic to the extracellular face of the plama membrane. These molecules serve as receptors for phagocytic cells that eliminate the apoptotic bodies. In contrast to necrosis, cell death by apoptosis does not result in the release of cellular contents, and therefore prevents the spread of intracellular pathogens and limits the inflammation caused by the dying cell. Apoptosis is not entirely immunologically silent, however, because antigen-presenting cells such as dendritic cells (DC), may acquire self- and foreign-antigens from apoptotic bodies and present these to T lymphocytes.

The genetic program that underlies apoptosis was first elucidated in the nematode, *Caenhorhabditis elegans (1)*. Eleven genes have been identified that are required for programmed cell death in this organism, but most of the principles of this process can be illustrated by considering how three key genes, *ced-3*, *ced-4*, and *ced-9* function. Importantly, these genes all have functional homologs in mammalian cells, and the basic mechanisms of apoptosis appear to have been conserved throughout evolution (*see* Fig. 1).

The product of the ced-3 gene is an aspartate-specific cysteine protease. Mammalian cells have a number of similar molecules, which are collectively called caspases *(2)*. These molecules exist in an inactive form in cells until apoptosis is initiated, at which time they are cleaved and become acti-

Table 1
Different Forms of Cell Death: Apoptosis vs Necrosis

	Apoptosis	Necrosis
Physiological role	Regulated elimination of cells	Pathological death of cells
Energy dependent	Yes	No
Key proteins	Caspases (cysteine proteases)	None
Condensation of nuclei and DNA degradation	Yes, chromatin cleaved into approx 180 bp fragments	No, degradation can occur but yields random-sized fragments
Disruption of plasma membrane	No, cell dissolves into multiple apoptotic bodies	Yes
Phagocytosis of dead cells	Yes	No
Release of intra-cellular pathogens	Limited	Yes
Processing of pro-inflammatory cytokines	Yes, especially IL-1 and IL-18	No, but release of cytoplasmic contents results in inflammation
Immunological consequence	Limited inflammation and T cell responses to antigens in apoptotic bodies? Involved in tolerance induction?	Inflammation

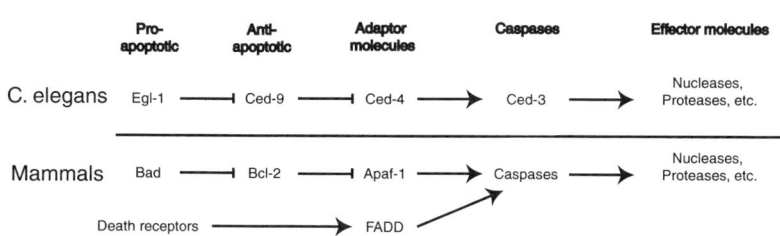

Fig. 1. Molecular basis of apoptosis. Only representative mammalian pro- and anti-apoptotic molecules are shown.

vated. The apoptosis signal is propagated and amplified by a caspase cascade where each activated casaspe in turn cleaves and activates a downstream component of the cascade. Finally, the terminal members of the caspase cascade activate a variety of effector molecules that are responsible for the cellular changes associated with apoptosis.

The activity of Ced-3, and caspases more generally, is largely regulated by Ced-9 and related molecules, such as Bcl-2 *(3)*. These block the activation of caspases and the apoptotic pathway by mechanisms that remain incompletely understood. Certain homologs of Ced-9 and Bcl-2, such as the *C. elegans* protein, Egl-1, and the mammalian proteins, Bad and Bax, have the opposite function. They promote apoptosis by binding to and inactivating Bcl-2. Therefore, whether a cell undergoes apoptotis or not is often dependent on the relative levels of the antiapoptotic and proapoptotic members of the Bcl-2 protein family.

Ced-4 and its mammalian homolog, APAF-1, function to initiate apoptosis by binding to caspases and bringing them together to form oligomers *(4)*. In these complexes, their low-level basal activity results in reciprocal cleavage and activation. Antiapoptotic molecules, like Ced-9 and Bcl-2, may function in part to block the formation of these caspase oligomers by binding to Ced-4. In mammalian cells, apoptosis can be initiated by a number of other molecules that bind caspases, most notably the death receptor proteins of the tumor necrosis factor receptor (TNF-R) family that are discussed later.

3. PASSIVE CELL DEATH AND ACTIVATION INDUCED CELL DEATH IN T CELLS

The ability to undergo programmed cell death is intrinsic to all cells of the immune system because they constitutively express the necessary effector molecules. However, the conditions and signals that cause lymphocytes to die vary greatly (*see* Fig. 2). After an infection has been cleared most of the protective lymphocytes die because the antigen to which they were responding has been eliminated and they no longer receive growth signals. Similarly, lymphocytes that do not develop normally die because they can not respond to extracellular signals that help keep healthy cells alive. This pathway of cell death is called passive cell death (or "death by neglect") because it occurs when lymphocytes are deprived of essential survival stimuli. However, lymphocytes can also be induced to undergo programmed cell death by chronic, or repetitive, antigen stimulation. This pathway of cell death is called activation-induced cell death (AICD) and serves to eliminate autoreactive cells.

Passive cell death and AICD are distinct not only in terms of their physiological roles, but also in how they are initiated and regulated (*see* Table 2). Lymphocytes are protected from passive cell death by antigen recognition, costimulation, and many cytokines, all of which promote cell survival by stimulating expression of anti-apoptotic proteins. Therefore, T cells undergo

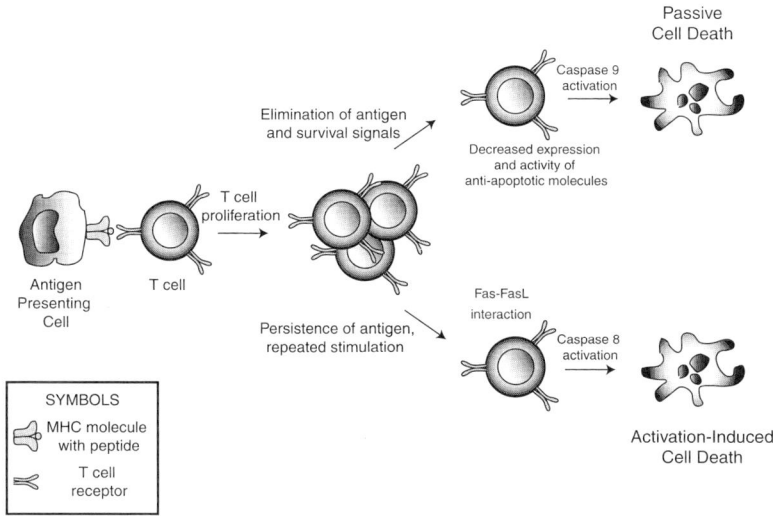

Fig. 2. Passive- and activation-induced cell death of T cells.

Table 2
**Different Pathways of Apoptosis in T Cells: Passive- vs
Activation-Induced Cell Death**

	Passive cell death ("death by neglect")	Activation-induced cell death
Physiological role	Homeostatic control of lymphocyte pool: loss of T cells that do not encounter antigen; elimination of activated T cells after infection has been cleared	Elimination of mature self-reactive lymphocytes
Induction	Absence of antigen and/or growth factors	Repeated antigenic stimulation
Sensitivity of naive and activated T cells	Both sensitive	Only activated cells sensitive
Role of antigen	Blocks	Induces
Role of IL-2	Blocks	Enhances
Role of other growth factors	Blocks	None
Role of Fas	None	Required to induce
Role of Bcl-2, Bcl-x	Blocks	None

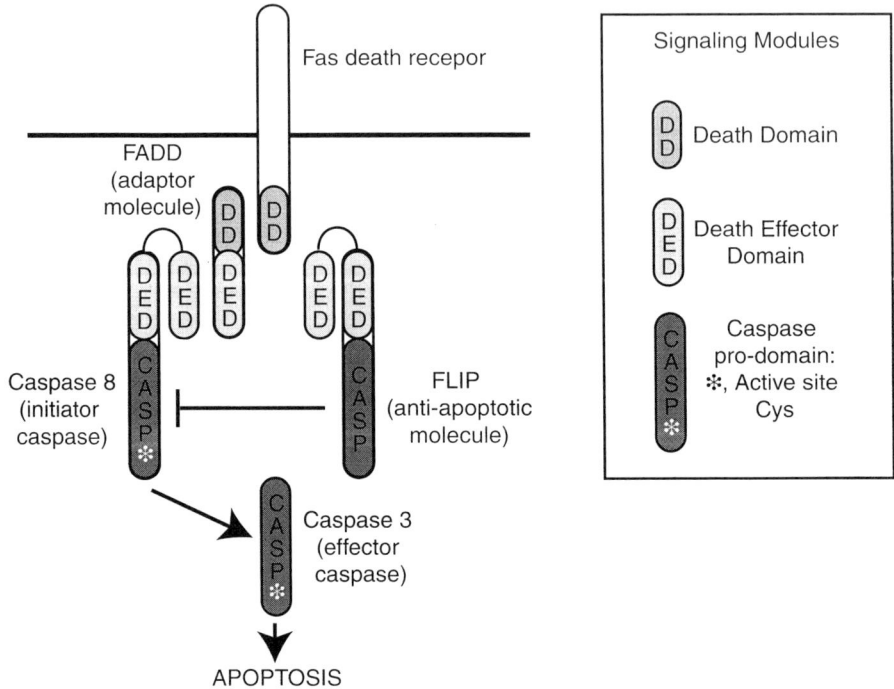

Fig. 3. Apoptosis signaling by Fas.

passive cell death when the level and activity of these antiapoptotic molecules, especially Bcl-2 and its related family members, drops below the threshold required to inhibit caspase activation. AICD, in contrast, is initiated by a specialized set of proteins that belong to the TNF-R family and are known as death receptors *(5)*. The best known of these, called Fas, is expressed on many cell types, including lymphocytes. Death receptors share a common feature, the presence in their cytoplasmic tails of a conserved motif called a death domain *(see* Fig. 3). These domains function as homotypic interaction modules that recruit intracellular adaptor molecules called FADD and TRADD to the crosslinked receptors upon ligation. These adaptor proteins in turn bind caspases via a distinct interaction motif called a death-effector domain. The types of caspases that are recruited to death receptors are called initiator caspases. By providing a direct link to caspase activation, death receptors can bypass the inhibition of cell death imposed by Bcl-2 in most cells. In fact, AICD can be induced in lymphocytes that express high levels of Bcl-2 and other proteins that block passive cell death *(6)*.

Although Fas is expressed constitutively on T cells, its ligand, FasL, is only induced on activated T cells that are responding to antigen *(see* Fig. 4) *(7)*.

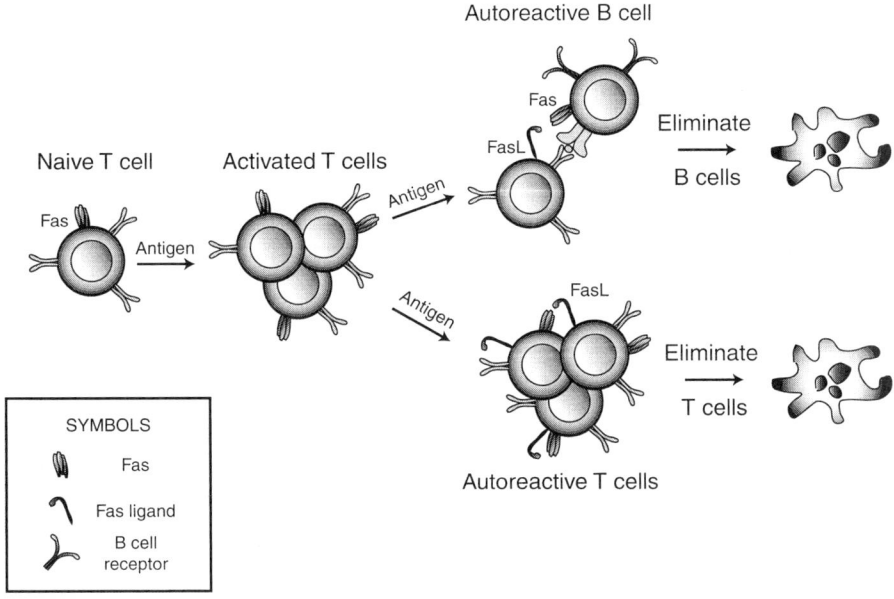

Fig. 4. Elimination of autoreactive B and T cells by Fas-mediated cell death.

Therefore, only activated T cells engage Fas and undergo AICD after exposure to antigen. Many autoreactive T cells are chronically stimulated by self-antigens, which is why they undergo AICD. FasL-expressing T cells are also responsible for eliminating other harmful cells, including autoreactive B cells and virally infected cells, by triggering Fas-mediated apoptosis (*see* Fig. 4) *(8,9)*. Because activated T cells express FasL during a protective immune response, the immune system has developed mechanisms to block AICD in useful cells. One molecule that can perform this function is called flice inhibitory protein (FLIP) *(10)*. FLIP is highly homologous to caspase 8, the first caspase that is recruited to death receptors and is responsible for initiating AICD. But FLIP is not catalytically active, and therefore functions as a competitive inhibitor of this caspase (Fig. 3). Importantly, FLIP is expressed at high levels in naive lymphocytes, as well as in activated lymphocytes that are resistant to AICD. Lymphocytes that lose FLIP expression following activation become sensitive to Fas-mediated AICD *(11)*. Therefore this molecule may serve as a switch between immunity and tolerance, protecting useful lymphocytes from apoptosis while allowing harmful cells to be eliminated. A number of viruses code for FLIP molecules, possibly to prevent the cells that they infect from being killed by AICD *(10)*.

4. CONSEQUENCES OF DISREGULATED CELL DEATH
IN THE IMMUNE SYSTEM

The pathophysiologic importance of passive cell death and AICD in the immune system has largely been defined using animal models with isolated defects in apoptosis. In transgenic mouse strains that overexpress the antiapoptotic molecules Bcl-2 or Bcl-x in B or T cells, the lymphocytes are resistant to passive cell death. These mice have increased numbers of lymphocytes and show prolonged responses to antigens *(3,6)*. In contrast, mice that lack these molecules or that carry transgenes for proapoptotic members of the Bcl-2 family, such as Bad, are more sensitive to passive cell death, and have decreased numbers of cells *(3,6,12)*. These experimental systems illustrate the role of passive cell death in maintaining homeostasis in the immune system, as well as regulating the magnitude and duration of immune responses to foreign antigens. In most cases, however, disrupting passive cell death does not affect immunological tolerance or cause autoimmunity by itself. Overexpression of Bcl-2 in B cells promotes the development of lupus-like autoimmunity in strains that are prone to autoimmune disease, probably because it increases B cell number and life-span rather than disrupting a mechanism for maintaining self-tolerance *(13)*.

The importance of AICD in maintaining tolerance to self antigens was established by studies of the autoimmune prone lpr (for lymphoproliferation) and gld (for generalized lymphoproliferation disease) mouse models. These strains develop a systemic autoimmune disease characterized by lymphadenopathy, the production of multiple autoantibodies, and nephritis, reminiscent of human systemic lupus erythematosus (SLE) *(14)*. The discovery that the autoimmunity in lpr mice resulted from a defect in the Fas gene, and, later, that gld mice carried a mutant FasL gene, provided the first molecular link between cell death and autoimmunity *(15)*. By breeding T or B cell receptor transgenic mice onto an lpr background, it became possible to follow Fas-deficient T and B cells as they responded to antigen. These systems showed that AICD was responsible for eliminating mature autoreactive lymphocytes as they responded to self-antigen *(16,17)*. More recently, AICD has been implicated in a human disease called autoimmune lymphoproliferative syndrome (ALPS), which is similar to the disease seen in lpr and gld mice. Many patients with this syndrome carry mutations in Fas, FasL, and at least one of the initiator caspases *(18,19)*.

5. REGULATION OF PASSIVE T CELL DEATH BY CYTOKINES

During an immune response, T cells, as well as other cell types, make cytokines that serve as growth and survival factors. Some of the most important of these are members of the interleukin-2 (IL-2) family, which includes IL-4, IL-7, IL-9, and IL-15, as well as IL-2. This group of cytokines share a common receptor component, called the common γ chain, but can also induce specific signals through unique receptor components *(20)*. The expression of these receptor components varies during T cell maturation and activation, so that immature T cells respond to IL-7, mature cells to IL-15, and activated cells to IL-2 and IL-4. Importantly, all cytokines of this family are able to protect T cells from passive cell death by inducing signaling pathways that increase the expression and activity of Bcl-2 and other antiapoptotic molecules, like AKT/protein kinase B *(see* Fig. 5) *(21,22)*. Mice that lack the common γ chain or IL-7 have greatly reduced numbers of immature T cells. The lack of IL-7 can be compensated by Bcl-2, suggesting that a major role of this cytokine is to protect immature lymphocytes from apoptosis *(23,24)*. In contrast, mice that are deficient in the unique α chain of the IL-15 receptor show decreased survival of mature T cells, implicating this cytokine in maintaining lymphocyte numbers *(25)*.

Naive and activated T cells are also protected from passive cell death by inflammatory cytokines, most notably IL-6, and interferon-α and -β *(26)*. These cytokines are secreted as part of the innate immune response to an infection and may function to promote T cell survival in inflammatory tissues. The mechanisms by which IL-6 and the interferons block passive cell death are not yet clear, but they appear to stimulate expression of Bcl-2 in T cells. Certain members of the TNF-R family, especially OX40 and 4-1BB, also can promote T cell survival. Because these molecules and their ligands are membrane-bound, they are traditionally thought of as costimulatory molecules *(27)*.

6. REGULATION OF AICD AND SELF-TOLERANCE BY CYTOKINES

In apparent contradiction to its role as an important T cell growth and survival factor, IL-2 also potentiates AICD. This is most noticeable in T cells from IL-2-deficient mice or mice that lack the α or β chain of the IL-2 receptor (IL-2R). These cells do not respond strongly to antigen stimulation in vitro, but do become activated. Activated IL-2-deficient cells, however, fail to upregulate FasL or downregulate FLIP, and do not undergo AICD when repeatedly stimulated *(see* Fig. 5) *(8)*. Both these molecular defects result from the failure to activate the IL-2-dependent transcription factor, Stat5 *(28)*. Stat5 is required to get high-level FasL expression on T cells and functions to inhibit the transcription of FLIP *(see* Fig. 5).

Most importantly, mice that are deficient in IL-2 accumulate activated T cells and develop autoimmunity *(8)*. This proves that IL-2 plays a nonredundant role in terminating T cell responses to self-antigens, whereas its role in promoting T cell growth and survival can be compensated by other cytokines. Superficially the autoimmune disease of IL-2-deficient mice appears similar to

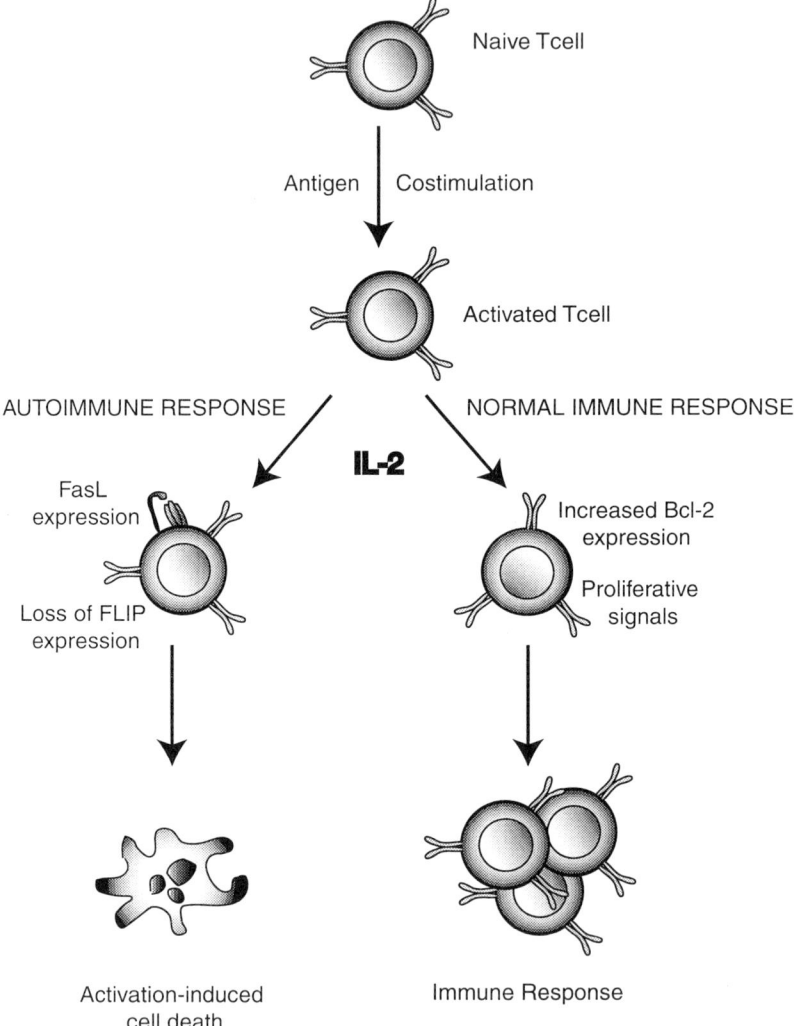

Fig. 5. Dual roles of IL-2 in T cell apoptosis and responses.

that of lpr and gld mice. All these mice accumulate mature lymphocytes in the peripheral lymphoid tissues and develop multiple autoantibodies including anti-double-stranded DNA antibodies. However, in contrast to lpr and gld mice, the most important autoantibodies in IL-2 knockout mice are directed against red blood cells and cause a fatal hemolytic anemia. Furthermore, the accumulating lymphocytes in IL-2-deficient animals are predominantly activated CD4$^+$ T cells, as opposed to the characteristic double negative (DN) (CD4$^-$CD8$^-$CD3$^+$) T cells that are responsible for the lymphadenopathy of lpr and gld mice. One reason for these differences may be that IL-2 is most important for regulating AICD of T cells, whereas in lpr and gld mice Fas-mediated elimination of both autoreactive T and B cells is defective. IL-2 may also serve other roles in addition to potentiating AICD that are important in the maintenance of self-tolerance. For instance, IL-2 may promote the development of regulatory T cells. IL-2-deficient T cells show defects in Th2 differentiation and IL-2 knockout mice also develop inflammatory bowel disease, a syndrome that is initiated by gut flora and occurs when regulatory T cells are absent *(29,30)*.

IL-2 has recently been implicated in the development of induced and spontaneous autoimmune diseases in mice, such as diabetes and experimental allergic encephalomyelitis (a mouse model for MS) *(31,32)*. In these disease models, a polymorphism of the IL-2 gene that decreases the stability of this cytokine appears to increase susceptibility to autoimmunity. It remains to be determined whether this less-stable variant of IL-2 is defective in promoting AICD or regulatory cell differentiation. The cell death-regulatory functions of IL-2 also are relevant in human T cells. Because a number of the autoimmune susceptibility loci identified in mice also appear to be involved in human disease, IL-2 may turn out to be involved more generally in self-tolerance and autoimmunity.

A second cytokine that can regulate AICD is IFN-γ. By activating the transcription factor Stat1, this cytokine increases the expression of caspase molecules, particularly those involved in Fas signaling (caspase 3 and 8) *(33)*. It is likely that this higher level of caspases makes T cells more sensitive to Fas crosslinking. In contrast to IL-2, IFN-γ deficiency does not lead to autoimmunity, but it does result in an accumulation of activated T cells following infection with viruses or mycobacteria *(34)*. Thus, IL-2 is produced rapidly following antigen recognition, and functions to stimulate T cell growth early in immune responses and to potentiate AICD if the responses persist, as with self-antigens. IFN-γ, on the other hand, is an effector cytokine that is secreted only after T cells have become activated. Therefore, IFN-γ may act to downregulate protective immune responses and prevent immune-mediated damage by promoting the elimination of activated T cells.

Certain Th2 cytokines, most notably IL-10 and transforming growth factor-β (TGF-β), have also been shown to modulate the sensitivity of T cells to AICD, usually decreasing it *(35,36)*. Interestingly, mice deficient in these cytokines show defects in immunological tolerance, although it is unclear that this is owing to a defect in cell death *(37,38)*. These observations suggest that the same factors that control T cell differentiation may also play a role in regulating the elimination of T cells by AICD.

7. CONCLUSION: DEFECTS IN CYTOKINE SIGNALING AND CELL DEATH THAT PREDISPOSE TO AUTOIMMUNITY

In this chapter, we have presented a summary of our current understanding of cell death regulation in T cells and how this relates to immunity and autoimmunity. A key concept is the existence of two distinct pathways of cell death in T cells: passive cell death and AICD. These different pathways of apoptosis play a central role in regulating distinct aspects of T cell responses. Passive cell death is important in regulating the number of T cells in the body, both before and after immune responses. When this form of apoptosis is defective, the consequence is either an accumulation of excess cells, which may lead to cancer, or a lack of cells, which may lead to immunodeficiencies. Defects in the cytokines that protect T cells from passive cell death or the receptors and signaling molecules that they use underlie a number of immunodeficiency syndromes in humans.

AICD, in contrast, functions to eliminate autoreactive lymphocytes and defects in this pathway of apoptosis lead to an increased susceptibility to autoimmune disease. IL-2, a cytokine that plays an important role in priming T cells for AICD, has been implicated as a susceptibility factor in a number of autoimmune diseases. Future research will further our understanding of how cytokines control T cell responses and tolerance by regulating their sensitivity to cell death.

REFERENCES

1. Hengartner, M. O. and Horvitz, H. R. (1994) Programmed cell death in Caenorhabditis elegans. *Curr. Opin. Genet. Dev.* **4,** 581–586.
2. Nicholson, D. W. and Thornberry, N. A. (1997) Caspases: killer proteases. *Trends Biochem. Sci.* **22,** 299–306.
3. Adams, J. M. and Cory, S. (1998) The Bcl-2 protein family: arbiters of cell survival. *Science* **281,** 1322–1326.
4. Yang, X., Chang, H. Y., and Baltimore, D. (1998) Essential role of CED-4 oligomerization in CED-3 activation and apoptosis. *Science* **281,** 1355–1357.
5. Nagata, S. (1997) Apoptosis by death factor. *Cell* **88,** 355–365.
6. Refaeli, Y., Van Parijs, L., and Abbas, A. K. (1999) Genetic models of abnormal apoptosis in lymphocytes. *Immunol. Rev.* **169,** 273–282.
7. Van Parijs, L., Ibraghimov, A., and Abbas, A. K. (1996) The roles of costimulation and Fas in T cell apoptosis and peripheral tolerance. *Immunity* **4,** 321–328.
8. Rathmell, J. C. and Goodnow, C. C. (1995) Autoimmunity. The Fas track. *Curr. Biol.* **5,** 1218–1221.
9. Shresta, S., Pham, C. T., Thomas, D. A., Graubert, T. A., and Ley, T. J. (1998) How do cytotoxic lymphocytes kill their targets? *Curr. Opin. Immunol.* **10,** 581–587.

10. Tschopp, J., Irmler, M., and Thome, M. (1998) Inhibition of fas death signals by FLIPs. *Curr. Opin. Immunol.* **10,** 552–558.

11. Van Parijs, L., Refaeli, Y., Abbas, A. K., and Baltimore, D. (1999) Autoimmunity as a consequence of retrovirus-mediated expression of C-FLIP in lymphocytes. *Immunity* **11,** 763–770.

12. Mok, C. L., Gil-Gomez, G., Williams, O., Coles, M., Taga, S., Tolaini, M., et al. Bad can act as a key regulator of T cell apoptosis and T cell development. *J. Exp. Med.* **189,** 575–586.

13. Strasser, A., Whittingham, S., Vaux, D. L., Bath, M. L., Adams, J. M., Cory, S,. and Harris, A. W. (1991) Enforced BCL2 expression in B-lymphoid cells prolongs antibody responses and elicits autoimmune disease. *Proc. Natl. Acad. Sci. USA* **88,** 8661–8665.

14. Cohen, P. L. and Eisenberg, R. A. (1991) Lpr and gld: single gene models of systemic autoimmunity and lymphoproliferative disease. *Annu. Rev. Immunol.* **9,** 243–269.

15. Nagata, S. and Suda, T. (1995) Fas and Fas ligand: lpr and gld mutations. *Immunol. Today* **16,** 39–43.

16. Rathmell, J. C., Cooke, M. P., Ho, W. Y., Grein, J., Townsend, S. E., Davis, M. M., et al. (1995) CD95 (Fas)-dependent elimination of self-reactive B cells upon interaction with CD4+ T cells. *Nature* **376,** 181–184.

17. Van Parijs, L., Peterson, D. A., and Abbas, A. K. (1998) The Fas/Fas ligand pathway and Bcl-2 regulate T cell responses to model self and foreign antigens. *Immunity* **8,** 265–274.

18. Straus, S. E., Sneller, M., Lenardo, M. J., Puck, J. M., and Strober, W. (1999) An inherited disorder of lymphocyte apoptosis: the autoimmune lymphoproliferative syndrome. *Ann. Intern. Med.* **130,** 591–601.

19. Wang, .J, Zheng, L., Lobito, A., Chan, F. K., Dale, J., Sneller, M., et al. (1999) Inherited human Caspase 10 mutations underlie defective lymphocyte and dendritic cell apoptosis in autoimmune lymphoproliferative syndrome type II. *Cell* **98,** 47–58.

20. Johnston, J. A., Bacon, C. M., Riedy, M. C., and O'Shea, J. J. (1996) Signaling by IL-2 and related cytokines: JAKs, STATs, and relationship to immunodeficiency. *J. Leukoc. Biol.* **60,** 441–452.

21. Van Parijs, L., Refaeli, Y., Lord, J. D., Nelson, B. H., Abbas, A. K., and Baltimore, D. (1999) Uncoupling IL-2 signals that regulate T cell proliferation, survival, and Fas-mediated activation-induced cell death. *Immunity* **11,** 281–288.

22. Nelms, K., Keegan, A. D., Zamorano, J., Ryan, J. J., and Paul, W. E. (1999) The IL-4 receptor: signaling mechanisms and biologic functions. *Annu. Rev. Immunol.* **17,** 701–738.

23. Maraskovsky, E., O'Reilly, L. A., Teepe, M., Corcoran, L. M., Peschon, J. J., and Strasser, A. (1997) Bcl-2 can rescue T lymphocyte development in interleukin-7 receptor-deficient mice but not in mutant rag-1-/- mice. *Cell* **89,** 1011–1019.

24. Akashi, K., Kondo, M., von Freeden-Jeffry, U., Murray, R., and Weissman, I. L. (1997) Bcl-2 rescues T lymphopoiesis in interleukin-7 receptor-deficient mice. *Cell* **89,** 1033–1041.

25. Lodolce, J. P., Boone, D. L., Chai, S., Swain, R. E., Dassopoulos, T., Trettin, S., and Ma, A. (1998) IL-15 receptor maintains lymphoid homeostasis by supporting lymphocyte homing and proliferation. *Immunity* **9,** 669–676.

26. Marrack, P., Mitchell, T., Bender, J., Hildeman, D., Kedl, R., Teague, K., and Kappler, J. (1998) T cell survival. *Immunol. Rev.* **165,** 279–285.

27. Watts, T. H. and DeBenedette, M. A. (1999) T cell co-stimulatory molecules other than CD28. *Curr. Opin. Immunol.* **11,** 286–293.

28. Van Parijs, L., Rafaeli, Y., Lord, J. D., Nelson, B. H., Abbas, A. K., and Baltimore, D. (1999) Uncoupling IL-2 signals that regulate T cell proliferation, survival, and Fas-mediated activation-induced cell death. *Immunity* **11,** 281–288.

29. Van Parijs, L., Biuckians, A., Ibragimov, A., Alt, F. W., Willerford, D. M., and Abbas, A. K. (1997) Functional responses and apoptosis of CD25 (IL-2R alpha)-deficient T cells expressing a transgenic antigen receptor. *J. Immunol.* **158,** 3738–3745.

30. MacDonald, T. T. (1994) Gastrointestinal inflammation. Inflammatory bowel disease in knockout mice. *Curr. Biol.* **4,** 261–263.

31. Denny, P., Lord, C. J., Hill, N. J., Goy, J. V., Levy, E. R., Podolin, P. L., et al. (1997) Mapping of the IDDM locus Idd3 to a 0.35-cM interval containing the interleukin-2 gene. *Diabetes* **46,** 695–700.

32. Encinas, J. A., Wicker, L. S., Peterson, L. B., Mukasa, A., Teuscher, C., Sobel, R., Weiner, H. L., et al. (1999) QTL influencing autoimmune diabetes and encephalomyelitis map to a 0.15-cM region containing Il2. *Nat. Genet.* **21,** 158–160.

33. Kumar, A., Commane, M., Flickinger, T. W., Horvath, C. M., and Stark, G. R. (1997) Defective TNF-alpha-induced apoptosis in STAT1-null cells due to low constitutive levels of caspases. *Science* **278,** 1630–1632.

34. Dalton, D. K., Pitts-Meek, S., Keshav, S., Figari, I. S., Bradley, A., and Stewart, T. A. (1993) Multiple defects of immune cell function in mice with disrupted interferon-gamma genes. *Science* **259,** 1739–1742.

35. Zhang, X., Giangreco, L., Broome, H. E., Dargan, C. M., and Swain, S. L. (1995) Control of CD4 effector fate: transforming growth factor beta 1 and interleukin 2 synergize to prevent apoptosis and promote effector expansion. *J. Exp. Med.* **182,** 699–709.

36. Zhang, X., Brunner, T., Carter, L., Dutton, R. W., Rogers, P., Bradley, L., et al. (1997) Unequal death in T helper cell (Th)1 and Th2 effectors: Th1, but not Th2, effectors undergo rapid Fas/FasL-mediated apoptosis. *J. Exp. Med.* **185,** 1837–1849.

37. Kuhn, R., Lohler, J., Rennick, D., Rajewsky, K., and Muller, W. (1993) Interleukin-10-deficient mice develop chronic enterocolitis. *Cell* **75,** 263–274.

38. Shull, M. M., Ormsby, I., Kier, A. B., Pawlowski, S., Diebold, R. J., Yin, M., et al. (1992) Targeted disruption of the mouse transforming growth factor-beta 1gene results in multifocal inflammatory disease. *Nature* **359,** 693–699.

7

Role of Chemokines and Their Receptors in the Induction and Regulation of Autoimmune Disease

Richard M. Ransohoff and William J. Karpus

1. CHEMOKINES AND CHEMOKINE RECEPTORS

1.1. Chemokines: Families and Nomenclature

Chemokines are a large superfamily of approximately 50 peptides. Although they are involved in diverse processes, their central and defining role in mammals appears to be action toward subpopulations of leukocytes *(1)*. This specificity is mediated by selective expression of chemokine receptors, heptahelical G-protein coupled membrane molecules. With time and further study, chemokines have now been implicated in developmental organogenesis, angiogenesis, neoplasia, differentiation, and a host of other physiological and pathological processes *(2,3)*. Considerable interest has been sparked by the discovery that several chemokine receptors are essential invasion coreceptors for human immunodeficiency virus (HIV)-1 and HIV-2 infection of human cells *(4,5)*.

Given the size and complexity of the chemokine family, organizing principles are essential for initiating focused meaningful study of their biology in both health and disease. Fortunately, some such principles are readily apparent. All elements with chemokine activity are small (10–15 kDa) and exhibit a conserved structure, which features a core globular β barrel established by three anti-parallel β-strands. This core is flanked by a highly basic C-terminal α helix and a short, relatively disordered N-terminal segment *(6)*. The N-terminal segment contains most or all of the structural information required for receptor specificity *(7)*. Therefore, naturally occurring proteolytic modifications of the N-terminal segments of chemokine peptides can dramatically change receptor affinity or specificity *(8–10)*. Furthermore,

From: *Cytokines and Autoimmune Diseases*
Edited by: V. K. Kuchroo, et al. © Humana Press Inc., Totowa, NJ

engineered modifications of the chemokine N-terminus can give rise to peptides with potent receptor-blocking activity *(11)*.

The core structures of chemokines are maintained in part by disulfide
bonds between cysteine resides that are positionally conserved *(6)*. For the
great majority of chemokine peptides, a recognizable structural characteristic is the distribution of four cysteines within the molecule. A conve-
nient informal terminology for the chemokines has been derived from the
observation that subfamilies of chemokine peptides are distinguished by
the organization of the cysteines near the N-terminus of the molecule.
Using this algorithm, four chemokine peptide families have been
described. In the first, or α-chemokine family, the initial two cysteines are
separated by a single residue. Thus, the α-chemokines are also known as
"CXC chemokines." In the β-chemokine family, the first two cysteines are
adjacent, giving rise to the term "CC chemokines." Lymphotactin, a peptide with all the characteristic features of a chemokine, has a single C residue near the N-terminus and defines the family of γ or "C chemokines."
The fourth family of chemokine elements is defined by a molecule termed
fractalkine, which is a unique component of the chemokine superfamily.
Fractalkine is expressed as a typical chemokine motif, tethered to the cell
membrane by a transmembrane anchor, and "presented" by a long mucin-
like stalk. The N-terminal cysteines of fractalkine are separated by three
residues and fractalkine defines the family of δ or "CX3C chemokines."
Beyond their structural similarities, the chemokine subfamilies exhibit
genetic association as well. Many CXC chemokines are encoded in a
multigene array on human chromosome four. Most, but not all, CC
chemokines are encoded in a similar large array on human chromosome
17. Lymphotactin and fractalkine are encoded elsewhere in the genome. A
substantial, current and practical chemokine website is maintained at:
http://cytokine.medic.kumamoto-u.jp/CFC/CK/chemokine.html.

A simplifying nomenclature for the chemokines and receptors has been
proposed and a current version is shown in Table 1 (modified from ref. *12*).
This scheme takes the chemokine subfamily name (e.g., CC or CX3C), adds
the designator "L" for ligand or "R" for receptor, and appends a unique
number. For ligands, the number indicates chronological order of characterization by molecular cloning. The ligand designations will be provided in
this review, for illustrative purposes, although the nomenclature is not
widely employed at present. The receptor nomenclature is more firmly
established. For the receptors, the order of numeration includes demonstration of molecular uniqueness; characterizing specific binding of ligand(s);
and documenting biological function (either calcium flux, chemotactic
response, or other signaling).

Table 1
The Chemokine Superfamily

Systematic name	Ligand (human)	Ligand (mouse)	Receptor(s)
C Family			
XCL1;2	Lymphotactin, SCM-1α ATAC; SCM-1β	Lymphotactin	XCR1
CC Family			
CCL1	I309	TCA-3, P500	CCR8
CCL2	MCP-1, MCAF	JE, MCP-1	CCR2
CCL3	MIP-1α, LD78α/β, AT 464.1/2, GOS19-1/2	MIP-1α	CCR1, CCR5
CCL4	MIP-1β, AT744.1, AT744.2, Act-2, G-26, HC21, H400, LAG-1	MIP-1β	CCR5
CCL5	RANTES	RANTES	CCR1, 3, 5
CCL6	?	C10, MRP-1	?
CCL7	MCP-3	NC28, FIC, MARC	CCR1, 2, 3
CCL8	MCP-2, HC14	MCP-2	CCR2, 3
CCL9, 10	MRP-2,CCF18, MIP-1γ	?	?
CCL11	Eotaxin	Eotaxin	CCR3
CCL12	?	MCP-5	CCR2
CCL13	MCP-4, NCC-1, CKβ-10	?	CCR2, 3
CCL14	HCC-1, HCC-3, NCC-2	?	CCR1
CCL15	HCC-2, MIP-1δ, NCC-3, MIP-5, Lkn-1	?	CCR1, 3
CCL16	HHC-4, NCC-4, LEC, LMC	LCC-1	CCR1
CCL17	TARC, dendrokine	TARC	CCR4
CCL18	DC-CK1, PARC, MIP-4, AMAC-1	?	?

(*continued*)

Table 1 *(continued)*

Systematic name	Ligand (human)	Ligand (mouse)	Receptor(s)
CCL19	MIP-3β, ELC, exodus-3, CKβ-11	MIP-3β	CCR7
CCL20	MIP-3α, LARC, exodus-1	MIP-3α	CCR6
CCL21	TCA4, exodus-2, SLC,	6Ckine	CCR7
CCL22	MDC, STCP-1, DCactin-β	ABCD-1	CCR4
CCL23	MPIF-1, MIP-3, CKβ-8, CKβ-8-1	?	CCR1
CCL24	Eotaxin-2, MPIF-2, CKβ-6	?	CCR3
CCL25	TECK	TECK	CCR9a,b
CCL26	Eotaxin-3	?	CCR3
CCL27	CTACK/ALP	CTAK, ALP	CCR10
CCL28	MEC	?	?
CXC Family			
CXCL1	GRO-1, GRO-α, MGSA-α	GRO (KC)	CXCR2, 1
CXCL2	GRO-2, GRO-β, MIP-2α, MGSA-β	GRO (KC)	CXCR2
CXCL3	GRO-3, GRO-β, MIP-2β	GRO (KC)	CXCR2
CXCL4	PF4	PF4var1, PF4alt	?
CXCL5	ENA-78	LIX	CXCR2
CXCL6	GCP-2	Ckα-3	CXCR1, 2
CXCL7	NAP-2	?	CXCR2
CXCL8	IL-8, MDNCF, NAP-1, NCF	?	CXCR1, 2
CXCL9	Mig, HuMig	Mig	CXCR3
CXCL10	IP-10	crg-2, mob-1	CXCR3
CXCL11	β-R1, I-TAC, H174	mI-TAC	CXCR3
CXCL12	SDF-1α, SDF-1β, PBSF	SDF-1α/β	CXCR4
CXCL13	BLC, BCA01	BLR1L, Angie	CXCR5
CXCL14	BRAK, bolekine	BRAK	?
CXCL15	?	Lungkine	?
CXCL16	?	?	CXCR6
CX3C Family			
CX3Cl1	Fractalkine	Fractalkine	CX3CR-1

1.2. Chemokines

1.2.1. CXC Chemokines

The CXC chemokines are a relatively diverse family with significant functional differences among subfamilies. Division into subfamilies is based on structural and functional characteristics. The prototype human CXC chemokine is CXCL8/interleukin 8 (IL-8) *(13)*. IL-8 is a neutrophil chemoattractant; structural analysis of several neutrophil-specific chemokines disclosed the presence of a conserved glutamate-leucine-arginine (ELR) motif near the N-terminus of the molecule. Subsequently, it was determined that all neutrophil-specific chemokines contained this motif and that CXC chemokines that failed to act toward neutrophils lacked it *(6,14,15)*. Therefore, the CXC chemokines are divided further into "ELR-positive" and "ELR-negative" subfamilies.

1.2.1.1. ELR-POSITIVE CXC CHEMOKINES

As noted earlier, these chemokines function toward neutrophils. There are seven ELR-positive CXC chemokines in the human system (CXCL1-CXCL3, CXCL5-CXCL8) and rodent orthologs have been described. The ELR motif defines the ability to bind to neutrophil-specific chemokine receptors *(14)*. In the human system, these receptors include CXCR1 and CXCR2. Mice lack both IL-8 and CXCR1.

A particularly interesting member of the ELR-positives CXC chemokine family is termed growth-regulated oncogene-α (GRO-α)/CXCL1. This chemokine has been discovered and studied in two completely different contexts: as a product related to the transformed state of cells; and as a typical neutrophil-specific ELR-positive CXC chemokine. KC, the mouse ortholog of GRO-α was initially cloned in 1982 in a differential hybridization experiment that was designed to identify platlet-derived growth factor (PDGF)-inducible genes in quiescent NIH 3T3 fibroblasts *(16)*. Several years thereafter, human GRO-α was identified, in studies that began with subtractive hybridization experiments to characterize genes that were highly expressed in tumorigenic Chinese hamster ovary (CHO) cell derivatives. The human homolog of one gene identified by this screen was termed "growth-regulated oncogene," after demonstrations that its transcription was stringently governed by growth conditions in non-neoplastic cells but loosened in tumor cell lines *(17)*. Subsequently, investigators studying a melanoma-cell autocrine growth factor (termed melanocyte growth stimulatory activity; MGSA) purified and cloned its cDNA and showed identity to human GRO-α *(18)*. Additionally, workers studying sarcomas induced in avian species by Rous sarcoma virus (RSV) identified a gene called CEF4 that was highly expressed in transformed chick fibroblasts *(19)*. With detailed sequence comparison, it was discovered that human GRO-α/MGSA was orthologous to murine KC and homologous to avian CEF4 *(20)*. More recently, it was determined that GRO-α provides a powerful proliferative signal for PDGF-stimulated oligodendrocyte progenitors *(21,22)*. At the same time, ELR-positive CXC chemokines have been implicated in many forms of neutrophilic inflammation and are considered potent mediators of angiogenesis *(23)*. These varied attributes have led to the suggestion that the principal physiological function of the three GRO peptides (CXCL1-CXCL3) is to promote wound-healing *(24)*.

1.2.1.2. ELR-NEGATIVE CXC CHEMOKINES

The ELR-negative CXC chemokines are a more diverse group. They include the first described chemokine peptide, platelet factor 4 (PF4)/ CXCL4 *(25)*. Despite its relative antiquity in this field, PF4 lacks a defined receptor *(26)*. In the context of immune-mediated inflammation, more salient roles are played by other non-ELR CXC chemokines including IP-10/ CXCL10, mig/CXCL9 and, possibly, β-R1/I-TAC/CXCL11 *(27)*. All these chemokines are ligands for a receptor termed CXCR3 *(28)* that is highly expressed on activated T cells *(29,30)*. To date, non-ELR CXC chemokines appear to be inert towards neutrophils *(31)*.

Another non-ELR CXC chemokine of considerable biological importance is stromal cell derived factor (SDF)-1 α/β/CXCL12. SDF-1, as its name implies, is expressed highly in bone marrow by stromal cells. However, SDF-1 is also expressed in a surprisingly large variety of other cells and tissues. Mutant mice that were rendered deficient for this chemokine (or for its receptor, CXCR4) accordingly showed a complex phenotype of impaired B cell lymphopoiesis, abnormal myelopoiesis, fatal ventricular septal defect, abnormal cerebellar organogenesis, and defective gastrointestinal vascularization *(32–40)*. SDF-1 and CXCR4 are considered representative of an ancestral chemokine/receptor pair that was initially committed to directing cell migration during embryonic organogenesis and subsequently was adapted for use by the migrating cells of the adult hematopoietic/immune system. It is of interest that a CXCR4 homolog described in the rainbow trout exhibits more than 80% similarity with the human protein *(41)*, consistent with a highly conserved functional role for this receptor.

A non-ELR CXC chemokine also plays an important role in B cell development by establishing lymph-node follicles. This chemokine, termed BLC/ CXCL13, is a ligand for CXCR5. Mice that were rendered deficient for CXCR5 failed to form appropriate architecture in secondary lymphoid organs because of loss of signaling by BLC through its receptor *(42)*.

1.2.2. CC Chemokines

CC chemokines constitute a large and diverse family (currently 28 human ligands) that signal to 11 defined receptors. For the most part, CC chemokines act towards cells that are implicated in adaptive and innate immune responses. These cells include the lymphocytes, monocytes, dendritic cells (DC), basophils, eosinophils, and mast T cells. Recent and elegant studies using gene-targeting strategies have implicated the CC chemokines in both organogenesis and function of the secondary lymphoid organs. At present, these experiments constitute the best indicators of the means by which chemokines direct T cell migration within an intact organism.

The CC chemokines can loosely be organized into functional subfamilies, as described later. However, because of complex, subtle biology and promiscuous ligand-receptor relationships, one cannot group the CC chemokines into functional subgroups as easily as one can do for the CXC chemokines.

1.2.2.1. MCPs

One group of CC chemokines sharing a certain degree of functional and structural similarity is represented by the monocyte chemoattractant proteins or MCPs. The first cloned MCP was the murine JE gene product, isolated in the same differential hybridization protocol that resulted in the identification of KC *(16)*. JE was later shown to exhibit identity with murine MCP-1 and high homology with human MCP-1/CCL2 *(43,44)*. The various MCPs were isolated in parallel in differential hybridization cloning experiments and by biochemical purification from cell-culture supernatants in studies designed to characterize monocyte chemoattractants *(45)*. Biochemical studies resulted in the isolation of activities in culture supernatants that were later shown to be MCP-1, MCP-2/CCL8, and MCP-3/CCL7 *(46,47)*. Cultures of human glioma cells were a particularly fertile source of MCPs *(48)*.

All MCPs exhibit potent chemoattractant activity toward monocytes. Several of the MCPs also act in vitro toward T cells *(49)*. The precise biological roles of the various MCPs remains to be defined fully. However, experiments using mice that were deleted for MCP-1 revealed a startling degree of biologically specific non-redundancy for this particular chemokine. In detailed studies, it was shown that MCP-1-deficient mice failed to accumulate monocytes in the peritoneal infiltrate that results from thioglycollate installation *(50,51)*. Furthermore, MCP-1-null mice exhibited impaired generation of T helper 2 (Th2) responses and tremendously retarded atherosclerosis *(1–4)*. Uncertain (but important) is the determination whether the phenotype of MCP-1-null mice results from the characteristics of regulation of expression of this chemokine or from structure-function attributes that were not evident in cell-culture studies. Significantly, the activities of all MCPs in vitro appear virtually identical *(47)*. Therefore, in vivo studies are essential for establishing function.

1.2.2.2. MIP–1

MIP-1α/CCL3 and MIP-1β/CCL4were initially identified biochemically as an activity termed macrophage inflammatory protein (MIP)-1 and later shown to contain two distinct components, as named earlier *(26)*. MIP-1α is a potent ligand for CCR1, while MIP-1β acts predominantly towards CCR5. MIP-1α also engages CCR3 and to a lesser extent CCR5. Both chemokines act toward monocytes and T cells. It is likely that MIP-1α also acts towards neutrophils in certain instances of inflammation in mice as suggested by in vitro studies and elegantly shown through the study of pulmonary inflammation in CCR1-deficient mice *(52)*. MIP-1α-deficient mice exhibited striking inability to clear a pulmonary challenge with influenza virus. Furthermore, such mice did not develop inflammatory myocarditis after infection with coxsackie B virus *(53,54)*.

MIP-1α is a potent and selective regulator of TH1 commitment by T cells in vitro as described below. Furthermore, antibodies to MIP-1α were used in the first demonstration that chemokines could function to regulate neuro-inflammatory disease such as experimental autoimmune encephalomyelitis (EAE) *(55)*.

1.2.2.3. RANTES

RANTES/CCL5 (regulated upon activation, normal T cell, expressed, and secreted) is a β-chemokine implicated in a wide variety of T cell-mediated inflammatory processes. This chemokine engages varied receptors, including CCR1, CCR3, and CCR5. Interestingly, CCR3 is expressed by Th2-committed T cells, while CCR5 is associated with Th1 responses *(56–61)*. Thus, RANTES may be involved in both Th1- and Th2-biased patterns of T cell-dependent inflammation, although its major function appears to involve promotion of Th1 and suppression of Th2 reactions *(62)*. In common with all chemokines, RANTES delivers chemotactic signals for directional migration and activating stimuli for integrin-mediated adhesion to cell-adhesion molecules (CAMs). Atypically, RANTES also mediates T cell-receptor independent proliferative events for T cells, at high concentrations *(63)*. Additionally, RANTES was shown to guide directional migration by dorsal root ganglion (DRG) neurons in vitro *(64)*. The receptor that transduces this effect is undefined, as neither MIP-1α (CCR1, CCR5 ligand) nor MIP-1β (CCR5 ligand) was functional in this assay *(64)*.

1.2.2.4. ELC, SLC

ELC/CCL19 and SLC/CCL21, in contrast to other CC chemokines described earlier, are expressed constitutively, primarily in secondary lymphoid organs. The specific means by which secondary lymphoid tissue chemokine (SLC) and ELC and their receptor, CCR7, participate in establishing secondary lymphoid organs have been recently reviewed in detail *(65,66)* and will be described briefly here and below. SLC was detected on high endothelial venules (HEV), by which naive T cells enter lymph nodes (LN). ELC was expressed within the T cell zones of LN, along with SLC. Several lines of genetic research led to the assignment of functional significance to these expression patterns. First, it was discovered that mice in which SLC and/or ELC expression patterns were disrupted also lacked appropriate organization of secondary lymphoid organs. Such mice included the paucity of LN T cell *(plt)* naturally occurring phenotype, that lacked expression of SLC, resulting in deficient formation of T cell zones in LN and spleen *(67)*. The *plt* mutation proved to result in deletion of one of two SLC genes, with the affected gene expressed preferentially in lymphoid tissues *(68)*. Engineered mutations in the lymphotoxin (LT)-α or -β and tumor necrosis factor receptor (TNF-R) 1 genes also led to varying patterns of disruption of organization of both T cell and B-cell zones in LN and spleen *(69)*. These defects proved to be determined by impaired expression of ELC and SLC (more prominent in LT-α or LT-β-deficiency than in TNF-R mutants), as well as BLC (observed with all mutations in the LT, TNF, or TNF-R genes). Recently, the alymphoplasia *(aly)* mutation, which also exhibits disordered lymphoid architecture, was shown to result from a point mutation in the nuclear factor-κ binding (NFκB)-inducing kinase (NIK) gene, thereby placing this element downstream of the TNF receptors in generating the chemokine expression required for secondary lymphoid organogenesis *(70)*.

1.3. Regulation of Chemokine Gene Expression

Regulation of cytokine gene expression is discussed in Chapter 1 by Glimcher and Rengarajan. Therefore, comments in this section will be restricted to chemokines.

As an overview, it is worthwhile to clarify two general patterns of chemokine expression: "constitutive" and "inflammatory." Chemokines such as SDF-1α and SLC are expressed under basal conditions in vivo and are designated constitutive chemokines. Peptides such as IP-10 and RANTES are strongly upregulated by inflammatory challenge in vivo and are considered to be inflammtory chemokines. Supporting these concepts, gene-targeted mice that are deficient for constitutive chemokines exhibit phenotypes of impaired organogenesis, as described earlier. However, it has become clear that constitutive chemokines can be upregulated by inflammatory challenge, and that inflammatory chemokines can be expressed under basal conditions. One particularly salient example is MCP-1, a typical inflammatory chemokine, which is expressed in secondary lymphoid organs and regulates commitment to the Th2 phenotype *(4)*.

The great majority of effort has been directed toward the understanding of regulation of inflammatory chemokine gene expression. One historical note: most if not all inflammatory chemokines were isolated at various times in differential hybridization experiments, using cytokine or growth factor-stimulated cells of various lineage. From this attribute, chemokines have been termed the "crab grass in every differential hybridization experiment." This historical fact also underscores the remarkably efficient and brisk transcriptional response of chemokine genes to inflammatory stimuli. Indeed, in many laboratories, chemokine gene promoters are utilized as model systems for the examination of transcriptional regulation.

The stimuli that regulate chemokine gene expression will readily suggest the regulatory principles that underlie this dramatic transcriptional response. It should be noted that most chemokine gene expression appears to be regulated at the transcriptional level and that relatively little information is available about post-transcriptional regulatory principles.

Returning to the more common theme, that of transcriptional regulation of chemokine genes, it has repeatedly been observed that individual inflammatory stimuli (such as interferon-γ [IFN-γ], tumor necrosis factor-α [TNF-α], IL-1, lipopolysaccharide [LPS]) induce such genes modestly but that combinations of these stimuli exert highly synergistic stimulatory effects. Examination of chemokine gene promoters reveals almost invariably that the promoters exhibit a large menu of stimulus-response *cis*-elements. These elements typically include interferon-stimulated response elements (ISRE), gamma activated sites (GAS elements), NFκB binding sites, AP-1 binding sites, and several others. In detailed structure-function analyses of these promoters, it is typically found that elimination of any one of the responding *cis*-elements from the promoter eliminates synergy and markedly reduces inducibility of promoter reporters bearing the mutation. Investigation of both murine and human IP-10 gene promoters has illustrated these concepts *(71–78)*. Interestingly, these two promoters contain three regulatory elements (one ISRE and two NFκB binding sites) whose sequence content and organization are absolutely conserved, while the remainder of the 5'-flanking sequence diverges markedly *(71)*.

In common with other cytokines genes chemokine messages frequently contain AU-rich regions in the 3'-UTR region, conferring instability and resulting in extremely rapid message turnover. Therefore, as a general state-ment, chemokine genes accumulate to high levels extremely rapidly, under transcriptional control; following dramatic accumulation, brisk decay of message levels is the rule. One prominent example of post-transcriptional regulation concerns the murine KC gene. Transcriptional upregulation of KC mRNA in murine macrophages by lipopolysaccharide (LPS) is sup-pressed by the cytokine IL-10, through a post-transcriptional mechanism that operates through a cluster of AU-rich elements *(79,80)*.

Clearly, there is much more information about the regulation of the inflammatory chemokines than the constitutively expressed chemokines. Elements that maintain high levels of SDF-1, for example, remain to be char-acterized. It is of considerable interest to note that maintenance of high levels of ELC and SLC transcripts in secondary lymphoid organs requires signaling by the lymphotoxins through TNF receptors and depends on the post-receptor kinase NIK *(69,70)*. Therefore, constitutive and inflammatory chemokine expression are regulated in this case by overlapping mechanisms *(81)*.

Translational control of chemokine expression has not been extensively characterized or described. Interestingly, post-translational regulatory control for chemokine function has been described in several cases. One particu-larly well-documented instance concerns the chemokine RANTES and the dipeptidyl dipeptidase, CD26. Using RANTES as a substrate, CD26 con-verts full-length RANTES (1–68), a potent ligand for CCR1, into truncated RANTES (3–68), which preferentially utilizes CCR5 *(9)*. Similar truncation of the CXC chemokine GCP-2/CXCL6 has no apparent effect on receptor utilization *(82)*.

A particularly parsimonious use of post-translational peptide-processing is illustrated by platelet basic protein (PBP), which gives rise to a proteolytic series including connective tissue activating peptide III (CTAP-III) and upon further cleavage to neutrophil activating peptide 2 (NAP-2). NAP-2/CXCL7 is a member of the ELR-positive CXC chemokine family and is a potent neutrophil-specific chemoattractant. However, absent proteolytic process-ing no neutrophil-directed chemoattractant activity is detected in prepara-tions of purified CTAP-III *(83,84)*.

1.4. Chemokine Receptors

1.4.1. Common Structure

Chemokine receptors belong to the superfamily of G-protein coupled receptors (GPCR). The GCPR are a large family of biologically important receptors with conserved structure and signaling properties. Perhaps the best-characterized family members are the adrenergic receptors and the retinal rhodopsins. GPCR exhibit a heptahelical disposition in the plasma membrane, with residues in the intramembrane helices being highly conserved within families. The N-terminal segments and extracellular loops one, two, and three constitute the ligand-binding domains of the receptors and vary, to impart ligand specificity. The intracellular loops and C-terminal tails of GPCR provide sites of association with signaling components, and vary, consistent with different signaling outputs of the various receptors. The GPCR are believed to be the largest superfamily of human genes, and constitute important targets for small-molecule therapeutics. Chemokine receptors belong to the family of group A GPCR, and to the subfamily of peptide-specific GPCR, thus being closely related to the receptors for C5a anaphylotoxin and the bacterial N-formylated peptides, such as N-formylmethionine-leucine-proline (fMLP). Useful information about GPCR can be obtained at the website: http://www.gpcr.org/7tm/html.

The juxtamembrane portion of the second intracellular loop of chemokine receptors contains a conserved DRYLAIV motif, which is found in all signaling chemokine receptors to date, and is a variant of the acidic residue-arginine-aromatic residue motif found at this position in all GPCR. Exceptions to this rule are the nonsignaling promiscuous chemokine receptor-like molecules, Duffy antigen receptor for chemokines (DARC) and D6 *(85–87)*. Both D6 and DARC bind many CC and CXC chemokines with low-nanomolar efficiency, despite their lack of signaling competence. D6 and DARC have provisionally been termed "chemokine-binding molecules" in preference to "chemokine receptors." Clearly, these observations strongly support the functional significance of the conserved DRYLAIV motif.

It is suspected that DARC and D6 exert nonsignaling functions such as immobilization of chemokines on endothelial surfaces, for "presentation" to passing leukocytes. DARC is differentially expressed on erythrocytes and endothelia, probably because of its adventitious function as the invasion receptor for *Plasmodium vivax,* a major human pathogen *(88,89).* Duffy is accordingly downregulated on erythrocytes of individuals from malaria-endemic areas, but is expressed on postcapillary venules even in people that are Duffy-negative on erythrocytes *(90,91).* Interestingly, DARC is expressed in the CNS on a population of cerebellar Purkinje cell neurons and is upregulated at the mRNA level in brain tissue of Multiple Sclerosis (MS) patients *(92–94).*

1.4.2. Nomenclature

A useful nomenclature for chemokine receptors has been established, as noted earlier. Molecular entities are assigned status as chemokine receptors upon demonstration that they represent a specific molecular species, that selective high-affinity ligand binding can be demonstrated and that signaling (preferentially with biological response) can be documented. Using this approach, there are at present 18 defined chemokine receptors (CCR1-10, CXCR1-1, XCR1, CX3CR1). Chemokine receptors are assigned to families by virtue of binding ligands from the structurally defined chemokine families. This nomenclature implies (which is indeed the case) that receptors preferentially bind ligands from individual families. Thus, CXCRs preferentially bind CXC chemokines, CCRs prefer to bind CC chemokines, and so forth. There are individual reports that CC chemokine bind CXC receptors, generally with high-nanomolar affinity and occasionally with effects that suggest antagonist function *(95)*. Despite these exceptions, the chemokine receptor nomenclature has been highly effective and useful.

1.4.3. Ligand-Receptor Relationships

Ligand-receptor relationships in the chemokine superfamily are complex. The receptors have been operationally subdivided according to the complexity of their relationships to ligands into various groups *(96)*. Thus, the private receptors (for example CXCR1) bind only a single ligand, in this case IL-8 (although it was recently reported that GCP-2/CXCL6 is also a full ligand at CXCR1). The public receptors (for example, CXCR2) bind multiple ligands (all seven ELR-positive CXC chemokines: IL-8, three GRO peptides, NAP-2, GCP-2, and ENA-78). The promiscuous receptors (DARC, D-6) bind multiple chemokines of several families, but do not signal or transduce biological effects. There is a substantial population of orphan receptors to which ligands have not yet been assigned but for which structural analysis indicates likely membership in the chemokine receptor family.

The fact that most chemokine receptors can respond to a diversity of ligands in vitro can lead to a confusing impression of redundancy in the chemokine system. Experiments in gene-targeted animals indicate that functional redundancy in vivo is not the rule. These disparate results of experiments in vitro and in vivo suggest that the apparent overabundance of chemokines and receptors is a reflection of intricate biological complexity and specificity *(97–99)*. At present, the most intellectually satisfying interpretation of chemokine ligand-receptor interactions holds that varying combinations of ligands and receptors can produce precisely tuned responses to a wide variety of environmental challenges *(100)*.

1.4.4. Virus-Encoded Chemokine Receptors and Ligands

There is a fascinating group of functionally competent chemokine receptors and chemokines encoded by viruses (primarily the herpesviridae) *(101,102)*. These virus-encoded chemokines and receptors probably play an important role in pathogenesis of primary viral infection *(103,104)*. Mechanisms of action include expression of receptors that bind and sequester chemokines within cells, limiting inflammatory responses. In some cases, these molecules may mediate unanticipated consequences of virus infection such as the development of Kaposi's sarcoma (KS) in individuals infected with HHV8, likely resulting from expression of the chemokine receptor encoded by ORF-74 *(105,106)*. Assignment of ligands for the virus-encoded chemokine receptors is clearly complicated, as biological readouts are not always readily available *(102,107,108)*. However, these receptors frequently bind multiple ligands from various chemokine families.

1.4.5. Regulation of Chemokine Receptor Expression

Target cells respond to chemokines only by virtue of expressing cognate receptors. Therefore, the regulation of the receptor expression is a critical checkpoint in defining how cells respond to chemokines in the environment. Leukocytes express chemokines receptors according to their lineage, their stage of differentiation, and their state of activation. One example comes from studies of T cells during activation and differentiation *(59,109)*. Naive, resting T cells express CXCR4 and CCR7. Upon activation, T cells rapidly upregulate CCR5 and CXCR3, with the latter receptor exhibiting sustained expression only in cells that are polarized towards Th1 phenotypic commitment *(57,59)*. T cells exposed to chronic activating stimuli will gradually upregulate CCR2. T cells that are polarized in a Th2 environment will express CCR3, CCR4, and CCR8 *(57–59)*.

Perhaps the most intricate and well-defined program of regulated chemokine expression is exhibited by DC *(65,109–112)*. Immature DC migrate from blood stream into tissue under the influence of high expression of CCR1, CCR2, and CCR5: receptors that respond to "inflammatory" chemokines. Such cells are competent for antigen ingestion and processing but not presentation. After antigen uptake, immature DC prepare to undergo reverse transmigration from tissue into blood and eventually to lymphoid organs. Along with other changes that indicate acquisition of the mature DC phenotype, these cells downregulate CCR1 and CCR5 to permit egress from the inflammatory site (where high concentrations of the ligands for these receptors are found). Mature DC upregulate CCR7, ligands for which are highly expressed in lymphoid organs. These cells pass from tissue into bloodstream and advance to afferent vessels from secondary lymphoid organs. This program of regulated chemokine receptor expression has been termed "weigh the anchor" (indicating the decrease in CCR1 and CCR5) followed by "hoist the sail" (alluding to increased CCR7 expression). These concepts have been elegantly explicated *(97)*.

1.4.6. Signaling

As might be expected from the diversity of biological responses mediated by chemokines, postreceptor signaling is complex, and this topic has been recently and ably reviewed *(113)*. Signals from chemokine receptors generate outputs that direct two cardinal biological responses: integrin activation and directional migration *(114)*. Integrin activation is dependent on calcium flux and MAP kinase activation, through "inside-out" signaling *(115)*. Cytoskeletal reorganization, uropod formation, and directional migration are dependent on calcium entry, G protein-coupled events, cytoplasmic GTPases including RhoA, as well as phospholipases C and D. Other functional responses (including proliferation and restraint of proliferation) appear to be dependent on these events as well but further require a variety of protein tyrosine kinases and phosphoinositol-3 kinase (PI3K) *(116,117)*.

One outstanding question in the chemokine receptor field is related to the G-protein-coupling for diverse responses in varied cells. It is clear that such diversity exists: Although early studies demonstrated that chemokine receptor signaling was virtually always pertusis-toxin sensitive (suggesting obligatory coupling to G_i), pertusis-toxin-insensitive responses to chemokine receptor stimulation have been unambiguously described *(118)*. Differential utiltization of G_α components by CXC and CC receptors has also been clearly demonstrated *(119)*. Furthermore, variation in G-protein coupling for individual receptors in different T cellular backgrounds has been described.

2. ROLES OF CHEMOKINES IN ORGAN-SPECIFIC AUTOIMMUNITY

2.1. Chemokines and Receptors in Adaptive Immune Responses

The functions of cytokines in governing immune responses in autoimmune diseases are covered in Part II of this book. This section will address new results and interpretations concerning the roles of chemokines in these processes. Findings from gene targeted mice, in vitro studies, cell-transfer studies, and a large variety of descriptive analyses of gene expression have culminated in a satisfying account of the roles of several chemokines and chemokine receptors in the generation of adaptive immune responses within secondary lymphoid organs such as lymph nodes. These concepts and the data that underlie them have recently been extensively and lucidly reviewed *(65,66,81,97,120,121)*.

In LN, DC charged with antigen must encounter naive T cells with cognate receptors. Naive T cells arrive in the T cell zones of LN through the action of CCR7. CCR7 initially engages SLC, which is highly expressed by the HEV, the distinctive vascular component of LN. Subsequently, after extravasation, naive T cells enter T cell zones and are retained there under the influence of high local concentrations of ELC and SLC again acting on CCR7.

As described earlier, immature DC enter tissue under the direction of CCR1 and CCR5. After uptake of antigen and achievement of the mature DC phenotype, these cells rapidly downmodulate all chemokine receptors, in part through engagement of CD40 *(110–112)*. Elimination of signaling from these receptors allows reverse transmigration from tissue into blood and is succeeded by gradual upregulation of CCR7. These DC, which are now fully competent APCs, migrate either through the blood or through the lymph into the T cell zones of LN under the influence of local high-level SLC and ELC concentrations. Therefore, through the action of CCR7 and its ligands, mature antigen-charged DC and naive T cells are brought into apposition in the T cell zones of LN. DC promote even closer contact, specifically with activated T cells by producing MDC, which acts on CCR4, expressed on activated but not naive T cells *(122,123)*. Upon activation by antigen, T cells downregulate CCR7 and acutely upregulate CXCR3. However, CXCR3 expression is sustained only on those T cells destined to become committed to the TH1 functional phenotype.

T cells that are activated in T cell zones but destined provide help for immunoglobulin synthesis may also upregulate CXCR5, which could render these T cells able to draw close to the B cell follicles of LN (under the influence of BLC *[124]*), there to provide help for B cell immunoglobin synthesis *(65)*. T cells that are destined to persist as Th2-committed helpers will persistently upregulate CCR3, CCR4, and CCR8. High levels of IP-10 and mig in sites of Th1-biased inflammatory responses are driven by the expression of IFN-γ and will serve to attract Th1-committed T cells through action on CXCR3 *(29,109)*. Complementary effects will promote the accumulation of Th2 cells through the action of eotaxin on CCR3; MDC on CCR4; and I309 on CCR8. Although RANTES engages both Th1- and Th2-associated receptors, its dominant effects seem to promote Th1 and inhibit Th2 expression *(62)*. Therefore, through the action of a limited number of chemokines and receptors, intricate, precise and efficient adaptive immune responses can be generated.

2.2. Role of Chemokines in Cytokine Expression and T Cell Differentiation

In addition to their roles as chemoattractants, several investigators have shown a role for chemokines in regulating T cell activation, cytokine production, and differentiation. Subsets of T cells are classified based upon the cytokines that they produce: Th1 cells produce IFN-γ, IL-2, and TNF-β, while Th2 cells produce IL-4, IL-5, and IL-10 *(125,126)*. Th1, but not Th2, cells have been shown to produce lymphotactin, MCP-1, and MIP-1α, whereas both subsets were capable of synthesizing MIP-1β in vitro *(127)*. Schrum et al. examined the response of human peripheral blood lymphocytes to parasitic extracts in addition to human Th1 and Th2 T cell clones and demonstrated that synthesis of MIP-1α, MIP-1β, and RANTES correlated with a Th1 cytokine-production profile *(128)*. In an experimental animal asthma model, transfer of Th1 and Th2 cells induced different chemokine expression *(129)*. By performing RNase protection assays, these workers demonstrated that lungs that received transferred Th2 cells expressed mainly eotaxin, whereas lungs that received Th1 transferred cells expressed lymphotactin and higher levels of IP-10, RANTES, and MCP-1. Collectively, these data suggest that differences exist in both cytokine and chemokine production between Th1 and Th2 cells. However, using IL-2 KO, STAT4 KO, IL-4 KO, and STAT6 KO, Herold et al. failed to find a relationship between T cell subset and MIP-1α production *(130)*.

The differentiation of Th0 into Th1 cells was shown to require IL-12, whereas differentiation into Th2 cells required IL-4 *(125)*. MIP-1α was associated with Th1-type granuloma formation, whereas MCP-1 was associated with Th2 type granuloma formation in a schistosomiasis model *(131,132)*. Additionally, although both MIP-1α and MCP-1 were able to increase IFN-γ production in mitogen-activated lymphocytes, only MCP-1 upregulated IL-4 production *(131)*. In antigen specific activation, MCP-1 increased and MIP-1α downregulated Th2 lymphocyte IL-4 production *(131)*. Recently it was shown that naive T cells from TCR-transgenic, RAG-1-deficient mice showed an enhanced IFN-γ production when incubated with MIP-1α and enhanced IL-4 production when incubated with MCP-1 *(133)*. Primary stimulation of T cells with an anti-TCR clonotypic antibody and chemokine, followed by secondary and tertiary stimulation with antibody alone, revealed enhanced IFN-γ production after MIP-1α stimulation and enhanced IL-4 production after MCP-1 stimulation in an OVA-specific TCR transgenic model *(133)*. Recently, MCP-1 has been shown to be important for in vivo T cell differentiation *(134)*. In this study, MCP-1 knockout mice failed to show antigen-specific Th2 commitment. In addition to inducing T cell differentiation, chemokines have been shown to regulate inflammatory cytokine production. Specifically, MCP-1 has been shown to downregulate IL-12 expression in the mucosa during oral-tolerance induction, thereby contributing to the T cell nonresponsive state *(135)*. Thus, chemokines not only induce differentiation of helper T cells, but can also participate in tissue-specific regulation of inflammatory cytokine expression.

2.3. Chemokine Receptors in T Cell Differentiation

Using in vitro polarized T cell lines, RNase protection assays, and calcium-mobilization assays, Sallusto et al. have identified a profile of chemokine receptors expressed on human Th1 and Th2 cells *(58,59)*. CCR3, originally described as a receptor on eosinophils and basophils for the chemokines eotaxin, eotaxin-2, RANTES, MCP-2, MCP-3, and MCP-4 *(136,137)*, was found selectively expressed on Th2 cells from human peripheral blood and also polarized Th2 lines expanded in vitro *(136)*. CCR4 was found on Th2 cells, but was also found on non-IL-4 producing cells *(57,59,138)*. These data suggest that T cell CCR3 expression correlates with the Th2 functional phenotype.

CXCR3, which is a receptor for IP-10, MIG, and I-TAC *(27,29,139)*, was expressed at higher levels on human Th1 cells compared to TH2 cells *(57,59)*. CCR5 expression has been demonstrated on human Th1, but not, Th2 clones *(56,57)*. However, Sallusto et al. *(59)* have found that CCR5 expression is transient and is expressed on T cells that possess an activated phenotype (CD86$^+$, L-selectin$^-$, CD45RO$^+$, CD45RA^{low}) and therefore is not necessarily a TH1 marker. When the regulation of CCR5 and CXCR3 expression was examined, it was noted that upon the removal of IL-2, CCR5 was decreased while CXCR3 expression remained elevated, suggesting that CCR5 is a marker for activated human T cells while CXCR3 is a marker for Th1 cells. These phenomena have not been demonstrated for mouse or rat T cells. However, Siveke and Hamann have shown that mouse Th subsets do respond preferentially to different chemoattractants *(140)*. Th1 cells selectively migrated towards MIP-1α, MIP-1β, and RANTES while both Th1 and Th2 cells migrated towards MCP-1 and SDF-1α with varying degrees of efficacy *(140)*.

2.4. Chemokines and EAE

Aspects of EAE are covered in Chapter 10 by Bettelli and Nicholson. This section will address the functions and expression patterns of chemokines and chemokine receptors in this important model disease. EAE is a CD4$^+$ Th1 cell mediated demyelinating disease of the central nervous system (CNS) used as an animal model for MS *(141)*. Clinically, EAE is characterized by progressive ascending hind-limb paralysis and periods of remission and relapses *(142)*. The disease can be actively induced in genetically-susceptible strains of animals by immunization with whole proteolipid protein (PLP) or with immunodominant peptides, such as PLP139-151 (for SJL/J mice) emulsified in complete Freund's adjuvant *(143)*. EAE can also be induced by the adoptive transfer of antigen-activated PLP139-151 specific T cells into naive susceptible recipients *(144)*, specifically demonstrating prototypical autoimmunity. Flow cytometric and immunohistologi-cal analysis show that EAE is characterized by an initial infiltration of anti-gen-specific and nonspecific CD4$^+$ and CD8$^+$ cells and an accumulation of recruited macrophages but not polymorphonuclear cells *(145–147)*. Recently, several groups have turned their attention to chemokine expres-sion and function during the course of the disease, to address how these molecules regulate EAE pathogenesis (*see* Table 2).

Several different investigators have shown that chemokine mRNA and protein levels correlated with the onset of EAE symptoms. Hulkower et al. *(148)* were the first to demonstrate the correlation between chemokine expression and EAE. Using the Lewis rat model, they observed that MCP-1 mRNA was expressed in the CNS at disease onset, and also that MCP-1 mRNA was not detectable when the animals entered remission. Ransohoff et al. *(149)* described expression of chemokine mRNA in the CNS of SJL/J mice with EAE. Using semi-quantitative reverse transcription-polymerase chain reaction (RT-PCR) and *in situ* hybridization they demonstrated that IP-10 and MCP-1 were expressed in the spinal cord. Godiska et al. *(150)* showed an upregulation of mRNA chemokine expression for RANTES, MIP-1β, MIP-1α, TCA-3, IP-10, MCP-1, KC, and MARC/MCP-3 just prior to the first appearance of clinical symptoms in a mouse model of EAE and that the chemokine levels remained elevated throughout the course of the disease. CNS expression of chemokine mRNA correlates with histological signs of inflammation and is not detectable before the earliest evidence of leukocyte infiltration *(151,152)*. In the early clinical stages of the Lewis rat model of EAE, Miyagishi et al. *(153)* found that RANTES and MIP-1α mRNA positive T cells were located in the perivascular and subpial regions. Glabinski et al. *(154)* also examined the source of chemokines in the CNS during EAE. Co-localization experiments using immunohistochemistry and *in situ* hybridization showed that MIP-1α and RANTES were expressed by infiltrating leukocytes, while IP-10 and MCP-1 were expressed only by astrocytes.

MIP-1α protein levels have been shown to be elevated in the CNS fol-lowing adoptive transfer of activated neuroantigen specific T cells *(155)* and it is also clear that MCP-1 protein levels increase with the development of the relapsing phase of disease *(155)*. Guided by these results, it has been possible to demonstrate the biological importance of chemokines in the CNS during EAE by the ability of in vivo anti-MIP-1α treatment to prevent acute clinical disease, and by the ability of anti-MCP-1 treatment to prevent relapsing disease *(155)*. The data demonstrating chemokine expression dur-ing the course of various EAE is models are summarized in Table 2.

Table 2
Summary of Chemokine Expression Patterns in Various Models of EAE

Disease induction		Initial attack[c]				Remission				Relapse			
Strain[a]	Antigen[b]	MCP-1	RANTES	MIP-1α	IP-10	MCP-1	RANTES	MIP-1α	IP-10	MCP-1	RANTES	MIP-1α	IP-10
SJL	PLP139-151/ CFA	++	++	+++	+++	+	+	+	+	++	++	+++	++
	PLP139-151 T cells	±	+	+++	ND	±	+	+++	ND	+++	+	+++	ND
SWXJ	PLP139-151/ CFA	+++	++	+++	+++	−	−	−	−	++	++	++	++
BALB/GKO	MBP/CFA	+++	ND	ND	−	ND	ND	ND	ND	ND	ND	ND	ND
PL/J	PLP43-64/ CFA	+++	ND	+++	ND	++	ND	++	ND	Nonrelapsing disease model			
LEWIS	MBP/CFA	+++	ND	ND	ND	−	ND	ND	ND	Nonrelapsing disease model			
	MBPT cells	+++	+	+++	++	ND	ND	ND	ND	Nonrelapsing disease model			
	S100βT cells	+	++	+	+	ND	ND	ND	ND	Nonrelapsing disease model			
C57BL/6	MOG35-55	++	+	−	+++	ND	ND	ND	ND	Nonrelapsing disease model			

[a]SWxJ, (SWR xSJL)F1; BALB/GKO, IFN-γ−/− mice on BALB/c background.

[b]PLP139-151/CFA, proteolipid protein 139-151 peptide in CFA; PLP43-64, proteolipid protein 43-64 peptide in CFA; MBP, myelin basic protein; S100β, astrocyte calcium-binding protein.

[c]MCP-1, monocyte chemotactic protein-1; RANTES, regulated on activation normal T cell expression and secreted; MIP-1α, macrophage inflammatory protein-1α; IP-10, IFN-γ inducible protein 10; −, undetectable; ±, equivocally detectable; + through +++, low-level through high-level expression; ND, not done.

A

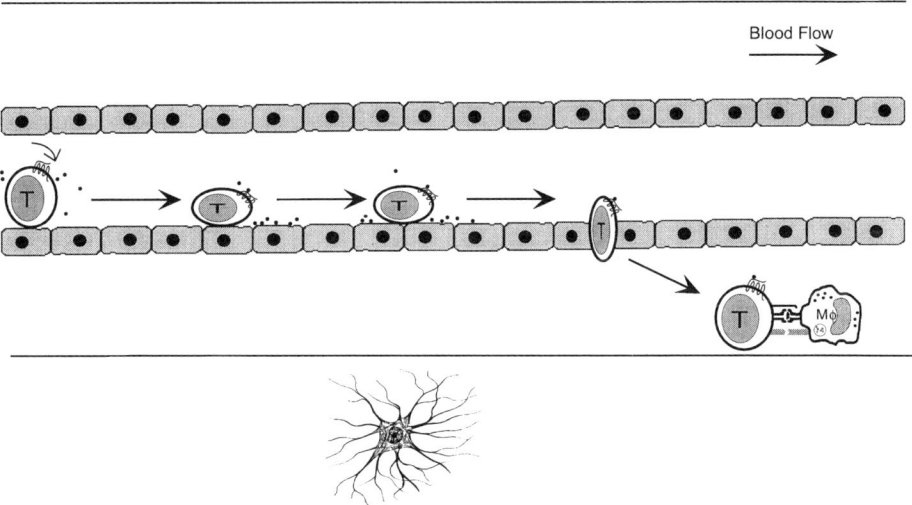

Fig. 1. Temporal and spatial chemokine expression governs CNS lymphocyte and monocyte accumulation. (**A**) Initial T cell infiltration into the CNS (*continued on next page*).

We hypothesize that CXCR3⁺ and CCR5⁺ T cells as well as CCR2⁺ macrophages are instrumental in the initiation of EAE. There is relatively little published information about the expression of chemokine receptors in EAE tissues; in one study, CCR2, CCR5, CXCR4, and CX3CR1 were increased in the CNS of Lewis rats displaying clinical symptoms of EAE *(156)*. Further studies in numerous labs are ongoing to determine the cell-specific expression of chemokine receptors during the course of clinical disease development and progression.

2.5. Chemokines and EAE: An Hypothesis

We postulate that differential spatial and temporal chemokine production by specific cell types serve as an important regulatory mechanism in the pathogenesis of EAE by directing mononuclear-cell (MNC) infiltration and trafficking within the target tissue. These concepts are summarized in Fig. 1. Figure 1A shows a cerebral microvessel, with intact blood-brain barrier (BBB); solid arrow indicates direction of flow. An activated T cell extravasates across BBB, and undergoes antigenic restimulation in the perivascular space. Reactivated T cells persist in CNS tissue compartment. Figure 1B shows an activated T cell/APC complex in the perivascular space producing inflammatory cytokines (solid dots) that may stimulate endothe-

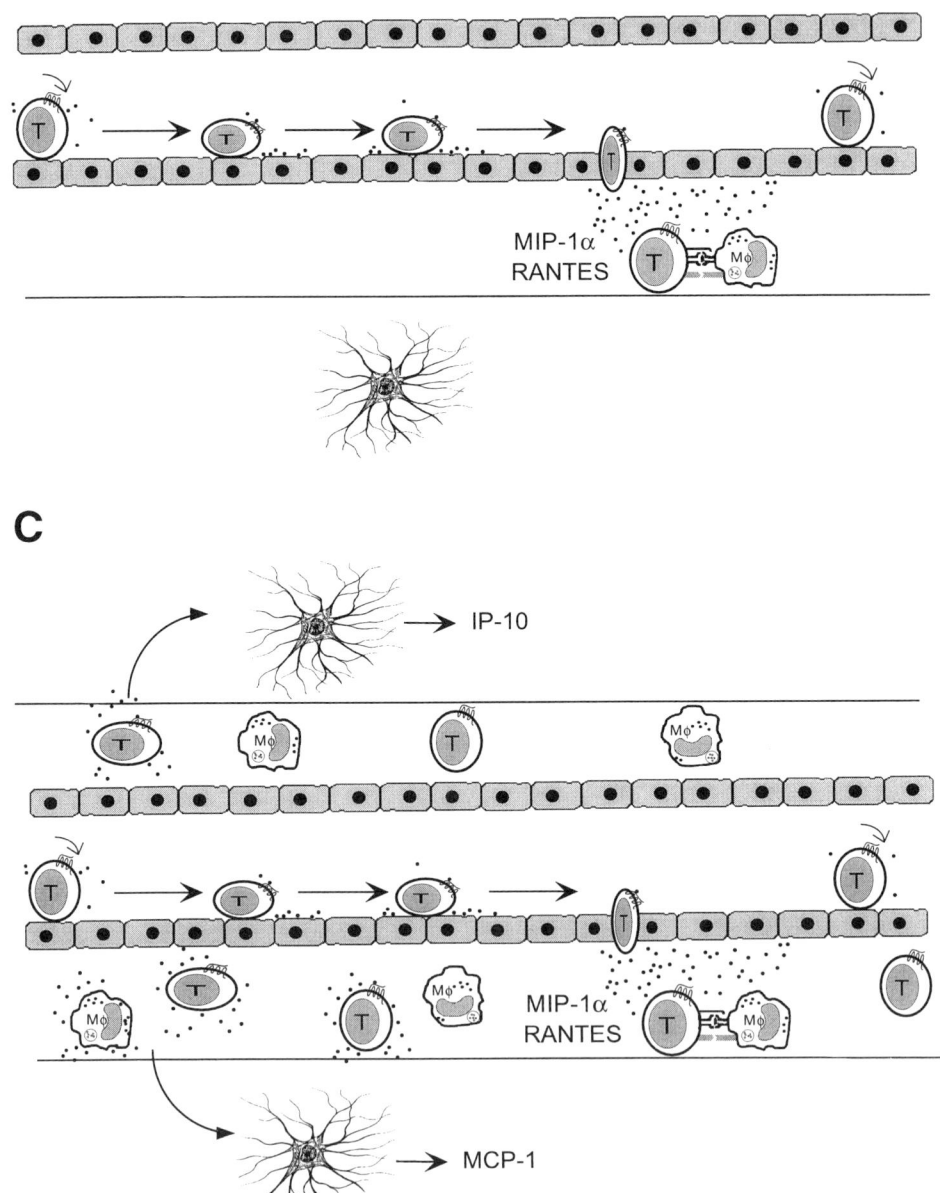

Fig. 1. (B) *(continued)* T cell restimulation in the perivascular space provides inflammatory stimulus for the direct and indirect expression of chemokines. **(C)** Chemokine expression in the perivascular space induces accumulation of T cells and monocytes.

D

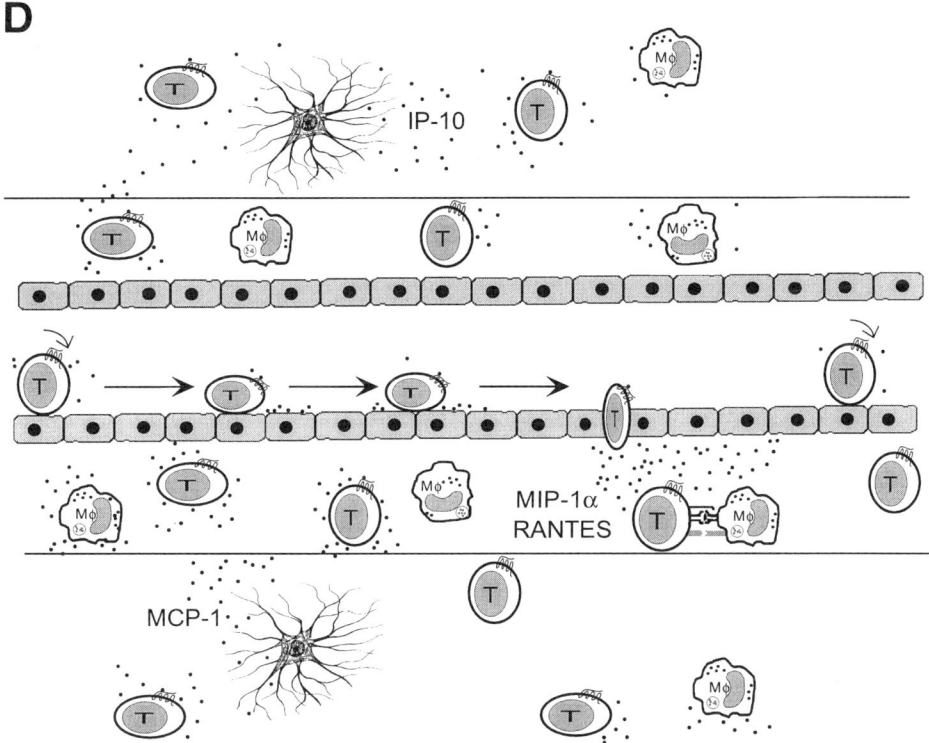

Fig. 1. (D) *(continued)* T cells induce CNS astrocytic production of chemokines resulting in lymphocyte and monocyte margination and invasion of the parenchyma.

lial production of cellular adhesion molecules and erode BBB function. Activated T cells and APC also express chemokines including MIP-1α and RANTES. Figure 1C demonstrates that the simultaneous presence of chemoattractants and focal endothelial activation results in accumulation of mononuclear inflammatory cells within perivascular space. Expression of MIP-1α and RANTES in the perivascular space serves to focus the inflammatory infiltrate toward the perivascular rather than parenchymal area. However, additional cytokine products of these MNCs (including IL-1, TNF-α, and IFN-γ) stimulate nearby astrocytes to express chemokines such as IP-10 and MCP-1. Figure 1D shows consequences of the tissue distribution of chemokines in EAE lesions. Once a significant inflammatory infiltrate has accumulated and activated astrocyte production of chemokines, macrophages begin to laminate at the outer border of the lesion and migrate into parenchyma along gradients of MCP-1 and related chemokines. Activated T cells invade parenchyma towards higher concentrations of IP-10. Many T cells remain in the perivascular space near higher levels of RANTES and MIP-1α. MCP-1 and IP-10 expression by activated astrocytes will subsequently be involved in the induction of further MNC infiltration. These secondarily recruited cells include antigen-specific T cells responsible for epitope spreading and episodes of relapsing disease as well as additional monocytes/macrophages, that mediate tissue injury.

REFERENCES

1. Baggiolini, M. (1998) Chemokines and leukocyte traffic. *Nature* **392(6676),** 565–568.
2. Rollins, B. J. (1997) Chemokines. *Blood* **90(3),** 909–928.
3. Zlotnik, A., Morales, J., and Hedrick, J. A. (1999) Recent advances in chemokines and chemokine receptors. *Crit. Rev. Immunol.* **19(1),** 1–47.
4. Bates, P. (1996) Chemokine receptors and HIV-1: an attractive pair? *Cell* **86,** 1–4.
5. Feng, Y., Broder, C. C., Kennedy, P. E., andBerger, E. A. (1996) HIV-1 entry cofactor: functional cDNA cloning of a seven-transmembrane G protein-coupled receptor. *Science* **272,** 872–877.
6. Clark-Lewis, I., Kim, K. S., Rajarathnam, K., Gong, J. H., Dewald, B., Moser, B., et al. (1995) Structure-activity relationships of chemokines. *J. Leukoc. Biol.* **5745(522),** 703–711.
7. Lusti-Narasimhan, M., Power, C. A., Allet, B., Alouani, S., Bacon, K. B., Mermod, J.-J., et al. (1995) Mutation of Leu25 and Val27 introduces CC chemokine activity into interleukin-8. *J. Biol. Chem.* **270,** 2716–2721.
8. Van Damme, J., Rampart, M., Conings, R., Decock, B., Van Osselaer, N., Willems, J., et al. (1990) The neutrophil-activating proteins interleukin 8 and β-thromboglobulin: *in vitro* and *in vivo* comparison of NH_2- terminally processed forms. *Eur. J. Immunol.* **20,** 2113–2118.
9. Oravecz, T., Pall, M., Roderiquez, G., Gorrell, M. D., Ditto, M., Nguyen, N. Y., et al. (1997) Regulation of the receptor specificity and function of the chemokine RANTES (regulated on activation, normal T cell expressed and secreted) by dipeptidyl peptidase IV (CD26)-mediated cleavage. *J. Exp. Med.* **186(11),** 1865–1872.
10. Struyf, S., De Meester, I., Scharpe, S., Lenaerts, J. P., Menten, P., Wang, J. M., et al. (1998) Natural truncation of RANTES abolishes signaling through the CC chemokine receptors CCR1 and CCR3, impairs its chemotactic potency and generates a CC chemokine inhibitor. *Eur. J. Immunol.* **28(4),** 1262–1271.
11. Proudfoot, A. E., Power, C. A., Hoogewerf, A. J., Montjovent, M. O., Borlat, F., Offord, R. E., et al. (1996) Extension of recombinant human RANTES by the retention of the initiating methionine produces a potent antagonist. *J. Biol. Chem.* **271(5),** 2599–2603.
12. Zlotnick, A. and Yoshie, O. (2000) Chemokines: a new classification system and their role in immunity. *Immunity* **12,** 121.

13. Baggiolini, M., Walz, A., and Kunkel, S. L. (1989) Neutrophil-activating peptide-1/interleukin 8, a novel cytokine that activates neutrophils. *J. Clin. Invest.* **84,** 1045–1049.
14. Clark-Lewis, I., Dewald, B., Geiser, T., Moser, B., and Baggiolini, M. (1993) Platelet factor 4 binds to interleukin 8 receptors and activates neutrophils when its N terminus is modified with Glu-Leu-Arg. *Proc. Natl. Acad. Sci. USA* **90(8),** 3574–3577.
15. Baggiolini, M., Dewald, B., and Moser, B. (1994) Interleukin-8 and related chemotactic cytokines—CXC and CC chemokines. *Adv. Immunol.* **55,** 97–179.
16. Cochran, B. J., Reffel, A. C., and Stiles, C. D. (1983) Molecular cloning of gene sequences regulated by platelet-derived growth factor. *Cell* **33,** 939–947.
17. Anisowicz, A., Bardwell, L., and Sager, R. (1987) Constitutive overexpression of a growth-regulated gene in transformed Chinese hamster and human cells. *Proc. Natl. Acad. Sci. USA* **84(20),** 7188–7192.
18. Richmond, A., Balentien, E., Thomas, H. G., Flaggs, G., Barton, D. E., Spiess, J., et al. (1988) Molecular characterization and chromosomal mapping of melanoma growth stimulatory activity, a growth factor structurally related to beta-thromboglobulin. *EMBO J.* **7(7),** 2025–2033.
19. Martins-Green, M. and Bissell, M. J. (1990) Localization of 9E3/CEF-4 in avian tissues: expression is absent in Rous sarcoma virus-induced tumors but is stimulated by injury. *J. Cell Biol.* **110(3),** 581–595.
20. Oquendo, P., Alberta, J., Wen, D. Z., Graycar, J. L., Derynck, R., and Stiles, C. D. (1989) The platelet-derived growth factor-inducible KC gene encodes a secretory protein related to platelet alpha-granule proteins. *J. Biol. Chem.* **264(7),** 4133–4137.
21. Robinson, S., Tani, M., Strieter, R. M., Ransohoff, R. M., and Miller, R. H. (1998) The chemokine growth-regulated oncogene-alpha promotes spinal cord oligodendrocyte precursor proliferation. *J. Neurosci.* **18(24),** 10457–10463.
22. Wu, Q., Miller, R., Ransohoff, R., Robinson, S., Bu, J., and Nishiyama, A. (2000) Elevated levels of the chemokine GRO-1 correlate with elevated oligodendrocyte progenitor proliferation in the jimpy mutant. *J. Neurosci.* **20,** 2609–2617.
23. Strieter, R. M., Polverini, P. J., Arenberg, D. A., and Kunkel, S. L. (1995) The role of CXC chemokines as regulators of angiogenesis. *Shock* **4(3),** 155–160.
24. Martins-Green, M. and Hanafusa, H. (1997) The 9E3/CEF4 gene and its product the chicken chemotactic and angiogenic factor (cCAF): potential roles in wound healing and tumor development. *Cytokine Growth Factor Rev.* **8(3),** 221–232.
25. Van Damme, J., Decock, B., Lenaerts, J. P., Conings, R., Bertini, R., and Mantovani, A. et al. (1989) Identification by sequence analysis of chemotactic factors for monocytes produced by normal and transformed cells stimulated with virus, double-stranded RNA or cytokine. *Eur. J. Immunol.* **19(12),** 2367–2373.
26. Wolpe, S. D. and Cerami, A. (1989) Macrophage inflammatory proteins 1 and 2: members of a novel superfamily of cytokines. *FASEB J.* **3(14),** 2565–2573.

27. Cole, K., Strick, C., Loetscher, M., Paradis, T., Ogborne, K., Gladue, R., et al. (1998) Interferon inducible T cell alpha chemattractant (I-TAC): a novel non-ELR CXC chemokine with potent activity on activated T cells through selective high affinity binding to CXCR3. *J. Exp. Med.* **187,** 2009–2021.
28. Loetscher, M., Gerber, B., Loetscher, P., Jones, S. A., Piali, L., Clark-Lewis, I., et al. (1996) Chemokine receptor specific for IP10 and mig: structure, function, and expression in activated T-lymphocytes. *J. Exp. Med.* **184(3),** 963–969.
29. Farber, J. M. (1997) Mig and IP-10: CXC chemokines that target lympho-cytes. *J. Leukoc. Biol.* **61(3),** 246–257.
30. Loetscher, M., Loetscher, P., Brass, N., Meese, E., and Moser, B. (1998) Lymphocyte-specific chemokine receptor CXCR3: regulation, chemokine binding and gene localization. *Eur. J. Immunol.* **28(11),** 3696–3705.
31. Dewald, B., Moser, B., Barella, L., Schumacher, C., Baggiolini, M., and Clark-Lewis, I. (1992) IP-10, a gamma-interferon-inducible protein related to interleukin-8, lacks neutrophil activating properties. *Immunol.Lett.* **32,** 81–84.
32. Nagasawa, T., Hirota, S., Tachibana, K., Takakura, N., Nishikawa, S., Kitamura, Y., et al. (1996) Defects of B-cell lymphopoiesis and bone-mar-row myelopoiesis in mice lacking the CXC chemokine PBSF/SDF-1. *Nature* **382(6592),** 635–638.
33. D'Apuzzo, M., Rolink, A., Loetscher, M., Hoxie, J. A., Clark-Lewis, I., Melchers, F., et al. (1997) The chemokine SDF-1, stromal cell-derived factor 1, attracts early stage B cell precursors via the chemokine receptor CXCR4. *Eur. J. Immunol.* **27(7),** 1788–1793.
34. Ma, Q., Jones, D., Borghesani, P. R., Segal, R. A., Nagasawa, T., Kishimoto, T., et al. (1998) Impaired B-lymphopoiesis, myelopoiesis, and derailed cer-ebellar neuron migration in CXCR4- and SDF-1-deficient mice. *Proc. Natl. Acad. Sci. USA* **95(16),** 9448–9453.
35. Zou, Y. R., Kottmann, A. H., Kuroda, M., Taniuchi, I., and Littman, D. R. (1998) Function of the chemokine receptor CXCR4 in haematopoiesis and in cerebellar development. *Nature* **393(6685),** 595–599.
36. Zhang, L., He, T., Talal, A., Wang, G., Frankel, S. S., and Ho, D.D. (1998) In vivo distribution of the human immunodeficiency virus/simian immunodefi-ciency virus coreceptors: CXCR4, CCR3, and CCR5. *J. Virol.* **72(6),** 5035–5045.
37. Ma, Q., Jones, D., and Springer, T. A. (1999) The chemokine receptor CXCR4 is required for the retention of B lineage and granulocytic precursors within the bone marrow microenvironment. *Immunity* **10(4),** 463–471.
38. Kawabata, K., Ujikawa, M., Egawa, T., Kawamoto, H., Tachibana, K., Iizasa, H., et al. (1999) A cell-autonomous requirement for CXCR4 in long-term lymphoid and myeloid reconstitution. *Proc. Natl. Acad. Sci. USA* **96(10),** 5663–5667.
39. McGrath, K. E., Koniski, A. D., Maltby, K. M., McGann, J. K., and Palis, J. (1999) Embryonic expression and function of the chemokine SDF-1 and its receptor, CXCR4. *Dev. Biol.* **213(2),** 442–456.
40. Tachibana, K., Hirota, S., Iizasa, H., Yoshida, H., Kawabata, K., Kataoka, Y., et al. (1998) The chemokine receptor CXCR4 is essential for vasculariza-tion of the gastrointestinal tract. *Nature* **393(6685),** 591–594.

41. Daniels, G. D., Zou, J., Charlemagne, J., Partula, S., Cunningham, C., and Secombes, C.J. (1999) Cloning of two chemokine receptor homologs (CXC-R4 and CC-R7) in rainbow trout Oncorhynchus mykiss. *J. Leukoc. Biol.* **65(5),** 684–690.

42. Forster, R., Mattis, A. E., Kremmer, E., Wolf, E., Brem, G., and Lipp, M. (1996) A putative chemokine receptor, BLR1, directs B cell migration to defined lymphoid organs and specific anatomic compartments of the spleen. *Cell* **87(6),** 1037–1047.

43. Rollins, B., Stier, P., Ernst, T., and Wong, G. (1989) The human homolog of the JE gene encodes a monocyte secretory protein. *Mol. Cell Biol.* **9(11),** 4687–4689.

44. Rollins, B. J. (1991) JE/MCP-1: an early-response gene encodes a monocyte-specific cytokine. *Cancer Cells* **3(12),** 517–524.

45. Rollins, B. J. (1996) Monocyte chemoattractant protein 1: a potential regulator of monocyte recruitment in inflammatory disease. *Mol. Med. Today* **2(5),** 198–204.

46. Van Damme, J., Proost, P., Lenaerts, J. P., and Opdenakker, G. (1992) Structural and functional identification of two human, tumor-derived monocyte chemotactic proteins (MCP-2 and MCP-3) belonging to the chemokine family. *J. Exp. Med.* **176(1),** 59–65.

47. Proost, P., Wuyts, A., and Van Damme, J. (1996) Human monocyte chemotactic proteins-2 and -3: structural and functional comparison with MCP-1. *J. Leukocyte Biol.* **59(1),** 67–74.

48. Yoshimura, T., Robinson, E. A., Tanaka, S., Appella, E., Kuratsu, J., and Leonard, E. J. (1989) Purification and amino acid analysis of two human glioma-derived monocyte chemoattractants. *J. Exp. Med.* **169,** 1449–1459.

49. Carr, M. W., Roth, S. J., Luther, E., Rose, S. S., and Springer, T.A. (1994) Monocyte chemoattractant protein 1 acts as a T-lymphocyte chemoattractant. *Proc. Natl. Acad. Sci. USA* **91,** 3652–3656.

50. Gu, L., Rutledge, B., Fiorillo, J., Ernst, C., Grewal, I., Flavell, R., et al. (1997) In vivo properties of monocyte chemoattractant protein-1. *J. Leukoc. Biol.* **62(5),** 577–580.

51. Lu, B., Rutledge, B. J., Gu, L., Fiorillo, J., Lukacs, N. W., Kunkel, S. L., et al. (1998) Abnormalities in monocyte recruitment and cytokine expression in monocyte chemoattractant protein 1-deficient mice. *J. Exp. Med.* **187(4),** 601–608.

52. Gerard, C., Frossard, J. L., Bhatia, M., Saluja, A., Gerard, N. P., Lu, B., et al. (1997) Targeted disruption of the beta-chemokine receptor CCR1 protects against pancreatitis-associated lung injury. *J. Clin. Invest.* **100(8),** 2022–2027.

53. Cook, D. N., Beck, M. A., Coffman, T. M., Kirby, S. L., Sheridan, J. F., Pragnell, I. B., et al. (1995) Requirement of MIP-1 alpha for an inflammatory response to viral infection. *Science* **269(5230),** 1583–1585.

54. Cook, D. N. (1996) The role of MIP-1 alpha in inflammation and hematopoiesis. *J. Leukoc. Biol.* **59(1),** 61–66.

55. Karpus, W. J., Lukacs, N. W., McRae, B. L., Strieter, R. M., Kunkel, S. L., and Miller, S. D. (1995) An important role for the chemokine macrophage inflammatory protein-1 alpha in the pathogenesis of the T cell-mediated

autoimmune disease, experimental autoimmune encephalomyelitis. *J. Immunol.* **155(10)**, 5003–5010.

56. Loetscher, P., Uguccioni, M., Bordoli, L., Baggiolini, M., Moser, B., Chizzolini, C., et al. (1998) CCR5 is characteristic of Th1 lymphocytes. *Nature* **391(6665)**, 344–345.

57. Bonecchi, R., Bianchi, G., Bordignon, P. P., D'Ambrosio, D., Lang, R., Borsatti, A., et al. (1998) Differential expression of chemokine receptors and chemotactic responsiveness of type 1 T helper cells (Th1s) and Th2s. *J. Exp. Med.* **187(1)**, 129–134.

58. Sallusto, F., Mackay, C. R., and Lanzavecchia, A. (1997) Selective expression of the eotaxin receptor CCR3 by human T helper 2 cells. *Science* **277(5334)**, 2005–2007.

59. Sallusto, F., Lenig, D., Mackay, C. R., and Lanzavecchia, A. (1998) Flexible programs of chemokine receptor expression on human polarized T helper 1 and 2 lymphocytes. *J. Exp. Med.* **187(6)**, 875–883.

60. Annunziato, F., Galli, G., Cosmi, L., Romagnani, P., Manetti, R., Maggi, E., et al. (1998) Molecules associated with human Th1 or Th2 cells. *Eur. Cytokine Netw.* **9(3 Suppl)**, 12–16.

61. Annunziato, F., Cosmi, L., Galli, G., Beltrame, C., Romagnani, P., Manetti, R., et al. (1999) Assessment of chemokine receptor expression by human Th1 and Th2 cells in vitro and in vivo. *J. Leukoc. Biol.* **65(5)**, 691–699.

62. Chensue, S. W., Warmington, K. S., Allenspach, E. J., Lu, B., Gerard, C., Kunkel, S. L., et al. (1999) Differential expression and cross-regulatory function of RANTES during mycobacterial (type 1) and schistosomal (type 2) antigen-elicited granulomatous inflammation. *J. Immunol.* **163(1)**, 165–173.

63. Bacon, K. B., Premack, B. A., Gardner, P., and Schall, T. J. (1995) Activation of dual T cell signaling pathways by the chemokine RANTES. *Science* **269(5231)**, 1727–1730.

64. Bolin, L. M., Murray, R., Lukacs, N. W., Strieter, R. M., Kunkel, S. L., Schall, T. J., et al. (1998) Primary sensory neurons migrate in response to the chemokine RANTES. *J. Neuroimmunol.* **81(1-2)**, 49–57.

65. Cyster, J. G. (1999) Chemokines and cell migration in secondary lymphoid organs. *Science* **286(5447)**, 2098–2102.

66. Cyster, J. G., Ngo, V. N., Ekland, E. H., Gunn, M. D., Sedgwick, J. D., and Ansel, K. M. (1999) Chemokines and B-cell homing to follicles. *Curr. Top. Microbiol. Immunol.* **246**, 87–92.

67. Gunn, M. D., Kyuwa, S., Tam, C., Kakiuchi, T., Matsuzawa, A., Williams, L. T., et al. (1999) Mice lacking expression of secondary lymphoid organ chemokine have defects in lymphocyte homing and dendritic cell localization. *J. Exp. Med.* **189(3)**, 451–460.

68. Vassileva, G., Soto, H., Zlotnik, A., Nakano, H., Kakiuchi, T., Hedrick, J. A., et al. (1999) The reduced expression of 6Ckine in the plt mouse results from the deletion of one of two 6Ckine genes. *J. Exp. Med.* **190(8)**, 1183–1188.

69. Ngo, V. N., Korner, H., Gunn, M. D., Schmidt, K. N., Riminton, D. S., Cooper, M. D., et al. (1999) Lymphotoxin alpha/beta and tumor necrosis factor

are required for stromal cell expression of homing chemokines in B and T cell areas of the spleen. *J. Exp. Med.* **189(2),** 403–412.

70. Shinkura, R., Kitada, K., Matsuda, F., Tashiro, K., Ikuta, K., Suzuki, M., et al. (1999) Alymphoplasia is caused by a point mutation in the mouse gene encoding NF-kappa b-inducing kinase. *Nat. Genet.* **22(1),** 74–77.
71. Majumder, S., Zhou, Z.-H. L., and Ransohoff, R. (1996) Transcriptional regulation of chemokine gene expression in astrocytes. *J. Neurosci. Res.* **45,** 758–769.
72. Narumi, S. and Hamilton, T. A. (1991) Inducible expression of murine IP-10 mRNA varies with the state of macrophage inflammatory activity. *J. Immunol.* **146,** 3038–3044.
73. Narumi, S., Wyner, L., Stoler, M., Tannenbaum, C., and Hamilton, T. (1992) Tissue specific expression of murine IP-10 mRNA following systemic treatment with interferon-g. *J. Leukoc. Biol.* **52,** 27–33.
74. Ohmori, Y. and Hamilton, T. A. (1994) Cell type and stimulus specific regulation of chemokine gene expression. *Biochem. Biophy. Res. Commun.* **198,** 590–596.
75. Ohmori, Y. and Hamilton, T. A. (1995) The interferon-stimulated response element and a kappa B site mediate synergistic induction of murine IP-10 gene transcription by IFN-gamma and TNF-alpha. *J. Immunol.* **154(10),** 5235–5244.
76. Wu, C., Ohmori, Y., Bandyopadhyay, S., Sen, G., and Hamilton, T. (1994) Interferon-stimulated response element and NF kappa B sites cooperate to regulate double-stranded RNA-induced transcription of the IP-10 gene. *J. Interferon. Res.* **14(6),** 357–363.
77. Majumder, S., Zhou, L. Z., Chaturvedi, P., Babcock, G., Aras, S., and Ransohoff, R. M. (1998) p48/STAT-1alpha-containing complexes play a predominant role in induction of IFN-gamma-inducible protein, 10 kDa (IP-10) by IFN-gamma alone or in synergy with TNF-alpha. *J. Immunol.* **161(9),** 4736–4744.
78. Kopydlowski, K. M., Salkowski, C. A., Cody, M. J., van Rooijen, N., Major, J., Hamilton, T. A., et al. (1999) Regulation of macrophage chemokine expression by lipopolysaccharide in vitro and in vivo. *J. Immunol.* **163(3),** 1537–1544.
79. Kim, H. S., Armstrong, D., Hamilton, T. A., and Tebo, J. M. (1998) IL-10 suppresses LPS-induced KC mRNA expression via a translation-dependent decrease in mRNA stability. *J. Leukoc. Biol.* **64(1),** 33–39.
80. Kishore, R., Tebo, J. M., Kolosov, M., and Hamilton, T. A. (1999) Cutting edge: clustered AU-rich elements are the target of IL-10-mediated mRNA destabilization in mouse macrophages. *J. Immunol.* **162(5),** 2457–2461.
81. Sedgwick, J. D., Riminton, D. S., Cyster, J. G., and Korner, I. (2000) Tumor necrosis factor: a master-regulator of leukocyte movement. *Immunol. Today* **21(3),** 110–113.
82. Rollins, B. (ed) (1999) *Chemokines and Cancer.* Humana Press, Totowa, NJ.
83. Harter, L., Petersen, F., Flad, H. D., and Brandt, E. (1994) Connective tissue-activating peptide III desensitizes chemokine receptors on neutrophils.

Requirement for proteolytic formation of the neutrophil-activating peptide 2. *J. Immunol.* **153(12)**, 5698–5708.

84. Iida, N., Haisa, M., Igarashi, A., Pencev, D., and Grotendorst, G. R. (1996) Leukocyte-derived growth factor links the PDGF and CXC chemokine families of peptides. *Faseb. J.* **10(11)**, 1336–1345.

85. Chaudhuri, A., Zbrzezna, V., Polyakova, J., Pogo, A., Hesselgesser, J., and Horuk, R. (1994) Expression of the Duffy antigen in K562 cells: Evidence that it is the human chemokine erythrocyte receptor. *J. Biol. Chem.* **269**, 7835–7838.

86. Lu, Z. H., Wang, Z. X., Horuk, R., Hesselgesser, J., Lou, Y. C., Hadley, T. J., et al. (1995) The promiscuous chemokine binding profile of the Duffy antigen/receptor for chemokines is primarily localized to sequences in the amino-terminal domain. *J. Biol. Chem.* **270(44)**, 26239–26245.

87. Nibbs, R. J. B., Wylie, S. M., Pragnell, I. B., and Graham, G. J. (1997) Cloning and characterization of a novel murine beta chemokine receptor, D6. Comparison to three other related macrophage inflammatory protein-1alpha receptors, CCR-1, CCR-3, and CCR-5. *J. Biol. Chem.* **272(19)**, 12,495–12,504.

88. Horuk, R., Chitnis, C. E., Darbonne, W. C., Colby, T. J., Rybicki, A., Hadley, T. J., et al. (1993) A receptor for the malarial parasite Plasmodium vivax: the erythrocyte chemokine receptor. *Science* **261(5125)**, 1182–1184.

89. Mallinson, G., Soo, K. S., Schall, T. J., Pisacka, M., and Anstee, D. J. (1995) Mutations in the erythrocyte chemokine receptor (Duffy) gene: the molecular basis of the Fya/Fyb antigens and identification of a deletion in the Duffy gene of an apparently healthy individual with the Fy(a-b-) phenotype. *Br. J. Haematol.* **90(4)**, 823–829.

90. Hadley, T. J., Lu, Z. H., Wasniowska, K., Martin, A. W., Peiper, S. C., Hesselgesser, J., et al. (1994) Postcapillary venule endothelial cells in kidney express a multispecific chemokine receptor that is structurally and functionally identical to the erythroid isoform, which is the Duffy blood group antigen. *J. Clin. Invest.* **94(3)**, 985–991.

91. Peiper, S. C., Wang, Z. X., Neote, K., Martin, A. W., Showell, H. J., Conklyn, M. J., et al. (1995) The Duffy antigen/receptor for chemokines (DARC) is expressed in endothelial cells of Duffy negative individuals who lack the erythrocyte receptor. *J. Exp. Med.* **181(4)**, 1311–1317.

92. Horuk, R., Martin, A., Hesselgesser, J., Hadley, T., Lu, Z. H., Wang, Z. X., et al. (1996) The Duffy antigen receptor for chemokines: structural analysis and expression in the brain. *J. Leukoc. Biol.* **59(1)**, 29–38.

93. Horuk, R., Martin, A. W., Wang, Z., Schweitzer, L., Gerassimides, A., Guo, H., et al. (1997) Expression of chemokine receptors by subsets of neurons in the central nervous system. *J. Immunol.* **158(6)**, 2882–2890.

94. Whitney, L. W., Becker, K. G., Tresser, N. J., Caballero-Ramos, C. I., Munson, P. J., Prabhu, V. V., et al. (1999) Analysis of gene expression in mutiple sclerosis lesions using cDNA microarrays. *Ann. Neurol.* **46(3)**, 425–428.

95. Soto, H., Wang, W., Strieter, R. M., Copeland, N. G., Gilbert, D. J., Jenkins, N. A., et al. (1998) The CC chemokine 6Ckine binds the CXC chemokine receptor CXCR3. *Proc. Natl. Acad. Sci. USA* **95(14)**, 8205–8210.

96. Premack, B. A. and Schall, T. J. (1996) Chemokine receptors: Gateways to inflammation and infection. *Nature Med.* **2**, 1174–1178.
97. Mantovani, A. (ed) (1999) *Chemokines.* Karger, Basel.
98. Mantovani, A. (1999) The chemokine system: redundancy for robust outputs. *Immunol. Today* **20(6)**, 254–257.
99. Broxmeyer, H. E. and Kim, C. H. (1999) Regulation of hematopoiesis in a sea of chemokine family members with a plethora of redundant activities. *Exp. Hematol.* **27(7)**, 1113–1123.
100. Gerard, C. (1999) Chemokine receptors and ligand specificity: understanding the enigma, in *Chemokines and Cancer.* (Rollins, B. J., ed.), Humana Press, Totowa, NJ, pp. 21–31.
101. Murphy, P. M. (1994) Molecular piracy of chemokine receptors by herpesviruses. Infect. *Agents Dis.* **3(2-3)**, 137–154.
102. Lalani, A. S., Barrett, J. W., and McFadden, G. (2000) Modulating chemokines: more lessons from viruses. *Immunol. Today* **21(2)**, 100–106.
103. Bodaghi, B., Jones, T. R., Zipeto, D., Vita, C., Sun, L., Laurent, L., et al. (1998) Chemokine sequestration by viral chemoreceptors as a novel viral escape strategy: withdrawal of chemokines from the environment of cytomegalovirus-infected cells. *J. Exp. Med.* **188(5)**, 855–866.
104. Howard, J., Justus, D. E., Totmenin, A. V., Shchelkunov, S., and Kotwal, G. J. (1998) Molecular mimicry of the inflammation modulatory proteins (IMPs) of poxviruses: evasion of the inflammatory response to preserve viral habitat. *J. Leukoc. Biol.* **64(1)**, 68–71.
105. Arvanitakis, L., Geras-Raaka, E., Varma, A., Gershengorn, M. C., and Cesarman, E. (1997) Human herpesvirus KSHV encodes a constitutively active G-protein-coupled receptor linked to cell proliferation. *Nature* **385(6614)**, 347–350.
106. Bais, C., Santomasso, B., Coso, O., Arvanitakis, L., Raaka, E. G., Gutkind, J.S., et al. (1998) G-protein-coupled receptor of Kaposi's sarcoma-associated herpesvirus is a viral oncogene and angiogenesis activator. *Nature* **391(6662)**, 86–89.
107. Rosenkilde, M. M., Kledal, T.N., Brauner-Osborne, H., and Schwartz, T. W. (1999) Agonists and inverse agonists for the herpesvirus 8-encoded constitutively active seven-transmembrane oncogene product, ORF-74. *J. Biol. Chem.* **274(2)**, 956–961.
108. Gershengorn, M. C., Geras-Raaka, E., Varma, A., and Clark-Lewis, I. (1998) Chemokines activate Kaposi's sarcoma-associated herpesvirus G protein-coupled receptor in mammalian cells in culture [see comments]. *J. Clin. Invest.* **102(8)**, 1469–72.
109. Sallusto, F., Lanzavecchia, A., and Mackay, C. R. (1998) Chemokines and chemokine receptors in T cell priming and Th1/Th2-mediated responses. *Immunol. Today* **19(12)**, 568–74.
110. Sallusto, F., Schaerli, P., Loetscher, P., Schaniel, C., Lenig, D., Mackay, C. R., et al. (1998) Rapid and coordinated switch in chemokine receptor expression during dendritic cell maturation. *Eur. J. Immunol.* **28(9)**, 2760–2769.

111. Sozzani, S., Allavena, P., D'Amico, G., Luini, W., Bianchi, G., Kataura, M., et al. (1998) Differential regulation of chemokine receptors during dendritic cell maturation: a model for their trafficking properties. *J. Immunol.* **161(3),** 1083–1086.

112. Sallusto, F., Palermo, B., Lenig, D., Miettinen, M., Matikainen, S., Julkunen, I., et al. (1999) Distinct patterns and kinetics of chemokine production regulate dendritic cell function. *Eur. J. Immunol.* **29(5),** 1617–1625.

113. Bacon, K. B. (1997) Analysis of signal transduction following lymphocyte activation by chemokines. *Methods Enzymol.* **288,** 340–361.

114. Campbell, J. J., Qin, S., Bacon, K. B., Mackay, C. R., and Butcher, E. C. (1996) Biology of chemokine and classical chemoattractant receptors: differential requirements for adhesion-triggering versus chemotactic responses in lymphoid cells. *J. Cell Biol.* **134(1),** 255–266.

115. Hynes, R. O. (1992) Integrins: versatility, modulation, and signaling in cell adhesion. *Cell* **69,** 11–25.

116. Wong, M.and Fish, E. N. (1998) RANTES and MIP-1alpha activate stats in T cells. *J. Biol. Chem.* **273(1),** 309–314.

117. Ganju, R. K., Dutt, P., Wu, L., Newman, W., Avraham, H., Avraham, S., et al. (1998) Beta-chemokine receptor CCR5 signals via the novel tyrosine kinase RAFTK. *Blood* **91(3),** 791–797.

118. Kelly, M. D., Naif, H. M., Adams, S. L., Cunningham, A. L., and Lloyd, A. R. (1998) Dichotomous effects of beta-chemokines on HIV replication in monocytes and monocyte-derived macrophages. *J. Immunol.* **160(7),** 3091–3095.

119. Bischoff, S. C., Krieger, M., Brunner, T., Rot, A., von Tscharner, V., Baggiolini, M., et al. (1993) RANTES and related chemokines activate human basophil granulocytes through different G protein-coupled receptors. *Eur. J. Immunol.* **23(3),** 761–767.

120. Melchers, F., Rolink, A. G., and Schaniel, C. (1999) The role of chemokines in regulating cell migration during humoral immune responses. *Cell* **99(4),** 351–354.

121. Cyster, J. G. (2000) Leukocyte migration: scent of the T zone. *Curr. Biol.* **10(1),** R30–33.

122. Imai, T., Chantry, D., Raport, C. J., Wood, C. L., Nishimura, M., Godiska, R., et al. (1998) Macrophage-derived chemokine is a functional ligand for the CC chemokine receptor 4. *J. Biol. Chem.* **273(3),** 1764–1768.

123. Tang, H. L. and Cyster, J. G. (1999) Chemokine up-regulation and activated T cell attraction by maturing dendritic cells. *Science* **284(5415),** 819–822.

124. Gunn, M. D., Ngo, V. N., Ansel, K. M., Ekland, E. H., Cyster, J. G., and Williams, L. T. (1998) A B-cell-homing chemokine made in lymphoid follicles activates Burkitt's lymphoma receptor-1. *Nature* **391(6669),** 799–803.

125. Abbas, A. K., Murphy, K. M., and Sher, A. (1996) Functional diversity of helper T lymphocytes. *Nature* **383,** 787–793.

126. Mosmann, T. R. and Coffman, R. L. (1989) Th1 and Th2 cells: different patterns of lymphokine secretion lead to different functional properties. *Annu. Rev. Immunol.* **7,** 145–174.

127. Bradley, L. M., Asensio, V. C., Schioetz, L. K., Harbertson, J., Krahl, T., Patstone, G., et al. (1999) Islet-specific Th1, but not Th2, cells secrete multiple chemokines and promote rapid induction of autoimmune diabetes. *J. Immunol.* **162(5)**, 2511–2520.

128. Schrum, S., Probst, P., Fleischer, B., and Zipfel, P. F. (1996) Synthesis of the CC-chemokines MIP-1α, MIP-1β, and RANTES is associated with a type 1 immune response. *J. Immunol.* **157**, 3598–3604.

129. Li, L., Xia, Y., Nguyen, A., Feng, L., and Lo, D. (1998) Th2-induced eotaxin expression and eosinophilia coexist with Th1 responses at the effector stage of lung inflammation. *J. Immunol.* **161(6)**, 3128–3135.

130. Herold, K. C., Lu, J., Rulifson, I., Vezys, V., Taub, D., Grusby, M. J., et al. (1997) Regulation of C-C chemokine production by murine T cells by CD28/B7 costimulation. *J. Immunol.* **159**, 4150–4153.

131. Chensue, S. W., Warmington, K. S., Lukacs, N. W., Lincoln, P. M., Burdick, M. D., Strieter, R. M., et al. (1995) Monocyte chemotactic protein expression during schistosome egg granuloma formation. Sequence of production, localization, contribution, and regulation. *Am. J. Pathol.* **146(1)**, 130–138.

132. Lukacs, N. W., Kunkel, S. L., Strieter, R. M., Warmington, K., and Chensue, S. W. (1993) The role of macrophage inflammatory protein 1a in Shistosoma mansoni egg-induced granulomatous inflammation. *J. Exp. Med.* **177**, 1551–1559.

133. Karpus, W. J., Lukacs, N. W., Kennedy, K. J., Smith, W. S., Hurst, S. D., and Barrett, T. A. (1997) Differential CC chemokine-induced enhancement of T helper cell cytokine production. *J. Immunol.* **158**, 4129–4136.

134. Gu, L., Tseng, S., Horner, R. M., Tam, C., Loda, M., and Rollins, B. J. (2000) Control of TH2 polarization by the chemokine monocyte chemoattractant protein-1. *Nature* **404(6776)**, 407–411.

135. Karpus, W. J, Kennedy, K. J., Kunkel, S. L., and Lukacs, N. W. (1998) Monocyte chemotactic protein 1 regulates oral tolerance induction by inhibition of T Helper Cell 1-related cytokines. *J. Exp. Med.* **187(5)**, 733–741.

136. Ponath, P. D., Qin, S., Post, T. W., Wang, J., Wu, L., Gerard, N. P., et al. (1996) Molecular cloning and characterization of a human eotaxin receptor expressed selectively on eosinophils. *J. Exp. Med.* **183(6)**, 2437–2448.

137. Uguccioni, M., Mackay, C. R., Ochensberger, B., Loetscher, P., Rhis, S., LaRosa, G. J., et al. (1997) High expression of the chemokine receptor CCR3 in human blood basophiles. Role in activation by eotaxin, MCP-4, and other chemokines. *J. Clin. Invest.* **100(5)**, 1137–1143.

138. Imai, T., Nagira, M., Takagi, S., Kakizaki, M., Nishimura, M., Wang, J., et al. (1999) Selective recruitment of CCR4-bearing Th2 cells toward antigen- presenting cells by the CC chemokines thymus and activation-regulated chemokine and macrophage-derived chemokine. *Int. Immunol.* **11(1)**, 81–88.

139. Luster, A. D. and Ravetch, J. V. (1987) Biochemical characterization of a gamma interferon-inducible cytokine (IP-10). *J. Exp. Med.* **166(4)**, 1084–1097.

140. Siveke, J. T. and Hamann, A. (1998) T helper 1 and T helper 2 cells respond differentially to chemokines. *J. Immunol.* **160(2)**, 550–554.

141. Arnason, B. G. (1983) Relevance of experimental allergic encephalomyelitis to multiple sclerosis. *Neurol. Clin.* **1**, 765–782.

142. McRae, B. L., Kennedy, M. K., Tan, L. J., Dal Canto, M. C., and Miller, S. D. (1992) Induction of active and adoptive chronic-relapsing experimental autoimmune encephalomyelitis (EAE) using an encephalitogenic epitope of proteolipid protein. *J. Neuroimmunol.* **38,** 229–240.

143. Tuohy, V. K., Sobel, R. A., Lu, Z., Laursen, R. A., and Lees, M. B. (1992) Myelin proteolipid protein: minimum sequence requirements for active induction of autoimmune encephalomyelitis in SWR/J and SJL/J mice. *J. Neuroimmunol.* **39,** 67–74.

144. Whitham, R. H., Bourdette, D. N., Hashim, G. A., Herndon, R. M., Ilg, R. C., Vandenbark, A. A., et al. (1991) Lymphocytes from SJL/J mice immunized with spinal cord respond selectively to a peptide of proteolipid protein and transfer relapsing demyelinating experimental autoimmune encephalomyelitis. *J. Immunol.* **146,** 101–107.

145. Cross, A. H., Cannella, B., Brosnan, C. F., and Raine, C. S. (1990) Homing to central nervous system vasculature by antigen-specific lymphocytes. I. Localization of C^{14}-labeled cells during acute, chronic, and relapsing experimental allergic encephalomyelitis. *Lab. Invest.* **63,** 162–170.

146. Hickey, W. F., Gonatas, N. K., Kimura, H., and Wilson, D. B. (1983) Identification and quantitation of T lymphocyte subsets found in the spinal cord of the Lewis rat during acute experimental allergic encephalomyelitis. *J. Immunol.* **131,** 2805–2809.

147. Pope, J. G., Karpus, W. J., VanderLugt, C., and Miller, S. D. (1996) Flow cytometric and functional analyses of central nervous system-infiltrating cells in SJL/J mice with Theiler's virus-induced demyelinating disease. *J. Immunol.* **156,** 4050–4058.

148. Hulkower, K., Brosnan, C. F., Aquino, D. A., Cammer, W., Kulshrestha, S., Guida, M. P., et al. (1993) Expression of CSF-1, c-fms, and MCP-1 in the central nervous system of rats with experimental allergic encephalomyelitis. *J. Immunol.* **150,** 2525–2533.

149. Ransohoff, R. M., Hamilton, T. A., Tani, M., Stoler, M. H., Shick, H. E., Major, J. A., et al. (1993) Astrocyte expression of mRNA encoding cytokines IP-10 and JE/MCP-1 in experimental autoimmune encephalomyelitis. FASEB *Journal* **7(6),** 592–600.

150. Godiska, R., Chantry, D., Dietsch, G. N., and Gray, P. W. (1995) Chemokine expression in murine experimental allergic encephalomyelitis. *J. Neuroimmunol.* **58(2),** 167–176.

151. Glabinski, A. R., Tani, M., Tuohy, V. K., Tuthill, R. J., and Ransohoff, R. M. (1995) Central nervous system chemokine mRNA accumulation follows initial leukocyte entry at the onset of acute murine experimental autoimmune encephalomyelitis. *Brain Behavior Immun.* **9(4),** 315–330.

152. Glabinski, A. R., Tuohy, V. K., and Ransohoff, R. M. (1998) Expression of chemokines RANTES, MIP-1alpha and GRO-alpha correlates with inflammation in acute experimental autoimmune encephalomyelitis. *Neuroimmunomodulation* **5(3-4),** 166–171.

153. Miyagishi, R., Kikuchi, S., Takayama, C., Inoue, Y., and Tashiro, K. (1997) Identification of cell types producing RANTES, MIP-1α, and MIP-1β in rat experimental autoimmune encephalomyelitis by in situ hybridization. *J. Neuroimmunol.* **77,** 17–26.

154. Glabinski, A. R., Tani, M., Strieter, R. M., Tuohy, V. K., and Ransohoff, R. M. (1997) Synchronous synthesis of α- and β-chemokines by cells of diverse lineage in the central nervous system of mice with relapses of chronic experimental autoimmune encephalomyelitis. *Am. J. Pathol.* **150,** 617–630.
155. Kennedy, K. J., Strieter, R. M., Kunkel, S. L., Lukacs, N. W., and Karpus, W. J. (1998) Acute and relapsing experimental autoimmune encephalomyelitis are regulated by differential expression of the CC chemokines macrophage inflammatory protein-1α and monocyte chemotactic protein-1. *J. Neuroimmunol.* **92,** 98–108.
156. Jiang, Y., Salafranca, M. N., Adhikari, S., Xia, Y., Feng, L., Sonntag, M. K., et al. (1998) Chemokine receptor expression in cultured glia and rat experimental allergic encephalomyelitis. *J. Neuroimmunol.* **86(1),** 1–12.

II

Cytokines: Role in Specific Autoimmune Diseases

8

Cytokines and Resistance to Organ Specific Autoimmune Disease

Benjamin M. Segal and Ethan M. Shevach

1. INTRODUCTION

Experiments in animals and humans over the past 20 years have demonstrated that autoreactive CD4[+] T cells are normal constituents of the T cell repertoire in healthy individuals. A diverse range of laboratory animals mount autoimmune responses following immunization with self proteins, such as Type II collagen and myelin basic protein (MBP) *(1–5)*. Furthermore, autoantigen-specific CD4[+] T cells are routinely detected among peripheral blood lymphocytes collected from healthy human volunteers. For example, in a number of studies T cell lines specific for myelin proteins, the presumed autoantigens targeted in multiple sclerosis (MS), have been propagated from blood samples obtained from asymptomatic controls *(6–14)*. Surprisingly, several investigators have found the precursor frequency of myelin-specific T cells to be comparable between healthy individuals and MS patients *(9–14)*. Collectively, these observations suggest that a significant number of autoreactive T cells ordinarily escape both negative selection in the thymus and clonal deletion in the periphery, and that their survival in the peripheral pool of mature T cells is not, in and of itself, predictive of autoimmune disease.

One explanation for the quiescence of autoreactive T cells in healthy individuals is that they remain "clonally ignorant" or oblivious to the existence of their target antigen, which is sequestered from immune surveillance behind an endothelial barrier. However, investigators have recently demonstrated that a number of candidate autoantigens, implicated in human as well as experimental autoimmune diseases, are actually expressed in secondary lymphoid tissues *(15–20)*. Nonetheless, autoimmune diseases are relatively rare. The solution to this apparent paradox is suggested by a body of research demonstrating that peripheral autoreactive CD4[+] T cells are tightly regu-

From: *Cytokines and Autoimmune Diseases*
Edited by: V. K. Kuchroo, et al. © Humana Press Inc., Totowa, NJ

lated by a complex cytokine network. In fact, a series of recent experiments suggest that "immunosuppressive" cytokines, such as interleukin-10 (IL-10) and transforming growth factor-β (TGF-β), are habitually secreted in naive animals to keep potential autoimmune-effector cells at bay *(21–23)*. These immunoregulatory cytokines are proving to be responsible, at least in part, for the high level of resistance exhibited by the majority of laboratory animals to experimentally induced autoimmune diseases, many of which require the administration of potent adjuvants, such as heat killed Mycobacteria, pertussis toxin, and/or immunostimulatory DNA sequences.

On the other hand, there is also evidence that a deficiency of "proinflammatory" cytokines could underlie resistance to autoimmunity in some circumstances. More and more is being learned about the specific cytokine requirements of autoreactive T cells for the acquisition and execution of pathogenic functions. As will be discussed later, the T helper (Th)1 polarizing monokine, IL-12, has emerged as an indispensable and nonredundant factor in the pathogenesis of organ specific autoimmune diseases *(24–26)*. In fact, environmental agents that trigger autoimmune exacerbations, including the bacterial products in the adjuvants used to induce experimental autoimmune diseases, appear to act by stimulating the production of IL-12, thereby leading to bystander activation of autoreactive T cells *(27)*. By logical extension, genetic and environmental factors that suppress IL-12 production by macrophages or dendritic cells (DC) or that dampen the IL-12 responsiveness of developing effector T cells, could raise resistance against organ-specific autoimmunity *(28,29)*.

One conclusion that can be drawn from the previous discussion is that susceptiblity to autoimmune disease is modulated by the cytokine milieu of the microenvironment(s) where autoimmune-effector cells are likely to be activated. Such sites include the target organ itself as well as secondary lymphoid tissues where autoreactive T cells could be stimulated by superantigens, molecular mimics, or ectopically expressed autoantigens. Of particular importance is the balance between proinflammatory/Th1-polarizing cytokines, such as IL-12, and immunosuppressive cytokines, such as IL-10 and TGF-β. In Subheading 2., we will review the data supporting the assertion that T cells must be polarized towards the Th1 lineage in order to mediate organ specific autoimmunity and, consequently, that IL-12 plays a central role in their development. Next, we will discuss the biological functions of IL-10 and TGF-β that could be used to inhibit Th1 effector cell differentiation and/or suppress autoimmunity at a later stage in pathogenesis. Finally, we will summarize the data supporting a role of IL-10- and TGF-β-dependent immunoregulatory circuits in resistance to "spontaneous" as well as actively induced organ specific autoimmunity.

2. ORGAN SPECIFIC AUTOIMMUNE DISEASES ARE INDUCED BY TH1 CD4⁺ T CELLS: ESSENTIAL ROLE OF IL-12 IN PATHOGENESIS

One of the most influential achievements in immunology over the past 30 years was the demonstration that CD4$^+$ T cells can be categorized into functional "Th" subsets based on their cytokine profiles *(30,31)*. In several experimental systems, immune responses to foreign peptides and even complex antigens (including whole microorganisms) were found to be dominated by CD4$^+$ T cells committed to a particular Th phenotype *(32–35)*. Subsequent studies revealed that either Th1 or Th2 anti-microbial responses could be protective depending on the nature of the pathogen *(36–41)*. By contrast, the autoreactive T cells capable of mediating organ specific autoimmune diseases exclusively fell into the Th1 subset *(42)*.

In several adoptive transfer models, including experimental autoimmune encephalomyelitis (EAE) in SJL and B10.PL mice, diabetes in NOD mice and uveitis in Lewis rats, a high correlation exists between the ability of autoantigen-specific T cells to mediate disease and their ability to produce IFN-γ, TNF-α and/or Lymphotoxin upon in vitro challenge *(43–50)*. On the other hand, lines and clones that recognize the same self-peptide/MHC complexes but are manipulated to produce Th2 rather than Th1 cytokines generally lose their disease-causing properties, and in some instances can act to suppress disease *(48,51–55)*. Furthermore, Th1 cytokine expression is upregulated in inflamed target organs and draining lymph nodes from laboratory animals with experimental autoimmune diseases (including collagen-induced arthritis [CIA], diabetes, inflammatory bowel disease [IBD], and encephalomyelitis) *(56–63)* as well as in biopsy and autopsy specimens from patients with the corresponding human ailments (such as rheumatoid arthritis [RA], Crohn's disease, juvenile onset insulin-dependent diabetes mellitus [IDDM], and MS) *(64–70)*. Systemic fluctuations in Th1 cytokines sometimes reflect fluctuations in the target organ and foreshadow disease activity. For example, MS patients have elevated levels of IL-12 in their blood as well as CSF *(71–74)*, whereas RA patients have elevated levels in blood and synovial fluid *(75)*. In the case of MS, elevations of intracellular IL-12 in circulating monocytes correlate with clinical and radiological exacerbations *(76)*.

In recent years, a more complex picture of the role of Th1 cytokines in organ specific autoimmune disease has emerged. It is now widely accepted that IL-12 signaling is crucial for the development and/or function of competent autoimmune effector cells (particularly in those diseases in which CD4$^+$ T cells play the predominant role) *(24,25)*. However, the role of individual Th1 effector cytokines has fallen into question. A review of earlier studies on the effects of neutralizing antibodies against IFN-γ or TNF-α in animal models of autoimmune diseases reveals frequent inconsistencies. For example, anti-IFN-γ was reported to suppress disease activity in some models of IBD, but to have no effect in others *(77,78)*. In one study blockade of TNF-α and Lymphotoxin-α abolished histological EAE, but in another it simply delayed inflammatory infiltration, and in yet another had no effect *(79–83)*. Perhaps the most erratic results have been obtained with anti-IFN-γ in the EAE model. Depending on the timing, strain, and autoantigen, IFN-γ neutralization could protect or, paradoxically, exacerbate the clinical course *(84–89)*.

Analyses of IFN-γ and IFN-γ receptor-deficient mice have yielded more consistent, though unexpected, results. In virtually all animal models of CD4+ T cell-mediated, organ specific autoimmunity thus far tested, IFN-γ and/or IFN-γ receptor knockout mice develop full-blown autoimmune disease with comparable, or even greater severity, than their wild-type counterparts. Specifically, they succumb to EAE, experimental autoimmune uveitis (EAU), CIA, adjuvant-induced arthritis, anti-glomerular basement membrane glomerulonephritis, experimental autoimmune thyroiditis (EAT), several models of inflammatory bowel disease, and diabetes in NOD mice *(90–103)*. The one exception is experimental autoimmune myasthenia gravis (EAMG), in which autoantibodies of the IgG2a subclass play the predominant role during the effector phase *(104)*. With regard to the EAE model, IFN-γ deficiency leads to increased susceptibility across a spectrum of different inbred strains, each challenged with a different myelin peptide or protein *(99–102)*. Similarly, TNF-α and/ or Lymphotoxin-α-deficient mice have been found to be at least as EAE-susceptible as their negative littermates, independent of the strain of origin *(105–109)*. Knockout mice with multiple cytokine deficiencies will have to be constructed to determine whether one Th1 effector cytokine compensates for the absence of another. Nonetheless, the collective data suggests that, although in certain animal models the abrupt blockade of individual Th1 effector cytokines may be therapeutic, as a general rule neither IFN-γ, TNF-α, or Lymphotoxin-α are indispensable for autoimmune pathogenesis.

The experience with IL-12 has been much more definitive. The literature has consistently demonstrated that the monokine plays an essential role in CD4+ T cell-mediated autoimmune pathogenesis *(24,25)*. Hence, the administration of recombinant IL-12 accelerates and/or intensifies EAE, CIA, diabetes in NOD mice, EAMG, and EAT *(110–117)*. Conversely, the administration of neutralizing antibodies against IL-12 protects otherwise susceptible inbred strains from the induction of EAE, inflammatory colitis, CIA, EAU, and EAT *(78,101,110,114,116,118–121)*. In addition, the administration of IL-12 antagonists prevents diabetes in NOD mice *(122)*. Even more impressively, established EAE and CIA are ameliorated by the administration of neutralizing antibodies against IL-12 during the effector phase *(110,121)*. Similarly, IL-12-deficient mice are completely resistant to EAE, EAU, CIA, EAT, and EAMG *(101,112,116,123,124)*. The one exception is diabetes in IL-12-deficient NOD mice *(125)*. However, this model differs from the others in that CD8+ T cells and antibodies play more of a substantive role in the pathogenic process.

Several experiments have directly compared the importance of IL-12 and IFN-γ in animal models of autoimmune disease. The results consistently demonstrate an obligatory role for IL-12, as opposed to IFN-γ, in pathogenesis. For example, neutralization of IL-12 suppresses established colitis in IL-10 deficient mice, whereas anti-IFN-γ has no detectable effect *(78)*. In two other experimental models of IBD, effector T cells from IFN-γ deficient mice, but not from STAT-4 deficient mice (which have blunted responses to IL-12), retain the ability to transfer disease *(97,126)*. Thyroglobulin-stimulated effector T cells from IFN-γ-deficient mice induce a more severe course of autoimmune thyroiditis following activation in the presence of recombinant IL-12 *(94)*. Most convincingly, the administration of neutralizing antibodies against IL-12 prevents the development of EAE and CIA in highly susceptible IFN-γ and IFN-γ receptor-deficient mice, respectively *(101,127)*. Hence, IL-12 can promote organ specific autoimmune disease by IFN-γ independent pathways. The overriding implication is that the most effective immunoregulatory mechanisms will target IL-12-mediated events, as opposed to effector cytokines further downstream.

3. ANTI-TH1/MACROPHAGE DEACTIVATING CYTOKINES AND SUPPRESSION OF AUTOIMMUNE PHENOMENA

Based on the previous discussion, it should come as no surprise that IL-10 and TGF-β are proving to play critical immunoregulatory roles in suppressing organ specific autoimmune diseases. Both cytokines have specific "anti-IL-12" effects. Shortly after the discovery of IL-10, a series of articles were published reporting that it suppressed cytokine production and antigen-specific proliferation by Th1 clones in vitro *(128–130)*. Conversely, the addition of anti-IL-10 neutralizing antibodies to primary lymph node cell cultures biased developing CD4+ T cells towards the Th1 pathway *(131)*. It was realized that most, if not all of these effects, were mediated indirectly through the modulation of antigen-presenting cells (APCs), because IL-10 was not as effective in accessory cell-independent systems *(132,133)*. Similarly, TGF-β was found to suppress Th1 differentiation through modulation of

APCs *(134,135)*. Indeed, it is now recognized that both cytokines directly suppress IL-12 secretion *(135–137)*, as well as expression of MHC Class II and costimulatory molecules *(132,138–140)*, by DC and/or macrophages. With respect to effects on costimulatory molecules, IL-10 downregulates B7 molecules *(141–145)* and TGF-β suppresses CD40 *(135,146)*. IL-10 and TGF-β each have direct biological effects on T cells as well. Both inhibit developing T cells from expressing the β2 subunit of the IL-12 receptor, thereby rendering them unresponsive to IL-12 and derailing Th1 differentiation *(147–150)*. In addition, TGF-β blocks IL-12 signal-transduction pathways *(151)*. Finally, IL-10 diminishes IL-2 and TNF-α secretion, even when T cells are stimulated under accessory cell-free conditions *(152–154)*, and TGF-β inhibits IL-2-dependent T cell proliferation, in part by downregulating the IL-2 receptor *(155)*.

IL-10- and TGF-β-mediated suppression of autoimmunity may involve more than the direct or indirect inhibition of effector T cells. Although in several animal models Th1 CD4$^+$ T cells initiate the inflammatory process, activated macrophages are believed to inflict the ultimate damage to host tissues, through production of free oxygen radicals and/ or TNF-α. In this regard, IL-10 and TGF-β both limit the production of nitric oxide (NO) and free oxygen radicals by monocytes-macrophages *(156–163)*. In addition, TGF-β hinders TNF-α secretion by these cell types *(161)* and IL-10 modulates the ability of macrophages to turnover the extracellular matrix (ECM) *(164,165)*.

4. ROLE OF ENDOGENOUS IMMUNOREGULATORY CYTOKINES IN PREVENTING "SPONTANEOUS" AUTOIMMUNITY

Much of the data substantiating the regulatory roles of IL-10 and TGF-β in maintaining "immune homeostasis" comes from experimental models of IBD. One of these models involves the transfer of CD45RB^{high} CD4$^+$ T cells isolated from naive BALB/c splenocytes into immunodeficient CB.17 SCID or RAG2 –/– mice. Inflammatory colitis invariably ensues within 3–5 wk of the transfer, but is prevented by cotransfer of the reciprocal CD45RB^{low} subpopulation *(166)*. This finding suggests that, in immunocompetent mice, CD45RB^{low} regulatory cells are continually engaged in the active suppression of CD45RB^{high} effector cells, thereby preventing the "spontaneous" development of colitis. The mechanism of suppression is dependent on the secretion of IL-10 and TGF-β, as supported by a wealth of circumstantial as well as direct evidence. First, the systemic administration of recombinant IL-10 (but not IL-4) inhibits CD45RB^{high} CD4+ T effector cells from inducing colitis *(77)*, while the administration of neutralizing antibodies against TGF-β or blocking antibodies against the IL-10 receptor abrogates protection by CD45RB^{low} regulatory T cells *(22,167)*. Furthermore, the biological functions of the CD4$^+$ T cell subsets can be reversed by genetically manipulating their IL-10 production patterns. For example, CD45RB^{low} T cells from IL-10 deficient mice not only fail to suppress colitis, but actually induce the disease when transferred alone into SCID recipients *(22)*. Conversely, CD45RB^{high} cells from transgenic mice expressing IL-10 under the IL-2 promoter not only fail to induce colitis in SCID recipients, but prevent the disease when coinjected with CD45RB^{high} T cells from control mice *(168)*. Hence, "forced" expression of IL-10 converts effector cells into regulatory cells, whereas deficient IL-10 expression converts regulatory cells into effectors.

Further evidence for the roles of endogenous IL-10 and TGF-β in suppressing spontaneous autoimmune phenomena comes from studies of cytokine-deficient mice. As one might predict, IL-10-deficient mice inevitably develop enterocolitis as they mature *(21)*. As in the reconstituted SCID model, the colitis appears to be mediated by a subset of Th1 CD4$^+$ effector cells. (The disease is transferred into Rag2$^{-/-}$ recipients by Th1-polarized CD4$^+$ cells harvested from the inflamed colons of adult IL-10 knockout mice and it is inhibited by neutralizing antibodies against IL-12 *[78,169–171]*.) The enterocolitis is not secondary to a developmental artifact because it is prevented by administration of recombinant IL-10 from birth *(172)*. Presumably, the autoimmune disease arises as a result of the functional absence of IL-10 producing regulatory T cells, analogous to the CD45RB^{low} subset that has been isolated from wild-type BALB/c splenocytes, as discussed previously.

Despite their pervasive developmental abnormalities, TGFβ1 knockout mice have also been informative with regard to endogenous immunoregulatory cytokine networks. At a young age (generally 2–3 wk), they develop multiorgan inflammatory infiltrates *(173)*. Concomitantly, autoantibodies appear in their sera and immune complexes appear in kidney glomeruli. This spontaneous autoimmune syndrome is driven by MHC Class II-restricted antigen presentation, because double knockout mice, that are deficient in MHC Class II as well as TGFβ1, are protected from autoimmune pathology *(174)*. Hence, autoreactive CD4$^+$ T cells play a key role in initiating the inflammatory process in the TGFβ1 single knockouts. By contrast, β2-microglobulin deficiency ameliorates, but does not abrogate, the autoimmune syndrome *(175)*. This suggests that CD8$^+$ T cells contribute to the autoimmune pathology, though in a less essential way than their CD4$^+$ counterparts.

In order to more accurately define the role of TGF-β in immune homeostasis, Gorelick and Flavell recently developed a transgenic approach to abrogate the TGF-β response exclusively in immune cells *(23)*. Specifically, they expressed a dominant-negative TGF-β receptor type II under the control of the CD4 promoter (which is expressed at some point in CD8$^+$ as well as CD4$^+$ T cells) thereby creating a mouse model whereby TGF-β signaling is blocked specifically in T cells. The phenotype of these transgenic mice is characterized by a wasting illness and diarrhea starting at 3–4 mo of age. Histological examination reveals marked-to-severe IBD, pulmonitis, and mild infiltration of the pancreas and kidneys. As in the TGFβ1 knockout, autoantibodies are found in the sera and immune complex deposits are found in the kidney glomeruli. Peripheral T cells in adult transgenic mice appear to have been activated by endogenous antigens. Lymph nodes are expanded to three times their normal size, and a high percentage of CD4$^+$ as well as CD8$^+$ cells express memory markers. Furthermore, unlike T cells harvested from naive wild-type mice, those from the transgenic produce effector cytokines (IFN-γ and IL-4) immediately upon in vitro activation, commensurate with a memory phenotype. These findings indicate that, if not for TGF-β-mediated suppression, a significant number of peripheral T cells in wild-type mice would inevitably enter an activated state without overt provocation. The development of multi-organ infiltrates in the transgenic mice implies that at least some of these TGF-β-inhibited T cells are autoreactive and would otherwise initiate spontaneous autoimmune disease.

In addition to IL-10 and TGF-β deficiency, a congenital absence of IL-2 results in the development of "spontaneous" enterocolitis *(176)*. This disease also appears to be IL-12 driven since Th1 CD4$^+$ T cells comprise the majority of the inflammatory infiltrate and IL-12 neutralizing antibodies are protective *(177,178)*. At first glance, the phenotype of the IL-2 knockout is somewhat surprising. IL-2 is the quintessential T cell growth factor. Hence one might expect widespread T cell anergy and, consequently, deficient autoreactive as well as foreign antigen-specific adaptive responses. The phenotype of IL-2 knockout mice may result from differences in the dependence of effector cells and regulatory cells on IL-2 for clonal expansion and/or survival. IL-12 can act as a growth factor for Th1 cells and in several systems has been shown to have anti-apoptotic effects *(179)*. It is possible that, in the absence of IL-2, the colitis-inducing cells are rescued by IL-12 signaling, whereas endogenous regulatory cells (which most likely do not express IL-12 receptors) do not have this recourse. In addition, IL-2 deficient mice have an absolute deficiency in the number of regulatory T cells that express the CD4$^+$ CD25$^+$ phenotype *(180)*. The selective advantage thereby gained by the effector cells results in their dominance and autoimmune pathology.

5. ROLE OF ENDOGENOUS IMMUNOREGULATORY CYTOKINES IN RESISTANCE TO ACTIVELY INDUCED AUTOIMMUNE DISEASES

In the last section we discussed the role of immunoregulatory cytokines in the prevention of "spontaneous" immune events in naive animals, not otherwise provoked. In this section, we will address their role in promoting resistance to organ specific autoimmune syndromes that are deliberately induced by active immunization with selected autoantigens combined with adjuvants. These models may simulate the physiological situation in humans when infectious illness triggers autoimmune exacerbations. The pathogen introduces a foreign antigen that mimics an autoantigen along with nonspecific immunomodulatory molecules that act as adjuvants (such as IL-12-stimulating bacterial DNA).

As in the case of "spontaneous" autoimmunity, the literature indicates that IL-10 and TGF-β are the predominant mediators used to control actively induced autoimmune syndromes. Hence, IL-10 deficient mice experience EAE and EAU at a greater incidence and severity than their wild-type counterparts *(101,181–183)*. This increased susceptibility does not represent a developmental artifact; adult wild-type mice treated with neutralizing antibodies against IL-10 experience an exacerbated clinical course similar to the knockouts *(101,183–185)*. IL-10 neutralization also increases susceptibility to experimental arthritis and diabetes *(186–189)*. By contrast, transgenic mice in which the IL-10 gene is under the control of the IL-2 promoter (targeting expression to T cells) or the MHC Class II promoter (targeting expression to APCs) are resistant to the induction of EAE and CD45RB^{low} CD4$^+$ T cell-mediated colitis, respectively *(168,190)*. We have previously stated that an IL-10/IL-12 immunoregulatory circuit controls susceptibility to autoimmune disease *(101)*. This was based on experiments that used neutralizing antibodies against IL-12 to prevent EAE. The protective effect of the antibodies was at least in part attributable to the emergence of IL-10 producing regulatory CD4$^+$ T cells. Our results suggest that during homeostasis a constant struggle exists between IL-12-mediated autoimmune processes and IL-10-mediated immunosuppression.

An extensive body of data demonstrates a similar role of TGF-β in immunoregulation. It is not practical to use TGFβ1-deficient mice in the study of actively induced autoimmune diseases because, as discussed earlier, they spontaneously develop rampant multi-organ inflammation at a young age and have relatively short life-spans. However, the neutralization of endogenous TGF-β in wild-type mice leads to an increase in the incidence and severity of EAE, CIA, and diabetes *(191–195)*.

The realization that organ specific autoimmune syndromes are Th1 mediated, leads many to speculate that endogenous IL-4 would also play an important immunoregulatory role in conferring resistance. IL-4 directly suppresses IL-12 production by DC *(136)*. It downregulates IL-12 receptor β2 expression (and therefore IL-12 responsiveness) by developing T cells under certain conditions *(196,197)*. Indeed, the administration of exogenous IL-4 (either as a recombinant cytokine or in an expression vector) has been shown to suppress EAE, several models of autoimmune arthritis, and diabetes in NOD mice *(186,188,198–204)*. IL-4 dependent pathways have also been implicated in the therapeutic effects of altered peptide ligands and oral tolerance *(54,55)*. Nonetheless, there is little convincing evidence that endogenous IL-4 participates in physiological immunoregulatory pathways. IL-4 deficient mice do not develop spontaneous colitis or any other autoimmune syndrome, for that matter. Furthermore, they resemble their wild-type counterparts with respect to incidence and severity of EAE and experimental diabetes *(101,182,205,206)*. CD4$^+$ CD45RB^{low} regulatory cells from IL-4 deficient, but not IL-10 deficient, donors are fully capable of suppressing IBD *(22,167)*. Neutralizing antibodies against IL-4 do not exacerbate diabetes in NOD mice *(207)*. Although some investigators found that anti-IL-4 treatment increases susceptibility to adjuvant induced arthritis and CIA *(208,209)*, others found it to be ineffective or to actually inhibit the development of disease *(188,210,211)*.

Endogenous IL-4 probably does not play as predominant a role in the regulation autoimmunity as IL-10 or TGF-β because of the conditions necessary for its production in vivo. The strongest promoter of Th2 differentiation is IL-4 itself and Th2-polarized CD4$^+$ T cells are the primary source of IL-4 *(33)*. Hence, this raises the quandry of how to induce IL-4 production *de novo* in the settings where autoimmune effector cells are activated. No such predicament arises when considering IL-10 and activated TGF-β as regulatory factors. Both are secreted by macrophage-monocytes and DC (as well as by regulatory T cells) in response to a broad range of nonspecific stimuli, including microbial products such as lipopolysaccharide (LPS) *(128,212–214)*. As noted earlier, infectious diseases often trigger autoimmune exacerbations, so such stimuli are likely to be present in the local microenvironment during effector-cell differentiation. In this way, regulatory pathways are set into motion at the inception of an autoimmune response. Furthermore, recent studies demonstrate that IL-10 production by APCs promotes the development of IL-10 and TGF-β-producing regulatory "Tr1" cells that can, in turn, perpetuate immunosuppression *(215)*. No such scenario can be painted using IL-4-dependent regulatory circuits.

6. QUALITATIVE DIFFERENCES IN CYTOKINE RESPONSES TO AUTOANTIGENS UNDERLIE GENETIC DIFFERENCES IN SUSCEPTIBILITY TO AUTOIMMUNE DISEASE

It has long been recognized that the relative susceptibility of inbred rodent strains to experimental autoimmune diseases generally correlates with their major histocompatibility complex (MHC) haplotype. This led to the practice of classifying MHC molecules as "permissive" or "nonpermissive" for the development of particular autoimmune syndromes. It was widely assumed that resistance resulted from a deficiency of MHC molecule/ autoantigen complexes that could positively select autoimmune-effector cells in the thymus and activate them in the periphery. However, this does not appear to always be the case. There are exceptional animals that bear a "permissive" MHC haplotype but are, nonetheless, resistant to autoimmune-disease induction. Moreover, lymphoproliferative and precursor-frequency analyses demonstrate that many of these resistant strains harbor a peripheral pool of autoantigen specific T cells that is comparable in size to that present in MHC-matched susceptible animals *(115,216,217)*.

In some instances, investigators have found a qualitative, as opposed to quantitative, difference in the autoimmune response mounted by resistant and susceptible strains, characterized by divergent patterns of cytokine production. Several generalities have emerged from such studies. First and foremost, autoimmune effector T cells from susceptible strains consistently express a Th1 phenotype, while innocuous T cells from resistant strains, with the same self peptide/MHC specificities, do not *(115,217–222)*. Th1 cytokines are upregulated within the target organs and draining lymph nodes of susceptible animals at peak disease. (This includes IFN-γ routinely and TNF-α frequently) *[59,60,223,224]*.) Moreover, T cells harvested from symptomatic donors produce the same proinflammatory Th1 cytokines upon challenge with the autoantigen ex vivo *(59,60,221,223–226)*. These Th1 effector cells are dependent on IL-12 for differentiation and/or biological functions; injection of susceptible animals with neutralizing antibodies against the monokine abrogates IFN-γ production and protects against the autoimmune disease *(101)*. Autoantigen-specific lymphoproliferation is preserved, suggesting that IL-12 neutralization acts by altering, rather than eliminating, the autoimmune response.

Conversely, the innocuous autoreactive T cells harvested from resistant animals generally produce significantly less IFN-γ and TNF-α than the effector cells from congenic susceptible mice, if any at all. Furthermore, Th1 cytokine expression is not upregulated in their target organs or draining lymph nodes following priming with autoantigen combined with adjuvants.

These observations are consistent across a spectrum of experimental autoimmune syndromes, including encephalomyelitis, uveitis, arthritis, neuritis, and myasthenia gravis *(115,217–221,223,225–227)*. In the EAE and EAU models, investigators have found that autoantigen-specific T cells from resistant animals with a permissive MHC haplotype differentiate along an autoimmune-effector lineage and acquire pathogenic properties following reactivation in the presence of exogenous IL-12 *(115,217)*. Hence, it can be confidently stated that non-MHC related genetic factors that influence the ability of autoreactive T cells to embark upon a Th1-differentation pathway modulate susceptiblity to autoimmune disease.

However, the literature is less exact in defining the cellular and molecular basis of resistance. For example, do resistant animals simply lack the "machinery" to mount an autoimmune Th1 response or is such a response actively suppressed by immunoregulatory pathways? In other words, does resistance represent a passive or an active immunological state? There is evidence supporting both sides and it may be that resistance is achieved by different means depending on the strain and even on the autoantigen.

Most of the evidence that genetically determined resistance to autoimmune disease results from active suppression is circumstantial. It is based on experiments where "immunosuppressive" cytokines (IL-10, TGF-β, and IL-4, either alone or in various combinations) have been detected in the target organ and/or draining lymph nodes of resistant rodents or in the supernatants of autoantigen-stimulated T cell lines ex vivo. For example, Maron and colleagues found that TGF-β and IL-10 are upregulated in the lymph nodes and CNS of EAE-resistant, I-A^s positive B10.S mice following immunization with a potentially encephalitogenic myelin peptide *(223)*. By contrast, only IFN-γ and IL-2 were detected in lymph nodes and CNS specimens from susceptible I-A^s positive SJL mice treated in the same manner. In parallel experiments they detected IL-4 and IL-10 in the lymph nodes and CNS of EAE-resistant, I-A^{g7}-positive strain III mice, but not in susceptible congenic NOD mice. Similarly, several investigators have detected TGF-β in T cells and in CNS specimens harvested from EAE-resistant, but not EAE-susceptible, rats sensitized against myelin antigens *(59,224,228)*. TGF-β expression has also been associated with strain-related resistance in experimental models of autoimmune neuritis and myasthenia gravis *(225,226)*. Finally, investigators have measured IL-4 production by autoantigen-primed splenocytes exclusively from mice that are resistant to arthritis *(221)* and IL-10 production by lymph-node cells exclusively from rats that are resistant to neuritis *(225)*. The skewing of autoimmune responses towards a Th1 or Th2 pathway may underlie gender-based, as well as strain-based, differences in susceptibility to organ-specific autoimmune diseases. Cua and colleagues found that EAE-resistant male SJL mice mount a Th2-polarized response against MBP (characterized by antigen-specific IL-4 production), while their EAE-susceptible female cohorts mount a polarized Th1 response (characterized by antigen-specific IFN-γ production) *(229)*.

However, these studies, while suggestive, prove nothing with regard to cause and effect. It is unclear if the "immunosuppressive" cytokines that were measured in the above studies are physiologically significant or simply represent an epiphenomenon. The importance of this distinction is perhaps best illustrated in the study reported by Maron and colleagues *(223)*. Despite the fact that TGF-β was detected in lymph nodes and brains of B10.S mice following sensitization with myelin peptides, neutralization of TGF-β in vivo did not overcome their resistance to EAE. On the other hand, in another study, EAE was induced in a normally resistant strain of rats by the injection of neutralizing antibodies against TGF-β at the time of sensitization *(228)*. To the authors' knowledge, a resistant strain has never been converted into a susceptible one by neutralization of IL-4 and/or IL-10 at the time of priming or at any point thereafter.

In contrast to the studies cited previously, others have not detected the production of immunosuppressive cytokines in autoantigen-sensitized "MHC permissive" animals that are resistant to autoimmune disease. In many of these experiments, the resistant animals were found to harbor significant numbers of autoreactive T cells based on autoantigen-specific lymphoproliferation and/or IL-2 or IL-3 production. However, they fail to mount a Th2, as well as a Th1, response. For example, Caspi and colleagues analyzed a panel of inbred rodent strains with varying degrees of susceptibility to autoimmune uveitis and found no consistent relationship between autoantigen-induced IL-4 production and resistance *(217,218,220)*. Similarly, we found that draining lymph nodes from EAE-resistant B10.S mice, immunized with an immunodominant MBP peptide, failed to secrete detectable IL-4 or IL-10 upon in vitro challenge *(115)*. Subsequent studies demonstrated that the MBP-reactive T cells from the B10.S mice, as opposed to those from susceptible SJL mice, have an antigen-specific defect in their capacity to upregulate CD40 ligand, induce the production of IL-12, and express functional IL-12 receptors. IL-12 receptor expression as well as encephalitogenicity of these cells could be restored by the addition of exogenous IL-12, but not by neutralization of either IL-4, IL-10, or TGF-β *(150)*. Hence, in this case resistance appears to result from a primary "Th1 defect" as opposed to active suppression. It should be noted that the different results obtained by ourselves and Maron et al. regarding the expression of TGF-β and IL-10 in B10.S mice could be owing to the fact that different myelin peptides were used as the targeted autoantigen. (We used the immunodominant peptide of MBP peptide; Maron used a peptide fragment of myelin oligo-dendroglial glycoprotein.) Nonetheless, as mentioned earlier, in neither case did neutralization of immunosuppressive cytokines reverse disease resistance. Finally, Kim and colleagues reported that the EAE-resistance of male SJL mice results from a gender-based defect in IL-12 production by accessory cells *(230)*. As opposed to Cua et al. *(229)*, they concluded that Th1 differentiation was blocked without immune deviation to a Th2 pathway.

It is possible that in some of the aforementioned studies active suppression is indeed responsible for disease resistance, but the investigators did not measure the pertinent immunoregulatory factors and/or analyze the pertinent subset of regulatory cells. Hence, Conboy et al. found that the resistance exhibited by B10.A mice to EAE is secondary to the production of a Th1 inhibitory soluble factor by splenic APCs *(219)*. Furthermore, this soluble factor is able to suppress the Th1 phenotype and encephaliogenicity of myelin-reactive T cell lines derived from B10.BR mice, which ordinarily are highly susceptible to disease induction. The immunosuppression is not inactivated by neutralization of either IL-10, IL-4, TGF-β, IFN-γ, TNF-α, or the natural IL-12 heterodimer antagonist, IL-12 p40 homodimer. As of now, the identity of the inhibitory molecule(s) remains unclarified. That is not to say that every case of resistance to autoimmune disease is mediated by accessory cell-derived suppressive factors. In our experiments, the innocuous phenotype of B10.S MBP-reactive T cells and the pathogenic phenotype of congenic SJL MBP-reactive T cells could not be reversed by mixing and matching APCs *(115)*.

7. CONCLUSION

Despite earlier assumptions to the contrary, it is now firmly established that autoreactive T cells are normal constituents of the peripheral repertoire in healthy individuals. Studies from several laboratories have demonstrated that, under certain circumstances, they have the potential to be transformed into autoimmune-effector cells following stimulation with IL-12. Consequently, during the course of evolution the immune system developed an intricate immunoregulatory network, largely dependent on the production of the "suppressive" cytokines, IL-10 and TGF-β, to block their pathogenic conversion. Genetic and environmental factors that upset the homeostatic balance maintained between the production of IL-12, on the one hand, and IL-10 and TGF-β on the other, modulate susceptibility to autoimmune disease. The challenge facing clincians and scientists in the future will be to tip the balance in favor of immunosuppression in an autoantigen-specific manner that does not compromise protective anti-microbial and anti-tumor Th1 responses.

REFERENCES

1. Courtenay, J. S., Dallman, M. J., Dayan, A. D., Martin, A, and Mosedale, B. (1980) Immunisation against heterologous type II collagen induces arthritis in mice. *Nature* **283(5748),** 666–668.
2. Fritz, R. B., Chou, C. C., and McFarlin, D. E. (1983) Induction of experimental allergic encephalomyelitis in PL/J and (SJL/J x PL/J)F1 mice by myelin basic protein and its peptides: localization of a second encephalitogenic determinant. *J. Immunol.* **130(1),** 191–194.
3. Stuart, J. M., Townes, A. S., and Kang, A. H. (1982) Nature and specificity of the immune response to collagen in type II collagen-induced arthritis in mice. *J. Clin. Invest.* **69(3),** 673–683.
4. Trentham, D. E., Townes, A. S., and Kang, A. H. (1977) Autoimmunity to type II collagen an experimental model of arthritis. *J. Exp. Med.* **146(3),** 857–868.
5. Zamvil, S. S. and Steinman, L. (1990) The T lymphocyte in experimental allergic encephalomyelitis. *Annu. Rev. Immunol.* **8,** 579–621.
6. Chou, Y. K., Vainiene, M., Whitham, R., Bourdette, D., Chou, C. H., Hashim, G., et al. (1989) Response of human T lymphocyte lines to myelin basic protein: association of dominant epitopes with HLA class II restriction molecules. *J. Neurosci. Res.* **23(2),** 207–216.
7. Martin, R., Utz, U., Coligan, J. E., Richert, J. R., Flerlage, M., Robinson, E., et al. (1992) Diversity in fine specificity and T cell receptor usage of the human CD4+ cytotoxic T cell response specific for the immunodominant myelin basic protein peptide 87-106. *J. Immunol.* **148(5),** 1359-1366.
8. Ota, K., Matsui M., Milford, E. L., Mackin, G. A., Weiner, H. L., and Hafler, D. A. (1990) T-cell recognition of an immunodominant myelin basic protein epitope in multiple sclerosis. *Nature* **346(6280),** 183–187.
9. Pette, M., Fujita, K., Kitze, B., Whitaker, J. N., Albert, E., Kappos, L., et al. (1990) Myelin basic protein-specific T lymphocyte lines from MS patients and healthy individuals. *Neurology* **40(11),** 1770–1776.
10. Martin, R., Jaraquemada, D., Flerlage, M., Richert, J., Whitaker, J., Long, E. O., et al. (1990) Fine specificity and HLA restriction of myelin basic protein-specific cytotoxic T cell lines from multiple sclerosis patients and healthy individuals. *J. Immunol.* **145(2),** 540–548.
11. Pelfrey, C. M., Tranquill, L. R., Vogt, A. B., and McFarland, H. F. (1996) T cell response to two immunodominant proteolipid protein (PLP) peptides in multiple sclerosis patients and healthy controls. *Mult. Scler.* **1(5),** 270–278.
12. Voskuhl, R. R., Martin, R., and McFarland, H. F. (1993) A functional basis for the association of HLA class II genes and susceptibility to multiple sclerosis: cellular immune responses to myelin basic protein in a multiplex family. *J. Neuroimmunol.* **42(2),** 199–207.
13. Voskuhl, R. R., Voskuhl, R. R., McFarlin, D. E., Tranquill, L. R., Deibler, G., Stone, R., et al. (1993) A novel candidate autoantigen in a multiplex family with multiple sclerosis: prevalence of T-lymphocytes specific for an MBP epitope unique to myelination. *J. Neuroimmunol.* **46(1-2),** 137–144.
14. Jingwu, Z., Medaer, R, Hashim, G. A., Chin, Y., van den Berg-Loonen, E., and Raus, J. C. (1992) Myelin basic protein-specific T lymphocytes in mul-

tiple sclerosis and controls: precursor frequency, fine specificity, and cyto-toxicity. *Ann. Neurol.* **32(3),** 330–338.

15. Fritz, R. B. and Zhao, M. L. (1996) Thymic expression of myelin basic pro-tein (MBP). Activation of MBP- specific T cells by thymic cells in the absence of exogenous MBP. *J. Immunol.* **157(12),** 5249–5523.

16. Mathisen, P. M., Pease, S., Garvey, J., Hood, L., and Readhead, C. (1993) Iden-tification of an embryonic isoform of myelin basic protein that is expressed widely in the mouse embryo. *Proc. Natl. Acad. Sci. USA* **90(21),** 10,125–10,129.

17. Pribyl, T. M., Campagnoni, C. W., Kampf, K., Kashima, T., Handley, V. W., McMahon, J., et al. (1993) The human myelin basic protein gene is included within a 179-kilobase transcription unit: expression in the immune and central nervous systems. *Proc. Natl. Acad. Sci. USA* **90(22),** 10,695–10,699.

18. Pribyl, T. M., Campagnoni, C. W., Kampf, K., Kashima, T., Handley, V. W., McMahon, J., et al. (1996) Expression of the myelin proteolipid protein gene in the human fetal thymus. *J. Neuroimmunol.* **67(2),** 125–130.

19. MacKenzie-Graham, A. J., Pribyl, T. M., Kim, S., Porter, V. R., Campagnoni, A. T., and Voskuhl, R. R. (1997) Myelin protein expression is increased in lymph nodes of mice with relapsing experimental autoimmune encephalomyelitis. *J. Immunol.* **159(9),** 4602–4610.

20. Voskuhl, R. R. (1998) Myelin protein expression in lymphoid tissues: impli-cations for peripheral tolerance. *Immunol. Rev.* **164,** 81–92.

21. Kuhn, R., Lohler, J., Rennick, D., Rajewsky, K., and Muller, W. (1993) Interleukin-10-deficient mice develop chronic enterocolitis. *Cell* **75(2),** 263–274.

22. Asseman, C., Mauze, S., Leach, M. W., Coffman, R. L., and Powrie, F. (1999) An essential role for interleukin 10 in the function of regulatory T cells that inhibit intestinal inflammation. *J. Exp. Med.* **190(7),** 995–1004.

23. Gorelik, L. and Flavell, R. A. (2000) Abrogation of TGFbeta signaling in T cells leads to spontaneous T cell differentiation and autoimmune disease. *Immunity* **12(2),** 171–181.

24. Caspi, R. R. (1998) IL-12 in autoimmunity. *Clin. Immunol. Immunopathol.* **88(1),** 4–13.

25. Trembleau, S., Germann, T., Gately, M. K., and Adorini, L. (1995) The role of IL-12 in the induction of organ-specific autoimmune diseases. *Immunol. Today* **16(8),** 383–386.

26. Seder, R. A., Kelsall, B. L., and Jankovic, D. (1996) Differential roles for IL-12 in the maintenance of immune responses in infectious versus auto-immune disease. *J. Immunol.* **157(7),** 2745–2748.

27. Segal, B. M., Klinman, D. M., and Shevach, E. M. (1997) Microbial prod-ucts induce autoimmune disease by an IL-12-dependent pathway. *J. Immunol.* **158(11),** 5087–5090.

28. Wu, C. Y., Wang, K., McDyer, J. F., and Seder, R. A. (1998) Prostaglandin E2 and dexamethasone inhibit IL-12 receptor expression and IL-12 responsiveness. *J. Immunol.* **161(6),** 2723–2730.

29. Bebo, B. F., Jr., Schuster, J. C., Vandenbark, A. A., and Offner, H. (1999) Androgens alter the cytokine profile and reduce encephalitogenicity of myelin-reactive T cells. *J. Immunol.* **162(1),** 35–40.

30. Cher, D. J. and Mosmann, T. R. (1987) Two types of murine helper T cell clone. II. Delayed-type hypersensitivity is mediated by TH1 clones. *J. Immunol.* **138(11),** 3688–3694.

31. Mosmann, T. R. and Coffman, R. L. (1989) TH1 and TH2 cells: different patterns of lymphokine secretion lead to different functional properties. *Annu. Rev. Immunol.* **7,** 145–173.

32. Tsicopoulos, A., Hamid, Q., Varney, V., Ying, S., Moqbel, R., Durham, S. R., et al. (1992) Preferential messenger RNA expression of Th1-type cells (IFN-gamma+, IL- 2+) in classical delayed-type (tuberculin) hypersensitivity reactions in human skin. *J. Immunol.* **148(7),** 2058–2061.

33. Seder, R. A. (1994) Acquisition of lymphokine-producing phenotype by CD4+ T cells. *J. Allergy Clin. Immunol.* **94(6 Pt 2),** 1195–1202.

34. Parronchi, P., Macchia, D., Piccinni, M. P., Biswas, P., Simonelli, C., Maggi, E., et al. (1991) Allergen- and bacterial antigen-specific T-cell clones established from atopic donors show a different profile of cytokine production. *Proc. Natl. Acad. Sci. USA* **88(10),** 4538–4542.

35. Del Prete, G. F., De Carli, M., Mastromauro, C., Biagiotti, R., Macchia, D., Falagiani, P., et al. (1991) Purified protein derivative of Mycobacterium tuberculosis and excretory- secretory antigen(s) of Toxocara canis expand in vitro human T cells with stable and opposite (type 1 T helper or type 2 T helper) profile of cytokine production. *J. Clin. Invest.* **88(1),** 346–350.

36. Bancroft, A. J., McKenzie, A. N., and Grencis, R. K. (1998) A critical role for IL-13 in resistance to intestinal nematode infection. *J. Immunol.* **160(7),** 3453–3461.

37. Else, K. J., Finkelman, F. D., Maliszewski, C. R., and Grencis, R. K. (1994) Cytokine-mediated regulation of chronic intestinal helminth infection. *J. Exp. Med.* **179(1),** 347–351.

38. Finkelman, F. D., Shea-Donohue, T., Goldhill, J., Sullivan, C. A., Morris, S. C., Madden, K. B., et al. (1997) Cytokine regulation of host defense against parasitic gastrointestinal nematodes: lessons from studies with rodent models. *Annu. Rev. Immunol.* **15,** 505–533.

39. Urban, J. F., Jr., Katona, I. M., Paul, W. E., and Finkelman, F. D. (1991) Interleukin 4 is important in protective immunity to a gastrointestinal nematode infection in mice. *Proc. Natl. Acad. Sci. USA* **88(13),** 5513–5517.

40. Scott, P., Pearce, E., Cheever, A. W., Coffman, R. L., and Sher, A. (1989) Role of cytokines and CD4+ T-cell subsets in the regulation of parasite immunity and disease. *Immunol. Rev.* **112,** 161–182.

41. Reiner, S. L. and Locksley, R. M. (1995) The regulation of immunity to Leishmania major. *Annu. Rev. Immunol.* **13,** 151–177.

42. Liblau, R. S., Singer, S. M., and McDevitt, H. O. (1995) Th1 and Th2 CD4+ T cells in the pathogenesis of organ-specific autoimmune diseases. *Immunol. Today* **16(1),** 34–38.

43. Ando, D. G., Clayton, J., Kono, D., Urban, J. L., and Sercarz, E. E. (1989) Encephalitogenic T cells in the B10. PL model of experimental allergic encephalomyelitis (EAE) are of the Th-1 lymphokine subtype. *Cell Immunol.* **124(1),** 132–143.

44. Baron, J. L., Madri, J. A., Ruddle, N. H., Hashim, G., and Janeway, C. A., Jr. (1993) Surface expression of alpha 4 integrin by CD4 T cells is required for their entry into brain parenchyma. *J. Exp. Med.* **177(1),** 57–68.

45. Bergman, B. and Haskins, K. (1994) Islet-specific T-cell clones from the NOD mouse respond to beta-granule antigen. *Diabetes* **43(2),** 197–203.
46. Haskins, K. and Wegmann, D. (1996) Diabetogenic T-cell clones. *Diabetes* **45(10),** 1299–1305.
47. Haskins, K. and McDuffie, M. (1990) Acceleration of diabetes in young NOD mice with a CD4+ islet-specific T cell clone. *Science* **249(4975),** 1433–1436.
48. Katz, J. D., Benoist, C., and Mathis, D. (1995) T helper cell subsets in insulin-dependent diabetes. *Science* **268(5214),** 1185–1188.
49. Powell, M. B., Mitchell, D., Lederman, J., Buckmeier, J., Zamvil, S. S., Graham, M., et al. (1990) Lymphotoxin and tumor necrosis factor-alpha production by myelin basic protein-specific T cell clones correlates with encephalitogenicity. *Intl. Immunol.* **2(6),** 539–544.
50. Savion, S., Oddo, S., Grover, S., and Caspi, R. R. (1994) Uveitogenic T lymphocytes in the rat: pathogenicity vs. lymphokine production, adhesion molecules and surface antigen expression. *J. Neuroimmunol.* **55(1),** 35–44.
51. van der Veen, R. C. and Stohlman, S. A. (1993) Encephalitogenic Th1 cells are inhibited by Th2 cells with related peptide specificity: relative roles of interleukin (IL)-4 and IL-10. *J. Neuroimmunol.* **48(2),** 213–220.
52. Nicholson, L. B., Greer, J. M., Sobel, R. A., Lees, M. B., and Kuchroo, V. K. (1995) An altered peptide ligand mediates immune deviation and prevents autoimmune encephalomyelitis. *Immunity* **3(4),** 397–405.
53. Khoruts, A., Miller, S. D., and Jenkins, M. K. (1995) Neuroantigen-specific Th2 cells are inefficient suppressors of experimental autoimmune encephalomyelitis induced by effector Th1 cells. *J. Immunol.* **155(10),** 5011–5017.
54. Chen, Y., Kuchroo, V. K., Inobe, J., Hafler, D. A., and Weiner, H. L. (1994) Regulatory T cell clones induced by oral tolerance: suppression of autoimmune encephalomyelitis. *Science* **265(5176),** 1237–1240.
55. Brocke, S., Gijbels, K., Allegretta, M., Ferber, I., Piercy, C., Blankenstein, T., et al. (1996)Treatment of experimental encephalomyelitis with a peptide analogue of myelin basic protein. *Nature* **379(6563),** 343–346.
56. Stasiuk, L. M., Abehsira-Amar, O., and Fournier, C. (1996) Collagen-induced arthritis in DBA/1 mice: cytokine gene activation following immunization with type II collagen. *Cell Immunol.* **173(2),** 269–275.
57. Shehadeh, N. N., LaRosa, F., and Lafferty, K. J. (1993) Altered cytokine activity in adjuvant inhibition of autoimmune diabetes. *J. Autoimmun.* **6(3),** 291–300.
58. Kennedy, M. K., Torrance, D. S., Picha, K. S., and Mohler, K. M. (1992) Analysis of cytokine mRNA expression in the central nervous system of mice with experimental autoimmune encephalomyelitis reveals that IL-10 mRNA expression correlates with recovery. *J. Immunol.* **149(7),** 2496–2505.
59. Issazadeh, S., Lorentzen, J. C., Mustafa, M. I., Hojeberg, B., Mussener, A., and Olsson, T. (1996) Cytokines in relapsing experimental autoimmune encephalomyelitis in DA rats: persistent mRNA expression of proinflammatory cytokines and absent expression of interleukin-10 and transforming growth factor-beta. *J. Neuroimmunol.* **69(1-2),** 103–115.
60. Issazadeh, S., Ljungdahl, A., Hojeberg, B., Mustafa, M., and Olsson, T. (1995) Cytokine production in the central nervous system of Lewis rats with

experimental autoimmune encephalomyelitis: dynamics of mRNA expression for interleukin-10, interleukin-12, cytolysin, tumor necrosis factor alpha and tumor necrosis factor beta. *J. Neuroimmunol.* **61(2),** 205–212.

61. Held, W., MacDonald, H. R., Weissman, I. L., Hess, M. W., and Mueller, C. (1990) Genes encoding tumor necrosis factor alpha and granzyme A are expressed during development of autoimmune diabetes. *Proc. Natl. Acad. Sci. USA* **87(6),** 2239–2243.

62. Hornquist, C. E., Lu, X., Rogers-Fani, P. M., Rudolph, U., Shappell, S., Birnbaumer, L., et al. (1997) G(alpha)i2-deficient mice with colitis exhibit a local increase in memory CD4+ T cells and proinflammatory Th1-type cytokines. *J. Immunol.* **158(3),** 1068–1077.

63. Bregenholt, S. and Claesson, M. H. (1998) Increased intracellular Th1 cytokines in scid mice with inflammatory bowel disease. *Eur. J. Immunol.* **28(1),** 379–389.

64. Windhagen, A. (1995) Expression of costimulatory molecules B7-1 (CD80), B7-2 (CD86), and interleukin 12 cytokine in multiple sclerosis lesions. *J. Exp. Med.* **182(6),** 1985–1996.

65. Simon, A. K., Seipelt, E., and Sieper, J. (1994) Divergent T-cell cytokine patterns in inflammatory arthritis. *Proc. Natl. Acad. Sci. USA* **91(18),** 8562–8566.

66. Pizarro, T. T., Michie, M. H., Bentz, M., Woraratanadharm, J., Smith, M. F., Foley, E., et al. (1999) IL-18, a novel immunoregulatory cytokine, is up-regulated in Crohn's disease: expression and localization in intestinal mucosal cells. *J. Immunol.* **162(11),** 6829–6835.

67. Parronchi, P., Romagnani, P., Annunziato, F., Sampognaro, S., Becchio, A., Giannarini, L., et al. (1997) Type 1 T-helper cell predominance and interleukin-12 expression in the gut of patients with Crohn's disease. *Am. J. Pathol.* **150(3),** 823–832.

68. Miltenburg, A. M., van Laar, J. M., de Kuiper, R., Daha, M. R., and Breedveld, F. C. (1992) T cells cloned from human rheumatoid synovial membrane functionally represent the Th1 subset. *Scand. J. Immunol.* **35(5),** 603–610.

69. Foulis, A. K., McGill, M., and Farquharson, M. A. (1991) Insulitis in type 1 (insulin-dependent) diabetes mellitus in man—macrophages, lymphocytes, and interferon-gamma containing cells. *J. Pathol.* **165(2),** 97–103.

70. Camoglio, L., Te Velde, A. A., Tigges, A. J., Das, P. K., and Van Deventer, S. J. (1998) Altered expression of interferon-gamma and interleukin-4 in inflammatory bowel disease. *Inflamm. Bowel. Dis.* **4(4),** 285–290.

71. Balashov, K. E., Smith, D. R., Khoury, S. J., Hafler, D. A., and Weiner, H. L. (1997) Increased interleukin 12 production in progressive multiple sclerosis: induction by activated CD4+ T cells via CD40 ligand. *Proc. Natl. Acad. Sci. USA* **94(2),** 599–603.

72. Comabella, M., Balashov, K., Issazadeh, S., Smith, D., Weiner, H. L., Khoury, S. J. (1997) Elevated interleukin-12 in progressive multiple sclerosis correlates with disease activity and is normalized by pulse cyclophosphamide therapy. *J. Clin. Invest.* **102(4),** 671–678.

73. Fassbender, K., Ragoschke, A., Rossol, S., Schwartz, A., Mielke, O., Paulig A., et al. (1998) Increased release of interleukin-12p40 in MS: association with intracerebral inflammation. *Neurology* **51(3)**, 753–758.

74. Nicoletti, F., Patti, F., Cocuzza, C., Zaccone, P., Nicoletti, A., Di Marco, R., et al. (1996) Elevated serum levels of interleukin-12 in chronic progressive multiple sclerosis. *J. Neuroimmunol.* **70(1)**, 87–90.

75. Kim, W. U., Min, S., Cho, M., Youn, J., Min, J., Lee, S., et al. (2000) The role of IL-12 in inflammatory activity of patients with rheumatoid arthritis (RA). *Clin. Exp. Immunol.* **119(1)**, 175–181.

76. van Boxel-Dezaire, A. H., Hoff, S. C., van Oosten, B. W., Verweij, C. L., Drager, A. M., Ader, H. J., et al. (1999) Decreased interleukin-10 and ncreased interleukin-12p40 mRNA are associated with disease activity and characterize different disease stages in multiple *Ann. Neurol.* **45(6)**, 695–703.

77. Powrie, F., Leach, M. W., Mauze, S., Menon, S., Caddle, L. B., and Coffman, R. L. (1994) Inhibition of Th1 responses prevents inflammatory bowel disease in scid mice reconstituted with CD45RBhi CD4+ T cells. *Immunity* **1(7)**, 553–562.

78. Davidson, N. J., Hudak, S. A., Lesley, R. E., Menon, S., Leach, M. W., Rennick, ?? (1998) IL-12, but not IFN-gamma, plays a major role in sustaining the chronic phase of colitis in IL-10-deficient mice. *J. Immunol.* **161(6)**, 3143–3149.

79. Ruddle, N. H., Bergman, C. M., McGrath, K. M., Lingenheld, E. G., Grunnet, M. L., Padula, S. J., et al. (1990) An antibody to lymphotoxin and tumor necrosis factor prevents transfer of experimental allergic encephalomyelitis. *J. Exp. Med.* **172(4)**, 1193–1200.

80. Selmaj, K., Walczak, A., Mycko, M., Berkowicz, T., Kohno, T., Raine, C. S. (1998) Suppression of experimental autoimmune encephalomyelitis with a TNF binding protein (TNFbp) correlates with down-regulation of VCAM-1/ VLA-4. *Eur. J. Immunol.* **28(6)**, 2035–2044.

81. Selmaj, K., Papierz, W., Glabinski, A., and Kohno, T. (1995) Prevention of chronic relapsing experimental autoimmune encephalomyelitis by soluble tumor necrosis factor receptor I. *J. Neuroimmunol.* **56(2)**, 135–141.

82. Willenborg, D. O., Fordham, S. A., Cowden, W. B., and Ramshaw, I. A. (1995) Cytokines and murine autoimmune encephalomyelitis: inhibition or enhancement of disease with antibodies to select cytokines, or by delivery of exogenous cytokines using a recombinant vaccinia virus system. *Scand. J. Immunol.* **41(1)**, 31–41.

83. Korner, H., Lemckert, F. A., Chaudhri, G., Etteldorf, S., and Sedgwick, J. D. (1997) Tumor necrosis factor blockade in actively induced experimental autoimmune encephalomyelitis prevents clinical disease despite activated T cell infiltration to the central nervous system. *Eur. J. Immunol.* **27(8)**, 1973–1981.

84. Lublin, F. D., Knobler, R. L., Kalman, B., Goldhaber, M., Marini, J., Perrault, M., et al. (1993) Monoclonal anti-gamma interferon antibodies enhance experimental allergic encephalomyelitis. *Autoimmunity* **16(4)**, 267–274.

85. Heremans, H., Dillen, C., Groenen, M., Martens, E., and Billiau, A. (1996) Chronic relapsing experimental autoimmune encephalomyelitis (CREAE) in mice: enhancement by monoclonal antibodies against interferon-gamma. *Eur. J. Immunol.* **26(10)**, 2393–2398.

86. Billiau, A., Heremans, H., Vandekerckhove, F., Dijkmans, R., Sobis, H., Meulepas, E., et al. (1988) Enhancement of experimental allergic encephalomyelitis in mice by antibodies against IFN-gamma. *J. Immunol.* **140(5),** 1506–1510.
87. Duong, T. T., St Louis, J., Gilbert, J. J., Finkelman, F. D., and Strejan, G. H. (1992) Effect of anti-interferon-gamma and anti-interleukin-2 monoclonal antibody treatment on the development of actively and passively induced experimental allergic encephalomyelitis in the SJL/J mouse. *J. Neuroimmunol.* **36(2-3),** 105–115.
88. Duong, T. T., Finkelman, F. D., and Strejan, G. H. (1992) Effect of interferon-gamma on myelin basic protein-specific T cell line proliferation in response to antigen-pulsed accessory cells. *Cell Immunol.* **145(2),** 311–323.
89. Duong, T. T., Finkelman, F. D., Singh, B., and Strejan, G. H. (1994) Effect of anti-interferon-gamma monoclonal antibody treatment on the development of experimental allergic encephalomyelitis in resistant mouse strains. *J. Neuroimmunol.* **53(1),** 101–107.
90. Jones, L. S., Rizzo, L. V., Agarwal, R. K., Tarrant, T. K., Chan, C. C., Wiggert, B., et al. (1997) IFN-gamma-deficient mice develop experimental autoimmune uveitis in the context of a deviant effector response. *J. Immunol.* **158(12),** 5997–6005.
91. Manoury-Schwartz, B., Chiocchia, G., Bessis, N., Abehsira-Amar, O., Batteux, F., Muller, S., et al. (1997) High susceptibility to collagen-induced arthritis in mice lacking IFN- gamma receptors. *J. Immunol.* **158(11),** 5501–5506.
92. Matthys, P., vermeire, K., Mitera, T., Heremans, H., Huang, s., Schols, D., et al. (1999) Enhanced autoimmune arthritis in IFN-gamma receptor-deficient mice is conditioned by mycobacteria in Freund's adjuvant and by increased expansion of Mac-1+ myeloid cells. *J. Immunol.* **163(6),** 3503–3510.
93. Vermeire, K., Heremans, H., Vandeputte, M., Huang, S., Billiau, A., and Matthys, P. (1997) Accelerated collagen-induced arthritis in IFN-gamma receptor-deficient mice. *J. Immunol.* **158(11),** 5507–5513.
94. Tang, H., Sharp, G. C., Peterson, K. P., and Braley-Mullen, H. (1998) IFN-gamma-deficient mice develop severe granulomatous experimental autoimmune thyroiditis with eosinophil infiltration in thyroids. *J. Immunol.* **160(10),** 5105–5112.
95. Ring, G. H., Dai, Z., Saleem, S., Baddoura, F. K., and Lakkis, F. G. (1999) Increased susceptibility to immunologically mediated glomerulonephritis in IFN-gamma-deficient mice. *J. Immunol.* **163(4),** 2243–2248.
96. Alimi, E., Huang, S., Brazillet, M. P., and Charreire, J. (1998) Experimental autoimmune thyroiditis (EAT) in mice lacking the IFN-gamma receptor gene. *Eur. J. Immunol.* **28(1),** 201–208.
97. Simpson, S. J., Shah, S., Comiskey, M., de Jong, Y. P., Wang, B., Mizoguchi, E., et al. (1998) T cell-mediated pathology in two models of experimental colitis depends predominantly on the interleukin 12/Signal transducer and activator of transcription (Stat)-4 pathway, but is not conditional on interferon gamma expression by T cells. *J. Exp. Med.* **187(8),** 1225–1234.
98. Hultgren, B., Huang, X., Dydbal, N., and Stewart, T. A. (1996) Genetic absence of gamma-interferon delays but does not prevent diabetes in NOD mice. *Diabetes* **45(6),** 812–817.

99. Ferber, I. A., Huang, X., Dybdal, N., and Stewart, T. A. (1996) Mice with a disrupted IFN-gamma gene are susceptible to the induction of experimental autoimmune encephalomyelitis (EAE). *J. Immunol.* **156(1)**, 5–7.

100. Krakowski, M. and Owens, T. (1996) Interferon-gamma confers resistance to experimental allergic encephalomyelitis. *Eur. J. Immunol.* **26(7)**, 1641–1646.

101. Segal, B. M., Dwyer, B. K., and Shevach, E. M. (1996) An interleukin (IL)-10/IL-12 immunoregulatory circuit controls susceptibility to autoimmune disease. *J. Exp. Med.* **187(4)**, 537–546.

102. Willenborg, D. O., Fordham, S., Bernard, C. C., Cowden, W. B., and Ramshaw, I. A. (1996) IFN-gamma plays a critical down-regulatory role in the induction and effector phase of myelin oligodendrocyte glycoprotein-induced autoimmune encephalomyelitis. *J. Immunol.* **157(8)**, 3223–3227.

103. Willenborg, D. O., Fordham, S. A., Staykova, M. A., Ramshaw, I. A., and Cowden, W. B. (1999) IFN-gamma is critical to the control of murine autoimmune encephalomyelitis and regulates both in the periphery and in the target tissue: a possible role for nitric oxide. *J. Immunol.* **163(10)**, 5278–5286.

104. Zhang, G. X., Xiao, B. G., Bai, X. F., van der Meide, P. H., Orn, A., and Link, H. (1999) Mice with IFN-gamma receptor deficiency are less susceptible to experimental autoimmune myasthenia gravis. *J. Immunol.* **162(7)**, 3775–3781.

105. Frei, K., Eugster, H. P., Bopst, M., Constantinescu, C. S., Lavi, E., and Fontana A. (1997) Tumor necrosis factor alpha and lymphotoxin alpha are not required for induction of acute experimental autoimmune encephalomyelitis. *J. Exp. Med.* **185(12)**, 2177–2182.

106. Liu, J., Marino, M. W., Wong, G., Grail, D., Dunn, A., Bettadapura, J., et al. (1998) TNF is a potent anti-inflammatory cytokine in autoimmune-mediated demyelination. *Nat. Med.* **4(1)**, 78–83.

107. Kassiotis, G., Pasparakis, M., Kollias, G., and Probert, L. (1999) TNF accelerates the onset but does not alter the incidence and severity of myelin basic protein-induced experimental autoimmune encephalomyelitis. *Eur. J. Immunol.* **29(3)**, 774–780.

108. Sean Riminton, D., et al. (1998) Challenging cytokine redundancy: inflammatory cell movement and clinical course of experimental autoimmune encephalomyelitis are normal in lymphotoxin-deficient, but not tumor necrosis factor-deficient, mice. *J. Exp. Med.* **187(9)**, 1517–1528.

109. Korner, H., Riminton, D. S., Strickland, D. H., Lemckert, F. A., Pollard, J. D., and Sedgwick, J. D. (1997) Critical points of tumor necrosis factor action in central nervous system autoimmune inflammation defined by gene targeting. *J. Exp. Med.* **186(9)**, 1585–1590.

110. Leonard, J. P., Waldburger, K. E., and Goldman, S. J. (1995) Prevention of experimental autoimmune encephalomyelitis by antibodies against interleukin 12. *J. Exp. Med.* **181(1)**, 381–386.

111. Germann, T., Szeliga, J., Hess, H., Storkel, S., Podlaski, F. J., Gately, M. K., et al. (1995) Administration of interleukin 12 in combination with type II collagen induces severe arthritis in DBA/1 mice. *Proc. Natl. Acad. Sci. USA* **92(11)**, 4823–4827.

112. Moiola, L., Galbiati, F., Martino, G., Amadio, S., Brambilla, E., Comi, G., et al. (1998) IL-12 is involved in the induction of experimental autoimmune myasthenia gravis, an antibody-mediated disease. *Eur. J. Immunol.* **28(8),** 2487–2497.

113. Joosten, L. A., , Lubberts, E., Helsen, M. M., and van den Berg,W. B. (1997) Dual role of IL-12 in early and late stages of murine collagen type II arthritis. *J. Immunol.* **159(8),** 4094–4102.

114. Parks, E., Strieter, R. M., Lukacs, N. W., Gauldie, J., Hitt, M., Graham, F. L., et al. (1998) Transient gene transfer of IL-12 regulates chemokine expression and disease severity in experimental arthritis. *J. Immunol.* **160(9),** 4615–4619.

115. Segal, B. M. and Shevach, E. M. (1996) IL-12 unmasks latent autoimmune disease in resistant mice. *J. Exp. Med.* **184(2),** 771–775.

116. Zaccone, P., Hutchings, P., Nicoletti, F., Penna, G., Adorini, L., and Cooke, A. (1999) The involvement of IL-12 in murine experimentally induced autoimmune thyroid disease. *Eur. J. Immunol.* **29(6),** 1933–1942.

117. Trembleau, S., Penna, G., Bosi, E., Mortara, A., Gately, M. K., and Adorini, L. (1995) Interleukin 12 administration induces T helper type 1 cells and accelerates autoimmune diabetes in NOD mice. *J. Exp. Med.* **181(2),** 817–821.

118. Neurath, M. F., Fuss I., Kelsall, B. L., Stuber, E., and Strober, W. (1995) Antibodies to interleukin 12 abrogate established experimental colitis in mice. *J. Exp. Med.* **182(5),** 1281–1290.

119. Malfait, A. M., Butler, D. M., Presky, D. H., Maini, R. N., Brennan, F. M., and Feldmann, M. (1998) Blockade of IL-12 during the induction of collagen-induced arthritis (CIA) markedly attenuates the severity of the arthritis. *Clin. Exp. Immunol.* **111(2),** 377–383.

120. Yokoi, H., Kato, K., Kezuka, T., Sakai, J., Usui, M., Yagita, H., et al. (1997) Prevention of experimental autoimmune uveoretinitis by monoclonal antibody to interleukin-12. *Eur. J. Immunol.* **27(3),** 641–646.

121. Butler, D. M., Malfait, A. M., Maini, R. N., Brennan, F. M., and Feldmann, M. (1999) Anti-IL-12 and anti-TNF antibodies synergistically suppress the progression of murine collagen-induced arthritis. *Eur. J. Immunol.* **29(7),** 2205–2212.

122. Trembleau, S., et al. Penna, G., Gregori, S., Gately, M. K., and Adorini, L. (1997) Deviation of pancreas-infiltrating cells to Th2 by interleukin-12 antagonist administration inhibits autoimmune diabetes. *Eur. J. Immunol.* **27(9),** 2330–2339.

123. McIntyre, K. W., Shuster, D. J., Gillooly, K. M., Warrier, R. R., Connaughton, S. E., Hall, L. B., et al. (1996) Reduced incidence and severity of collagen-induced arthritis in interleukin-12-deficient mice. *Eur. J. Immunol.* **26(12),** 2933–2938.

124. Tarrant, T. K., Silver, P. B., Chan, C. C., Wiggert, B., and Caspi, R. R. (1998) Endogenous IL-12 is required for induction and expression of experimental autoimmune uveitis. *J. Immunol.* **161(1),** 122–127.

125. Trembleau, S., Penna, G., Gregori, S., Chapman, H. D., Serreze, D. V., Magram, J., and Adorini, L. (1999) Pancreas-infiltrating Th1 cells and diabetes develop in IL-12-deficient nonobese diabetic mice. *J. Immunol.* **163(5),** 2960–2968.

126. Claesson, M. H., Bregenholt, S., Bonhagen, K., Thoma, S., Moller, P., Grusby, M. J., et al. (1999) Colitis-inducing potency of CD4+ T cells in immunodeficient, adoptive hosts depends on their state of activation, IL-12 responsiveness, and CD45RB surface phenotype. *J. Immunol.* **162(6),** 3702–3710.

127. Matthys, P., Vermeire, K., Mitera, T., Heremans, H., Huang, S., and Billiau, A. (1998) Anti-IL-12 antibody prevents the development and progression of collagen-induced arthritis in IFN-gamma receptor-deficient mice. *Eur. J. Immunol.* **28(7),** 2143–2151.

128. de Waal Malefyt, R., Abrams, J., Bennett, B., Figdor, C. G., and de Vries, J. E. (1991) Interleukin 10(IL-10) inhibits cytokine synthesis by human monocytes: an autoregulatory role of IL-10 produced by monocytes. *J. Exp. Med.* **174(5),** 1209–1220.

129. Fiorentino, D. F., Bond M. W., and Mosmann, T. R. (1989) Two types of mouse T helper cell. IV. Th2 clones secrete a factor that inhibits cytokine production by Th1 clones. *J. Exp. Med.* **170(6),** 2081–2095.

130. Vieira, P., de Waal-Malefyt, R., Dang, M. N., Johnson, K. E., Kastelein, R., Fiorentino, D. F., et al. (1991) Isolation and expression of human cytokine synthesis inhibitory factor cDNA clones: homology to Epstein-Barr virus open reading frame BCRFI. *Proc. Natl. Acad. Sci. USA* **88(4),** 1172–1176.

131. Hsieh, C. S., Heimberger, A. B., Gold, J. S., O'Garra, A., and Murphy, K. M. (1992) Differential regulation of T helper phenotype development by interleukins 4 and 10 in an alpha beta T-cell-receptor transgenic system. *Proc. Natl. Acad. Sci. USA* **89(13),** 6065–6069.

132. de Waal Malefyt, R., Haanen, J., Spits, H., Roncarolo, M. G., te Velde, A., Figdor, C., et al. (1991) Interleukin 10 (IL-10) and viral IL-10 strongly reduce antigen-specific human T cell proliferation by diminishing the antigen-presenting capacity of monocytes via downregulation of class II major histocompatibility complex expression. *J. Exp. Med.* **174(4),** 915–924.

133. Fiorentino, D. F., Zlotnik, A., Vieira, P., Mosmann, T. R., Howard, M., Moore, K. W., et al. (1991) IL-10 acts on the antigen-presenting cell to inhibit cytokine production by Th1 cells. *J. Immunol.* **146(10),** 3444–3451.

134. King, C., Davies, J., Mueller, R., Lee, M. S., Krahl, T., Yeung B., et al. (1998) TGF-beta1 alters APC preference, polarizing islet antigen responses toward a Th2 phenotype. *Immunity* **8(5)** 601–613.

135. Takeuchi, M., Alard, P., and Streilein, J. W. (1998) TGF-beta promotes immune deviation by altering accessory signals of antigen-presenting cells. *J. Immunol.* **160(4),** 1589–1597.

136. Koch, F., Stanzl, U., Jennewein, P., Janke, K., Heufler, C., Kampgen, E., et al. (1996) High level IL-12 production by murine dendritic cells: upregulation via MHC class II and CD40 molecules and downregulation by IL-4 and IL-10. *J. Exp. Med.* **184(2),** 741–746.

137. D'Andrea, A., Aste-Amezaga, M., Valiante, N. M., Ma, X., Kubin, M., and Trinchieri, G. (1993) Interleukin 10 (IL-10) inhibits human lymphocyte interferon gamma-production by suppressing natural killer cell stimulatory factor/IL-12 synthesis in accessory cells. *J. Exp. Med.* **178(3),** 1041–1048.

138. Huang, X. R., Kitching, A. R., Tipping, P. G., and Holdsworth, S. R. (2000) Interleukin-10 inhibits macrophage-induced glomerular injury. *J. Am. Soc. Nephrol.* **11(2)**, 262–269.

139. Mottonen, M., Isomaki, P., Saario, R., Toivanen, P., Punnonen, J., and Lassila, O. (1998) Interleukin-10 inhibits the capacity of synovial macrophages to function as antigen-presenting cells. *Br. J. Rheumatol.* **37(11)**, 1207–1214.

140. Czarniecki, C. W., Chiu, H. H., Wong, G. H., McCabe, S. M., and Palladino, M. A. (1988) Transforming growth factor-beta 1 modulates the expression of class II histocompatibility antigens on human cells. *J. Immunol.* **140(12)**, 4217–4223.

141. Mitra, R. S., Judge, T. A., Nestle, F. O., Turka, L. A., and Nickoloff, B. J. (1995) Psoriatic skin-derived dendritic cell function is inhibited by exogenous IL-10. Differential modulation of B7-1 (CD80) and B7-2 (CD86) expression. *J. Immunol.* **154(6)**, 2668–2677.

142. Willems, F., Marchant, A., Delville, J. P., Gerard, C., Delvaux, A., Velu, T., et al. (1994) Interleukin-10 inhibits B7 and intercellular adhesion molecule-1 expression on human monocytes. *Eur. J. Immunol.* **24(4)**, 1007–1009.

143. Ding, L., Linsley, P. S., Huang, L. Y., Germain, R. N., and Schevach, E. (1993) IL-10 inhibits macrophage costimulatory activity by selectively inhibiting the up-regulation of B7 expression. *J. Immunol.* **151(3)**, 1224–1234.

144. Ding, L. and Shevach, E. M. (1992) IL-10 inhibits mitogen-induced T cell proliferation by selectively inhibiting macrophage costimulatory function. *J. Immunol.* **148(10)**, 3133–3139.

145. Buelens, C., Willems, F., Delvaux, A., Pierard, G., Delville, J. P., Velu, T., et al. (1995) Interleukin-10 differentially regulates B7-1 (CD80) and B7-2 (CD86) expression on human peripheral blood dendritic cells. *Eur. J. Immunol.* **25(9)**, 2668–2672.

146. Nguyen, V. T., Walker, W. S. and Benveniste, E. N. (1998) Post-transcriptional inhibition of CD40 gene expression in microglia by transforming growth factor-beta. *Eur. J. Immunol.* **28(8)**, 2537–2548.

147. Wu, C., Warrier, R. R., Wang, X., Presky, D. H., and Gately, M. K. (1997) Regulation of interleukin-12 receptor beta1 chain expression and interleukin-12 binding by human peripheral blood mononuclear cells. *Eur. J. Immunol.* **27(1)**, 147–154.

148. Pardoux, C., Ma, X., Gobert, S., Pellegrini, S., Mayeux, P., Gay, F., et al. (1999) Downregulation of interleukin-12 (IL-12) responsiveness in human T cells by transforming growth factor-beta: relationship with IL-12 signaling. *Blood* **93(5)**, 1448–1455.

149. Gorham, J. D., Guler, M. L., Fenoglio, D., Gubler, U., and Murphy, K. M. (1998) Low dose TGF-beta attenuates IL-12 responsiveness in murine Th cells. *J. Immunol.* **161(4)**, 1664–1670.

150. Chang, J. T., Shevach, E. M. and Segal, B. M. (1999) Regulation of interleukin (IL)-12 receptor beta2 subunit expression by endogenous IL-12: a critical step in the differentiation of pathogenic autoreactive T cells. *J. Exp. Med.* **189(6)**, 969–978.

151. Bright, J. J. and Sriram, S. (1998) TGF-beta inhibits IL-12-induced activation of Jak-STAT pathway in T lymphocytes. *J. Immunol.* **161(4)**, 1772–1777.

152. de Waal Malefyt, R., Yssel, H. and de Vries, J. E. (1993) Direct effects of IL-10 on subsets of human CD4+ T cell clones and resting T cells. Specific inhibition of IL-2 production and proliferation. *J. Immunol.* **150(11),** 4754–4765.

153. Taga, K., Mostowski, H. and Tosato, G. (1993) Human interleukin-10 can directly inhibit T-cell growth. *Blood* **81(11),** 2964–2971.

154. Taga, K. and Tosato, G. (1992) IL-10 inhibits human T cell proliferation and IL-2 production. *J. Immunol.* **148(4),** 1143–1148.

155. Kehrl, J. H., Wakefield, L. M., Roberts, A. B., Jakowlew, S., Alvarez-Mon, M., Derynck, R., et al. (1986) Production of transforming growth factor beta by human T lymphocytes and its potential role in the regulation of T cell growth. *J. Exp. Med.* **163(5),** 1037–1050.

156. Bogdan, C., Vodovotz, Y. and Nathan, C. (1991) Macrophage deactivation by interleukin 10. *J. Exp. Med.* **174(6),** 1549–1555.

157. Bogdan, C. and Nathan, C. (1993) Modulation of macrophage function by transforming growth factor beta, interleukin-4, and interleukin-10. *Ann. NY Acad. Sci.* **685,** 713–739.

158. Chaves, M. M., Silvestrini, A. A., Silva-Teixeira, D. N., and Nogueira-Machado, J. A. (1996) Effect in vitro of gamma interferon and interleukin-10 on generation of oxidizing species by human granulocytes. *Inflamm. Res.* **45(7),** 313–315.

159. Cenci, E., Romani, L., Mencacci, A., Spaccapelo, R., Schiaffella, E., Puccetti, P., et al. (1993) Interleukin-4 and interleukin-10 inhibit nitric oxide-dependent macrophage killing of Candida albicans. *Eur. J. Immunol.* **23(5),** 1034–1038.

160. Oswald, I. P., Wynn, T. A., Sher, A., and James, S. L. (1992) Interleukin 10 inhibits macrophage microbicidal activity by blocking the endogenous production of tumor necrosis factor alpha required as a costimulatory factor for interferon gamma-induced activation. *Proc. Natl. Acad. Sci. USA* **89(18),** 8676–8680.

161. Tsunawaki, S., Sporn, M., Ding, A., and Nathan, C. (1988) Deactivation of macrophages by transforming growth factor-beta. *Nature* **334(6179),** 260–262.

162. Vodovotz, Y. and Bogdan, C. (1994) Control of nitric oxide synthase expression by transforming growth factor-beta: implications for homeostasis. *Prog. Growth. Factor. Res.* **5(4),** 341–351.

163. Vodovotz, Y., Bogdan, C., Paik, J., Xie, Q. W., and Nathan, C. (1993) Mechanisms of suppression of macrophage nitric oxide release by transforming growth factor beta. *J. Exp. Med.* **178(2),** 605–613.

164. Mertz, P. M., DeWitt, D. L., Stetler-Stevenson, W. G., and Wahl, L. M. (1994) Interleukin 10 suppression of monocyte prostaglandin H synthase-2. Mechanism of inhibition of prostaglandin-dependent matrix metalloproteinase production. *J. Biol. Chem.* **269(33),** 21,322–21,329.

165. Lacraz, S., Nicod, L. P., Chicheportiche, R., Welgus, H. G., and Dayer, J. M. (1995) IL-10 inhibits metalloproteinase and stimulates TIMP-1 production in human mononuclear phagocytes. *J. Clin. Invest.* **96(5),** 2304–2310.

166. Powrie, F., Leach, M. W., Mauze, S., Caddle, L. B., and Coffman, R. L. (1993) Phenotypically distinct subsets of CD4+ T cells induce or protect from chronic intestinal inflammation in C. B-17 scid mice. *Intl. Immunol.* **5(11),** 1461–1471.

167. Powrie, F., Carlino, J., Leach, M. W., Mauze, S., and Coffman, R. L. (1996) A critical role for transforming growth factor-beta but not interleukin 4 in the suppression of T helper type 1-mediated colitis by CD45RB(low) CD4+ T cells. *J. Exp. Med.* **183(6),** 2669–2674.

168. Hagenbaugh, A., Sharma, S., Dubinett, S. M., Wei, S. H., Aranda, R., Cheroutre, H., et al. (1997) Altered immune responses in interleukin 10 transgenic mice. *J. Exp. Med.* **185(12),** 2101–2110.

169. Rennick, D. M., Fort, M. M. and Davidson, N. J. (1997) Studies with IL-10-/- mice: an overview. *J. Leukoc. Biol.* **61(4),** 389–396.

170. Davidson, N. J., Fort, M. M., Muller, W., Leach, M. W., and Rennick, D. M. (2000) Chronic colitis in IL-10-/- mice: insufficient counter regulation of a Th1 response. *Intl. Rev. Immunol.* **19(1),** 91–121.

171. Davidson, N. J., Leach, M. W., Fort, M. M., Thompson-Snipes, L., Kuhn, R., Muller, W., et al. (1996) T helper cell 1-type CD4+ T cells, but not B cells, mediate colitis in interleukin 10-deficient mice. *J. Exp. Med.* **184(1),** 241–251.

172. Berg, D. J., Davidson, N., Kuhn, R., Muller, W., Menon, S., Holland, G., et al. (1996) Enterocolitis and colon cancer in interleukin-10-deficient mice are associated with aberrant cytokine production and CD4(+) TH1-like responses. *J. Clin. Invest.* **98(4),** 1010–1020.

173. Shull, M. M., Ormsby, I., Kier, A. B., Pawlowski, S., Diebold, R. J., Yin, M., et al (1992) Targeted disruption of the mouse transforming growth factor-beta 1 gene results in multifocal inflammatory disease. *Nature* **359(6397),** 693–699.

174. Letterio, J. J., Geiser, A. G., Kulkarni, A. B., Dang, H., Kong, L., Nakabayashi, T., et al. (1996) Autoimmunity associated with TGF-beta1-deficiency in mice is dependent on MHC class II antigen expression. *J. Clin. Invest.* **98(9),** 2109–2119.

175. Kobayashi, S., Yoshida, K., Ward, J. M., Letterio, J. J., Longenecker, G., Yaswen, L., et al. (1999) Beta 2-microglobulin-deficient background ameliorates lethal phenotype of the TGF-beta 1 null mouse. *J. Immunol.* **163(7),** 4013–4019.

176. Sadlack, B., Merz, H., Schorle, H., Schimpl, A., Feller, A. C., and Horak I. (1993) Ulcerative colitis-like disease in mice with a disrupted interleukin-2 gene. *Cell* **75(2),** 253–261.

177. Autenrieth, I. B., Bucheler, N., Bohn, E., Heinze, G., and Horak, I. (1997) Cytokine mRNA expression in intestinal tissue of interleukin-2 deficient mice with bowel inflammation. *Gut* **41(6),** 793–800.

178. Ehrhardt, R. O., Ludviksson, B. R., Gray, B., Neurath, M., and Strober, W. (1997) Induction and prevention of colonic inflammation in IL-2-deficient mice. *J. Immunol.* **158(2),** 566–573.

179. Fuss, I. J., Marth, T., Neurath, M. F., Pearlstein, G. R., Jain, A., and Strober, W. (1999) Anti-interleukin 12 treatment regulates apoptosis of Th1 T cells in experimental colitis in mice. *Gastroenterology* **117(5),** 1078–1088.

180. Papiernik, M., de Moraes, M. L., Pontoux, C., Vasseur, F., and Penit, C. (1998) Regulatory CD4 T cells: expression of IL-2R alpha chain, resistance to clonal deletion and IL-2 dependency. *Intl. Immunol.* **10(4),** 371–378.

181. Samoilova, E. B., Horton, J. L. and Chen, Y. (1998) Acceleration of experimental autoimmune encephalomyelitis in interleukin-10-deficient mice: roles of interleukin-10 in disease progression and recovery. *Cell Immunol.* **188(2),** 118–124.

182. Bettelli, E., Das, M. P., Howard, E. D., Weiner, H. L., Sobel, R. A., and Kuchroo, V. K. (1998) IL-10 is critical in the regulation of autoimmune encephalomyelitis as demonstrated by studies of IL-10- and IL-4-deficient and transgenic mice. *J. Immunol.* **161(7),** 3299–2306.

183. Rizzo, L. V., Xu, H., Chan, C. C., Wiggert, B., and Caspi, R. R. (1998) IL-10 has a protective role in experimental autoimmune uveoretinitis. *Intl. Immunol.* **10(6),** 807–814.

184. Crisi, G. M., Santambrogio, L., Hochwald, G. M., Smith, S. R., Carlino, J. A., Thorbecke, G. J. (1995) Staphylococcal enterotoxin B and tumor-necrosis factor-alpha-induced relapses of experimental allergic encephalomyelitis: protection by transforming growth factor-beta and interleukin-10. *Eur. J. Immunol.* **25(11),** 3035–3300.

185. Cannella, B., Gao, Y. L., Brosnan, C., Raine, C. S. (1996) IL-10 fails to abrogate experimental autoimmune encephalomyelitis. *J. Neurosci. Res.* **45(6),** 735–746.

186. Lubberts, E., Joosten, L. A., van Den Bersselaar, L., Helsen, M. M., Bakker, A. C., van Meurs, J. B., et al. (1998) Regulatory role of interleukin 10 in joint inflammation and cartilage destruction in murine streptococcal cell wall (SCW) arthritis. More therapeutic benefit with IL-4/IL-10 combination therapy than with IL-10 treatment alone. *Cytokine* **10(5),** 361–369.

187. Kasama, T., Strieter, R. M., Lukacs, N. W., Lincoln, P. M., Burdick, M. D., and Kunkel, S. L. (1995) Interleukin-10 expression and chemokine regulation during the evolution of murine type II collagen-induced arthritis. *J. Clin. Invest.* **95(6),** 2868–2876.

188. Joosten, L. A., Lubberts, E., Durez, P., Helsen, M. M., Jacobs, M. J., Goldman, M., et al. (1997) Role of interleukin-4 and interleukin-10 in murine collagen-induced arthritis. Protective effect of interleukin-4 and interleukin-10 treatment on cartilage destruction. *Arthritis. Rheum.* **40(2),** 249–260.

189. Singer, S. M., Tisch, R., Yang, X. D., Sytwu, H. K., Lublau, R., and McDevitt, H. O. (1998) Prevention of diabetes in NOD mice by a mutated I-Ab transgene. *Diabetes* **47(10),** 1570–1577.

190. Cua, D. J., Groux, H., Hinton, D. R., Stohlman, S. A., and Coffman, R. L. (1999) Transgenic interleukin 10 prevents induction of experimental autoimmune encephalomyelitis. *J. Exp. Med.* **189(6),** 1005–1010.

191. Johns, L. D. and Sriram, S. (1993) Experimental allergic encephalomyelitis: neutralizing antibody to TGF beta 1 enhances the clinical severity of the disease. *J. Neuroimmunol.* **47(1),** 1–7.

192. Han, H. S., Jun, H. S., Utsugi, T., and Yoon, J. W. (1996) A new type of CD4+ suppressor T cell completely prevents spontaneous autoimmune dia-

betes and recurrent diabetes in syngeneic islet- transplanted NOD mice. *J. Autoimmun.* **9(3)**, 331–339.

193. Racke, M. K., Cannella, B., Albert, P., Sporn, M., Raine, C. S., and McFarlin, D. E. (1992) Evidence of endogenous regulatory function of transforming growth factor-beta 1 in experimental allergic encephalomyelitis. *Intl. Immunol.* **4(5)**, 615–620.

194. Santambrogio, L., Hochwald, G. M., Leu, C. H., and Thorbecke, G. J. (1993) Antagonistic effects of endogenous and exogenous TGF-beta and TNF on autoimmune diseases in mice. *Immunopharmacol. Immunotoxicol.* **15(4)**, 461–478.

195. Thorbecke, G. J., Shah, R., Leu, C. H., Kuruvilla, A. P., Hardison, A. M., and Palladino, M. A. (1992) Involvement of endogenous tumor necrosis factor alpha and transforming growth factor beta during induction of collagen type II arthritis in mice. *Proc. Natl. Acad. Sci. USA* **89(16)**, 7375–7379.

196. Szabo, S. J., Jacobson, N. G., Dighe, A. S., Gubler, U., and Murphy, K. M. (1995) Developmental commitment to the Th2 lineage by extinction of IL-12 signaling. *Immunity* **2(6)**, 665–675.

197. Szabo, S. J., Dighe, A. S., Gubler, U., and Murphy, K. M. (1997) Regulation of the interleukin (IL)-12R beta 2 subunit expression in developing T helper 1 (Th1) and Th2 cells. *J. Exp. Med.* **185(5)**, 817–824.

198. Shaw, M. K., Lorens, J. B., Dhawan, A., DalCanto, R., Tse, H. Y., Tran, A. B., et al. (1997) Local delivery of interleukin 4 by retrovirus-transduced T lymphocytes ameliorates experimental autoimmune encephalomyelitis. *J. Exp. Med.* **185(9)**, 1711–1714.

199. Racke, M. K., Bonomo, A., Scott, D. E., Cannella, B., Levine, A., Raine, C. S., et al. (1994) Cytokine-induced immune deviation as a therapy for inflammatory autoimmune disease. *J. Exp. Med.* **180(5)**, 1961–1966.

200. Piccirillo, C. A. and Prud'homme, G. J. (1999) Prevention of experimental allergic encephalomyelitis by intramuscular gene transfer with cytokine-encoding plasmid vectors. *Human Gene Ther.* **10(12)**, 1915–1922.

201. Furlan, R., Poliani, P. L., Galbiati, F., Bergami, A., Grimaldi, L. M., Comi G., et al. (1998) Central nervous system delivery of interleukin 4 by a nonreplicative herpes simplex type 1 viral vector ameliorates autoimmune demyelination. *Human Gene Ther.* **9(17)**, 2605–2617.

202. Rapoport, M. J., Jaramillo, A., Zipris, D., Lazarus, A. H., Serreze, D. V., Leiter, E. H., et al (1993) Interleukin 4 reverses T cell proliferative unresponsiveness and prevents the onset of diabetes in nonobese diabetic mice. *J. Exp. Med.* **178(1)**, 87–99.

203. Tominaga, Y., Nagata, M., Yasuda, H., Okamoto, N., Arisawa, K., Moriyama, H., et al. (1998) Administration of IL-4 prevents autoimmune diabetes but enhances pancreatic insulitis in NOD mice. *Clin. Immunol. Immunopathol.* **86(2)**, 209–218.

204. Lubberts, E., Joosten, L. A., van Den Bersselaar, L., Helsen, M. M., Bakker, A. C., van Meurs, J. B., et al. (1999) Adenoviral vector-mediated overexpression of IL-4 in the knee joint of mice with collagen-induced arthritis prevents cartilage destruction. *J. Immunol.* **163(8)**, 4546–4556.

205. Liblau, R., Steinman, L. and Brocke, S. (1997) Experimental autoimmune encephalomyelitis in IL-4-deficient mice. *Intl. Immunol.* **9(5),** 799–803.

206. Wang, B., et al. (1998) Interleukin-4 deficiency does not exacerbate disease in NOD mice. *Diabetes* **47(8),** 1207–1211.

207. Xiang, M., Zaccone, P., Di Marco, R., Harris, R., Magro, G., Di Mauro, M., et al. (1999) Failure of exogenously administered interferon-gamma or blockage of endogenous interleukin-4 with specific inhibitors to augment the incidence of autoimmune diabetes in male NOD mice. *Autoimmunity* **30(2),** 71–80.

208. Yoshino, S. and Yoshino, J. (1998) Enhancement of T-cell-mediated arthritis in mice by treatment with a monoclonal antibody against interleukin-4. *Cell Immunol.* **185(2),** 153–157.

209. Yoshino, S. (1998) Effect of a monoclonal antibody against interleukin-4 on collagen-induced arthritis in mice. *Br. J. Pharmacol.* **123(2),** 237–242.

210. Hesse, M., Bayrak, S. and Mitchison, A. (1996) Protective major histocompatibility complex genes and the role of interleukin-4 in collagen-induced arthritis. *Eur. J. Immunol.* **26(12),** 3234–3237.

211. Jacobs, M. J., van den Hoek, A. E., van Lent, P. L., van de Loo, F. A., van de Putte, L. B., and van den Berg, W. B. (1994) Role of IL-2 and IL-4 in exacerbations of murine antigen-induced arthritis. *Immunology* **83(3),** 390–396.

212. Durez, P., Abramowicz, D., Gerard, C., Van Mechelen, M., Amraoui, Z., Dubois C., et al. (1993) In vivo induction of interleukin 10 by anti-CD3 monoclonal antibody or bacterial lipopolysaccharide: differential modulation by cyclosporin A. *J. Exp. Med.* **177(2),** 551–555.

213. Grotendorst, G. R., Smale, G. and Pencev, D. (1989) Production of transforming growth factor beta by human peripheral blood monocytes and neutrophils. *J. Cell Physiol.* **140(2),** 396–402.

214. Assoian, R. K, Fleurdelys, B. E., Stevenson, H. C., Miller, P. J., Madtes, D. K., Raines, E. W., et al. (1987) Expression and secretion of type beta transforming growth factor by activated human macrophages. *Proc. Natl. Acad. Sci. USA* **84(17),** 6020–6024.

215. Groux, H., O'Garra, A., Bigler, M., Rouleau, M., Antonenko, S., de Vries J. E., et al. (1997) A CD4+ T-cell subset inhibits antigen-specific T-cell responses and prevents colitis. *Nature* **389(6652),** 737–742.

216. Sun, D., Whitaker, J. N. and Wilson, D. B. (1999) Regulatory T cells in experimental allergic encephalomyelitis. III. Comparison of disease resistance in Lewis and Fischer 344 rats. *Eur. J. Immunol.* **29(4),** 1101–1106.

217. Caspi, R. R., (1996) Genetic susceptibility to experimental autoimmune uveoretinitis in the rat is associated with an elevated Th1 response. *J. Immunol.* **157(6),** 2668–2675.

218. Caspi, R. R., Sun, B., Agarwal, R. K., Silver, P. B., Rizzo, L. V., Chan, C. C., et al. (1997) T cell mechanisms in experimental autoimmune uveoretinitis: susceptibility is a function of the cytokine response profile. *Eye* **11(Pt 2),** 209–212.

219. Conboy, I. M., (1997) Novel genetic regulation of T helper 1 (Th1)/Th2 cytokine production and encephalitogenicity in inbred mouse strains. *J. Exp. Med.* **185(3),** 439–451.

220. Sun, B., Rizzo, L. V., Sun, S. H., Chan, C. C., Wiggert, B., Wilder, R. L., et al. (1997) Genetic susceptibility to experimental autoimmune uveitis involves more than a predisposition to generate a T helper-1-like or a T helper-2-like response. *J. Immunol.* **159(2),** 1004–1011.

221. Mussener, A., Lorentzen, J. C., Kleinau, S., and Klareskog, L. (1997) Altered Th1/Th2 balance associated with non-major histocompatibility complex genes in collagen-induced arthritis in resistant and non- resistant rat strains. *Eur. J. Immunol.* **27(3),** 695–699.

222. Weissert, R., (1998) MHC haplotype-dependent regulation of MOG-induced EAE in rats. *J. Clin. Invest.* **102(6),** 1265–1273.

223. Maron, R., Hancock, W. W., Slavin, A., Hattori, M., Kuchroo, V., and Weiner, H. L. (1999) Genetic susceptibility or resistance to autoimmune encephalomyelitis in MHC congenic mice is associated with differential production of pro- and anti-inflammatory cytokines. *Intl. Immunol.* **11(9),** 1573–1580.

224. Kjellen, P., Issazadeh, S., Olsson, T., and Holmdahl, R. (1998) Genetic influence on disease course and cytokine response in relapsing experimental allergic encephalomyelitis. *Intl. Immunol.* **10(3),** 333–340.

225. Zhu, J., Zou, L. P., Bakhiet, M., and Mix, E. (1998) Resistance and susceptibility to experimental autoimmune neuritis in Sprague-Dawley and Lewis rats correlate with different levels of autoreactive T and B cell responses to myelin antigens. *J. Neurosci. Res.* **54(3),** 373–381.

226. Zhang, G. X., Zou, L. P., Bakhiet, M., and Mix, E. (1996) Autoreactive T cell responses and cytokine patterns reflect resistance to experimental autoimmune myasthenia gravis in Wistar Furth rats. *Eur. J. Immunol.* **26(11),** 2552–2558.

227. Lenz, D. C., Wolf, N. A. and Swanborg, R. H. (1999) Strain variation in autoimmunity: attempted tolerization of DA rats results in the induction of experimental autoimmune encephalomyelitis. *J. Immunol.* **163(4),** 1763–1768.

228. Cautain, B., Damoiseaux, J., Bernard, I., Fournie, E., van Brenda Vriesman, P., Druet, P., et al. (1999) Non-MHC determined resistance of Brown-Norway rats to develop experimental allergic encephalomyelitis is mediated by the endogenous production of transforming growth factor-beta. *Transplant Proc.* **31(3),** 1602–1603.

229. Cua, D. J., Hinton, D. R., and Stohlman, S. A. (1995) Self-antigen-induced Th2 responses in experimental allergic encephalomyelitis (EAE)-resistant mice. Th2-mediated suppression of autoimmune disease. *J. Immunol.* **155(8),** 4052–4059.

230. Kim, S. and Voskuhl, R. R. (1999) Decreased IL-12 production underlies the decreased ability of male lymph node cells to induce experimental autoimmune encephalomyelitis. *J. Immunol.* **162(9),** 5561–5568.

9

The Role of Cytokines in Induction and Regulation of Autoimmune Uveitis

Rachel R. Caspi

1. INTRODUCTION

Uveitis is a generic term that encompasses a variety of intraocular inflammations. Noninfectious uveitis, affecting an otherwise intact eye, is believed to have an autoimmune or immune-mediated origin. It can affect the front, middle, or back part of the eye, and is then termed anterior, intermediate, and posterior uveitis, respectively. A schematic drawing of a human eye is shown in Fig. 1. The uveitic conditions that affect the back of the eye where the photoreceptor cells are located are particularly likely to adversely affect vision. These sight-threatening diseases can be mostly confined to the eye, such as sympathetic ophthalmia or birdshot retinochoroidopathy, or they can be part of a more generalized systemic syndrome where the eye is one of a number of organs involved, such as Behçet's disease, sarcoidosis, or Vogt-Koyanagi-Harada syndrome *(1)*. It is estimated that collectively posterior uveitic diseases are responsible for about 10% of the severe visual handicap in the United States.

Experimental autoimmune uveoretinitis (EAU) is a cell-mediated autoimmune disease model that targets the neural retina and serves as an experimental equivalent to posterior uveitic diseases in the human. EAU can be induced in susceptible animal species by immunization with retinal antigens or their fragments, and in mice and rats also by infusion of retinal antigen-specific T cell lines and clones. A number of proteins derived from the photoreceptor cell layer, among them the interphotoreceptor retinoid-binding protein (IRBP), the retinal soluble antigen (S-Ag), recoverin, rhodopsin, and its illuminated form opsin were found to be pathogenic and to cause essentially identical pathology *(2)*. Typically, these are evolutionarily highly conserved proteins involved in the visual cycle. The microanatomy of normal and uveitic retina of a mouse immunized with IRBP is shown in Fig. 2.

From: *Cytokines and Autoimmune Diseases*
Edited by: V. K. Kuchroo, et al. © Humana Press Inc., Totowa, NJ

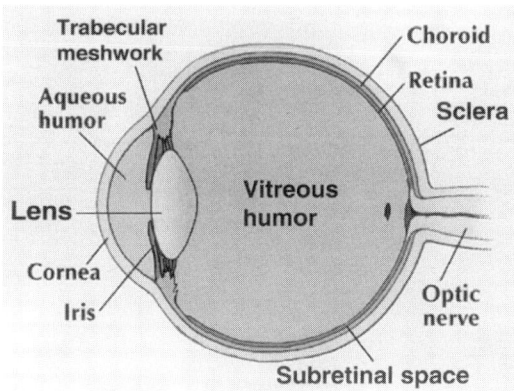

Fig. 1. Schematic of a cross-section of a human eye.

Susceptible animal species include rodents as well as primates, which makes this model useful not only for basic studies of immune mechanisms but also for preclinical testing of therapeutic modalities. Although the antigens driving human uveitis are still unknown, uveitis patients frequently display strong cellular responses to retinal antigens that are uveitogenic in animals, and it is therefore believed that the findings in animal models can be extrapolated to the human *(1–4)*. A recently described autoimmune model of mostly anterior uveitis, reminiscent of Vogt-Koyanagi-Harada disease, can be induced with ocular melanin (reviewed in ref. *5*). Although cytokine-related mechanisms have not been studied extensively, they appear similar to those of EAU.

The healthy eye represents a unique, immunologically privileged environment. Immune privilege is manifested as lack of "normal" immune recognition of antigens placed in the eye. Foreign tissues placed in the eye are not rejected and foreign antigens injected into the eye elicit a deviant immune response that is characterized by suppressed cellular immunity of the delayed hypersensitivity type, and humoral immunity primarily of noncomplement-binding antibody isotypes, a phenomenon known as ACAID (anterior chamber-associated immune deviation). The processes that lead to the establishment and preservation of the immunologically privileged status of the eye are multilayered and complex. The eye becomes closed off from the immune system early in ontogeny. Like the brain, the eye resides behind blood-tissue barrier. Tight junctions between adjacent vascular endothelial cells and epithelial cells of the various ocular structures limit entry not only of cells but even of small protein molecules into the eye. Ocular fluids drain directly into the blood through a structure at the angle of

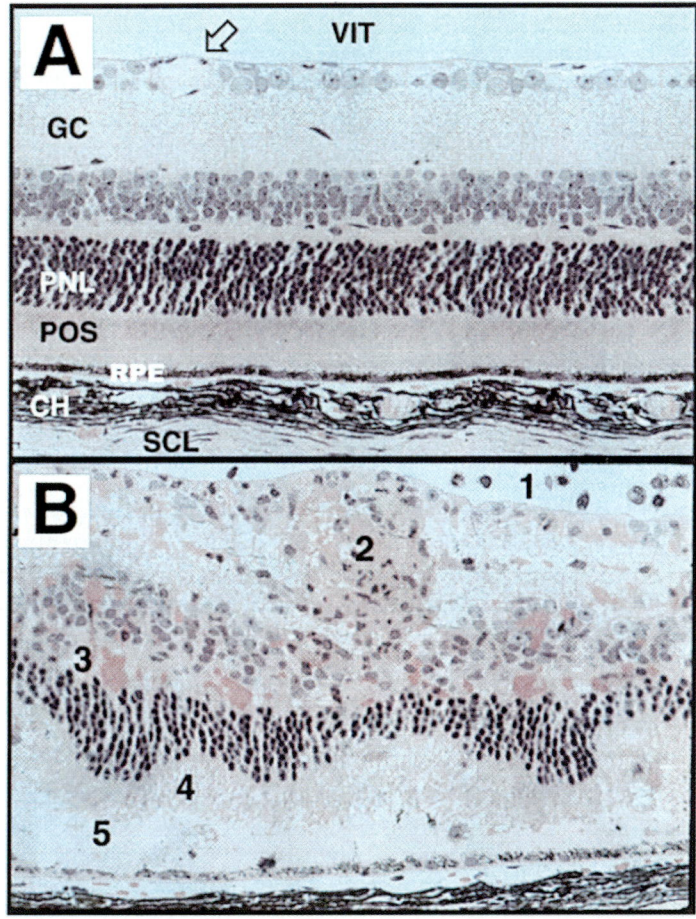

Fig. 2. Normal and uveitic eye—mouse. (**A**) Normal retina. VIT, vitreous; GC, ganglion cell layer; PNR, photoreceptor nuclear layer; POS, photoreceptor outer segments; RPE, retinal pigment epithelium; CH, choroid; SCL, sclera. Note retinal vessel (empty arrow). (**B**) Uveitic retina. Note 1, vitritis; 2, vasculitis; 3, retinal hemorrhage; 4, photoreceptor folding; 5, retinal detachment. Hematoxylin and eosin. Original magnification, ×400.

the iris and the cornea known as trabecular meshwork (*see* Fig. 1 for schematic), thus bypassing the lymphatic system and the elicitation of conventional immunity. In addition, the interior of the eye represents a profoundly immunosuppressive environment that among other things prevents Tcell activation, proliferation, and interferon-γ (IFN-γ) production, as well as the release of NO by macrophages. This is a result of the combined action of suppressive cytokines and soluble factors, as well as contact-dependent mechanisms, that will be discussed ahead (reviewed in refs. *6–8*).

The eye is exquisitely sensitive to presence of inflammatory cytokines: inoculation of either tumor necrosis factor-α (TNF-α), interleukin-1 (IL-1), IL-6, IL-8, granulocyte-macrophage colony-stimulating facotr (GM-CSF), or IFN-γ into the eye induces uveitis within hours *(9)*. It has been proposed that an ocular environment nonpermissive to the induction and expression of cellular immunity has developed during evolution in response to the need to preserve vision in the face of a variety of proinflammatory physical and microbial insults. Vision is dependent probably more than any other function of the body on the absolute integrity of the anatomical structures involved, and good vision is a most powerful selective pressure. Evolution has, therefore, favored mechanisms that preserve the integrity of the tissue by inhibiting and/or channeling destructive inflammatory processes into pathways less damaging to vision *(7,8)*.

The relative isolation of the eye from the immune system raises the question whether, and how, does the immune system "see" the ocular antigens themselves? Are they sufficiently available intrathymically during ontogeny and peripherally during postnatal life to eliminate or control autoreactive repertoires? Egwuagu et al. *(10)* presented evidence for expression of the retinal S-Ag and IRBP in the thymus of mice and rats, and correlated it to susceptibility of these strains to induction of uveitis by immunization with these antigens. However, it is not clear how effective this level of expression is in supporting negative selection, because even for antigens that are well represented in the thymus the negative selection process is not 100% efficient. Peripheral tolerance induction through presentation on "nonprofessional" antigen-presenting cells (APCs) in the absence of costimulation is probably limited, because the antigens in question are largely limited to the eye, which becomes isolated from the immune system early in ontogeny. However, retinal antigens are expressed also in the pineal gland ("third eye"), which has no blood-organ barrier. It is therefore reasonable to infer that some level of tolerance exists to retina-specific antigens. Nevertheless, the findings that retinal antigen-specific lymphocytes can be easily cultured from peripheral blood of healthy animals and humans, and that ocular autoimmunity is easily induced in experimental animals, indicate that tolerance to retinal antigens is incomplete. Recent data from our laboratory, showing that mice expressing the retinal antigen IRBP extraocularly on a class II promoter are highly resistant to EAU induced with an IRBP-derived epitope, demonstrate directly that the normally restricted expression of this retinal antigen does not support efficient self-tolerization *(11)*.This is further supported by the report of Koevary et al. that intrathymic injection of S-Ag prevents development of EAU in Lewis rats *(12)*. Thus, on the one hand, evolution has taken pains to limit the access and to control the interaction of the immune system with ocular components. On the other hand, the very isolation that protects the eye from the immune system, also prevents efficient development of tolerance to ocular antigens, so that when integrity of the blood-tissue barriers is disrupted, lymphocytes from the periphery—that have not been rendered tolerant—can enter the eye, and autoimmunity may ensue.

2. CYTOKINES IN THE HEALTHY EYE AND THEIR RELATION TO IMMUNE PRIVILEGE

A number of cytokines, for the most part produced by the ocular tissues themselves, have been identified in the eye, and additional ones are probably yet to be discovered. The ocular fluid that has been best-studied, owing mainly to its accessibility, is the aqueous humor (AH). However, there is diffusion of molecules among the different compartments of the eye, so that many if not most of the substances identified in the aqueous are also present in other compartments. Indeed, immune privilege also has been shown to exist in the vitreous cavity as well as in the subretinal space *(8)*.

Perhaps the most prominent and well studied among the suppressive ocular cytokines is transforming growth factor-$\beta 2$ (TGF-$\beta 2$) *(13)*. The eye contains surprisingly large amounts of this cytokine, mostly in latent but also in active form, and it accounts for most of the direct immunoinhibitory activity of aqueous humor. TGF-$\beta 2$ is the isoform that appears to be typical of immune privileged sites. Not only the eye, but also the cerebrospinal fluid (CSF) and the amniotic fluid contain large amounts of TGF-$\beta 2$ *(13–16)*. AH-derived TGF-$\beta 2$ not only inhibits lymphocyte function, but—at least in the case of responses to soluble protein Ags such as ovalbumin (OVA)— also acts to endow ocular APCs with inhibitory properties that are central to the induction of the ACAID response, the deviant immune response mentioned earlier that is elicited to antigens presented through the eye. Furthermore, TGF-β alters the properties of conventional APC (peritoneal exudate cells), that would normally be able to prime T cells towards the T helper (Th)1 pathway. When incubated with OVA in the presence of biological fluids derived from one of these privileged sites or with purified TGF-$\beta 2$, these APCs produce IL-10 instead of IL-12 during antigen processing, and promote differentiation of antigen specific T cells towards the Th2 phenotype *(17,18)*. Finally, TGF-β-altered APC induce generation of ACAID-specific CD8[+] regulatory cells that suppress delayed type hypersensitivity (DTH) responses to OVA by a unique mechanism involving migration of the ACAID-inducing APC into the spleen and local production of MIP-2 by them, recruitment of CD1-restricted natural killer T (NKT) cells into the spleen, and induction of IL-10 production by these recruited NKT cells, that presumably acts to promote differentiation of ACAID regulatory T cells *(19–21)*.

Other cytokines/soluble factors found in the eye include macrophage migration inhibitory factor (MIF), IL-1 receptor antagonist (IL-1RA), alpha melanocyte stimulating hormone (α-MSH), vasoactive intestinal peptide (VIP), calcitonin gene-related peptide (CGRP) and free cortisol *(7,8)*. The combined activities of these different cytokines and soluble factors in concert are responsible for the immunoinhibitory effects of ocular fluids on T cells. Thus, the anti-proliferative effect is mediated mainly by TGF-β2 and VIP, whereas inhibition of IFN-γ synthesis is owing to α-MSH. CGRP is primarily responsible for inhibition of nitric oxide (NO) production by macrophages, and inhibition of target-cell killing by NK cells is accomplished by TGF-β2 and MIF. In contrast, killing by cytotoxic T cells is not inhibited by AH, underscoring the selectivity of the ocular environment in favor of those effector mechanisms that do not result in widespread and nonselective tissue damage.

An integral part of the unique immunological environment of the eye, and working in part through cytokine responses, is expression of FasL on ocular tissues. The demonstration of constitutive expression of FasL as an important component of immune privilege in general has first been demonstrated in the eye, and subsequently extended to other immunologically privileged tissues *(6,22)*. Studies by Ferguson et al. *(23,24)* utilizing injection of virus-infected or TNP-derivatized syngeneic spleen cells into the anterior chamber have revealed that the role of FasL in ocular immune privilege is twofold: (1) it promotes apoptosis of infiltrating lymphocytes, and thus has a direct role in eliminating pathogenic effector cells from the eye; (2) the cells that have been signaled to die promote induction of systemic ACAID to the antigen they carry. The process of apoptosis triggers IL-10 production by the affected cells. Phagocytes that ingest the IL-10-laden apoptotic cells display an altered APC function and prime antigen-specific T cells for immune deviation. Although it is possible that the interaction between apoptotic T cells and APCs might take place in the eye, apoptotic bodies (presumably derived from the T cells injected into the eye) are subsequently found in the blood; it is thought that they reach the spleen and encounter resident APCs there. This phenomenon could be conceptualized to represent the fate of autoreactive T cells that have infiltrated the eye and have come in contact with ocular antigens.

It is interesting to note the different but parallel mechanisms operating in ACAID induction to soluble (OVA) and cell-bound antigen (TNP-coupled

T cells). The latter involves an obligate step of apoptotic death of antigen-bearing cells and their concomitant IL-10 production. However, in both cases cells—either APCs or apoptotic T cells—exit the eye and go to the spleen, but in the case of soluble antigen they are modified macrophages, and in the case of particulate antigen they are apoptotic T cells. In both cases, tolerogenic antigen presentation is accomplished by modified APC, which in the case of soluble Ag have been affected by TGF-β2 in the eye, and in the case of particulate Ags have been affected by apoptotic T cell-produced IL-10. In both cases production of IL-10 is required, but in the former it is accomplished by attracting IL-10 producing NKT cells, and in the latter the apoptotic T cells themselves serve as the source of the cytokine. Thus, the oculo-splenic axis, the participation of functionally altered APC, and the obligate role of IL-10 represent common themes of the two pathways.

That immune privilege and the ACAID phenomenon may be relevant to controlling ocular autoimmunity was demonstrated by Hara et al., who showed prevention, as well as reversal, of EAU by induction of IRBP-specific ACAID using injections of the soluble IRPB into the anterior chamber *(25)*. Unexpectedly, however, recent work from our laboratory has demonstrated that expression of FasL on ocular tissues does not appear to reduce susceptibility to induction of EAU *(25a)*. This was evidenced by the finding that FasL deficient (lpr) mice, lethally irradiated and reconstituted with wild-type bone marrow, were just as susceptible to EAU as the FasL-competent the wild-type when challenged with a uveitogenic IRBP regimen. Thus, local mechanisms of immune privilege do not afford protection against a strong disease-inducing stimulus, but protection can be achieved by a state of systemic immune deviation through directed manipulation of these mechanisms. Given that the intensity of most natural environmental triggers probably falls short of an experimental uveitogenic regimen, the immune privilege and the ACAID phenomenon may well serve to raise the threshold of resistance, and may partly compensate for the apparently limited effectiveness of central and peripheral tolerance in eliminating self-reactive T cell repertoires capable of recognizing retinal antigens.

3. CYTOKINES AND UVEITIS

3.1. Genetics and the Effector Response

EAU in the wild-type host is associated with a Th1 response. IL-12p40 deficient mice, that produce no functional IL-12 and are unable to mount a Th1 response, as well as wild-type mice treated with neutralizing anti-IL-12 antibodies fail to develop EAU *(26* and Silver et al., unpublished data).

Mice   **Rats**

Parameter	BALB/c	A/J	AKR	B10.A	BALB/k	C57BL/10	F344	Lewis
H-2	d	a	k	a	k	b	r	l
I-A	d	k	k	k	k	b	l	l
EAU Scores	−	+	−	+++	++	++	±	+++
LNC prolif.	+	+	++	++	+	++	++	++
IL-4	++	+	−	−	−	−	±	±
IFN-γ	−	−	−	+++	++	+++	±	+++
IgG2a / IgG1	1	2a	2a	2a	2a or 1	2a	ND	ND
Th1 / Th2	Th2	?	?	Th1	Th1	Th1	?	Th1

Fig. 3. EAU susceptibility and immunological responses of genetically defined mouse and rat strains. Animals were given a uveitogenic regimen of IRBP (mice) or its major pathogenic peptide (rats). Draining lymph node cells were explanted into culture after 12–16 d and were stimulated with the immunizing antigen. Cytokines in 48 h supernatants and anti-IRBP Ig subclasses in the serum were assayed by enzyme-linked immunosorbent assay (ELISA), except for IL-4 in rats which was assessed in stimulated cells by reverse transcription polymerase chain reaction (RT-PCR). EAU was evaluated by Histopathology.

Genetically susceptible strains of rats and mice are dominant Th1 responders to the uveitogenic antigen, whereas EAU-resistant strains are likely to be low Th1 responders, or overt Th2 responders *(27,28)*. In this context, it is notable that pertussis toxin, which breaks EAU resistance in genetically nonsusceptible strains, at the same time causes polarization of their cytokine response towards Th1 *(29)*. The chart in Fig. 3 shows an analysis of the cytokine response phenotype vs susceptibility to EAU induced by IRPB or its peptide, in a series of inbred mouse and rat strains. Interestingly, the Th1-low response pattern associated with resistance does not have to be achieved through a dominant Th2 response to the uveitogen. Genotypes with a "null" response—that is, low in both Th1-type and Th2-type cytokines, such as the F344 rat and the AKR mouse—are as resistant to EAU induction as the Th2-biased BALB/c mouse. This indicates that control of the pathogenic Th1 response does not require having a response skewed towards the Th2 pathway. Additional factors (either anti-inflammatory such as TGF-β, or proinflammatory such as TNF-α, that might be superimposed on the Th1/Th2 response pattern, undoubtedly contribute to the complex nature of the regulatory mechanisms that determine susceptibility or resistance to ocular autoimmune disease.

In keeping with the genetic predisposition towards Th1 as a factor in susceptibility, uveitogenic T cell lines and clones are Th1-like in terms of their cytokine profile. Furthermore, primary T cell populations that make IFN-γ are uveitogenic, whereas those that make little or no IFN-γ are not, however, they can be converted to a pathogenic, IFN-γ producing phenotype by culture with IL-12 *(26,27,30)*. In contrast, a Th2 response is counterregulatory, in that experimentally skewing the developing response toward Th2, by early treatment with IL4+IL-10 or by injections of mercuric chloride, can protect from development of disease *(31,32)*. However, a Th2-like effector response may also lead to severe tissue damage. An example is induction of EAU in IFN-γ knockout mice, that do not mount a normal Th1 response owing to their inability to produce the prototypic Th1 effector cytokine, IFN-γ. These mice develop EAU at least as readily as wild-type mice, but tissue damage is effected by a distinct mechanism, showing many characteristics of a deviant, Th2-like response *(33)*. IFN-γ deficient mice exhibit an antigen-specific response high in IL-5, IL-10, and IL-6, and do not upregulate inducible nitric oxide synthase (iNOS) (whose regulation is strongly IFN-γ driven). Unlike the wild type, their inflammatory infiltrate is dominated by polymorphonuclear leukocytes and contains a large proportion of eosinophils, strikingly reminiscent of an immediate hypersensitivity-like reaction (Fig. 4). Data in the EAE model showed that adoptive transfer of Th2 clones to immunodeficient (SCID) mice can lead to severe tissue damage having a similar allergic-like pathology *(34)*. Thus, an unopposed Th2 response can be as destructive to the tissue as a Th1 response.

Interestingly, however, IL-12 deficient animals that also develop a Th2-like response to the uveitogenic protein, are highly resistant to EAU *(26)*. Furthermore, IFN-γ knockout mice treated with neutralizing antibodies to IL-12 fail to develop EAU. This indicates that IL-12 plays a role that is independent of IFN-γ and that IL-12, rather than IFN-γ, is a necessary cytokine for differentiation of uveitogenic effector T cells, irrespective of their particular cytokine profile.

3.2. Regulatory Cytokines in Control of EAU

Control of EAU by regulatory cytokines is accomplished at multiple levels. As an example, TGF-β and IL-10, which have a role in immune privilege, may intervene at a level that prevents the initiation of processes leading to autoimmune tissue attack. Th2 response, which under normal circumstances is counterregulatory, can prevent development of a pathogenic effector response when a perturbation has already occurred. Finally, if a pathogenic response phenotype has become established and has precipitated tissue damage, it must be downregulated to bring about remission or recovery.

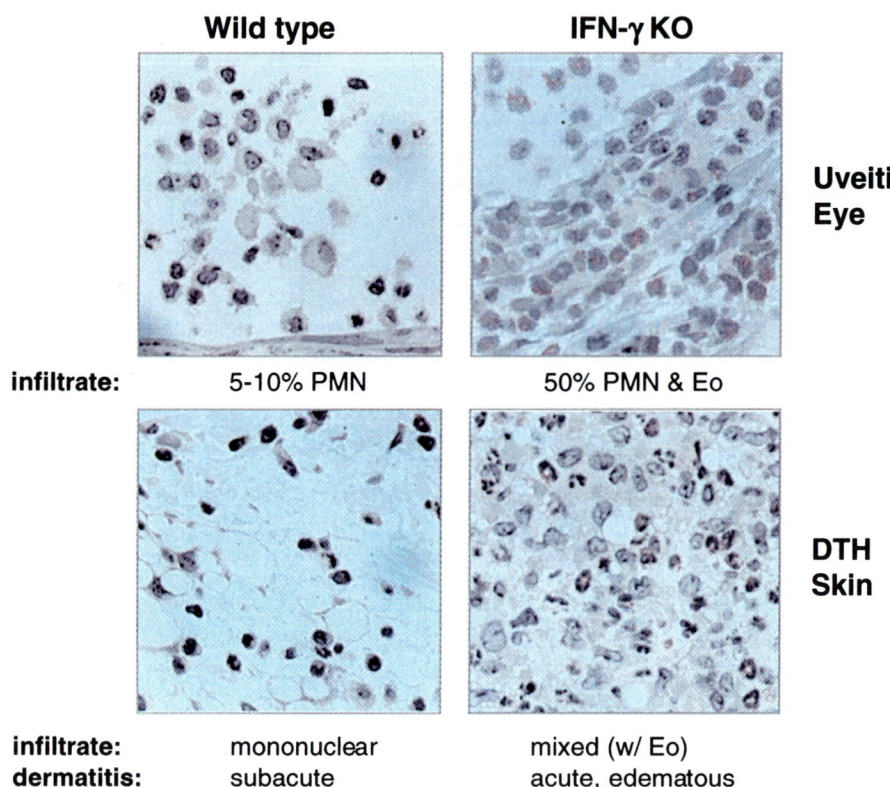

Wild type   **IFN-γ KO**

Uveitic Eye

infiltrate: 5-10% PMN   50% PMN & Eo

DTH Skin

infiltrate: mononuclear   mixed (w/ Eo)
dermatitis: subacute   acute, edematous

Fig. 4. Cellular composition of inflammatory infiltrate typical of EAU in IFN-γ KO mice. Shown are sections through the eye (vitreous infiltrate) and through the DTH lesion in wild-type and IFN-γ knockout mouse. Note numerous eosinophils (Eo) in IFN-γ knockout infiltrate, vs their paucity in wild-type. Hematoxylin and eosin. Original magnification ×400.

3.3. IL-4 and IL-10

Data derived from in vivo treatment of EAU-susceptible mice given a uveitogenic regimen of IRBP with recombinant IL-4 and IL-10 showed that early treatment with IL-4 alone did not affect EAU. Early treatment with IL-10 downregulated disease scores and inhibited the Th1-type cytokines, but without deviating the immune response towards Th2. However, combined IL4+IL-10 treatment shifted the cytokine profile towards Th2 and was synergistic in terms of protection from disease *(31)*. This might indicate that achieving immune deviation in a Th1-predisposed host requires a concomitant suppression of the genetically dominant Th1 response. Interestingly,

Ramanathan et al. *(35)* reported exacerbation of EAU and augmentation of the Th1 response in rats in Lewis rats, which are strongly predisposed to Th1, by treatment with IL-4.

Several lines of evidence suggest that IL-10 might constitute one of the mechanisms mediating natural recovery from EAU *(31)*. Administration of exogenous IL-10 was able to prevent EAU, whereas administration of anti-IL-10 exacerbated disease. IL-10 is one of only a few cytokines able to inhibit the function of fully differentiated uveitogenic Th1 cells in culture, and expression IL-10 mRNA in uveitic mouse eyes was seen to rise during the resolution phase of EAU. Recent data, showing higher expression of IL-10 mRNA in eyes of EAU-resistant than EAU-susceptible rat strains, suggested that basal levels of IL-10 are present in the healthy eye and can affect susceptibility to disease *(36)*. As mentioned earlier, IL-10 also appears to be one of the obligate mediators of the ACAID phenomenon, supporting the notion that endogenous IL-10 could be involved not only in recovery, but also in prevention of ocular autoimmunity *(17,24)*.

3.4. TGF-β

As discussed above, TGF-β is inextricably linked with regulation of immunological responses in the eye, and to the eye. In addition to its central role in ocular immune privilege it may also affect systemic responses involved in EAU. Mice given a uveitogenic immunization during pregnancy develop reduced EAU scores compared to nonpregnant controls, and their antigen-specific cytokine responses indicated a selective reduction of Th1 immunity *(37)*. Interestingly, pregnant mice given an infusion of IRBP-primed lymphoid cells from nonpregnant donors also developed reduced EAU, suggesting that not only the generation, but also the function of mature uveitogenic effector T cells, is inhibited by pregnancy. Because pregnant mice have elevated serum levels of TGF-β (but not of IL-10), these effects may be secondary to supranormal systemic levels of this cytokine. Interestingly, female patients suffering from autoimmune uveitis are reported to experience a temporary remission of their symptoms during pregnancy. We hypothesize that TGF-β might cause inhibition of Th1 cells at least in part through antagonizing the effects of IL-12. This is suggested by in vitro experiments showing reduction of IL-12 driven IFN-γ production and IL-12Rβ2 mRNA accumulation in IRBP-primed lymph node cells cultured in the presence of TGF-β (Xu et al., unpublished results).

TGF-β may also have a role in helping to downregulate inflammation in the eye that has already developed EAU *(38)*. Loss of ability of AH to inhibit T cell proliferation coincides with onset of EAU and elevated titers of IL-6, which counteracts the suppressive effects of TGF-β. However, within a week, the aqueous reexpressed its ability to suppress T cell proliferation, owing to high levels of blood-derived TGF-β1 and eye-derived TGF-β2 in the absence of IL-6. It sees a reasonable assumption that the restoration of the immunosuppressive ocular microenvironment may help to turn off inflammation at the tissue level. Interestingly, high levels of IL-6 in the eye were found to be correlated with severity of endotoxin-induced uveitis (9), implicating IL-6 as an important inflammatory mediator in the eye. Thus, a regulatory circuit that shuts off IL-6 and prevents it from counteracting the effects TGF-β, which then antagonizes the effects IL-12 and promotes IL-10 secretion, may be involved in resolution of EAU.

3.5. Negative Regulation by IL-12 and IFN-γ

The local effects of IFN-γ within the eye are unquestionably proinflammatory (9). However, systemic effects of this cytokine appear to be exactly opposite. Treatment of wild-type mice with neutralizing antibodies to IFN-γ exacerbates disease, whereas treatment with recombinant IFN-γ ameliorates it. Furthermore, IFN-γ knockout mice are more susceptible than wild-type to EAU induced with a uveitogenic peptide or with limiting doses of IRBP, and in contrast to the wild-type, develop a chronic relapsing disease (39,40, and Silver et al., unpublished results).

Insights into the mechanism underlying the protective systemic effects of IFN-γ were recently provided by a series of experiments, initially designed to confirm the role of the Th1 response in EAU. Because genetic resistance to EAU appeared connected to a low Th1 response (Fig. 3), we expected that treatment with IL-12 would permit EAU development in resistant strains by shifting their response towards Th1. Unexpectedly, treatment of mice given a uveitogenic regimen of IRBP in complete Freund's adjuvant with 100 ng/d of IL-12 for the first 5 d after immunization not only did not enhance EAU in resistant strains, but in fact completely inhibited its development in susceptible strains (41). Treated mice had nanogram levels of circulating IFN-γ in the serum, evidence of enhanced apoptosis in the draining lymph nodes, and their subsequent antigen-specific responses, especially IFN-γ production, were suppressed. In a series of experiments using IFN-γ-deficient, iNOS-deficient, and Bcl-2 transgenic mice, which are all poorly protected by IL-12, it was possible to delineate a seqeuence of events whereby administration of IL-12 causes systemic hyperinduction of IFN-γ. This mediates protection at least in part by activation of iNOS and production of NO, which in turn triggers Bcl-2-related apoptotic deletion of antigen-specific T cells as they are being primed (Fig. 5). Existence of additional IFN-γ-driven mechanisms besides NO-driven apoptosis, such as TNF or Fas/FasL-driven apoptosis, as well as other antiproliferative mechanisms, are suggested by

Genotype	Wild Type	IFN-γ KO	iNOS KO	Bcl-2 TG
% protection by IL-12	100	0	35	75

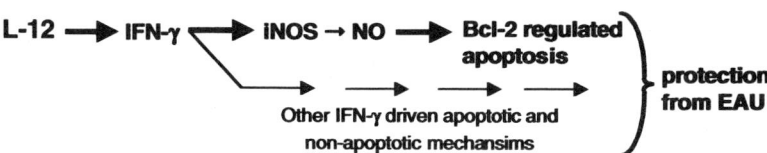

Fig. 5. Control of EAU by excess IFN-γ and the proposed pathway. Mice were immunized with a uveitogenic regimen of IRBP and were injected once daily with 100 μg of recombinant murine IL-12 for the first 5 d after immunization. EAU was evaluated by histopathology 21 d after immunization.

the progressive reduction in interference with protection at each step following IFN-γ in this proposed pathway . Interestingly, the same IL-12 treatment started on d 7 after immunization is not protective, indicating that regulation by excess systemic IFN-γ is only effective during initial priming, but is ineffective against effector cells that have already been generated. We propose that regulation of the Th1 response by excess systemic IFN-γ is a regulatory mechanism to control Th1 responses in general, by preventing recruitment of additional lymphocytes into the effector pool when a strong cellular response, signified by high levels of inflammatory cytokines such as IL-12 and IFN-γ, is already present. The in vivo relevance of this pathway is supported by the observation that IFN-γ and iNOS knockout mice, both of which cannot use this type of regulation, are highly susceptible to EAU and have elevated cellular responses to IRBP *(33,40,42)*.

3.6. Chemokines

Research on chemokines in uveitis is limited. Thus far, no chemokines have been described that are uniquely or preferentially expressed in the eye. The uninflamed eye does not express detectable chemokine mRNA species. However, chemokines such as IL-8, MCP-1, RANTES, GRO, and IP-10 are produced in the eye under inflammatory conditions. At least in some cases, they can be shown to be associated with, and presumably are produced by, the ocular tissues themselves *(43–45)*. Explanted retinal pigment epithelial cells stimulated with cytokines produce copious amounts of MCP-1 and IL-8 *(46)*.

That chemokines are necessary for expression of EAU is shown by the dependence of disease induction on chemokine-receptor signaling. Pertussis toxin is known to ADP-ribosylate and inactivate Gi proteins, which are involved in chemokine signaling. Incubation of uveitogenic T cells with pertussis toxin before their infusion into recipients, or treatment of recipients themselves with pertussis toxin, completely prevents induction of adoptively transferred EAU. The effect is dependent on the ADP-ribosylating activity of pertussis toxin, and the in vitro treated cells, as well as lymphoid cells from treated animals, fail to migrate to chemokines in chemotaxis chambers *(47)*. Thus, blockade of chemokine receptor signaling aborts disease induction by disruption of cell migration and infiltration into the target organ. The effectiveness of this process in preventing disease raises the notion of blocking chemokine signaling as a potential therapeutic approach to uveitis.

4. IMMUNOTHERAPEUTIC STRATEGIES BASED ON MODULATING CYTOKINES OR CYTOKINE RECEPTORS: CLINICAL TRIALS

4.1. Immune-Deviation Strategies of Therapy and Oral Tolerance

The existence of Th1-low, nonpathogenic response phenotypes that were discussed earlier, raises the notion of evoking a nonpathogenic response as a means of preventing a pathogenic one. In animal models, deviating the response to the immunizing retinal antigen towards the Th2 phenotype by directed immunomodulation has resulted in protection from disease *(31,32)*. Although an unopposed Th2-like effector response can be as destructive to the tissue as a Th1-like response *(33,34)*, this has mostly been seen in immunologically abnormal or immunocompromised hosts. An attractive way to deviate the immune response is by oral tolerance induced by antigen feeding. Oral tolerance as an immunotherapeutic strategy has recently gained attention and been explored experimentally and clinically in a number of autoimmune diseases, including uveitis *(48)*, and is discussed more fully elsewhere in this volume.

Two distinct, nonmutually exclusive mechanisms that mediate oral tolerance have been described: clonal anergy or deletion of the antigen-specific cells and active suppression by regulatory cells secreting IL-4, IL-10, and TGF-β. Which of these two major mechanisms of tolerance will predominate is affected by the antigen dose and the feeding regimen *(48–50)*. In EAU, cytokine-mediated tolerance has been shown to require the ability to produce both IL-4 and IL-10. Mice deficient in either one fail to develop oral tolerance dependent on regulatory cytokines, although they are unimpaired in their ability to develop oral tolerance mediated by anergy/deletion *(51)*. This may indicate that IL-4 and IL-10 are needed at different stages of the oral-tolerance process. Based on these results, and on the effects of in vivo administration of IL-4 and IL-10 described earlier *(31)*, we have hypothesized that IL-4 is required to induce the regulatory cells, whereas IL-10 may be important as an effector cytokine in controlling the expression of EAU.

Based on the encouraging results in animals and a pilot trial in two uveitis patients given oral therapy with retinal S-Ag *(52)*, a double-masked placebo-controlled clinical trial was recently performed in which uveitis patients were fed purified bovine S-Ag, crude retinal extract, or a mixture of both *(53)*. The trial gave encouraging results, however, it has not been confirmed that the beneficial effects on disease in fact involved regulatory cytokines. Notably, however, the crude retinal extract seemed to worsen the disease compared to the placebo when fed alone, and to abrogate the therapeutic benefit of S-Ag therapy when the two were given together *(53)*. The possibility has been raised that an oral tolerance regimen will "backfire," and induce pathology instead of tolerance *(54,55)*. Although in clinical trials of oral tolerance in rheumatoid arthritis (RA) or multiple sclerosis (MS) such a complication has not been noted, the negative effect of the crude retinal extract in the uveitis patients raises a note of caution.

4.2. Targeting IL-2 Receptor Positive Cells

The pathogenic effector T cells in EAU, and presumably in human uveitis, are Th1-type and express IL-2 receptors. Early experiments in the rat EAU model, using a chimeric protein composed of IL-2 and pseudomonas exotoxin, showed the efficacy of this type of approach *(56)*. This approach was subsequently validated in a primate model of EAU by using humanized monoclonal antibodies (MAbs) to the α-chain of the IL-2 receptor and the β-chain shared by the IL-2 and IL-15 receptors *(57)*. Finally, an open label clinical trial was performed in which 10 patients with severe sight-threatening uveitis were treated with infusions of humanized anti-IL-2 receptor α chain antibody for the period of 1 yr. This therapy prevented expression of disease in 8 of 10 patients, with noted improvements in visual acuity *(58)*. This is an excellent bench-to-bedside example how basic studies in an animal model can lead to improved understanding of the mechanisms of disease and result in a successful clinical treatment paradigm.

REFERENCES

1. Nussenblatt, R. B., Whitcup, S. M., and Palestine, A. G. (1996) *Uveitis: Fundamentals and Clinical Practice.* Mosby-Year Book, Inc., St. Louis, MO.
2. Gery, I. and Streilein, J. W. (1994) Autommunity in the eye and its regulation. *Curr. Opin. Immunol.* **6,** 938–945.

3. Caspi, R. R. (1994) Experimental autoimmune uveoretinitis: rat and mouse, in *Animal Models for Autoimmune Diseases: A Guidebook*. (Cohen, I. R. and Miller, A., eds.), Academic Press, pp. 57–81.
4. Gery, I., Mochizuki, M., and Nussenblatt, R. B. (1986) Retinal specific antigens and immunopathogenic processes they provoke. *Prog. Retinal Res.* **5,** 75–109.
5. Smith, J. R., Hart, P. H., and Williams, K. A. (1998) Basic pathogenic mechanisms operating in experimental models of acute anterior uveitis. *Immunol. Cell Biol.* **76,** 497–512.
6. Ferguson, T. A. and Griffith, T. S. (1997) A vision of cell death: insights into immune privilege. *Immunol. Rev.* **156,** 167–184.
7. Streilein, J. W. (1999) Regional immunity and ocular immune privilege. *Chem. Immunol.* **73,** 11–38.
8. Streilein, J. W. (1999) Immunologic privilege of the eye. *Springer Semin. Immunopathol.* **21,** 95–111.
9. Kijlstra, A. (1997) Cytokines: their role in uveal disease. *Eye* **11,** 200–205.
10. Egwuagu, C. E., Charukamnoetkanok, P., and Gery, I. (1997) Thymic expression of autoantigens correlates with resistance to autoimmune disease. *J. Immunol.* **159,** 3109–3112.
11. Xu, H., Wawrousek, E. F., Redmond, T. M., Nickerson, J. M., Wiggert, B., Chan, C. C., and Caspi, R. R. (2000) Transgenic expression of an immunologically privileged retinal antigen extraocularly enhances self tolerance and abrogates susceptibility to autoimmune uveitis. *Eur. J. Immunol.* **30,** 272–278.
12. Koevary, S. B. and Caspi, R. R. (1997) Prevention of experimental autoimmune uveoretinitis by intrathymic S-antigen injection. *Ocul. Immunol. Inflamm.* **5,** 165–172.
13. Cousins, S. W., McCabe, M. M., Danielpour, D., and Streilein, J. W. (1991) Identification of transforming growth factor-beta as an immunosuppressive factor in aqueous humor. *Invest. Ophthalmol. Vis. Sci.* **32,** 2201–2211.
14. Granstein, R. D., Staszewski, R., Knisely, T. L., Zeira, E., Nazareno, R., Latina, M., and Albert, D. M. (1990) Aqueous humor contains transforming growth factor-beta and a small (less than 3500 daltons) inhibitor of thymocyte proliferation. *J. Immunol.* **144,** 3021–3027.
15. Wilbanks, G. A. and Streilein, J. W. (1992) Fluids from immune privileged sites endow macrophages with the capacity to induce antigen-specific immune deviation via a mechanism involving transforming growth factor-beta. *Eur. J. Immunol.* **22,** 1031–1036.
16. Altman, D. J., Schneider, S. L., Thompson, D. A., Cheng, H. L., and Tomasi, T. B. (1990) A transforming growth factor beta 2 (TGF-beta 2)-like immunosuppressive factor in amniotic fluid and localization of TGF-beta 2 mRNA in the pregnant uterus. *J. Exp. Med.* **172,** 1391–1401.
17. D'Orazio, T. J. and Niederkorn, J. Y. (1998) A novel role for TGF-beta and IL-10 in the induction of immune privilege. *J. Immunol.* **160,** 2089–2098.
18. Takeuchi, M., Alard, P., and Streilein, J. W. (1998) TGF-beta promotes immune deviation by altering accessory signals of antigen-presenting cells. *J. Immunol.* **160,** 1589–1597.

19. Sonoda, K. H., Exley, M., Snapper, S., Balk, S. P., and Stein-Streilein, J. (1999) CD1-reactive natural killer T cells are required for development of systemic tolerance through an immune-privileged site. *J. Exp. Med.* **190,** 1215–1226.

20. Faunce, D. E., Sonoda, K. H., and Stein-Streilein, J. (2001) MIP-2 recruits NKT cells to the spleen during tolerance induction. *J. Immunol.* **166,** 313–321.

21. Sonada, K. H., Faunce, D. E., Taniguchi, M., Exley, M., Balk, S., and Stein-Streilein, J. (2001) NK T cell derived IL-10 is essential for the differentiation of antigen-specific T regulatory cells in systemic tolerance. *J. Immunol.* **166,** 42–50.

22. Guller, S. and LaChapelle, L. (1999) The role of placental Fas ligand in maintaining immune privilege at maternal-fetal interfaces. *Semin. Reprod. Endocrinol.* **17,** 39–44.

23. Griffith, T. S., Yu, X., Herndon, J. M., Green, D. R., and Ferguson, T. A. (1996) CD95-induced apoptosis of lymphocytes in an immune privileged site induces immunological tolerance. *Immunity* **5,** 7–16.

24. Gao, Y., Herndon, J. M., Zhang, H., Griffith, T. S., and Ferguson, T. A. (1998) Antiinflammatory effects of CD95 ligand (FasL)-induced apoptosis. *J. Exp. Med.* **188,** 887–896.

25. Hara, Y., Caspi, R. R., Wiggert, B., Chan, C. C., and Streilein, J. W. (1992) Use of ACAID to suppress interphotoreceptor retinoid binding protein- induced experimental autoimmune uveitis. *Curr. Eye Res.* **11,** 97–100.

25a. Wahlsten, J. L., Gitchell, H. L., Chan, C. C., Wiggert, B., and Caspi, R. R. (2000) Fas and Fas ligand expressed on cells of the immune system, not on the target tissue, control induction of experimental autoimmune uveitis. *J. Immunol.* **165,** 5480–5486.

26. Tarrant, T. K., Silver, P. B., Chan, C. C., Wiggert, B., and Caspi, R. R. (1998) Endogenous IL-12 is required for induction and expression of experimental autoimmune uveitis. *J. Immunol.* **161,** 122–127.

27. Caspi, R. R., Silver, P. B., Chan, C. C., Sun, B., Agarwal, R. K., Wells, J., et al. (1996) Genetic susceptibility to experimental autoimmune uveoretinitis in the rat is associated with an elevated Th1 response. *J. Immunol.* **157,** 2668–2675.

28. Sun, B., Rizzo, L. V., Sun, S. H., Chan, C. C., Wiggert, B., Wilder, R. L., and Caspi, R. R. (1997) Genetic susceptibility to experimental autoimmune uveitis involves more than a predisposition to generate a T helper-1-like or a T helper-2- like response. *J. Immunol.* **159,** 1004–1011.

29. Silver, P. B., Chan, C. C., Wiggert, B., and Caspi, R. R. (1999) The requirement for pertussis to induce EAU is strain-dependent: B10.RIII, but not B10.A mice, develop EAU and Th1 responses to IRBP without pertussis treatment. *Invest. Ophthalmol. Vis. Sci.* **40,** 2898–2905.

30. Xu, H., Rizzo, L. V., Silver, P. B., and Caspi, R. R. (1997) Uveitogenicity is associated with a Th1-like lymphokine profile: cytokine-dependent modulation of primary and committed T cells in EAU. *Cell. Immunol.* **178,** 69–78.

31. Rizzo, L. V., Xu, H., Chan, C. C., Wiggert, B., and Caspi, R. R. (1998) IL-10 has a protective role in experimental autoimmune uveoretinitis. *Intl. Immunol.* **10,** 807–814.

32. Saoudi, A., Kuhn, J., Huygen, K., de Kozak, Y., Velu, T., Goldman, M., et al. (1993) TH2 activated cells prevent experimental autoimmune uveoretinitis, a TH1-dependent autoimmune disease. *Eur. J. Immunol.* **23,** 3096–3103.

33. Jones, L. S., Rizzo, L. V., Agarwal, R. K., Tarrant, T. K., Chan, C. C., Wiggerrt, B., and Caspi, R. R. (1997) Interferon gamma-deficient mice develop experimental autoimmune uveitis in the context of a deviant effector response. *J. Immunol.* **158,** 5997–6005.

34. Lafaille, J. J., Keere, F. V., Hsu, H. L., Baron, J. L., Haas, W., Raine, C. S., and Tonegawa, S. (1997) Myelin basic protein-specific T helper 2 (Th2) cells cause experimental autoimmune encephalomyelitis in immunodeficient hosts rather than protect them from the disease. *J. Exp. Med.* **186,** 307–312.

35. Ramanathan, S., de Kozak, Y., Saoudi, A., Goureau, O., Van der Meide, P. H., Druet, P., and Bellon, B. (1996) Recombinant IL-4 aggravates experimental autoimmune uveoretinitis in rats. *J. Immunol.* **157,** 2209–2215.

36. Sun, B., Sun, S.-H., Chan, C. C., and Caspi, R. R. (2000) Evaluation of in vivo cytokine expression in EAU-susceptible and resistant rats: a role for IL-10 in resistance? *Exp. Eye. Res.* **70,** 493–502.

37. Agarwal, R. K., Chan, C. C., Wiggert, B., and Caspi, R. R. (1999) Pregnancy ameliorates induction and expression of experimental autoimmune uveitis. *J. Immunol.* **162,** 2648–2654.

38. Ohta, K., Wiggert, B., Yamagami, S., Taylor, S. W., and Streilein, J. W. (2000) Analysis of immunomodulatory activities of aqueous humor from eyes of mice with experimental autoimmune uveitis. *J. Immunol.* **164,** 1185–1192.

39. Avichezer, D., Chan, C. C., Silver, P. B., Wiggert, B., and Caspi, R. R. (2000) Residues 1-20 of IRBP and whole IRBP elicit different uveitogenic and immunological responses in interferon gamma deficient mice. *Exp. Eye Res.* **71,** 111–118.

40. Rizzo, L. V., Vallochi, A. L., Schlesinger, D., Martins, M. C., and Belfort Jr., R. (2000) The role of inflammatory and anti-inflammatory cytokines in the progression of experimental autoimmune uveitis. AAI/CIS Annual Meeting, Seattle, WA. *FASEB J.* **14,** A997. (Abstract # 52.24).

41. Tarrant, T. K., Silver, P. B., Wahlsten, J. L., Rizzo, L. V., Chan, C. C., Wiggert, B., and Caspi, R. R. (1999) Interleukin 12 protects from a T helper type 1-mediated autoimmune disease, experimental autoimmune uveitis, through a mechanism involving interferon gamma, nitric oxide, and apoptosis. *J. Exp. Med.* **189,** 219–230.

42. Silver, P. B., Tarrant, T. K., Chan, C. C., Wiggert, B., and Caspi, R. R. (1999) Mice deficient in inducible nitric oxide synthase are susceptible to experimental autoimmune uveoretinitis. *Invest. Ophthalmol. Vis. Sci.* **40,** 1280–1284.

43. Mo, J. S., Matsukawa, A., Ohkawara, S., and Yoshinaga, M. (2000) CXC chemokine GRO is essential for neutrophil infiltration in LPS-induced uveitis in rabbits. *Exp. Eye Res.* **70,** 221–226.

44. Crane, I. J., Kuppner, M. C., McKillop-Smith, S., Knott, R. M., and Forrester, J. V. (1998) Cytokine regulation of RANTES production by human retinal pigment epithelial cells. *Cell Immunol.* **184,** 37–44.

45. Guex-Crosier, Y., Wittwer, A. J., and Roberge, F. G. (1996) Intraocular production of a cytokine (CINC) responsible for neutrophil infiltration in endotoxin induced uveitis. *Br. J. Ophthalmol.* **80,** 649–653.

46. Elner, V. M., Burnstine, M. A., Strieter, R. M., Kunkel, S. L., and Elner, S. G. (1997) Cell-associated human retinal pigment epithelium interleukin-8 and

monocyte chemotactic protein-1: immunochemical and in-situ hybridization analyses. *Exp. Eye Res.* **65,** 781–789.

47. Su, S. B., Silver, P. B., Zhang, M. F., Chan, C. C., and Caspi, R. R. (2001) Pertussis toxin inhibits induction of tissue specific autoimmune disease by disrupting G-protein coupled signals. *J. Immunol.,* in press.

48. Weiner, H. L. (1997) Oral tolerance: immune mechanisms and treatment of autoimmune diseases. *Immunol. Today* **18,** 335–343.

49. Gregerson, D. S., Fling, S. P., Obritsch, W. F., Merryman, C. F., and Donoso, L. A. (1989) Identification of T cell recognition sites in S-antigen: dissociation of proliferative and pathogenic sites. *Cell Immunol.* **123,** 427–440.

50. Rizzo, L. V., Miller-Rivero, N. E., Chan, C. C., Wiggert, B., Nussenblatt, R. B., and Caspi, R. R. (1994) Interleukin-2 treatment potentiates induction of oral tolerance in a murine model of autoimmunity. *J. Clin. Invest.* **94,** 1668–1672.

51. Rizzo, L. V., Morawetz, R. A., Miller-Rivero, N. E., Choi, R., Wiggert, B., Chan, C. C., et al. (1999) IL-4 and IL-10 are both required for the induction of oral tolerance. *J. Immunol.* **162,** 2613–2622.

52. Nussenblatt, R. B., Whitcup, S. M., de Smet, M. D., Caspi, R. R., Kozhich, A. T., Weiner, H. L., et al. (1996) Intraocular inflammatory disease (uveitis) and the use of oral tolerance: a status report. *Ann. NY Acad. Sci.* **778,** 325–337.

53. Nussenblatt, R. B., Gery, I., Weiner, H. L., Ferris, F. L., Shiloach, J., Remaley, N., et al. (1997) Treatment of uveitis by oral administration of retinal antigens: results of a phase I/II randomized masked trial. *Am. J. Ophthalmol.* **123,** 583–592.

54. Blanas, E., Carbone, F. R., Allison, J., Miller, J. F., and Heath, W. R. (1996) Induction of autoimmune diabetes by oral administration of autoantigen. *Science* **274,** 1707–1709.

55. Xiao, B. G. and Link, H. (1997) Mucosal tolerance: a two-edged sword to prevent and treat autoimmune diseases. *Clin. Immunol. Immunopathol.* **85,** 119–128.

56. Roberge, F. G., Lorberboum-Galski, H., Le Hoang, P., de Smet, M., Chan, C. C., Fitzgerald, D., and Pastan, I. (1989) Selective immunosuppression of activated T cells with the chimeric toxin IL-2-PE40. Inhibition of experimental autoimmune uveoretinitis. *J. Immunol.* **143,** 3498–3502.

57. Guex-Crosier, Y., Raber, J., Chan, C. C., Kriete, M. S., Benichou, J., Pilson, R. S., et al. (1997) Humanized antibodies against the alpha-chain of the IL-2 receptor and against the beta-chain shared by the IL-2 and IL-15 receptors in a monkey uveitis model of autoimmune diseases. *J. Immunol.* **158,** 452–458.

58. Nussenblatt, R. B., Fortin, E., Schiffman, R., Rizzo, L., Smith, J., Van Veldhuisen, P., et al. (1999) Treatment of noninfectious intermediate and posterior uveitis with the humanized anti-Tac mAb: a phase I/II clinical trial. *Proc. Natl. Acad. Sci. USA* **96,** 7462–7466.

10

Pathogenic and Regulatory Cytokines in Experimental Autoimmune Encephalomyelitis

Estelle Bettelli and Lindsay B. Nicholson

1. INTRODUCTION

Experimental autoimmune encephalomyelitis (EAE) is a T cell mediated disease that shares many clinical and histological features with multiple sclerosis (MS) *(1,2)*. The disease is characterized by ascending paralysis accompanied by demyelination and a general inflammation in the central nervous system (CNS) *(3)*. EAE is induced in different species by immunization with myelin antigens such as myelin basic protein (MBP), myelin proteolipid protein (PLP), and myelin oligodendrocyte glycoprotein (MOG), or by adoptive transfer of T cells specific for these myelin antigens. Upon immunization with myelin antigens or peptides derived from them, autoreactive T cells are activated in the periphery and traffic through the blood brain barrier (BBB) into the CNS. In the CNS, these autoreactive T cells come in contact with antigen presenting cells (APCs) such as perivascular macrophages, microglial cells, or astrocytes, which are able to present myelin antigens in the context of their MHC class II molecules. In this inflammatory microenvironment, T lymphocytes and other cells express cytokines and chemokines, which both promote and regulate the pathogenic process.

Myelin antigen-reactive helper T cells are sufficient to induce EAE, because the elimination of MBP-reactive $Ly1^+$ but not $Ly2^+$ cells prevents transfer of EAE *(4)*, and monoclonal antibodies (MAbs) specific for $CD4^+$ T cells can inhibit and/or reverse ongoing disease *(5,6)*. Direct evidence for the role of $CD4^+$ T cells in EAE induction came from adoptive transfer studies in which MBP-, PLP-, and MOG-reactive $CD4^+$ T cell lines or clones were shown to induce encephalomyelitis and paralysis following transfer

From: *Cytokines and Autoimmune Diseases*
Edited by: V. K. Kuchroo, et al. © Humana Press Inc., Totowa, NJ

(7–10). The work of several groups confirmed that disease was caused by antigen-specific type 1 T helper cells (Th1), which characteristically produce interleukin-2 (IL-2), interferon-γ (IFN-γ), and lymphotoxin-α (LT-α) and which elicit delayed-type hypersensitivity (DTH) responses and activate macrophages *(8,11)*. Type 2 Th cells (Th2), on the other hand, which produce IL-4 and other cytokines such as IL-10, IL-5, and IL-13, and are especially important for IgE production and eosinophilic inflammation, were not found among T cell clones causing disease in immunocompetent mice. Because Th1 and Th2 cells crossregulate each other, the hypothesis that Th2 cytokines and myelin antigen-reactive Th2 cells may protect from disease was investigated by a number of groups. These experiments found that the production of Th1 cytokines by myelin antigen-specific cells alone is not sufficient to guarantee the development of disease *(8,11)*. On the other hand, it was possible to demonstrate that myelin antigen specific cells that secrete Th2 cytokines can protect animals from EAE, but not all such cells do so, and in immunodeficient mice MBP-specific Th2 cells can cause neuroinflammation and clinical disease *(12)*. Therefore, despite some exceptions, in EAE there are specific cytokines that are usually associated with disease progression and other cytokines that are usually associated with prevention and/or recovery from disease. What are the different functions of these cytokines?

Cytokines play many roles in EAE. They affect differentiation of T cells, the activation and recruitment of other lymphocytes, macrophages, monocytes, and resident APCs, and they may be directly toxic to tissues in the CNS. They also modulate the inflammatory process and reduce tissue damage or terminate an active inflammatory response. Appreciation of the diverse and important contribution of these molecules has prompted detailed analysis of the role of many individual cytokines in EAE.

Active EAE is usually induced by subcutaneous immunization with myelin-derived proteins or peptides, emulsified in complete Freund's Adjuvant (CFA), and given with pertussis toxin. The time-course of disease varies somewhat with different antigens and mouse strains. Using PLP-derived peptides, SJL mice are clinically normal during the induction phase for a period of 7–10 d following immunization *(13)*. They then enter the effector phase, lose weight, and 1–2 d later develop an ascending paralysis whose initial clinical manifestation is a limp tail. Histological examination of the CNS reveals an influx of lymphocytes prior to the development of clinical disease. Clinical disease reaches a peak 2–3 d after onset, and then usually remits. Mice relapse 15–20 d after their initial episode of disease. In other strains of mice, disease may become chronic and not remit. In this chapter, we have discussed these distinct phases separately (Fig. 1). Certain cytokines

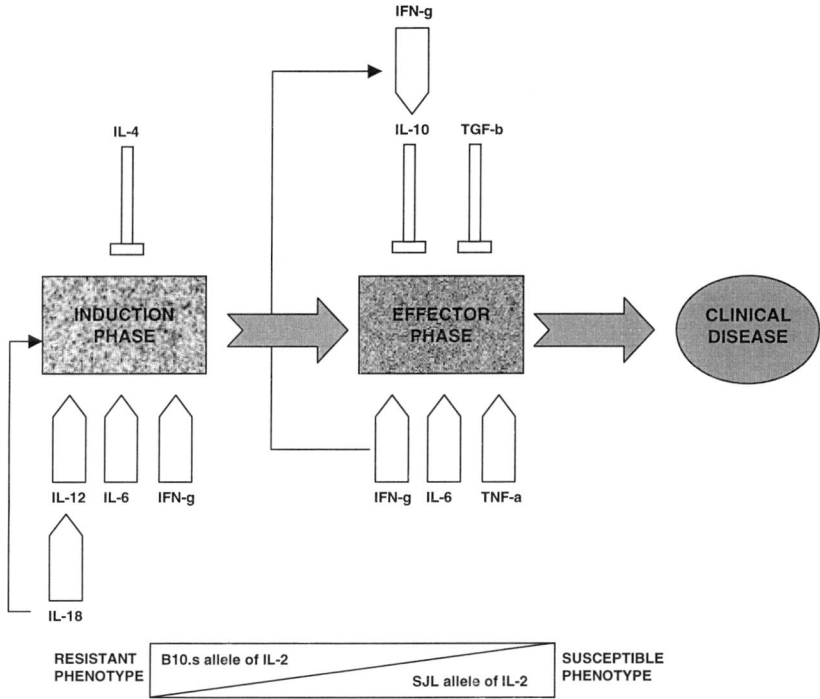

Fig. 1. Cytokines in the induction and effector phases of EAE. In EAE, the balance of effects of cytokines changes between the induction phase and the effector phase. In the induction phase, signals stimulating differentiation along the Th1 pathway from IL-12 (and IL-18) are crucial. Differentiation to the Th2 phenotype is associated with protection, but other factors may also be important. In the effector phase, disease is induced by cells secreting Th1 cytokines, but these cytokines may also induce their own regulation by stimulating the production of IL-10 and other regulatory cytokines. Different alleles of cytokines (all of which are functional) may pre-dispose animals to be more or less susceptible to disease. IL-2 is the best-characterized example of this type of effect.

may have a dominant role in the different stages of disease, and other cytokines may have several opposing functions on the disease as it progresses. When cytokines are neutralized or removed the clinical outcome depends on the relative importance of these different roles.

2. CYTOKINES IN INDUCTION

During the induction phase, antigen-specific T cells expand and differentiate into effector cells of different phenotypes. This priming process occurs in lymph nodes draining the sites of immunization. Cytokines are important at this stage as growth factors and as differentiation factors.

Two major differentiation factors have been identified: IL-12, which polarizes cells along the Th1 pathway, and IL-4, which is important for the generation of Th2 cells. It is now established that IL-12, a cytokine produced mainly by monocytes/macrophages, but also by dendritic cells (DC), promotes the differentiation of naive T cells into Th1 cells *(14,15)*. IL-12 mRNA expression was detected in the CNS of mice or rats before or during EAE onset and decreased upon clinical remission *(16,17)*. The administration of IL-12 to SJL mice increases disease severity and enhances Th1 responses, whereas treatment of animals with anti-IL-12 antibodies is able to attenuate disease *(18,19)*. Interestingly, IL-12-treated mice have an increased number of activated nitric oxide synthase (NOS)[+] macrophages within perivascular CNS lesions but no increased number of T cells within the CNS *(20)*. This would suggest that despite its role in promoting Th1 and IFN-γ production by T cells, IL-12 may contribute to EAE pathology by increasing free radicals. Indeed, NO has a cytotoxic effect on oligodendrocytes, which leads to myelin destruction, and contributes to astrocytes-reactive-glyosis *(21)*. Recently, C57Bl/6 IL-12[−/−] mice have been found to be resistant to MBP-induced EAE *(20)*. Taken together, these results suggest that IL-12 is necessary for EAE induction. IL-18 (IFN-γ-inducing factor; IGIF) works in synergy with IL-12 *(22)*. In human systems it has been shown to enhance Th1 differentiation *(23)*, and in experiments using murine cells, IL-1, and IL-1α had reciprocal effects on Th1 and Th2 cells which were mediated in part by their ability to induce NF-κB p50/p65 activation *(24)*. In rats, neutralizing antibodies for IL-18 inhibited the development of EAE, and splenic T cells from treated rats showed changes in the ratio of IL-4:IFN-γ following activation compared with control animals *(25)*.

IL-4 is produced by activated Th2 cells, mast cells, NK cells, and basophils, and seems to be the cytokine necessary for the differentiation of Th cells into the Th2 lineage *(26,27)*, and for regulating isotype switching in B cells by stimulating the production of IgG1 and IgE *(28)*. Although IL-4 is crucial for normal Th2 differentiation, blocking or knocking out this cytokine has only modest effects on disease. Direct administration of recombinant IL-4 usually reduces the severity of EAE *(29)*, and a T cell hybridoma transduced to express IL-4 has also been shown to ameliorate MBP-induced EAE in (PL/J X SJL) F1 mice *(30)*. In contrast Liblau et al. found that IL-4[−/−] mice on the PL/J background develop similar disease compared to control *(31)*, whereas we and others found that IL-4[−/−] mice (on the C57Bl/6 background) develop a slightly exacerbated disease *(32)*. Therefore, although the absence of IL-4 probably does increase EAE, in contrast to IL-12 its absence does not have a dramatic effect on the disease phenotype. This may be because although IL-12 is crucial in the development of pathogenic cells, once they have been induced there are multiple downstream regulatory events, some of which are IL-4-independent.

IL-6 is produced by activated T cells upon antigen stimulation. It is also produced by B cells, macrophages, endothelial cells, and fibroblasts *(33)*. Several studies have implied that IL-6 may play a role in the pathogenicity of EAE. First, the upregulation of IL-6 mRNA correlates with the severity of EAE *(34)*. In addition, the overexpression of IL-6 in the CNS of mice increases BBB permeability and causes neurological symptoms *(35,36)*. In one report, anti-IL-6 antibody administration was shown to prevent EAE *(37)*. However, another report showed that anti-IL-6 injections have no significant effect on the disease development and that infection of mice with a vaccinia virus producing recombinant IL-6 could inhibit EAE *(38)*. In another system, IL-6 was proposed to have anti-inflammatory effects in part by downregulating TNF-α secretion *(39)*. IL-6$^{-/-}$ mice have been generated and studied by different groups, who find that these mice are resistant to the development of EAE *(40–42)*. A small decrease in recombinant MOG (rMOG)-specific Tcell proliferation was observed in IL-6$^{-/-}$ mice compared to control mice, and MOG 35-55-specific T cells derived from IL-6$^{-/-}$ mice were unable to transfer disease to a wild-type recipient, suggesting that in the absence of IL-6, the function of pathogenic T cells is impaired in vivo. This hypothesis is supported by the fact that MOG35-55 specific T cells derived from wild-type mice induce disease on transfer into IL-6$^{-/-}$ mice. Although a lower anti-MOG antibody response was also observed in IL-6$^{-/-}$ mice, this seems to reflect a generally lower production of antibody in IL-6$^{-/-}$ mice and probably does not explain the resistance to EAE of these mice. The previous results suggest a role for IL-6 in the generation of pathogenic T cells. This is difficult to reconcile with a report describing IL-6 as a differentiating factor for Th2 cells, which in immunocompetent animals have not been shown to induce EAE.

IL-2 is a critical T cell growth factor *(43)*. Early studies of IL-2 in EAE found that IL-2 could enhance disease *(44)*, an effect consistent with a nonspecific role supporting cell expansion. More recent genetic studies have found that different alleles of *il2* have a significant effect on disease susceptibility both in EAE and also in diabetes *(45,46)*. The mechanism for this is presently uncertain, but may relate to the half-life of the different forms of the cytokine. As well as acting as a growth factor, IL-2 acts on activated T cells to prime them for activation-induced cell death *(47)*, and changes in its half-life may alter the size of effector-cell populations as the immune response progresses. Therefore, following priming, the size of the effector population may be critical in determining susceptibility to clinical disease because it determines the number of cells that progress to the effector phase.

3. CYTOKINES IN THE EFFECTOR PHASE

There are many processes in the effector phase of disease in which cytokines are likely to play a role. Activated lymphocytes must traffic from the draining lymph nodes at the site of immunization to the CNS where they have to cross the BBB. Within the CNS and its draining lymph nodes, they will encounter APCs loaded with peptides derived from myelin antigens, which will result in further activation, cell expansion, and the release of chemokines and effector cytokines. Tissue damage arises through the effects of edema, through direct toxic effects on the myelin sheath and the BBB of specific cytokines, and the effects of other inflammatory mediators induced or potentiated by cytokines, and later by Th1-dependent, complement-fixing antibodies. Finally regulation of the immune response within the CNS occurs by downmodulation of antigen presentation, increased cell death, and the deactivation of lymphocytes and APCs by cells in the inflammatory microenvironment secreting regulatory cytokines. Present evidence suggests that few, if any, of these processes are critically dependent on a single cytokine. This complexity may explain why the deletion of effector cytokines has proven to have rather unpredictable effects in vivo, because it is the overall balance of the milieu that determines the outcome of disease.

The most important regulatory cytokines described to date are IL-10 and TGF-β. In the mouse system, IL-10 is produced by Th2 and Th0 CD4$^+$ T cell clones but not by Th1 cells *(48)*, although it has been reported that some human CD4$^+$ T cells can secrete both IL-10 and IFN-γ *(49)*. Mouse B cells (especially the Ly1 B cell subset) also produce IL-10, but the major source of IL-10 seems to be activated macrophages *(48)*. Although controversial, IL-10 does not seem to play a direct role in the differentiation of T cells toward the Th1 or Th2 subset *(50)*. IL-10 does appear to inhibit Th1 cells and its effects appear to be mediated to a large extent via inhibition of IL-12 synthesis by APCs. Conflicting results have been obtained when recombinant IL-10 or anti-IL-10 antibodies have been injected in vivo. While Rott et al. found that administration of IL-10 during the induction phase of EAE in rats could suppress the clinical signs of the disease *(51)*, Cannella et al. showed that injection of IL-10 in mice worsened its clinical course *(52)*. Intracranial injection of soluble rIL-10 or plasmid containing a retroviral promoter-directed IL-10 cDNA at day 12 after active immunization did not suppress EAE *(53)*. However, when an encephalitogenic PLP139-151 specific T cell clone transfected with IL-10 was injected into animals, the onset of EAE could be inhibited *(54)*. We and others *(32,55)*, using MOG35-55 as the encephalitogenic antigen, have reported that IL-10$^{-/-}$ mice on the C57Bl/6 background develop a more severe EAE than wild-type mice. While analyzing the mechanism by which IL-10$^{-/-}$ mice develop such a severe disease, we found that T cells from these mice exhibit a stronger MOG35-55 specific proliferation, produce more proinflammatory cytokines (IFN-γ and TNF-α), and induce very severe disease upon transfer into unimmunized mice. We also showed that mice transgenic for IL-10 under the CD2 promoter are completely resistant to EAE induction. These results were confirmed by Cua et al., who showed that CD4$^+$ T cells from EAE-resistant IL-10 transgenic mice (human IL-10 is expressed under the control of the MHC class II promotor: MHC IIp-hIL-10) produced reduced levels of IFN-γ compared to controls *(56)*. If neutralizing antibodies to IL-10 were added to the culture, however, MBP-specific T cells from hIL-10 transgenic mice produced IFN-γ levels similar to those of the controls. Taken together, these results suggest that IL-10 may not substantially inhibit the development of pathogenic Th1 cells but plays a critical role in limiting disease progression, by inhibiting their effector function and cytokine production, presumably via effects on APCs. The source of the IL-10 produced during these immunoregulatory processes remains an interesting subject. Clearly, IL-10 can be produced by APCs such as macrophages as well as by CD4$^+$ T cells. Segal et al. reported that the disease-promoting effects of IL-12 were antagonized by IL-10 produced by antigen-nonspecific CD4$^+$ T cells *(20)*. In addition, EAE induced by adoptive transfer of MBP-specific T cells could be inhibited by cotransfer of KLH-specific Th2 cells and subcutaneous immunization with keyhole limpit hemocyanin (KLH) *(57)*. Using anti-IL10 and anti-IL-10R neutralizing antibodies, the authors showed that the protection was mediated by KLH-specific T cells producing IL-10 *(57)*. Recent studies in other experimental systems have also shown that the inhibitory effects of IL-10 may also be owing to the induction of a regulatory T cell population. Groux et al. *(58)* reported that cell culture with IL-10 gives rise to CD4$^+$ T cell clones, which themselves produce high levels of IL-10 with little or no IL-4 or IL-2. These T cells suppress the proliferation of CD4$^+$ T cells and prevent colitis when transferred into SCID mice. The authors designated these IL-10-producing T cells as Tr1, a unique subset of regulatory T cells that have the capacity to suppress Ag-specific immune responses and actively downregulate autoimmune responses in vivo. The role of IL-4 and IL-10 has been compared. Taken together, the results of several studies suggest that IL-4, although important, is not as critical as IL-10 in regulating disease progression. Moreover, when IL-10 and IL-4 were injected together, IL-4 seem to abrogate the inhibitory effect of IL-10 on disease progression *(59)*.

TGF-β has been shown to inhibit proliferation of T and B lymphocytes *(60)* and to inhibit the effect or the production of IFN-γ, TNF-α, TNF-β, and IL-2 *(61)*. The cytokine exhibits a dual role on monocytes/macrophages. TGF-β has a chemotactic effect and induces the expression of inflammatory mediators such as IL-1 and TNF-α by monocytes. On the other hand, TGF-β exerts a deactivating effect once the monocytes are differentiated into macrophages, e.g., suppressing peroxide release by these cells *(62)*. Treatment with anti-TGF-β antibody exacerbated clinical signs of EAE *(63–65)*, whereas administration of TGF-β in animals reduces the severity of disease *(63,66)*. The important role of TGF-β in the regulation of EAE is also supported by data from animals made tolerant by feeding myelin antigens (*see* Chapter 11 by Weiner). T cells producing TGF-β appeared in rats spontaneously recovered from disease and seemed to inhibit IFN-γ production by encephalitogenic T cells, suggesting that TGF-β may exert a direct downregulatory role on pathogenic T cells in the natural remission of disease *(66)*. The oral administration of MBP in rats or in mice suppresses EAE, and TGF-β has an essential role in this process *(67,68)*. Feeding MBP to mice gives rise to regulatory T cells called Th3 cells, which release TGF-β and are able to protect animals from actively induced EAE *(67,69,70)*. This downregulation of neuroinflammation by regulatory cytokines appears to reduce CNS damage, because neutralizing both IL-10 and TGF-β exacerbates disease.

Immunohistochemical studies and analysis of mRNA expression in the CNS shows that regulatory cytokines are usually detected after the appearance of proinflammatory Th1 cytokines in the CNS, although there is some debate in the literature regarding the relative importance of IL-4 and IL-10 *(34,71,72)*. It has also been shown by these techniques that IL-12 and proinflammatory cytokines such as IFN-γ and TNF-α peak before disease onset and correlate with EAE severity. This raises the possibility that the induction of effective regulation is in some way dependent on the presence of a normal proinflammatory response. Indirect support for this hypothesis comes from experiments examining the role of IFN-γ in EAE.

IFN-γ produced by T cells, which have entered the CNS, has profound effects on the resident APCs. IFN-γ induces upregulation of MHC and adhesion molecules on cerebrovascular endothelial cells, which facilitate the trafficking of T cells across the BBB *(73)*. It also induces the expression of costimulatory molecules on macrophages and CNS resident cells such as microglia and astrocytes, which can then perpetuate CNS inflammation and demyelination by the presentation of autoantigen *(74)*. IFN-γ is the signature cytokine of Th1 cells, but the pathogenic role of this cytokine (as opposed to the Th1 cells it defines) in EAE is complex. Although some studies have reported a direct pathogenic role for IFN-γ *(8)*, much recent data in the murine system demonstrates that the absence of IFN-γ and signaling through the IFN-γR exacerbates disease. First, the administration of neutralizing antibodies to IFN-γ leads to an exacerbation of the disease in different strains of mice *(44,75–77)*. Similarly, the injection of IFN-γ decreases the severity of EAE in mice *(75,77)*. Second, the analysis of IFN-γ$^{-/-}$ and IFN-γR$^{-/-}$ show that these mice develop a similar or exacerbated disease compared to their littermate controls *(78–80)*. Moreover, the treatment of IFN-γ$^{-/-}$ mice with anti-IL-12 antibodies prevents EAE in these mice *(20)*. The transfer of MOG-reactive T cells from IFN-γR$^{-/-}$ into IFN-γR$^{-/-}$ recipients induced severe disease with no recovery, whereas the same cells transferred into wild-type mice induced similar disease, but all the animals recovered. One interpretation of these results would be that IFN-γR$^{-/-}$ MOG-specific T cells both induce disease and then stimulate a negative feedback via their production of IFN-γ, which downregulates the inflammatory process and allows the mice to recover *(80,81)*. One obvious candidate effector molecule for this process is IL-10.

TNF-α is a cytokine that is secreted by many cell types and is often associated with the Th1 phenotype in the mouse model of EAE. Lymphotoxin-α (LT-α, also called TNF-β) is secreted by T cells and is also a Th1 cytokine. Like IFN-γ, these cytokines have been associated with the encephalitogenic capacity of Th1 cells. Consistent with this observation, the administration of neutralizing antibodies to TNF-α or LT-α decreased the severity of disease *(82)*. LT-α$^{-/-}$ mice on the C57Bl/6 background immunized with MOG35-55 develop a less severe disease than control *(83)*. The analysis of TNF-α$^{-/-}$ is more controversial. In one study, TNF-α$^{-/-}$ mice generated directly on the C57Bl/6 background develop a disease similar in severity to their control littermates but with a later onset *(84)*. In another study, where the TNF-α$^{-/-}$ mice had to be backcrossed on the C57Bl/6 background, the authors did not find any delayed onset but observed that TNF-α$^{-/-}$ mice develop a more severe disease than the controls *(85)*. However, because the TNF-α gene is located within the major histocompatibility complex (MHC) locus, these mice may still retain genes such as the MHC, which could have influenced the outcome of the disease. More recently TNF-α$^{-/-}$ LT-α$^{-/-}$ double knockout mice backcrossed on the SJL background were found to develop a disease similar to control mice *(86)*. Because of the location of the TNF-α gene, and because TNF-α$^{-/-}$ animals lack peripheral secondary lymphoid organs, it is difficult to interpret these results. It does seem reasonable to conclude from these studies that neither TNF-α nor LT-α are necessary for the induction of disease, supporting the hypothesis that in the effector phase, multiple overlapping pathways initiate clinical disease as well as disease regulation.

TNF-α and IFN-γ have direct cytopathic effects on CNS resident cells. They are able to induce oligodendrocyte apoptosis in vitro, which can result in demyelination in vivo *(87,88)*. IFN-γ as well as TNF-α induces the expression of iNOS in macrophages, which leads to the production of NO by these cells. NO, itself, has a cytotoxic effect effect on oligodendrocytes leading to myelin destruction, and contributes to astrocyte-reactive gliosis *(21)*. In order to understand the direct role of these cytokines on the CNS, several transgenic mice have been generated, in which the expression of a particular cytokine is controlled by a CNS resident cell-specific promoter. The results of IFN-γ or TNF-α overexpression in the CNS seem to depend on the level of cyokine produced. Mice with a low copy number of either transgene did not show evidence of spontaneous pathology or glial reactivity. However, mice expressing high copy number of TNF-α develop spontaneous demyelinating pathology.

4. CYTOKINES AND ANTIBODIES

Cytokines can help B cells make antibodies and also influence isotype switching. Anti-CNS antibodies can clearly have a role in disease in at least some models of EAE. Initial experiments in the Lewis rat demonstrated that MOG-specific autoantibodies contributed to the severity and the immuno-pathology of EAE *(89,90)*. In this model, the transfer of MBP-specific T cell lines induced an inflammatory response in the CNS with an increased permeability of the BBB but a moderate demyelination *(90)*. However, the transfer of MBP-specific T cells in association with an injection of a MOG-specific MAb 8-18C5, augmented the clinical signs of EAE and primary demyelination *(89)*. In SJL mice, which develop a chronic relapsing EAE, 8-18C5 antibody injection into mice in remission induced a fatal relapse *(91)*. Based on these results, it was proposed that after T cells specific for different myelin antigens have infiltrated the CNS and initiated inflammation and the opening of the BBB, auto-antibodies against myelin antigens (especially MOG) can penetrate the CNS and mediate demyelination. Based on these results and work from other groups, it was proposed that the antibodies, which mediate demyelination, are complement fixing *(92–94)*. This attracts macrophages that destroy oligodrocytes and release complement and inflammatory cytokines. Results from other groups suggest that B cells or antibodies may also play a protective role in EAE by influencing cytokine production and mediating immune deviation. Treatment of MBP immunized Lewis rats with the encephalitogenic peptide of MBP covalently linked to mouse anti-rat Ig D, protected these animals from EAE. It was suggested that the antibody-peptide conjugate targets the peptide to B cells, which induces a Th2-type cytokine response, which controls the encephalitogenic

Th1 response and reduces the level of leukocyte infiltration into the CNS *(95,96)*. In marmosets, immunization with MOG induces a form of EAE in which MOG-specific antibodies play a critical role in mediating demyelination *(97)*. Furthermore, immunized animals, when injected intraperitonealy with soluble antigen, were protected from acute clinical disease. This regimen increases MOG-specific antibodies in these animals and shifts the cytokine profile toward a Th2-like phenotype. However, the MOG-tolerized animals developed a lethal acute disease after withdrawal of the tolerization treatment. Based on these observations, the authors speculate that the Th2 immune response induced by MOG tolerization promotes an anti-MOG antibody response that enhances demyelination. However, it is not clear whether the pathogenic autoantibodies are Th1- or Th2-dependent. Finally, recent studies in B cell-deficient mice favor a limited role for B cells and antibodies in EAE progression and pathology because these mice still develop clinical disease *(98,99)*. So, although myelin specific antibodies can be directly responsible for demyelination, they are not necessary for EAE to develop and whether B cells and their products regulate the T cell repertoire remains an open question.

5. INTERVENTION IN EAE DIRECTED AT CYTOKINES

The clear evidence that in experimental models the application or removal of specific cytokines, or the introduction of lymphocytes secreting specific cytokines, can profoundly impact the clinical course of EAE, raises the possibility of deliberate intervention targeted at these normal immunoregulatory circuits. Although such strategies have been investigated in animal models, they have yet to be tested in a clinical setting, and shown to be applicable to MS.

One problem with this approach, as discussed earlier, is that the underlying mechanisms are complex and their dependencies are poorly understood. The simple paradigm that CNS autoantigen-specific Th1 cells cause disease, and that Th2 cells of the same specificity protect from disease, has been challenged by the failure of all myelin antigen-specific clones to cause disease *(1)* and by the failure of transgenic Th2 MBP-specific cells to protect in the predicted fashion *(12)*. In other systems *(100)*, Th2 cells can clearly confer protection on transfer, but the necessity for individual Th2 cytokines was not demonstrated by the stringent test of selectively neutralizing the action of specific Th2 cytokines in the protected animals. Furthermore, the antigen receptors on the protective T cells were found to be drawn from a different precursor population than pathogenic T cells *(101)*. Finally, the genetic background of the animal model can profoundly influence the outcome of therapy. These observations raise the possibility that the secretion of Th2 cytokines might be a marker for a protective subset of T cells, or that they might be necessary but not sufficient to confer protection.

A second problem with the current state of the field is that there are few techniques to analyze the interplay of several cytokines in the development and regulation of the immune response. Perhaps the best methods in this regard are immunohistochemical studies *(68)*, which can identify the presence of multiple specific cytokines within the lesions of animals developing EAE, and can follow the disease through time, allowing one to correlate the appearance of specific cytokines with the clinical state of the animals. However, this approach is limited in its ability to resolve the cell of origin of many of these cytokine mediators, and it does not have the power to determine how the different cells act on each other.

But, even without a detailed picture of the interplay between different cells types, it is possible to identify a number of strategies that have been successful, at least in experimental models, in modulating disease, and whose mechanisms are believed at least in part to involve alterations of the cytokine milieu. These encompass changing the genetic background in which disease arises *(102)* (*see* Chapter 8 by Segal and Shevach); the route of antigen administration (discussed by Weiner in Chapter 11); modulation of the conditions of T cell activation either by altering costimulation *(100)* or using altered peptide ligands (APLs) *(103,104)*; and finally the administration, blocking, or removal of specific cytokines from the immunizing environment.

Disease susceptibility can be manipulated by introgressing stretches of chromosome from one mouse strain into another. These techniques are expensive and time-consuming, but have allowed investigators to identify regions within chromosomes that are specifically associated with susceptibility or resistance to disease *(105–107)*. These analyses have been carried out in a number of different mouse strains and for a number of autoimmune diseases, and have raised the possibility that there are common genes that contribute to susceptibility to multiple diseases *(108,109)*. The loci for many of these susceptibility genes may overlap with genes that are associated with resistance to infectious disease. The best-characterized autoimmune-susceptibility locus to date is the locus containing the gene for the cytokine IL-2, and other cytokine loci are under active investigation in similar studies. One intriguing region, which has been associated with disease, is on chromosome 11, where there is a cluster of Th2 cytokines genes *(105)*.

Current estimates of the number of individual genes involved in susceptibility to autoimmune disease are in the range of 10–20 genes *(110)*. It seems likely that susceptibility genes will fall into three classes: (1) genes for which specific alleles confer susceptibility to multiple autoimmune diseases; (2) genes for which specific alleles confer relative susceptibility to one autoimmune disease but relative resistance to another; and (3) genes for which certain alleles confer susceptibility to a single autoimmune diseases but that have no association with other diseases. Understanding how the differences in function of allelic variants of these same proteins influences disease is likely to provide important insights into how these diseases can be manipulated pharmacologically.

The use of ligands, which interfere with the normal activation of autopathogenic cells, has produced interesting insights into the importance of different crossreactive populations in EAE *(111)*. In these studies protection has been associated with T cells secreting Th2 cytokines *(100)*, but other factors may be of equal importance *(108)*. In experiments performed in our laboratory in the PLP system, SJL mice immunized with PLP 139–151 in the presence of anti-B7.1, or immunized with APLs derived from PLP 139–151 (Q144, a tryptophan to glutamine substitution at position 144 and L144/ R147, a tryptophan to leucine substitution at position 144 and a histidine to arginine substitution at position 147) developed populations of PLP 139–151 reactive T cells that were able to confer protection from clinical disease on transfer into naive hosts *(103,112)*. These cells were of a Th0 and Th2 phenotype and this immune deviation appeared to be critical to their ability to protect from disease. That is, protection was associated with T cells that recognized PLP 139–151 but secreted Th2 cytokines, and the protective capacity of these cells was demonstrated by transfer experiments in a number of systems. The question then arose as to whether the population of PLP 139–151-specific T cells that protected mice from EAE was derived from the same precursors that caused disease or were derived from different cells. When protection was induced with analog peptides, we observed that the resulting T cells were much more crossreactive than the population of PLP 139–151-specific disease-causing cells, and on these grounds they were different cells. However, it is possible that two T cell clones expressing the same TCR may show variation in their patterns of crossreactivity *(113)*. To investigate directly if the protective population of T cells induced by APLs or anti-B7-1 used TCRs with the same properties as disease-inducing cells, we mapped how the TCRs of the protective Th2 clones recognized peptide. Using a panel of PLP 139–151 alanine-substituted peptides, we found that there was less dependence on position 144 in these Th2 clones compared with the encephalitogenic Th1 clones, and a greater dependence on positions 141 and 142 (Fig. 2) *(114)*. The same analysis carried out on cells derived from animals immunized with Q144 came to similar conclusions, although these cells appeared to have an additional requirement for position 147 (Fig. 2). From this data, we conclude that as well as showing differences in cytokine phenotype, pathogenic and protective cells carry TCRs that can be distinguished on functional grounds. Therefore it remains possible that the factors that determine the selection of the two different reper-

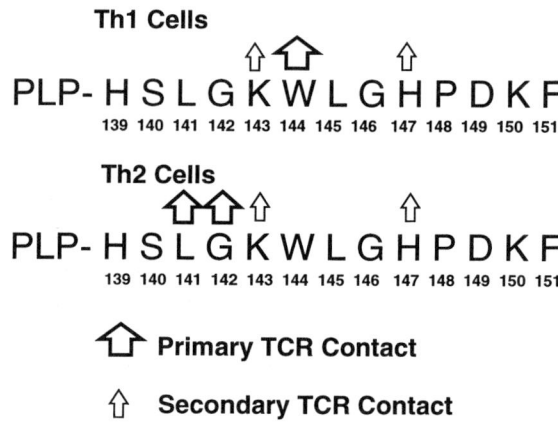

Fig. 2. Pathogenic and protective peptide motifs in the PLP 139-151 system. The pattern of peptide recognition by the TCRs of pathogenic Th1 and protective Th2 cells is different. These cells may be drawn from different precursor populations that may influence their effects in vivo.

toires also influence differentiation and that the observation represents an association but not a causal relationship.

Expansion of one repertoire that is dependent on W144 in the center of the peptide and appears to differentiate predominantly along the Th1 pathway, induces EAE. The other repertoire is more dependent on the N-terminal residues L141/G142 and this repertoire preferentially differentiates along the Th2 pathway and regulates EAE. Although the pathogenic W144-reactive repertoire is induced by self-antigen, the protective L141/G142 repertoire is induced by APLs that have substitutions at position 144, or by immunization in the presence of anti-B7-1. These two PLP 139–151-specific repertoires may play a crucial role in balancing the immune responses to autoantigen and in preventing autoimmunity in the animal. Preferential expansion of one or other repertoire may result in autoimmunity or inhibition/prevention of autoimmune disease. Clearly the administration of cytokines such as IL-4 in vivo can lead to protection, but how far this also involves the selection of pathogenic over protective repertoires is not known. The expansion of autoreactive cells, associated with Th2 cytokine production, has been shown in other systems to depend on the presence of the autoantigen in the periphery, and can also be modulated by the nature of the APC. More detailed understanding of the generation and maintenance of lymphocytes involved in these processes and their expression of cytokines will likely be important in a general understanding of autoimmune disease.

Interventions targeted at blocking various cell-surface molecules (CD4, CD30, and CD2) have been shown to affect T cell phenotype in a number of models. In human T cells crosslinking CD30 favors the development of the Th2 phenotype in vitro *(115)*, whereas in mice, anti-CD2 MAbs enhanced the production of Th2-dependent antibodies *(116)*. In rats, a nondepleting anti-CD4 monoclonal antibody induced a Th2 response in vitro, which correlated with the effect of this antibody on EAE *(117)* and as discussed earlier, targeting antigen to B cells using anti-rat IgD was shown to skew immune responses towards a Th2 phenotype and protect animals from developing EAE *(96)*.

Cell-surface markers have also been used to identify populations of regulatory cells. In mice CD45RB and CD25 have both been used to identify cells that precipitate or protect from autoimmune disease *(118–120)*. Both IL-10 *(121)*, and TGF-β *(122,123)* have been found to be important effectors of immunoregulation by these cells in some experimental systems, however, other contact-dependent mechanisms of regulation are also thought to be important. The role of these cells in EAE is uncertain.

The future of cytokine research in EAE is very exciting. The advances made in cloning and characterizing individual cytokines over the last two decades is gradually leading to a much more sophisticated understanding of the subtle interplay between these immune mediators in the inflammatory milieu. Studies have begun to define the delicate balance between cytokines that exacerbate and ameliorate disease, and how cytokines of each type interact and recruit their own regulators. In other studies discussed elsewhere, the intracellular molecules, which mediate signals from cytokine receptors, are also being unraveled and there is therefore a rich mix of candidate molecules that are potential targets for intervention. Future advances will require refining techniques that can address specific questions about interactions between cells of the immune system, and between cells of the immune system and the CNS, in vivo. As genome-wide scanning and candidate-gene analysis identify key players in determining autoimmune susceptibility and resistance, we will need to be able to examine the function that the proteins these genes encode have in relation to each other. Such multiparameter analysis will be critical to a detailed understanding of the autoimmune process. Then as the characteristics of regulatory cells, and the roles of the cytokines that they secrete become better understood, immunomodulatory therapy will progress to treatment targeted to specific cytokines and cytokine receptors, and to the cells that secrete them.

REFERENCES

1. Zamvil, S. S. and Steinman, L. (1990) The T lymphocyte in experimental allergic encephalomyelitis. *Annu. Rev. Immunol.* **8**, 579–621.
2. Wekerle, H. (1993) Experimental autoimmune encephalomyelitis as a model of immune-mediated CNS disease. *Curr. Opin. Neurobiol.* **3**, 779–784.
3. Sobel, R. A., Blanchette, B. W., Bhan, A. K., and Colvin, R. B. (1984) The immunopathology of experimental allergic encephalomyelitis. I. Quantitative analysis of inflammatory cells in situ. *J. Immunol.* **132**, 2393–2401.
4. Pettinelli, C. B. and McFarlin, D. E. (1981) Adoptive transfer of experimental allergic encephalomyelitis in SJL/J mice after in vitro activation of lymph node cells by myelin basic protein: requirement for Lyt 1+ 2- T lymphocytes. *J. Immunol.* **127**, 1420–1423.
5. Brostoff, S. W. and Mason, D. W. (1984) Experimental allergic encephalomyelitis: successful treatment in vivo with a monoclonal antibody that recognizes T helper cells. *J. Immunol.* **133**, 1938-1942.
6. Waldor, M. K., Sriram, S. Hardy, S. Herzenberg, L. A Lanier, L. Lim, M. and Steinman, L. (1985) Reversal of experimental allergic encephalomyelitis with monoclonal antibody to a T-cell subset marker. *Science* **227**, 415–417.
7. Ben-Nun, A., Wekerle, H., and Cohen, I. R. (1981) The rapid isolation of clonable antigen-specific T lymphocyte lines capable of mediating autoimmune encephalomyelitis. *Eur. J. Immunol.* **11**, 195–199.
8. Baron, J. L., Madri, J. A., Ruddle, N. H., Hashim, G., and Janeway, Jr., C. A. (1993) Surface expression of alpha 4 integrin by CD4 T cells is required for their entry into brain parenchyma. *J. Exp. Med.* **177**, 5768.
9. Kuchroo, V. K., Sobel, R. A., Laning, J. C., Martin, C. A., Greenfield, E., Dorf, M. E., and Lees, M. B. (1992) Experimental allergic encephalomyelitis mediated by cloned T cells specific for a synthetic peptide of myelin proteolipid protein. Fine specificity and T cell receptor V beta usage. *J. Immunol.* **148**, 3776–3782.
10. Mendel, I., Kerlero de Rosbo, N., and Ben-Nun, A. (1995) A myelin oligodendrocyte glycoprotein peptide induces typical chronic experimental autoimmune encephalomyelitis in H-2b mice: fine specificity and T cell receptor V beta expression of encephalitogenic T cells. *Eur. J. Immunol.* **25**, 1951–1959.
11. Kuchroo, V. K., Martin, C. A., Greer, J. M., Ju, S. T., Sobel, R. A., and Dorf, M. E. (1993) Cytokines and adhesion molecules contribute to the ability of myelin proteolipid protein-specific T cell clones to mediate experimental allergic encephalomyelitis. *J. Immunol.* **151**, 4371–4382.
12. Lafaille, J. J., Van de Keere, F., Hsu, A. L., Baron, J. L., Haas, W., Raine, C. S., and Tonegawa, S. (1997) Myelin basic protein-specific T helper 2 (Th2) cells cause experimental autoimmune encephalomyelitis in immunodeficient hosts rather than protect them from the disease. *J. Exp. Med.* **186**, 307–312.

13. Sobel, R. A. and Kuchroo, V. K. (1992) The immunopathology of acute allergic encephalomyelitis induced with myelin proteolipid protein. *J. Immunol.* **149,** 1444–1451.

14. Hsieh, C. S., Macatonia, S. E., Tripp, C. S., Wolf, S. F., O'Garra, A., and Murphy, K. M. (1993) Development of TH1 CD4+ T cells through IL-12 produced by Listeria- induced macrophages. *Science* **260,** 547–549.

15. Seder, R. A., Gazzinelli, R., Sher, A., and Paul, W. E. (1993) Interleukin 12 acts directly on CD4+ T cells to enhance priming for interferon gamma production and diminishes interleukin 4 inhibition of such priming. *Proc. Natl. Acad. Sci. USA* **90,** 10,188–10,192.

16. Issazadeh, S., Ljungdahl, A., Hojeberg, B., Mustafa, M., and Olsson, T. (1995) Cytokine production in the central nervous system of Lewis rats with experimental autoimmune encephalomyelitis: dynamics of mRNA expression for interleukin-10, interleukin-12, cytolysin, tumor necrosis factor alpha and tumor necrosis factor beta. *J. Neuroimmunol.* **61,** 205–212.

17. Bright, J. J., Musuro, B. F., Du, C., and Sriram. S. (1998) Expression of IL-12 in CNS and lymphoid organs of mice with experimental allergic encephalitis. *J. Neuroimmunol.* **82,** 22–30.

18. Leonard, J. P., Waldburger, K. E., and Goldman, S. J. (1995) Prevention of experimental autoimmune encephalomyelitis by antibodies against interleukin 12. *J. Exp. Med.* **181,** 381–386.

19. Leonard, J. P., Waldburger, K. E., and Goldman, S. J. (1996) Regulation of experimental autoimmune encephalomyelitis by interleukin- 12. *Ann. NY Acad. Sci.* **795,** 216–226.

20. Segal, B. M., Dwyer, B. K., and Shevach, E. M. (1998) An interleukin (IL)-10/IL-12 immunoregulatory circuit controls susceptibility to autoimmune disease. *J. Exp. Med.* **187,** 537–546.

21. Merrill, J. E., Ignarro, L. J., Sherman, M. P., Melinek, J., and Lane, T. E. (1993) Microglial cell cytotoxicity of oligodendrocytes is mediated through nitric oxide. *J. Immunol.* **151,** 2132–2141.

22. Ahn, H. J., Maruo, S., Tomura, M., Mu, J., Hamaoka, T., Nakanishi, K., et al. (1997) A mechanism underlying synergy between IL-12 and IFN-gamma-inducing factor in enhanced production of IFN-gamma. *J. Immunol.* **159,** 2125–2131.

23. Micallef, M. J., Ohtsuki, T., Kohno, K., Tanabe, F., Ushio, S., Namba, M., et al. (1996) Interferon-gamma-inducing factor enhances T helper 1 cytokine production by stimulated human T cells: synergism with interleukin-12 for interferon-gamma production. *Eur. J. Immunol.* **26,** 1647–1651.

24. Robinson, D., Shibuya, K., Mui, A., Zonin, F., Murphy, E., Sana, T., et al. (1997) IGIF does not drive Th1 development but synergizes with IL-12 for interferon-gamma production and activates IRAK and NFkappaB. *Immunity* **7,** 571–581.

25. Wildbaum, G., Youssef, S., Grabie, N., and Karin. N. (1998) Neutralizing antibodies to IFN-gamma-inducing factor prevent experimental autoimmune encephalomyelitis. *J. Immunol.* **161,** 6368–6374.

26. Swain, S. L., Weinberg, A. D., English, M., and Huston, G. (1990) IL-4 directs the development of Th2-like helper effectors. *J. Immunol.* **145**, 3796–3806.
27. Seder, R. A., Paul, W. E., Davis, M. M., and Fazekas de St. Groth, B. (1992) The presence of interleukin 4 during in vitro priming determines the lymphokine-producing potential of CD4+ T cells from T cell receptor transgenic mice. *J. Exp. Med.* **176**, 1091–1098.
28. Kuhn, R., Rajewsky, K., and Muller, W. (1991) Generation and analysis of interleukin-4 deficient mice. *Science* **254**, 707–710.
29. Racke, M. K., Bonomo, A., Scott, D. E., Cannella, B., Levine, A., Raine, C. S., et al. (1994) Cytokine-induced immune deviation as a therapy for inflammatory autoimmune disease. *J. Exp. Med.* **180**, 1961–1966.
30. Shaw, M. K., Lorens, J. B., Dhawan, A., DalCanto, R., Tse, H. Y., Tran, A. B., et al. (1997) Local delivery of interleukin 4 by retrovirus-transduced T lymphocytes ameliorates experimental autoimmune encephalomyelitis. *J. Exp. Med.* **185**, 1711–1714.
31. Liblau, R., Steinman, L., and Brocke, S. (1997) Experimental autoimmune encephalomyelitis in IL-4-deficient mice. *Intl. Immunol.* **9**, 799–803.
32. Bettelli, E., Das, M. P., Howard, E. D., Weiner, H. L., Sobel, R. A., and Kuchroo, V. A. (1998) IL-10 is critical in the regulation of autoimmune encephalomyelitis as demonstrated by studies of IL-10- and IL-4-deficient and transgenic mice. *J. Immunol.* **161**, 3299–3306.
33. Taga, T. and Kishimoto, T. (1997) Gp130 and the interleukin-6 family of cytokines. *Annu. Rev. Immunol.* **15**, 797–819.
34. Kennedy, M. K., Torrance, D. S., Picha, K. S., and Mohler, K. M. (1992) Analysis of cytokine mRNA expression in the central nervous system of mice with experimental autoimmune encephalomyelitis reveals that IL-10 mRNA expression correlates with recovery. *J. Immunol.* **149**, 2496–2505.
35. Brett, F. M., Mizisin, A. P., Powell, H. C., and Campbell, I. L. (1995) Evolution of neuropathologic abnormalities associated with blood-brain barrier breakdown in transgenic mice expressing interleukin-6 in astrocytes. *J. Neuropathol. Exp. Neurol.* **54**, 766–775.
36. Campbell, I. L., Abraham, C. R., Masliah, E., Kemper, P., Inglis, J. D., Oldstone, M. B., and Mucke, L. (1993) Neurologic disease induced in transgenic mice by cerebral overexpression of interleukin 6. *Proc. Natl. Acad. Sci. USA* **90**, 10,061–10,065.
37. Gijbels, K., Brocke, S., Abrams, J. S., and Steinman, L. (1995) Administration of neutralizing antibodies to interleukin-6 (IL-6) reduces experimental autoimmune encephalomyelitis and is associated with elevated levels of IL-6 bioactivity in central nervous system and circulation. *Mol. Med.* **1**, 795–805.
38. Willenborg, D. O., Fordham, S. A., Cowden, W. B., and Ramshaw, I. A. (1995) Cytokines and murine autoimmune encephalomyelitis: inhibition or enhancement of disease with antibodies to select cytokines, or by delivery of exogenous cytokines using a recombinant vaccinia virus system. *Scand. J. Immunol.* **41**, 31–41.
39. Fattori, E., Cappelletti, M., Costa, P., Sellitto, C., Cantoni, L., Carelli, M., et al. (1994) Defective inflammatory response in interleukin 6-deficient mice. *J. Exp. Med.* **180**, 1243–1250.

40. Mendel, I., Katz, A., Kozak, N., Ben-Nun, A., and Revel, M. (1998) Interleukin-6 functions in autoimmune encephalomyelitis: a study in gene-targeted mice. *Eur. J. Immunol.* **28,** 1727–1737.

41. Okuda, Y., Sakoda, S., Bernard, C. C., Fujimura, H., Saeki, Y., Kishimoto, T., and Yanagihara, T. (1998) IL-6-deficient mice are resistant to the induction of experimental autoimmune encephalomyelitis provoked by myelin oligodendrocyte glycoprotein. *Intl. Immunol.* **10,** 703–708.

42. Samoilova, E. B., Horton, J. L., Hilliard, B., Liu, T. S., and Chen, Y. (1998) IL-6-deficient mice are resistant to experimental autoimmune encephalomyelitis: roles of IL-6 in the activation and differentiation of autoreactive T cells. *J. Immunol.* **161,** 6480–6486.

43. Smith, K. A. (1988) Interleukin-2: inception, impact, and implications. *Science* **240,** 1169–1176.

44. Duong, T. T., St. Louis, J., Gilbert, J. J., Finkelman, F. D., and Strejan, G. H. (1992) Effect of anti-interferon-gamma and anti-interleukin-2 monoclonal antibody treatment on the development of actively and passively induced experimental allergic encephalomyelitis in the SJL/J mouse. *J. Neuroimmunol.* **36,** 105–115.

45. Encinas, J. A., Wicker, L. S., Peterson, L. B., Mukasa, A., Teuscher, C., Sobel, R., et al. (1999) QTL influencing autoimmune diabetes and encephalomyelitis map to a 0.15-cM region containing Il2. *Nat. Genet.* **21,** 158–160.

46. Podolin, P. L., Denny, P., Lord, C. J., Hill, N. J., Todd, J. A., Peterson, L. B., et al. (1997) Congenic mapping of the insulin-dependent diabetes (*Idd*) gene, Idd10, localizes two genes mediating the Idd10 effect and eliminates the candidate Fcgr1. *J. Immunol.* **159,** 1835–1843.

47. Van Parijs, L., Refaeli, Y., Lord, J. D., Nelson, B. H., Abbas, A. K., and Baltimore, D. (1999) Uncoupling IL-2 signals that regulate T cell proliferation, survival, and Fas-mediated activation-induced cell death. *Immunity* **11,** 281–288.

48. Mosmann, T. R. (1994) Properties and functions of interleukin-10. *Adv. Immunol.* **56,** 1–26.

49. Pohl-Koppe, A., Balashov, K. E., Steere, A. C., Logigian, E. L., and Hafler, D. A. (1998) Identification of a T cell subset capable of both IFN-gamma and IL-10 secretion in patients with chronic Borrelia burgdorferi infection. *J. Immunol.* **160,** 1804–1810.

50. Romani, L., Mencacci, A., Grohmann, U., Mocci, S., Mosci, P., Puccetti, P., and Bistoni, F. (1992) Neutralizing antibody to interleukin 4 induces systemic protection and T helper type 1-associated immunity in murine candidiasis. *J. Exp. Med.* **176,** 19–25.

51. Rott, O., Fleischer, B., and Cash, E. (1994) Interleukin-10 prevents experimental allergic encephalomyelitis in rats. *Eur. J. Immunol.* **24,** 1434–1440.

52. Cannella, B., Gao, Y. L., Brosnan, C., and Raine, C. S. (1996) IL-10 fails to abrogate experimental autoimmune encephalomyelitis. *J. Neurosci. Res.* **45,** 735–746.

53. Croxford, J. L., Triantaphyllopoulos, K., Podhajcer, O. L., Feldmann, M., Baker, D., and Chernajovsky, Y. (1998) Cytokine gene therapy in experi-

mental allergic encephalomyelitis by injection of plasmid DNA-cationic liposome complex into the central nervous system. *J. Immunol.* **160,** 5181–5187.

54. Mathisen, P. M., Yu, M., Johnson, J. M., Drazba, J. A., and Tuohy, V. K. (1997) Treatment of experimental autoimmune encephalomyelitis with genetically modified memory T cells. *J. Exp. Med.* **186,** 159–164.

55. Samoilova, E. B., Horton, J. L., and Chen, Y. (1998) Acceleration of experimental autoimmune encephalomyelitis in interleukin-10-deficient mice: roles of interleukin-10 in disease progression and recovery. *Cell Immunol.* **188,** 118–124.

56. Cua, D. J., Groux, H., Hinton, D. R., Stohlman, S. A., and Coffman, R. L. (1999) Transgenic interleukin 10 prevents induction of experimental autoimmune encephalomyelitis. *J. Exp. Med.* **189,** 1005–1010.

57. Stohlman, S. A., Pei, L., Cua, D. J., Li, Z., and Hinton, D. R. (1999) Activation of regulatory cells suppresses experimental allergic encephalomyelitis via secretion of IL-10. *J. Immunol.* **163,** 6338–6344.

58. Groux, H., O'Garra, A., Bigler, M., Rouleau, M., Antonenko, S., de Vries, J. E., and Roncarolo, M. G. (1997) A CD4+ T-cell subset inhibits antigen-specific T-cell responses and prevents colitis. *Nature* **389,** 737–742.

59. Nagelkerken, L., Blauw, B., and Tielemans, M. (1997) IL-4 abrogates the inhibitory effect of IL-10 on the development of experimental allergic encephalomyelitis in SJL mice. *Intl. Immunol.* **9,** 1243–1251.

60. Kehrl, J. H., Wakefield, L. M., Roberts, A. B., Jakowlew, S., Alvarez-Mon, M., Derynck, R., et al. (1986) Production of transforming growth factor beta by human T lymphocytes and its potential role in the regulation of T cell growth. *J. Exp. Med.* **163,** 1037–1050.

61. Espevik, T., Figari, I. S., Shalaby, M. R., Lackides, G. A., Lewis, G. D., Shepard, H. M., and Palladino, Jr., M. A. (1987) Inhibition of cytokine production by cyclosporin A and transforming growth factor beta. *J. Exp. Med.* **166,** 571–576.

62. Tsunawaki, S., Sporn, M., Ding, A., and Nathan, C. (1988) Deactivation of macrophages by transforming growth factor-beta. *Nature* **334,** 260–262.

63. Kuruvilla, A. P., Shah, R., Hochwald, G. M., Liggitt, H. D., Palladino, M. A., and Thorbecke, G. J. (1991) Protective effect of transforming growth factor beta 1 on experimental autoimmune diseases in mice. *Proc. Natl. Acad. Sci. USA* **88,** 2918–2921.

64. Racke, M. K., Cannella, B., Albert, P., Sporn, M., Raine, C. S., and McFarlin, D. E. (1992) Evidence of endogenous regulatory function of transforming growth factor-beta 1 in experimental allergic encephalomyelitis. *Intl. Immunol.* **4,** 615–620.

65. Johns, L. D., Flanders, K. C., Ranges, G. E., and Sriram, S. (1991) Successful treatment of experimental allergic encephalomyelitis with transforming growth factor-beta 1. *J. Immunol.* **147,** 1792–1796.

66. Racke, M. K., Dhib-Jalbut, S., Cannella, B., Albert, P. S., Raine, C. S., and McFarlin, D. E. (1991) Prevention and treatment of chronic relapsing experimental allergic encephalomyelitis by transforming growth factor-beta 1. *J. Immunol.* **146,** 3012–3017.

67. Chen, Y., Kuchroo, V. K., Inobe, J., Hafler, D. A., and Weiner, H. L. (1994) Regulatory T cell clones induced by oral tolerance: suppression of autoimmune encephalomyelitis. *Science* **265,** 1237–1240.

68. Khoury, S. J., Hancock, W. W., and Weiner, H. L. (1992) Oral tolerance to myelin basic protein and natural recovery from experimental autoimmune encephalomyelitis are associated with downregulation of inflammatory cytokines and differential upregulation of transforming growth factor beta, interleukin 4, and prostaglandin E expression in the brain. *J. Exp. Med.* **176,** 1355–1364.

69. Miller, A., Lider, O., Roberts, A. B., Sporn, M. B., and Weiner, H. L. (1992) Suppressor T cells generated by oral tolerization to myelin basic protein suppress both in vitro and in vivo immune responses by the release of transforming growth factor beta after antigen-specific triggering. *Proc. Natl. Acad. Sci. USA* **89,** 421–425.

70. Chen, Y., Inobe, J., Kuchroo, V. K., Baron, J. L., Janeway, Jr., C. A., and Weiner, H. L. (1996) Oral tolerance in myelin basic protein T-cell receptor transgenic mice: suppression of autoimmune encephalomyelitis and dose-dependent induction of regulatory cells. *Proc. Natl. Acad. Sci. USA* **93,** 388–391.

71. Merrill, J. E., Kono, D. H., Clayton, J., Ando, D. G., Hinton, D. R., and Hofman, F. M. (1992) Inflammatory leukocytes and cytokines in the peptide-induced disease of experimental allergic encephalomyelitis in SJL and B10.PL mice. *Proc. Natl. Acad. Sci. USA* **89,** 574–578.

72. Begolka, W. S., Vanderlugt, C. L., Rahbe, S. M., and Miller, S. D. (1998) Differential expression of inflammatory cytokines parallels progression of central nervous system pathology in two clinically distinct models of multiple sclerosis. *J. Immunol.* **161,** 4437–4446.

73. Dore-Duffy, P., Balabanov, R., Rafols, J., and Swanborg, R. H. (1996) Recovery phase of acute experimental autoimmune encephalomyelitis in rats corresponds to development of endothelial cell unresponsiveness to interferon gamma activation. *J. Neurosci. Res.* **44,** 223–234.

74. Tan, L., Gordon, K. B., Mueller, J. P., Matis, L. A., and Miller, S. D. (1998) Presentation of proteolipid protein epitopes and B7-1-dependent activation of encephalitogenic T cells by IFN-gamma-activated SJL/J astrocytes. *J. Immunol.* **160,** 4271–4279.

75. Billiau, A., Heremans, H., Vandekerckhove, F., Dijkmans, R., Sobis, H., Meulepas, E., and Carton, H. (1988) Enhancement of experimental allergic encephalomyelitis in mice by antibodies against IFN-gamma. *J. Immunol.* **140,** 1506–1510.

76. Duong, T. T., Finkelman, F. D., Singh, B., and Strejan, G. H. (1994) Effect of anti-interferon-gamma monoclonal antibody treatment on the development of experimental allergic encephalomyelitis in resistant mouse strains. *J. Neuroimmunol.* **53,** 101–107.

77. Lublin, F. D., Knobler, R. L., Kalman, B., Goldhaber, M., Marini, J., Perrault, M., et al. (1993) Monoclonal anti-gamma interferon antibodies enhance experimental allergic encephalomyelitis. *Autoimmunity* **16,** 267–274.

78. Ferber, I. A., Brocke, S., Taylor-Edwards, C., Ridgway, W., Dinisco, C., Steinman, L., et al. (1996) Mice with a disrupted IFN-gamma gene are sus-

ceptible to the induction of experimental autoimmune encephalomyelitis (EAE). *J. Immunol.* **156,** 5–7.

79. Krakowski, M. and Owens, T. (1996) Interferon-gamma confers resistance to experimental allergic encephalomyelitis. *Eur. J. Immunol.* **26,** 1641–1646.

80. Willenborg, D. O., Fordham, S., Bernard, C. C., Cowden, W. B., and Ramshaw. I. A. (1996) IFN-gamma plays a critical down-regulatory role in the induction and effector phase of myelin oligodendrocyte glycoprotein-induced autoimmune encephalomyelitis. *J. Immunol.* **157,** 3223–3227.

81. Willenborg, D. O., Fordham, S. A., Staykova, M. A., Ramshaw, I. A., and Cowden, W. B. (1999) IFN-gamma is critical to the control of murine autoimmune encephalomyelitis and regulates both in the periphery and in the target tissue: a possible role for nitric oxide. *J. Immunol.* **163,** 5278–5286.

82. Ruddle, N. H., Bergman, C. M., McGrath, K. M., Lingenheld, E. G., Grunnet, M. L., Padula, S. J., and Clark, R. B. (1990) An antibody to lymphotoxin and tumor necrosis factor prevents transfer of experimental allergic encephalomyelitis. *J. Exp. Med.* **1723,** 1193–1200.

83. Suen, W. E., Bergman, C. M., Hjelmstrom, P., and Ruddle, N. H. (1997) A critical role for lymphotoxin in experimental allergic encephalomyelitis. *J. Exp. Med.* **186,** 1233–1240.

84. Korner, H., Riminton, D. S., Strickland, D. H., Lemckert, F. A., Pollard, J. D., and Sedgwick, J. D. (1997) Critical points of tumor necrosis factor action in central nervous system autoimmune inflammation defined by gene targeting. *J. Exp. Med.* **186,** 1585–1590.

85. Liu, J., Marino, M. W., Wong, G., Grail, D., Dunn, A., Bettadapura, J., et al. (1998) TNF is a potent anti-inflammatory cytokine in autoimmune-mediated demyelination. *Nat. Med.* **4,** 78–83.

86. Frei, K., Eugster, H. P., Bopst, M., Constantinescu, C. S., Lavi, E., and Fontana, A. (1997) Tumor necrosis factor alpha and lymphotoxin alpha are not required for induction of acute experimental autoimmune encephalomyelitis. *J. Exp. Med.* **185,** 2177–2182.

87. Selmaj, K. and Raine, C. S. (1988) Tumor necrosis factor mediates myelin damage in organotypic cultures of nervous tissue. *Ann. NY Acad. Sci.* **540,** 568–570.

88. Selmaj, K., Raine, C. S., Farooq, M., Norton, W. T., and Brosnan, C. F. (1991) Cytokine cytotoxicity against oligodendrocytes. Apoptosis induced by lymphotoxin. *J. Immunol.* **147,** 1522–1529.

89. Linington, C., Bradl, M., Lassmann, H., Brunner, C., and Vass, K. (1988) Augmentation of demyelination in rat acute allergic encephalomyelitis by circulating mouse monoclonal antibodies directed against a myelin/oligodendrocyte glycoprotein. *Am. J. Pathol.* **130,** 443–454.

90. Lassmann, H., Brunner, C., Bradl, M., and Linington, C. (1988) Experimental allergic encephalomyelitis: the balance between encephalitogenic T lymphocytes and demyelinating antibodies determines size and structure of demyelinated lesions. *Acta. Neuropathol.* **75,** 566–576.

91. Schluesener, H. J., Sobel, R. A., Linington, C., and Weiner, H. L. (1987) A monoclonal antibody against a myelin oligodendrocyte glycoprotein induces

relapses and demyelination in central nervous system autoimmune disease. *J. Immunol.* **139,** 4016–4021.

92. Linington, C. and Lassmann, H.(1987) Antibody responses in chronic relapsing experimental allergic encephalomyelitis: correlation of serum demyelinating activity with antibody titre to the myelin/oligodendrocyte glycoprotein (MOG). *J. Neuroimmunol.* **17,** 61–69.

93. Linington, C., Morgan, B. P., Scolding, N. J., Wilkins, P., Piddlesden, S., and Compston, D. A. (1989) The role of complement in the pathogenesis of experimental allergic encephalomyelitis. *Brain* **112,** 895–911.

94. Piddlesden, S. J., Lassmann, H., Zimprich, F., Morgan, B. P., and Linington, C. (1993) The demyelinating potential of antibodies to myelin oligodendrocyte glycoprotein is related to their ability to fix complement. *Am. J. Pathol.* **143,** 555–564.

95. Day, M. J., Tse, A. G., Puklavec, M., Simmonds, S. J., and Mason, D. W. (1992) Targeting autoantigen to B cells prevents the induction of a cell-mediated autoimmune disease in rats. *J. Exp. Med.* **175,** 655–659.

96. Saoudi, A., Simmonds, S., Huitinga, I., and Mason, D. (1995) Prevention of experimental allergic encephalomyelitis in rats by targeting autoantigen to B cells: Evidence that the protective mechanism depends on changes in the cytokine response and migratory properties of the autoantigen-specific T cells. *J. Exp. Med.* **182,** 335–344.

97. Genain, C. P., Nguyen, M. H., Letvin, N. L., Pearl, R., Davis, R. L., Adelman, M., et al. (1995) Antibody facilitation of multiple sclerosis-like lesions in a nonhuman primate. *J. Clin. Invest.* **96,** 2966–2974.

98. Wolf, S. D., Dittel, B. N., Hardardottir, F., and Janeway, Jr., C. A. (1996) Experimental autoimmune encephalomyelitis induction in genetically B cell-deficient mice. *J. Exp. Med.* **184,** 2271–2278.

99. Litzenburger, T., Fassler, R., Bauer, J., Lassmann, H., Linington, C., Wekerle, H., and Iglesias, A. (1998) B lymphocytes producing demyelinating autoantibodies: development and function in gene-targeted transgenic mice. *J. Exp. Med.* **188,** 169–180.

100. Kuchroo, V. K., Das, M. P., Brown, J. A., Ranger, A. M., Zamvil, S. S., Sobel, R. A., et al. (1995) B7-1 and B7-2 costimulatory molecules activate differentially the Th1/Th2 developmental pathways: application to autoimmune disease therapy. *Cell* **80,** 707–718.

101. Prabhu Das, M., Nicholson, L. B., Greer, J. M., and Kuchroo, V. K. (1997) Auto-pathogenic Th1 and protective Th2 clones differ in their recognition of the autoantigenic peptide of myelin proteolipid protein. *J. Exp. Med.* **186,** 867–876.

102. Encinas, J. A., Weiner, H. L., and Kuchroo, V. K. (1996) Inheritance of susceptibility to experimental autoimmune encephalomyelitis. *J. Neurosci. Res.* **45,** 655–669.

103. Nicholson, L. B., Greer, J. M., Sobel, R. A., Lees, M B., and Kuchroo, V. K. (1995) An altered peptide ligand mediates immune deviation and prevents autoimmune encephalomyelitis. *Immunity* **3,** 397–405.

104. Brocke, S., Gijbels, K., Allegretta, M., Ferber, I., Piercy, C., Blankenstein, T., et al. (1996) Treatment of experimental encephalomyelitis with a peptide analogue of myelin basic protein. *Nature* **379,** 343–346.

105. Baker, D., Rosenwasser, O. A., O'Neill, J. K., and Turk, J. L. (1995) Genetic analysis of experimental allergic encephalomyelitis in mice. *J. Immunol.* **155,** 4046-4051.

106. Butterfield, R. J., Sudweeks, J. D., Blankenhorn, E. P., Korngold, R., Marini, J. C., Todd, J. A., et al. (1998) New genetic loci that control susceptibility and symptoms of experimental allergic encephalomyelitis in inbred mice. *J. Immunol.* **161,** 1860–1867.

107. Encinas, J. A., Lees, M. B., Sobel, R. A., Symonowicz, C., Greer, J. A., Shovlin, C. L., et al. (1996) Genetic analysis of susceptibility to experimental autoimmune encephalomyelitis in a cross between SJL/J and B10.S mice. *J. Immunol.* **157,** 2186–2192.

108. Teuscher, C., Hickey, W. F., Grafer, C. M., and Tung, K. S. (1998) A common immunoregulatory locus controls susceptibility to actively induced experimental allergic encephalomyelitis and experimental allergic orchitis in BALB/c mice. *J. Immunol.* **160,** 2751–2756.

109. Becker, K. G., Simon, R. M., Bailey-Wilson, J. E., Freidlin, B., Biddison, W.E., McFarland, H. F., and Trent, J. M. (1998) Clustering of non-major histocompatibility complex susceptibility candidate loci in human autoimmune diseases. *Proc. Natl. Acad. Sci. USA* **95,** 9979–9984.

110. Wicker, L. and Wekerle, H. (1995) Autoimmunity. *Curr. Opin. Immunol.* **7,** 783–785.

111. Wraith, D. C., McDevitt, H. O., Steinman, L., and Acha-Orbea, H. (1989) T cell recognition as the target for immune intervention in autoimmune disease. *Cell* **57,** 709–715.

112. Nicholson, L. B., Waldner, H., Carrizosa, A. M., Sette, A., Collins, M., and Kuchroo, V. K. (1998) Heteroclitic proliferative responses and changes in cytokine profile induced by altered peptides: implications for autoimmunity. *Proc. Natl. Acad. Sci. USA* **95,** 264–269.

113. Nicholson, L. B., Anderson, A. C., and Kuchroo, V. K. (2000) Tuning T cell activation threshold and effector function with cross-reactive peptide ligands. *Intl. Immunol.* **12,** 205–213.

114. Nicholson, L. B., Carrizosa, A. M., and Kuchroo, V. K. (1998) Pathogenic versus protective repertoires in autoimmune disease: tuning the balance. *Immunologist* **6,** 151–157.

115. Del Prete, G., De Carli, M., D'Elios, M. M., Daniel, K. C., Almerigogna, F., Alderson, M., et al. (1995) CD30-mediated signaling promotes the development of human T helper type 2-like T cells. *J. Exp. Med.* **182,** 1655–1661.

116. Biancone, L., Andres, G., Ahn, H., Lim, A., Dai, C., Noelle, R., et al. (1996) Distinct regulatory roles of lymphocyte costimulatory pathways on T helper type 2-mediated auto immune disease. *J. Exp. Med.* **183,** 1473–1481.

117. Stumbles, P. and Mason, D. (1995) Activation of CD4+ T cells in the presence of a nondepleting monoclonal antibody to CD4 induces a Th2-type response in vitro. *J. Exp. Med.* **182,** 5–13.

118. Groux, H. and Powrie, F. (1999) Regulatory T cells and inflammatory bowel disease. *Immunol. Today* **20,** 442–445.

119. Thornton, A. M. and Shevach. E. M. (1998) CD4+CD25+ immunoregulatory T cells suppress polyclonal T cell activation in vitro by inhibiting interleukin 2 production. *J. Exp. Med.* **188,** 287–296.

120. Takahashi, T., Kuniyasu, Y., Toda, M., Sakaguchi, N., Itoh, M., Iwata, M., Shimizu, J., and Sakaguchi, S. (1998) Immunologic self-tolerance maintained by CD25+CD4+ naturally anergic and suppressive T cells: induction of autoimmune disease by breaking their anergic/suppressive state. *Intl. Immunol.* **10,** 1969–1980.

121. Asseman, C., Mauze, S., Leach, M. W., Coffman, R. L., and Powrie, F. (1999) An essential role for interleukin 10 in the function of regulatory T cells that inhibit intestinal inflammation. *J. Exp. Med.* **190,** 995–1004.

122. Seddon, B. and Mason, D. (1999) Regulatory T cells in the control of autoimmunity: the essential role of transforming growth factor beta and interleukin 4 in the prevention of autoimmune thyroiditis in rats by peripheral CD4(+)CD45RC- cells and CD4(+)CD8(-) thymocytes. *J. Exp. Med.* **189,** 279–288.

123. Powrie, F., Carlino, J., Leach, M. W., Mauze, S., and Coffman, R. L. (1996) A critical role for transforming growth factor-β but not interleukin 4 in the suppression of T helper type 1-mediated colitis by CD45RB low CD4+ T cells. *J. Exp. Med.* **183,** 2669–2674.

11

Role of Cytokines in Multiple Sclerosis and in Mucosal Tolerance

Howard L. Weiner

1. MULTIPLE SCLEROSIS

Although the etiology and pathogenesis of multiple sclerosis (MS) may still be considered by many to be "unknown," the working hypothesis of most investigators is that MS is a cell-mediated autoimmune disease directed against central nervous system (CNS) myelin and is related in some way to a viral infection *(1)*. Multiple sclerosis means "many scars" and is clearly not an appropriate definition of the disease process. MS is best-defined as "recurrent inflammation of CNS white matter leading to myelin destruction and progressive neurologic impairment." The major question that then must be addressed is what causes this specific and recurrent inflammation and how can it be regulated.

The pathologic picture of MS is one consistent with cell-mediated immune damage to the myelin sheath *(2–4)*. Inflammation is associated with increased expression of IFN-γ, endothelial-cell activation with expression of class II and adhesion molecules, and macrophage-mediated destruction of myelin via receptor-mediated endocytosis. IL-12 expression and B7.1 upregulation in the active lesions are consistent with a Th1-type or cell-mediated autoimmune process *(5)*. The picture is consistent with a delayed-type hypersensitivity (DTH) type response in the CNS. In support of this, cellular reactivity against several myelin antigens (myelin basic protein [MBP], myelin proteolipid protein [PLP], myelin oligodentdrocyte glyco-protein [MOG]) has been demonstrated in the peripheral blood and cere-brospinal fluid (CSF) of MS patients *(6–8)*. These are identical to cells that cause an MS-like disease in the animal model of MS, experimental allergic encephalomyelitis (EAE), and since they have been found in MS patients, they can be considered pathogenic cells capable of cell-mediated CNS inflammation. In some instances there may be large number of myelin

From: *Cytokines and Autoimmune Diseases*
Edited by: V. K. Kuchroo, et al. © Humana Press Inc., Totowa, NJ

Table 1
Multiple Sclerosis as a Th1-Type Cell-Mediated Autoimmune Disease

Exacerbation of MS induced by administration of IFN-γ
Elevated production of IFN-γ and TNF in blood and CNS
Increased production of IL-12 in progressive MS
Presence of IL-12 and B7.1 in MS lesions
Similarities of MS to EAE, which is a Th1 cell-mediated autoimmune disease

autoreactive cells *(9)*. Autoantibodies to myelin antigens have also been demonstrated in MS *(10)*, and although they do not appear to be important in initiating the disease they could play an important secondary role in the disease process by causing demyelination. For example, in animals, antibody against MOG has been shown to enhance demyelination when inflammation is present *(11,12)* although alone, these antibodies have minimal pathologic effects. To date, anti-MOG antibodies have not been consistently demonstrated in patients with MS though there may be other antibodies that play a role in the process. Thus, the primary immunologic and pathologic event that causes MS is the generation of Th1 type CD4[+] cells that become activated, secrete interferon-γ (IFN-γ) and other proinflammatory cytokines, and are specific for antigens in the myelin sheath (*see* Table1). Although CD8[+] cells could also theoretically participate in CNS inflammation, this has not been demonstrated and defects in CD8[+] cells may be related to altered immunoregulation in the disease.

For many years, it was felt that identification of "the" autoantigen in MS would be the key to understanding and treating the disease. This theory was analogous to the demonstration that the acetylcholine receptor was the primary autoantigen in myasthenia gravis. This is no longer a valid assumption because it has now been demonstrated that even though CNS inflammation may be initiated by a cell-meditated attack against a specific myelin antigen such as MBP, there is spreading of immune reactivity to other antigens in the target organ. This has been shown in animal models of EAE *(13–15)* and in another prototypic organ-specific autoimmune disease, diabetes in the nonobese diabetic (NOD) mouse *(16,17)*. Indeed in MS, reactivity to multiple myelin autoantigens has been demonstrated *(6–8,18)* and in the NOD mouse model of diabetes similar spreading of autoreactivity has been demonstrated with reactivity to insulin, glutamic acid decarboxylase (GAD), heat-shock proteins, and other islet antigens *(19)*. In MS, it is possible that spreading of reactivity among antigens and their epitopes may be responsible for causing different attacks of the disease. Furthermore, other

Table 2
Class of Immune Response

	Th1	Th2	Th3
Cytokine[a]	IFN-γ	IL-4	TGF-β
Help	DTH/ IgG2a	IgG1/IgE	IgA
Suppression	Th2	Th1	Th1/2
Immunity[b]	Cell-mediated	Humoral	Mucosal

[a]The primary cytokine associated with each class of immune response is presented. In vivo, there can also be mixed cytokine patterns.

[b]Different types of immunity are favored by each type of T cell, but are not exclusive. Thus, although secretion of TGF-β is favored in mucosal immunity, it is seen as part of systemic immunity as well, and Th3 responses involve cells that may secrete IL-4 and IL-10. TR1 cells are a recently described class of regulatory cells that primarily secrete IL-10 *(25)*.

cells such as γδ cells may be recruited to the CNS once inflammation has been initiated and also participate in the pathologic inflammatory process *(20,21)*. Thus, there is no single autoantigen that is the target of an autoimmune attack, but reactivity to multiple myelin antigens. This makes therapy directed at eliminating specific cells that react to only one myelin antigen or that have a unique T cell receptor (TCR) problematic.

There must be a triggering event or a series of triggering events that initiate the disease. The immune system evolved to protect the host against environmental pathogens and in MS the immune system is misdirected in an organ specific fashion and attacks myelin components in the CNS. Thus, the initiation of the disease involves sensitization initiated by an infectious process that also confers specificity for myelin components and this occurs via infectious agents that have components that crossreact with myelin antigens or by a self-limited infection of the brain that releases myelin antigens and results in sensitization.

A major advance in our understanding of the function and regulation of the immune response is an understanding of the type or "class" of immune response that is induced (*see* Table 2). T-helper (Th)1-type responses are characterized by IFN-γ secretion, and are important in the generation of DTH responses and in immune responses against viruses. Th1-type responses also induce cell-mediated autoimmune diseases in animals such as EAE and by inference Th1 type responses against myelin antigens would induce MS in humans. Administration of IFN-γ to MS patients caused worsening of disease *(22)*. Th1 responses, however, are important in protection against certain parasitic infections (e.g., Leishmaniasis) *(23)*. Th2 type responses are

Table 3
Factors that Influence the Class of Immune Responses

Route of antigen exposure
Type of antigen
Genetics of the host
Environmental exposure
Adjuvant
Local milieu

characterized by IL-4 secretion, regulate Th1-type responses, and IL-4 administration is protective in EAE *(24)*. CD4$^+$ regulatory T cells that suppress Th1 responses and primarily secrete IL-10 have also recently been described *(25)*. Th3 type responses are characterized by TGF-β secretion and are preferentially induced following mucosal presentation of antigen *(26)*. Furthermore, natural recovery from EAE is associated with the appearance of cells that secrete TGF-β *(27,28)*. According to this paradigm, the response of a nonsusceptible individual exposed to a myelin antigen is either not to respond or to generate a Th2 or Th3 response that is nonpathogenic and protective, whereas in patients with MS, a pathogenic Th1-type response is generated. Thus, the central concept that underlies whether MS is initiated and perpetuated and that forms the basis for treatment is the class of immune response (*see* Table 3).

Major histocompatibility complex (MHC) linkage to MS is well known with DR2 being the most closely linked factor associated with MS *(29)*. MHC may be linked to disease in several ways: (1) it could determine the ability of a person to generate pathogenic autoreactive T cells by determining which myelin peptides are presented to T cells; (2) it could determine the shape of the T cell repertoire at the time of T cell development during thymic ontogeny and during peripheral deletion; (3) it could determine the class of immune response based on the binding affinity of peptides in the MHC groove. Of note is that HLA-DR2 is linked to increased production of lymphotoxin and TNF-α (Th1-type cytokines) by T cells *(30)*. However, it is also clear than non-MHC genes are important in determining the class of immune response to myelin antigens. For example, in animal models there are non-MHC linked genes which determine whether an animal is susceptible or not to EAE. B10.S and SJL mice are both H-2^s, yet only SJL animals are susceptible to EAE *(31)*. It appears that susceptibility is determined by the class of immune response generated as when SJL are immunized with MOG or MBP in complete Freund's adjuvant (CFA), Th1-type T cells are induced, whereas when B10.S animals are immunized in an identical fashion, Th2 and Th3 cells are induced *(32)*. The importance of non-MHC genes in determining the class of immune response and susceptibility or resistance to autoimmunity has also been observed in the collagen arthritis model *(33)*. Another non-MHC linked immune factor that can influence the class of immune response is the type of costimulation that occurs when antigen is presented by an antigen-presenting cell (APC) to a T cell *(34)*. A recent study supports the hypothesis that MS patients may be genetically predisposed to Th1 responses because they have less IgE-mediated allergic diseases that represent a Th2 mediated disease *(35)*.

Other factors beside genetics must play a role in MS because it is known that identical twins are not 100% concordant for MS *(36)*. Even though identical twins raised in the same house are exposed to a similar environment, their exposure to infectious agents is not identical and this differential environmental exposure accounts for the nonconcordance rate. Differential environmental exposure impacts on the development of MS by creating an immune milieu that leads to a Th1 vs a Th2 or Th3 response against myelin antigens. As discussed earlier, environmental antigens may also lead to the generation of myelin crossreactive populations of memory cells. In addition, the age at which an individual is exposed to environmental agents may also play an important role in generating different classes of immune responses against myelin antigens. In this regard, there is some evidence that MS may be related to a viral infection that occurs at a certain time in childhood *(37)*. Also, it is known that there are seasonal variations in MS attacks *(38)* and we have recently found that progressive MS patients, but not controls, have increased anti-CD3 induced IFN-γ secretion in winter months *(39)*.

Defects in immune regulation have been described in MS but have never been completely understood, in part because of our incomplete understanding of immune regulation and tolerance maintenance. These defects include a number of defects in antigen-nonspecific suppressor mechanisms *(40,41)*. However, a generalized defect of immune regulation or tolerance in MS does not explain the specificity of the autoimmune responses against myelin antigens, or the lack of generalized autoimmunity in MS. It may be, however, that defects in regulation or tolerance are simply related to regulation of the class of immune response generated (Th1 vs Th2/Th3) or the state of immune activation of T cells in MS patients. Theoretically, there could also be defects related to innate immune responses that could also determine class of immune response or affect mechanisms associated with deletion.

MS is not a localized disease of the CNS, but one that is driven by the movement of cells from the peripheral immune system into the CNS *(42)*.

Thus, immune abnormalities related to the disease process can be identified and monitored in the peripheral blood of MS patients. Activated T cells are present both in the peripheral blood and the CNS of MS patients (43–45). However, local immune responses may subsequently be established in the CNS, one of the best-characterized being the local production of immunoglobulin. In addition, there may be local activation of microglia. Nonetheless, migration of cells into the nervous system plays a crucial role in initiating and perpetuating the disease, especially in earlier stages of the diseases.

MS is not a uniform disease, but one with different subtypes. For example, sub-types of MS may be related to immune reactivity against different myelin antigens, e.g., MBP vs PLP vs MOG. Studies in the EAE model suggest that differences in lesion distribution in MS may reflect differences in the myelin specificity of autoreactive T cells (46). In addition, there may be different disease subtypes related to immune-response genes and sub-types related to an individual's unique environmental exposure. Also spinal MS and primary progressive MS may represent a specifically unique sub-type (47). The existence of different subtypes complicates the investigation and treatment of the disease.

One of the clinical features of relapsing remitting MS is that patients generally recover from an attack. This implies that there are natural regulatory mechanisms that are affecting the immune process to the benefit of the host. In the EAE model, immune mechanisms associated with recovery include apoptosis of pathogenic T cells (48) and a class switch from Th1 to Th2/Th3 responses (27,49,50). Evidence for a class switch during recovery from attacks is beginning to accumulate in MS as well. For example, patients who are in a recovery stage from an acute attack appear to have an increase in IL-10-secreting PLP-reactive cells (51). Understanding these natural regulatory mechanisms and determinindetermining ways to augment them is likely to help the disease process.

When MS changes from the relapsing-remitting to the chronic progressive form, T cells enter a state of chronic activation. It is the chronic progressive form of MS that usually leads to disability. There is recent evidence that changes in the immune system occur when patients change from the relapsing remitting to the chronic progressive form of the disease. These changes involve the emergence of activated T cells which drive the immune system toward a Th1 bias. Specifically, T cells from patients with progressive forms of MS differentiate into cells that drive non T cells to produce IL-12, a powerful inducer of Th1-type responses (52) and may be independent of costimulation requirements. We have also found an increase in IL-12 secreting monocytes in progressive MS (53). These results are important as

Table 4
EAE and Immune Therapy of MS

Activation of myelin-reactive T cells in the peripheral immune system
Migration of cells into the CNS
Recruitment of additional cells
Release of inflammatory mediators
Sensitization to new antigens in the CNS
Suppression of autoimmune response
Tissue repair

they demonstrate that there is a basic difference in the peripheral immune system in progressive vs relapsing-remitting MS. By inference, there may be different responses to immunomodulatory therapy in relapsing remitting vs chronic progressive patients. More important, these results imply that the study of MS should not only involve the investigation of what initiates the disease, but what occurs when the disease switches from the relapsing-remitting to the progressive form. It is also likely that changes within the CNS itself occur in the progressive form such as the development of axonal atrophy and localized CNS immune responses.

If one assumes that MS is a cell-mediated CNS autoimmune disease directed against myelin components, it is then analogous to EAE *(54)*. EAE involves a well-defined series of immunologic events leading to myelin destruction and occurs in relapsing and progressive forms (*see* Table 4). Interruption of this pathway at different stages in the cascade has an ameliorating effect on EAE. Although imperfect, EAE has served as an important working model for testing treatment approaches prior to clinical trials in MS. One of the major differences between treatment of MS and EAE is that many treatments tested in EAE are given at a restricted time during the course of EAE or prior to immunization. Also, EAE is studied in inbred strains of animals, whereas MS occurs in an outbred population. Furthermore, treatment of MS requires chronic therapy of an immune system that may already be activated or in a state of differentiation. One of the unexplained differences between EAE and MS is the protective role of IFN-γ in EAE under some circumstances *(55–57)*, although defects in IFN-γ suppression by CD8 cells have been observed in progressive MS *(57)*. Nonetheless, EAE remains an important model for the study of mechanisms by which cell-mediated immunity against myelin antigens causes myelin damage and can be regulated.

In the past it has been argued that there were no effective treatments for MS. It has now become clear that there are numerous immune-modulating treatments that can affect the disease process, albeit imperfectly and not under all circumstances *(58)*. A treatment may have a positive effect on MS even though all trials may not have demonstrated a positive clinical effect. Differences may relate to dosage schedules and differential responses in patient subgroups. For example we have found that patients with primary progressive MS do not respond as well to pulse cyclophosphamide *(59)*. Antibiotics would not benefit all patients with pneumonia in a trial that mixed both viral and bacterial pneumonia. MS is different than other CNS diseases such as amyotrophic lateral sclerosis (ALS) in which there are not many drugs that can impact on the disease process. Thus, it is important to consider MS as a disease in which immunomodulatory drugs can affect the disease process and to understand the manner in which these drugs positively impact on the disease. Furthermore, it is unlikely that each of these drugs is acting differently but that these drugs act through a limited number of pathways that ultimately impact on one final common pathway.

If MS is a Th1 cell-mediated disease, then an increase in Th1-type myelin-reactive cells would be associated with worsening of disease and Th2- or Th3-type myelin-reactive cells would have an ameliorating effect on the disease process. This is the theoretical basis for treatment with oral tolerance *(60)*, which increases Th3-type myelin-reactive cells *(61)* or altered peptide ligand that increases Th2-type myelin-reactive cells *(62)*. Thus, one could postulate that effective treatment of MS will relate to the balance of Th2 + Th3/Th1 myelin-reactive cells. Nonetheless, even if a treatment affects this balance, it must do so with a strong enough biologic effect to impact on the disease process, something that argues for combination therapy.

Because of bystander suppression, knowledge of "the" antigen in MS is not required for antigen-specific therapy to be beneficial in the disease. Regulatory cells that are specific for an autoantigen secrete anti-inflammatory cytokines when they encounter the autoantigen in the target tissue and thus will suppress inflammation in the organ under attack independent of the autoantigen. This has been termed bystander suppression *(63)* and has been demonstrated in a number of animal models. Thus, in the EAE model one can suppress PLP-induced EAE by feeding MBP *(64)*. Also in the lymphocytic chrroriomeningitis virus (LCMV) viral model of diabetes, the LCMV protein is expressed in the pancreatic islets on the insulin promoter. When animals are infected with the virus, viral-specific immune responses result in diabetes. Feeding insulin generates insulin-specific regulatory cells that suppress the viral-induced diabetes by migrating to the islets, reacting with insulin, and secreting anti-inflammatory cytokines *(65)*. Oral MBP can decrease stroke size in rat models by increasing TGF-β levels in the brain and suppressing inflammation associated with stroke *(66)*. Although bystander suppression was initially described in association with mucosally induced regulatory cells, any immune manipulation that induces a class switch and Th2 or Th3 regulatory cells would have the same effect. It has been argued that this is one of the mechanisms by which copolymer 1 is effective, viz., copolymer 1 induces Th2-type cells that crossreact with MBP *(67)*. Also altered peptide ligands that induce IL-4 and TCR vaccination may also act via this mechanism *(62)*. Bystander suppression solves the conundrum of having to know what the autoantigen is for antigen-specific therapy.

For the most part, there is no "antigen nonspecific" therapy. Effective treatment must ultimately affect antigen-specific myelin-reactive cells. I would argue that most treatments that affect the disease process ultimately impact on antigen-specific myelin-reactive cells either by decreasing IFN-γ secreting or increasing Th2 of Th3 myelin-reactive cells. Thus, even "antigen-nonspecific" immunomodulatory treatments have their effect by affecting the balance of Th1 vs Th2/3 myelin-reactive cells in the nervous system. For example, we have found that IFN-β causes a class switch by decreasing anti-CD3 induced IFN-γ secretion and increasing IL-4 secretion *(68)* and IFN-β has also been shown to increase IL-10 *(69)*. Unexpectedly, we have also found that cyclophosphamide, thought to be a general immunosuppressant, induces a marked immune deviation with an increase in IL-4 and TGF-β and a decrease in IFN-γ and IL-12 *(53)*. In addition, there is an increase of IL-4 secreting MBP- and PLP-specific cells in cyclophosphamide-treated patients *(70)*.

It has sometimes been assumed that if a treatment is found for MS it should help all patients. However, a very important treatment concept in MS is that there will be responders and nonresponders to each "effective" therapy. Thus, because an individual patient does not respond to a particular treatment does not mean that the treatment is ineffective. Furthermore, because the disease is heterogeneous, one of the most important aims of clinical and immunologic research in MS is to understand why people are responders or nonresponders. For example, in our studies of pulse cyclophosphamide, we recently found that the shorter the length of time a person is chronic progressive correlates with whether they respond to therapy *(59)*. Furthermore, as with any disease process in medicine, it would be expected that the disease would be easiest to arrest at early stages and that later stages would be less responsive to therapy.

2. MUCOSAL TOLERANCE

Tolerance has been defined as a lack of response to self but a more appropriate definition of tolerance is any mechanism by which a potentially injurious immune response is prevented, suppressed, or shifted to a non-injurious class of immune response. Thus, tolerance is related to productive self-recognition rather than blindness of the immune system to its autocomponents.

Oral tolerance, in this sense, is of unique immunologic importance becuase it is a continuous natural immunologic event driven by exogenous antigen. Owing to their privileged access to the internal milieu, antigens that continuously contact the mucosa represent a frontier between foreign and self-components. Thus, oral tolerance is an immunological mechanism that evolved to treat external agents that gain access to the body via a natural route as internal components that then become part of self. Given this, it would seem logical that autoimmune diseases caused by an inappropriate response to self-antigens might ultimately be treated by presenting such autoantigens to the mucosal surface where they can be dealt with in a noninjurious (noninflammatory) immunologic environment.

It is now clear that oral tolerance is an active immunologic process and is mediated by more than one mechanism. Low doses of antigen administration favor the induction of active cellular regulation, whereas higher doses favor the induction of anergy or deletion. Although important principals regarding oral tolerance were described in the 1970s and 1980s, most of these early studies of oral tolerance did not distinguish dose effects. Thus, the feeding protocols (dose and frequency) used in the early studies must be carefully delineated when interpreting their results. In many respects the term "oral tolerance" is an inadequate immunologic term as it has primarily been used to define the occurrence of systemic hyporesponsiveness when an animal is immunized after oral antigen administration. We now realize that "oral tolerance" is a complex process that involves suppression of some immune responses and the induction of others. Thus, an understanding of oral tolerance and its use for the treatment of autoimmune or inflammatory diseases involves defining the basic immunologic events that occur when antigen encounters the gut-associated lymphoid tissue (GALT). Antigen may act directly at the level of the GALT or have an effect following absorption. In this regard, "oral tolerance" and "mucosal immunization" are part of one immunologic continuum and are ultimately explained in the context of how an APC interacts with a T cell in the GALT and the factors that modulate and regulate this response. Thus, in addition to antigen dose, the nature of the antigen, the innate immune system, the genetic background and immunological status of the host, and mucosal adjuvants influence the immunologic outcome following oral antigen administration.

2.1. Cytokine Milieu and the Induction of Oral Tolerance

The inductive phase of oral tolerance occurs when antigens encounter the GALT, a well-developed immune network consisting of lymphoid nodules termed Peyer's patches (PP), villi containing epithelial cells, intraepithelial lymphocyte (IELs), and lymphocytes scattered throughout the lamina propria. Although dietary antigens are degraded by the time they reach the small intestine, studies in humans and rodents have indicated that degradation is partial and that some intact antigen is absorbed, especially when large doses of antigen are fed *(71,72)*. High-dose oral antigen may result in systemic antigen presentation, which induces hyporesponsiveness either via clonal T-cell anergy or clonal deletion.

It is generally believed that in low-dose antigen-fed animals, oral tolerance is induced in the gut, with a major component occurring in the Peyer's patches. Several cells capable of antigen presentation exist in the GALT. These include macrophages, dendritic cells, B cells, and epithelial cells. Dendritic cells have been shown as the major intestinal APC that can acquire and process orally administered antigen *(73)*. Epithelial cells may preferentially trigger the activation of CD8+ regulatory T cells. In the rat, these epithelial cell-induced CD8+ T cells are antigen-specific *(74)*, whereas in the human they were found to be antigen nonspecific *(75)*. MHC- class II positive intestinal epithelial cells from 2, 4-dinitrochlorobenzene (DNCB)-fed mice could induce anergy of DNCB-primed T cells *(76)*. Recently, it has been shown that lamina propria cells (LPC) may serve as APCs for oral tolerance *(77)*. Presentation of Ag by LPC stimulated high levels of IFN-γ and TGF-β and adoptive transfer of Ag-pulsed LPC induced oral tolerance to that antigen in the recipients *(77)*. However, the type of APC responsible for the effect of LPC was not resolved.

Th2 cells are preferentially generated in the GALT *(78,79)*, and their differentiation depends on the cytokine microenvironment to which Th precursor cells are exposed during their activation *(80)*. If IL-12 is present during activation, Th1 cell-differentiation occurs, whereas IL-4 induces Th2 cell differentiation. The intestinal mucosa has high basal levels of IL-4, IL-10, and TGF-β expression and shortly after oral administration of antigen, their expression is upregulated *(81)*. This cytokine microenvironment may be crucial for the induction of Th2 or Th3 (TGF-β secreting cells) in the gut. Dendritic cells (DC) from PP preferentially stimulate Th0 clones to produce large amounts of IL-4, whereas DC from spleen induce high IFN-γ production *(82)*. There is also evidence that DC may be involved in oral-tolerance induction because the expansion of DC in vivo with Flt3 ligand enhances oral tolerance *(83)*. It is possible that dendritic cells, the most potent APC in activating resting T cells, under the influence of gut cytokine milieu, present antigen for Th2 or Th3 cell differentiation.

APCs provide costimulatory signals needed for T cell activation. B7.1 and B7.2 are the most important costimulatory molecules. B7.2 has been

Table 5
Modulation of Oral Tolerance

Augments	Decreases
IL-2	IFN-γ
IL-4	IL-12
IL-10	CT
Anti-IL-12 Ab	Anti-MCP-1
TGF-β	Anti-γδ Ab
INF-β	GVH
CTB	Anti-B7.2 MAb (low
Flt-3 ligand	dose tolerance)
LPS	
Multiple emulsions	

Abbreviations: Ab, antibody; CT, cholera toxin; CTB, choleran toxin B subunit; GVH, graft-vs-host; IFN, interferon; IL, interleukin; LPS, lipopolysaccharide; MCP, monocyte chemotactic protein 1.

shown to be critical for Th2 type cell differentiation *(84)*. In vivo in the EAE model, injection of anti-B7.2 but not anti-B7.1 inhibited the induction of oral tolerance to low-dose (0.5 mg) but not high-dose MBP (20 mg). On the other hand, we have also found that CTLA-4 stimulation is important for high-dose oral tolerance *(85)*. Class II molecules on the APC also appear to be critical for the induction of oral tolerance because oral tolerance can not be induced in class II-deficient mice *(86)*.

2.2. Cytokines and the Modulation of Oral Tolerance

A number of factors have been reported to modulate oral tolerance. As oral tolerance has usually been defined in terms of Th1 responses, anything that suppress Th1 and/or enhances Th2 or Th3 cell development would enhance oral tolerance *(see* Table 5). Th3 cells appear to use IL-4 as one of its growth /differentiation factors *(87)*. Seder have also recently found that IL-4, and TGF-β, may serve to promote growth of TGF-β-secreting cells *(88)*. Thus, IL-4 administration intraperitoneally (i.p.) enhances low-dose oral tolerance to MBP in the EAE model and is associated with increased fecal IgA anti-MBP antibodies *(87)*. Oral IL-10 and IL-4 can also enhance oral tolerance when coadministered with antigen *(89)* and cytokines have also been administered by the nasal route *(90)*. Large doses of IFN-γ given i.p. abrogate oral tolerance *(91)*, anti-IL-12 enhances oral tolerance and is associated both with increased TGF-β production and T cell apoptosis *(92)*, and subcutaneous administration of IL-12 reverses mucosal tolerance *(93)*. In the uveitis model, i.p. IL-2 potentiates oral tolerance and is associated with increased production of TGF-β, IL-10, and IL-4 *(94)*. Oral but not subcutaneous lipopolysaccaride (LPS) enhances oral tolerance to MBP *(95)* and is associated with increased expression of IL-4 in the brain. Oral IFN-β synergizes with the induction of oral tolerance in SJL/PLJ mice fed low doses of MBP *(96)* Cholera toxin (CT) is one of the most potent mucosal adjuvants, and feeding CT abrogates oral tolerance when fed with an unrelated protein antigen *(97)*. However, when a protein is coupled to recombinant cholera toxin B subunit (CTB) and given orally, there is enhancement of peripheral immune tolerance *(98)*. Oral administration of corneal epithelial cells markedly enhanced the corneal allograft survival *(99)*. Antibody to chemokine monocyte chemotactic protein 1 (MCP-1) abrogates oral tolerance *(100)*. Oral antigen delivery using a multiple emulsion system also enhances oral tolerance *(101)*. γδ T cells may have important role in oral tolerance induction because it seems more difficult to induce oral tolerance in animals depleted of such cells *(102,103)* or in δ chain-deficient animals *(104)*. The steroid hormone dehydroepiandrosterone (DHEA) breaks intranasally induced tolerance *(105)* and diesel exhaust particles block induction of oral tolerance in mice *(106)*. In the arthritis model, administration of TGF-β or dimaprid (a histamine type 2 receptor agonist) i.p., both of which are believed to promote the development of immunoregulatory cells, enhances the induction of oral tolerance to collagen II even after the onset of arthritis *(107)*.

ACKNOWLEDGMENTS

Supported by NIH grants NS23132, AI43458 a grant from the National Multiple Sclerosis Society, The Foundation for Neurological Diseases, and The Nancy Davis Center Without Walls.

REFERENCES

1. Martin, R., McFarland, H. F., and McFarlin, D. E. (1992) Immunological aspects of demyelinating diseases. *Annu. Rev. Immunol.* **10,** 153–187.
2. Raine, C. S. (1994) The Dale McFarlin memorial lecture. The immunology of the MS lesion. *Ann. Neurol.* **36,** S61–S72.
3. Prineas, J. W. (1996) Pathology of multiple sclerosis, in *Handbook of Multiple Sclerosis*, vol. 10. (Cook, S. D., ed.), Marcel Dekker, Inc., Newark, NJ p. 233.
4. Lassmann, H. (1983) *Comparative Neuropathology of Chronic Experimental Allergic Encephalomyelitis and Multiple Sclerosis.* Springer-Verlag, Berlin.
5. Windhagen, A., Newcombe, J., Dangond, F., Strand, C., Woodroofe, M. N., Cuzner, M. L., and Hafler, D. A (1995) Expression of costimulatory molecules B7-1 (CD80), B7-2 (CD86), and interleukin 12 cytokine in multiple sclerosis lesions. *J. Exp. Med.* **182,** 1985–1996.

6. Olsson, T., Wang, W.-Z., Höjeberg, B., Kostulas, V., Jiang, Y.-P., Anderson, G., et al. (1990) Autoreactive T-lymphocytes in multiple sclerosis determined by antigen-induced secretion of interferon-gamma. *J. Clin. Invest.* **86,** 981–985.

7. Allegretta, M., Nicklas, J., Sriram, S., and Albertini, R. (1990) T cells responsive to myelin basic protein in patients with multiple sclerosis. *Science* **247,** 718–721.

8. Zhang, J., Markovic, S., Raus, J., Lacet, B. Weiner, H. L., and Hafler, D. A. (1993) Increased frequency of IL-2 responsive T cells specific for myelin basic protein and proteolipid protein in peripheral blood and cerebrospinal fluid of patients with multiple sclerosis. *J. Exp. Med.* **179,** 973–984.

9. Bieganowska, K. D., Ausubel, L. J., Modabber, Y., Slovik, E., Messersmith, W., and Hafler, D. A. (1997) Direct ex vivo analysis of activated, fas-sensitive autoreactive T cells in human autoimmune disease. *J. Exp. Med.* **185,** 1585–1594.

10. Warren, K. G., Catz, I., Johnson, E., and Mielke, B. (1994) Anti-myelin basic protein and anti-proteolipid protein specific forms of multiple sclerosis. *Ann. Neurol.* **35,** 280–289.

11. Linington, C., Bradi, M., Lassmann, H., Brunner, C., and Vass, K. (1988) Augmentation of demyelination in rat acute allergic encephalomyelitis by circulating mouse monclonal antibodies directed against a myelin/oligodendrocyte glycoprotein. *Am. J. Pathol.* **130,** 443–454.

12. Schluesener, H., Sobel, R., Linington, C., and Weiner, H. L. (1987) A monoclonal antibody against a myelin oligodendrocyte glycoprotein induces relapses and demyelination in CNS autoimmune disease. *J. Immunol.* **139,** 4016–4021.

13. Lehmann, P., Forsthuber, T., Miller, A., and Sercarz, E. (1992) Spreading of T-cell autoimmunity to cryptic determinants of an autoantigen. *Nature* **358,** 155–157

14. McCarron, R., Fallis, R., and McFarlin, D. (1990) Alterations in T-cell antigen specificity and class II restriction during the course of chronic relapsing experimental allergic encephlomyelitis. *J. Neuroimmunol.* **29,** 73–79.

15. Cross, A. H., Tuohy, V. K., and Raine, C. S. (1993) Development of reactivity to new myelin antigens during chronic relapsing autoimmune demyelination. *Cell. Immunol.* **146,** 261–269.

16. Kaufman, D. I., Clare-Salzler, M., Tian, J., Forsthuber, T., Ting, G. S. P., Robinson, P., et al. (1993) Spontaneous loss of T-cell tolerance to glutamic acid decarboxylase in murine insulin-dependent diabetes. *Nature* **366,** 69–72.

17. Tisch, R., Yang, X.-D., Singer, S. M., Liblau, R. S., Fugger, L., and McDevitt, H. O. (1993) Immune response to glutamic acid decarboxylase correlates with insulitis in non-obese diabetic mice. *Nature* **366,** 72–75.

18. Kerlero de Rosbo, N., Milo, R., Lees, M. B., Burger, D., Bernard, C. C. A., and Ben-Nun, A. (1993) Reactivity to myelin antigens in multiple sclerosis: peripheral blood lymphocytes respond predominantly to myelin oligodendrocyte glycoprotein. *J. Clin. Invest.* **92,** 2602–2608.

19. Harrison, L. C. (1992) Islet cell antigens in insulin-dependent diabetes: Pandora's box revisited. *Immunol. Today* **13**, 348–352.

20. Shimonkevitz, R., Colburn, C., Burnham, J., Murray, R. S., and Kotzin, B. L. (1993) Clonal expansion of activated gamma/delta T cells in recent onset multiple sclerosis. *Proc. Natl. Acad. Sci. USA* **90**, 923–927.

21. Wucherpfennig, K. W., Newcombe, J., Kebby, C., Cuzner, M. L., and Hafler, D. A. (1992) Gamma/delta T-cell receptor repertoire in acute demyelinating multiple sclerosis lesions. *Proc. Natl. Acad. Sci. USA* **89**, 4588–4592.

22. Panitch, H. S., Hirsch, R. L., Haley, A. S., and Johnson, K. P. (1987) Exacerbations of multiple sclerosis in patients treated with gamma interferon. *Lancet* **1**, 893–895.

23. Seder, R. A. and Paul, W. E. (1994) Lymphocytes responses and cytokines. *Cell* **76**, 241–251.

24. Racke, M. K., Bonomo, A., Scott, D. E., Cannella, B., Levine, A., Raine, C. S., et al. (1994) Cytokine-induced immune deviation as a therapy for inflammatory autoimmune disease. *J. Exp. Med.* **180**, 1961–1966.

25. Groux, H., O'Garra, A., Bigler, M., Rouleau, M., Antonenko, S., de Vries, J. E., and Roncarolo, M. G. (1997) A CD4+ T-cell subset inhibits antigen-specific T-cell responses and prevents colitis. *Nature* **389**, 737–742.

26. Chen, Y., Kuchroo, V. K., Inobe, J.-I., Hafler, D. A., and Weiner, H. L. (1994) Regulatory T-cell clones induced by oral tolerance: suppression of autoimmune encephalomyelitis. *Science* **265**, 1237–1240.

27. Khoury, S. J., Hancock, W. W., and Weiner, H. L. (1992) Oral tolerance to myelin basic protein and natural recovery from experimental autoimmune encephalomyelitis as associated with downregulation of inflammatory cytokines and differential upregulation of transforming growth factor β, interleukin 4, and prostaglandin E expression in the brain. *J. Exp. Med.* **176**, 1355–1364.

28. Karpus, W. and Swanborg, R. (1991) CD4+ suppressor cells inhibit the function of effector cells of experimental autoimmune encephalomyelitis through a mechanism involving transforming growth factor beta. *J. Immunol.* **146**, 1163–1168.

29. Steinman, L. (1992) Multiple sclerosis and its animal models: the role of the major histocompatibility complex and the T-cell receptor repertoire. *Semin. Immunopathol.* **14**, 79–93.

30. Zipp, F., Weber, F., Huber, S., Sotgiu, S., Czlonkowska, A., Holler, E., et al. (1995) Genetic control of multiple sclerosis: increased production of lymphotoxin and tumor necrosis factor-α by HLA-DR2+ T cells. *Ann. Neurol.* **38**, 723–730.

31. Segal, B. M. and Shevach, E. M. (1996) IL-12 unmasks latent autoimmune disease in resistant mice. *J. Exp. Med.* **184**, 771–775.

32. Maron, R., Hancock, W. W., Slavin, A., Hattori, M., Kuchroo, V., and Weiner, H. L. (1999) Genetic susceptibility or resistance to autoimmune encephalomyelitis in MHC congenic mice is associated with differential production of pro- and anti-inflammatory cytokines. *Intl. Immunol.* **11**, 1573–1580.

33. Mussener, A., Lorentzen, J. C., Kleinau, S., and Klareskog, L. (1997) Altered Th1/Th2 balance associated with non-major histocompatibility complex

genes in collagen-induced arthritis in resistant rat strains. *Eur. J. Immunol.* **27,** 695–699.

34. Kuchroo, V., Prabhu Das, M., Brown, J. A., Ranger, A. M., Zamvil, S. S., Sobel, R. A., et al. (1995) B7-1 and B7-2 costimulatory molecules differentially activate the Th1/Th2 developmental pathways: application to autoimmune disease therapy. *Cell* **80,** 707–718.

35. Oro, A. S., Guarino, T. J., Driver, R., Steinman, L., and Umetsu, D. T. (1996) Regulation of disease susceptibility: decreased prevalence of IgE- mediated allergic disease in patients with multiple sclerosis. *J. Allergy Clin. Immunol.* **97,** 1402–1408.

36. Sadovnick, A. D., Rice, G. P., and Armstrong, H. (1993) A population-based study of multiple sclerosis in twins: update. *Ann. Neurol.* **33,** 281–285.

37. Kurtzke, J. F. (1985) Epidemiology of multiple sclerosis., in *Handbook of Clinical Neurology,* vol. 3. (Vinken, P. J., Bruyn, G. W., Klawans, H. L., et al., eds.), Elsevier Science, New York, pp. 259–274.

38. Bamford, C. R., Sibley, W. A., and Thies, C. (1983) Seasonal variation of multiple sclerosis exacerbations in Arizona. *Neurology* **33,** 697–701.

39. Balashov, K. E., Olek, M. J., Smith, D. R., Khoury, S. J., and Weiner, H. L. (1998) Seasonal variation of interferon-gamma production in progressive multiple sclerosis. *Ann. Neurol.* **44,** 824–828.

40. Antel, J., Arnason, B., and Medof, M. (1978) Suppressor cell function in multiple sclerosis: correlation with clinical disease activity. *Ann. Neurol.* **5,** 338–342.

41. Hafler, D. A. and Weiner, H. L. (1995) Immunologic mechanisms and therapy in multiple sclerosis. *Immunol. Rev.* **144,** 75–107.

42. Hafler, D. A. and Weiner, H. L. (1987) In vivo labeling of peripheral blood T cells using monoclonal antibodies: rapid traffic into cerebrospinal fluid in multiple sclerosis. *Ann. Neurol.* **22,** 89–93.

43. Bongioanni, P. and Meucci, G. (1997) T-cell tumor necrosis factor-alpha receptor binding in patients with multiple sclerosis. *Neurology* **48,** 826–831.

44. Noronha, A., Toscas, A., and Jensen, M. A. (1990) Interferon beta augments suppressor cell function in multiple sclerosis. *Ann. Neurol.* **27,** 207–210.

45. Hafler, D., Fox, D., Manning, M., Schlossman, S., Reinherz, E., and Weiner, H. (1985) In vivo activated T lymphocytes in the peripheral blood and cerebrospinal fluid of patients with multiple sclerosis. *N. Engl. J. Med.* **312,** 1405–1411.

46. Berger, T., Weerth, S., Kojima, K., Linington, C., Wekerle, H., and Lassmann, H. (1997) Experimental autoimmune encephalomyelitis: the antigen specificity of T lymphocytes determines the topography of lesions in the central and peripheral nervous system. *Lab. Invest.* **76,** 355–364.

47. Revesz, T., Kidd, D., Thompson, A. J., Barnard, R. O., and McDonald, W. I. (1994) A comparison of the pathology of primary and secondary progressive multiple sclerosis. *Brain* **117,** 759–765.

48. Schmied, M., Breitschopf, H., Gold, R., Zischler, H., Rothe, G., Wekerle, H., and Lassmann, H. (1993) Apoptosis of T lymphocytes in experimental autoimmune encephalomyelitis. Evidence for programmed cell death as a mechanism to control inflammation in the brain. *Am. J. Pathol.* **143,** 446–452.

49. Kennedy, M. K., Torrance, D. S., Picha, K. S., and Mohler, K. M. (1992) Analysis of cytokine mRNA expression in the central nervous system of mice with experimental autoimmune encephalomyelitis reveals that IL-10 mRNA expression correlates with recovery. *J. Immunol.* **149,** 2496–2505.

50. Chen, Y., Hancock, W. W., Marks, R., Gonnella, P. A., and Weiner, H. L. (1998) Mechanisms of recovery from experimental allergic encephalomyelitis: T-cell deletion and immune deviation in myelin basic protein T-cell receptor transgenic mice. *J. Neuroimmunol.* **82,** 149–159.

51. Correale, J., Gilmore, W., McMillan, M., Li, S., McCarthy, K., Le, T., and Weiner, L P. (1995) Patterns of cytokine secretion by autoreactive proteolipid protein-specific T-cell clones during the course of multiple sclerosis. *J. Immunol.* **154,** 2959–2968.

52. Balashov, K. E., Smith, D. R., Khoury, S. J., Hafler, D. A., and Weiner, H. L. (1997) Increased IL-12 production in progressive multiple sclerosis: induction by activated CD4+ T cells via CD40 ligand. *Proc. Natl. Acad. Sci. USA* **94,** 599–603.

53. Comabella, M., Balashov, K., Issazadeh, S., Smith, D., Weiner, H. L., and Khoury, S. J. (1998) Elevated interleukin-12 in progressive multiple sclerosis correlates with disease activity and is normalized by pulse cyclophosphamide therapy. *J. Clin. Invest.* **102,** 671–678.

54. Martin, R. and McFarland, H. F. (1995) Immunological aspects of experimental allergic encephalomyelitis and multiple sclerosis. *Crit. Rev. Clin. Lab. Sci.* **32,** 121–182.

55. Lublin, F. D., Knobler, R. L., Kalman, B., Goldhaber, M., Marini, J., Perrault, M., et al. (1993) Monoclonal anti-gamma interferon antibodies enhance experimental allergic encephalomyelitis. *Autoimmunity* **16,** 267–274.

56. Ferber, I. A., Brocke, S., Taylor-Edwards, C., Ridgway, W., Dinisco, C., Steinman, L., Dalton, D., and Fathman, C. G. (1996) Mice with disrupted IFN-γ gene are susceptible to the indcution of experimental autoimmune encephalomyelitis (EAE). *J. Immunol.* **156,** 5–7.

57. Billiau, A., Heremans, H., Vandekerckhove, F., Dijkmans, R., Sobis, H., Meulepas, E., and Carton, H. (1988) Enhancement of experimental allergic encephalomyelitis by antibodies against IFN-γ. *J. Immunol.* **140,** 1506–1510.

58. Weiner, H., Hohol, M., Khoury, S., Dawson, D., and Hafler, D. (1995) Therapy for MS. *Neurol. Clin.* **13,** 173–196.

59. Hohol, M. J., Olek, M. J., Orav, E. J., Stazzone, L., Hafler, D. A., Khoury, S. J., et al. (1999) Treatment of progressive multiple sclerosis with pulse cyclophosphamide/methylprednisolone: response to therapy is linked to the duration of progressive disease. *Mult. Scler.* **5,** 403–409.

60. Weiner, H. L. (1997) Oral tolerance: immune mechanisms and treatment of autoimmune diseases. *Immunol. Today* **18,** 335–343.

61. Fukaura, H., Kent, S. C., Pietrusewicz, M. J., Khoury, S. J., Weiner, H. L., and Hafler, D. A. (1996) Induction of circulating myelin basic protein and proteolipid protein-specific transforming growth factor-beta1-secreting Th3 T cells by oral administration of myelin in multiple sclerosis patients. *J. Clin. Invest.* **98,** 70–77.

62. Nicholson, L., Greer, J., Sobel, R., Lees, M., and Kuchroo, V. (1995) An altered peptide ligand mediates immune deviation and prevents EAE. *Immunity* **3**, 397–405.

63. Miller, A., Lider, O., and Weiner, H. L. (1991) Antigen-driven bystander suppression following oral administration of antigens. *J. Exp. Med.* **174**, 791–798.

64. Al-Sabbagh, A., Miller, A., Santos, L. M. B., and Weiner, H. L. (1994) Antigen-driven tissue-specific suppression following oral tolerance: orally administered myelin basic protein suppresses proteolipid induced experimental autoimmune encephalomyelitis in the SJL mouse. *Eur. J. Immunol.* **24**, 2104–2109.

65. Von Herrath, M. G., Dyrberg, T., and Oldstone, M. B. A. (1996) Oral insulin treatment suppresses virus-induced antigen-specific destruction of beta cells and prevents autoimmune diabetes in transgenic mice. *J. Clin. Invest.* **98**, 1324–1331.

66. Becker, K. J., McCarron, R. M., Ruetzler, C., Laban, O., Sternberg, E., Flanders, K. C., and Hallenbeck, J. M. (1997) Immunologic tolerance to myelin basic protein decreases stroke size after transient focal cerebral ischemia. *Proc. Natl. Acad. Sci. USA* **94**, 10,873–10,878.

67. Aharoni, R., Teitelbaum, D., Sela, M., and Arnon, R. (1997) Copolymer 1 induces T cells of the T helper type 2 that crossreact with myelin basic protein and suppress experimental autoimmune encephalomyelitis. *Proc. Natl. Acad. Sci. USA* **94**, 10,821–10,826.

68. Smith, D. R., Balashov, K. E., Hafler, D. A., Khoury, S. J., and Weiner, H. L. (1997) Immune deviation following pulse cyclophosphamide/methylprednisolone treatment of multiple sclerosis: increased interleukin-4 production and associated eosinophilia. *Ann. Neurol.* **42**, 313–318.

69. Rudick, R., Ransohoff, R., and Peppler, R. (1996) Interferon beta induces IL-10 expression: relevance to multiple sclerosis. *Ann. Neurol.* **40**, 618–627.

70. Takashima, H., Smith, D. R., Fukaura, H., Khoury, S. J., Hafler, D. A., and Weiner, H. L. (1998) Pulse cyclophosphamide plus methylprednisolone induces myelin-antigen-specific IL-4-secreting T cells in multiple sclerosis patients. *Clin. Immunol. Immunopathol.* **88**, 28–34.

71. Bruce, M. G. and Ferguson, A. (1986) Oral tolerance to ovalbumin in mice: studies of chemically modified and 'biologically filtered' antigen. *Immunology* **57**, 627–630.

72. Bruce, M. G. and Ferguson, A. (1987) Oral tolerance induced by gut-processed antigen. *Adv. Exp. Med. Biol.* **216A**, 721–731.

73. Liu, L. M. and MacPherson, G. G. (1993) Antigen acquisition by dendritic cells: intestinal dendritic cells acquire antigen administered orally and can prime naive T cells in vivo. *J. Exp. Med.* **177**, 1299–1307.

74. Bland, P. W. and Warren, L. G. (1986) Antigen presentation by epithelial cells of the rat small intestine. II Selective induction of suppressor T cells. *Immunology* **58**, 9–14.

75. Mayer, L. and Shlien, R. (1987) Evidence for function of Ia molecules on gut epithelial cells in man. *J. Exp. Med.* **166**, 1471–1483.

76. Galliaerde, V., Desvignes, C., Peyron, E., and Kaiserlian, D. (1995) Oral tolerance to haptens: intestinal epithelial cells from 2,4-dinitrochlorobenzene-fed mice inhibit hapten-specific T-cell activation in vitro. *Eur. J. Immunol.* **25,** 1385–1390.

77. Harper, H. M., Cochrane, L., and Williams, N. A. (1996) The role of small intestinal antigen-presenting cells in the induction of T-cell reactivity to soluble protein antigens: association between aberrant presentation in the lamina propria and oral tolerance. *Immunology* **89,** 449–456.

78. Daynes, R., Araneo, B., Dowell, T., Huang, K., and Dudley, D. (1990) Regulation of murine lymphokine production in vivo. III. The lymphoid tissue microenvironment exerts regulatory influences over T helper cell function. *J. Exp. Med.* **171,** 979–996.

79. Xu-Amano, J., Aicher, W. K., Taguchi, T., Kiyono, H., and McGhee, J. R. (1992) Selective induction of Th_2 cells in murine Peyer's patches by oral immunization. *Intl. Immunol.* **4,** 433–445.

80. Abbas, A. K., Murphy, K. M., and Sher, A. (1996) Functional diversity of helper T lymphocytes. *Nature* **383,** 787–793.

81. Gonnella, P. A., Chen, Y., Inobe, J.-i., Quartulli, M., and Weiner, H. L. (1998) In situ immune response in gut associated lymphoid tissue (GALT) following oral antigen in TcR transgenic mice. *J. Immunol.* **160,** 4708–4718.

82. Everson, M. P., Lemak, D. G., McGhee, J. R., and Beagley, K. W. (1997) FACS-sorted spleen and Peyer's patch dendritic cells induce different responses in Th0 clones. *Adv. Exp. Med. Biol.* **417,** 357–362.

83. Viney, J. L., Mowat, A. M., O'Malley, J. M., Williamson, E., and Fanger, N. A. (1998) Expanding dendritic cells in vivo enhances the induction of oral tolerance. *J. Immunol.* **160,** 5815–5825.

84. Freeman, G. J., Boussiotis, V. A., Anumanthan, A., Bernstein, G. M., Ke, K.-Y., Rennert, P. D., et al. (1995) B7-1 and B7-2 do not deliver identical costimulatory signals, since B7-2 but not B7-1 preferentially costimulates the initial production of IL-4. *Immunity* **2,** 523–532.

85. Samoilova, E. B., Horton, J. L., Zhang, H., Khoury, S. J., Weiner, H. L., and Chen, Y. (1998) CTLA4 is required for the induction of high dose oral tolerance. *Intl. Immunol.* **10,** 491–498.

86. Desvignes, C., Bour, H., Nicolas, J. F., and Kaiserlian, D. (1996) Lack of oral tolerance but oral priming for contact sensitivity to dinitrofluorobenzene in major histocompatibility complex class II-deficient mice and in CD4+ T-cell-depleted mice. *Eur. J. Immunol.* **26,** 1756–1761.

87. Inobe, J., Slavin, A. J., Komagata, Y., Chen, Y., Liu, L., and Weiner, H. L. (1998) IL-4 is a differentiation factor for transforming growth factor-beta secreting Th3 cells and oral administration of IL-4 enhances oral tolerance in experimental allergic encephalomyelitis. *Eur. J. Immunol.* **28,** 2780–2790.

88. Seder, R. A., Marth, T., Sieve, M. C., Strober, W., Letterio, J. J., Roberts, A. B., and Kelsall, B. (1998) Factors involved in the differentiation of TGF-β-producing cells from naive CD4+ T cells: IL-4 and IFN-γ have opposing effects, while TGF-β positively regulates its own production. *J. Immunol.* **160,** 5719–5728.

89. Slavin, A. J., Maron, R., Garcia, G., Gonnella, P., and Weiner, H. L. (1998) Oral administration of IL-4 and IL-10 enhance the induction of low dose oral tolerance. *FASEB J.* **II,** A599.

90. Xiao, B. G., Bai, X. F., Zhang, G. X., and Link, H. (1998) Suppression of acute and protracted-relapsing experimental allergic encephalomyelitis by nasal administration of low-dose IL-10 in rats. *J. Neuroimmunol.* **84,** 230–237.

91. Zhang, Z. and Michael, J. G. (1990) Orally inducible immune unresponsiveness is abrogated by IFN-γ treatment. *J. Immunol.* **144,** 4163–4165.

92. Marth, T., Strober, W., and Kelsall, B. L. (1996) High dose oral tolerance in ovalbumin TCR-transgenic mice: Systemic neutralization of IL-12 augments TGF-β secretion and T-cell apoptosis. *J. Immunol.* **157,** 2348–2357.

93. Claessen, A. M., von Blomberg, B. M., De Groot, J., Wolvers, D. A., Kraal, G., and Scheper, R. J., (1996) Reversal of mucosal tolerance by subcutaneous administration of interleukin-12 at the site of attempted sensitization. *Immunology* **88,** 363–367.

94. Rizzo, L. V., Miller-Rivero, N. E., Chan, C.-C., Wiggert, B., Nussenblatt, R. B., and Caspi, R. R. (1994) Interleukin-2 treatment potentiates induction of oral tolerance in a murine model of autoimmunity. *J. Clin. Invest.* **94,** 1668–1672.

95. Khoury, S. J., Lider, O., al-Sabbagh, A., and Weiner, H. L. (1990) Suppression of experimental autoimmune encephalomyelitis by oral administration of myelin basic protein. III. Synergistic effect of lipopolysaccharide. *Cell. Immunol.* **131,** 302–310.

96. Nelson, P. A., Akselband, Y., Dearborn, S. M., al-Sabbagh, A., Tian, Z. J., Gonnella, P. A., et al. (1996) Effect of oral beta interferon on subsequent immune responsiveness. *Ann. NY Acad. Sci.* **778,** 145–155.

97. Elson, C. O. and Ealding, W. (1984) Cholera toxin feeding did not induce oral tolerance in mice and abrogated oral tolerance to an unrelated protein antigen. *J. Immunol.* **133,** 2892–2897.

98. Sun, J.-B., Holmgren, C., and Czerkinsky, C. (1994) Cholera toxin B subunit: an efficient transmucosal carrier-delivery system for induction of peripheral immunological tolerance. *Proc. Natl. Acad. Sci. USA* **91,** 10,795–10,799.

99. Ma, D., Mellon, J., and Niederkorn, J. Y. (1997) Oral immunisation as a strategy for enhancing corneal allograft survival. *Br. J. Ophthalmol.* **81,** 778–784.

100. Karpus, W. J., Kennedy, K. J., Kunkel, S. L., and Lukacs, N. W. (1998) Monocyte chemotactic protein 1 regulates oral tolerance induction by inhibition of T helper cell1-related cytokines. *J. Exp. Med.* **187,** 733–741.

101. Elson, C. O., Tomasi, M., Dertzbaugh, M. T., Thaggard, G., Hunter, R., and Weaver, C. (1996) Oral antigen delivery by way of a multiple emulsion system enhances oral tolerance. *Ann. NY Acad. Sci.* **778,** 156–162.

102. Ke, Y., Pearce, K., Lake, J. P., Ziegler, H. K., and Kapp, J. A. (1997) Gamma delta T lymphocytes regulate the induction and maintenance of oral tolerance. *J. Immunol.* **158,** 3610–3618.

103. Mengel, J., Cardillo, F., Aroeira, L. S., Williams, O., Russo, M., and Vaz, N. M., (1995) Anti-γδ T-cell antibody blocks the induction and maintenance of oral tolerance to ovalbumin in mice. *Immunolol. Lett.* **48,** 97–102.

104. Spahn, T. W. and Weiner, H. L. (1998) γδ T cells are necessary for low dose but not high dose oral tolerance. *FASEB J.* **12,** A597.
105. Wolvers, D. A., Bakker, J. M., Bagchus, W. M., and Kraal, G. (1998) The steroid hormone dehydroepiandrosterone (DHEA) breaks intranasally induced tolerance, when administered at time of systemic immunization. *J. Immunol.* **89,** 19–25.
106. Yoshino, S., Ohsawa, M., and Sagai, M. (1998) Diesel exhaust particles block induction of oral tolerance in mice. *J. Pharmacol. Exp. Ther.* **287,** 679–683.
107. Thorbecke, G. J., Schwarcz, R., Leu, J., Huang, C., and Simmons, W. J. (1999) Modulation by cytokines of induction of oral tolerance to type II collagen. *Arthritis Rheum.* **42,** 110–118.

12

Cytokines and Human Type 1 Diabetes

Sally C. Kent, Vissia Viglietta, and David A. Hafler

1. INTRODUCTION

Although the immunological- and cytokine-mediated events preceding the development of full-blown Type 1 diabetes in the nonobese diabetic (NOD) mouse model are becoming better known, the events preceding disease in humans are less well-characterized. In human Type 1 diabetes, much effort has focused on establishing criteria for disease-development risk, which include genetic associations and the presence of autoantibodies. The contribution of human leukocyte antigen (HLA) alleles for susceptibility (HLA-DR3, HLA-DR4) or resistance (HLA-DQ8) to disease have been studied (reviewed in refs. *1–4*). The diagnostic use of autoantibodies titers to isleT cell antigens such as glutamic acid decarboxylase (GAD) 65, insulin, and other antigens provide a risk assessment for disease onset *(5)*. These markers, along with metabolic measurements, allow clinicians to track patients who are likely to develop disease and to provide support when disease development is imminent.

Although the genetic contribution to disease and the autoreactive B lymphocyte secretion of autoantibodies as disease predictors are known, the reactivity and function of autoreactive T cells in human Type 1 diabetes is controversial and not well-characterized. In this review, we will discuss the data that exists for human Type 1 diabetes in regard to influence of cytokine on immune function and disease initiation/progression. These data include the cytokine-mediated destruction of β-islet cells, the presence of cytokines in the serum of patients and a reinterpretation of those data, the T cell-functional information available, especially with respect to cytokine secretion phenotype of autoreactive T cells, and the potential regulation of the autoimmune response by a subset of T cells, natural killer (NK) T cells.

From: *Cytokines and Autoimmune Diseases*
Edited by: V. K. Kuchroo, et al. © Humana Press Inc., Totowa, NJ

2. CYTOKINE-MEDIATED DESTRUCTION OF β ISLET CELLS

There is evidence to suggest that lymphocytes and macrophages play a crucial role in mediating β cell damage and causing insulin-dependent diabetes mellitus (IDDM). β cell destructive insulitis is associated with increased expression of proinflammatory cytokines (interleukin-1 [IL-1], tumor necrosis factor-α [TNF-α], and interferon-α [IFN-α]) and type 1 cytokines (IFN-γ, TNF-β, IL-2, and IL-12), whereas nondestructive (benign) insulitis is associated with increased expression of type 2 cytokines (IL-4 and IL-10) and the type 3 cytokines (TGF-β) *(6,7)*. A mononuclear cell (MNC) infiltrate, which includes T lymphocytes and macrophages, is a characteristic feature of the islets of Langherans at diagnosis. T lymphocytes could be directly responsible for β cell damage, or they could provoke injury through recruitment of macrophages. Macrophages are the first cells to appear in considerable number during insulitis in animal models of diabetes. Both T cells and macrophages operate and interact through the release of cytokines, which influence the type and magnitude of immune response.

According to a proposed pathogenetic model, the antigen presenting cells are activated and induced to produce cytokines after β cell protein release. These proteins are taken up by antigen-presenting cells (APC) in the islets and are processed to antigenic peptides and as such presented by major histocompatibility complex (MHC) class II molecules on the cell surface. This activates the APC to secrete monokines, IL-1 and TNF, and upregulate costimulatory signals, which induce the transcription of a series of lymphokines genes in T helper (Th) lymphocytes, recognizing the antigenic peptide *(8)*. One of these lymphokines is IFN-γ, which in a feedback loop stimulates the APC to increase the expression of MHC class II molecules and IL-1 and TNF. IL-1 secretion potentiated by TNF-α and IFN-γ is cytotoxic for the β cell through the induction of free radicals in the islets *(9)*. As part of β cell destructive mechanisms, some β cell proteins are damaged and presented to the immune system, thereby amplifying the autodestructive response.

Different approaches have been used to understand the role of these cytokines in the pathogenesis of Type 1 diabetes, both in the animal models and humans. Evidence from human studies to support the role of cytokines in β cell destruction in insulin-dependent diabetes mellitus is scarce. This evidence is derived from: (1) evaluating their expression in the insulitis lesion, (2) studying their effects on isolated islets, (3) studying the effects of their systemic administration in mice, and (4) detecting their levels in the serum of diabetic patients.

Several studies demonstrated marked expression of IL-1, TNF-α, IFN-γ, and IL-6 mRNA in the insulitis infiltrate of nonobese diabetic (NOD) and biobreeding (BB) islets in vivo. IL-1, IFN-γ, and IL-6 proteins have also been demonstrated in NOD islets. TNF-α secreted by activated immune cells in animal models of Type 1 diabetes was found to be higher than in nondiabetes-prone animals, and basal and stimulated serum TNF-α levels were much higher in prediabetic BB rats and NOD mice as compared to control animals. Another proinflammatory cytokine, IFN-α, has been detected in β cells of human subjects with recent onset Type 1 diabetes and the level of mRNA expression is increased significantly in the pancreata of IDDM patients as compared with control human pancreata *(8)*, whereas the expression of other interferon species (β, γ) is not significantly altered *(10,11)*. Also, islet expression of IFN-α precedes insulitis and diabetes in BB rats. These findings suggest the IFN-α production could be induced by initial β cell stress that allows the recruitment of immune system cells, which could also damage the IFN-α-producing islet β cells.

Many functional experiments have been performed to evaluate the effects of IL-1 and TNF species on both animal model and human pancreatic islets even though cytokine applications to islets may not mimic the molecular pathology of the pancreatic insulitis lesion in vivo. These studies show that IL-1 selectively inhibits β cell secretion of insulin and not α cell secretion of glucagon in separated preparations of islet endocrine cells. The cytodestructive effect of IL-1 on β cells in whole islet preparations and not on purified β cells suggests that non β cells in whole islets may contribute to IL-1 induced β cell damage, via additional cytokines such as TNF-α and other inflammatory mediators such as free radicals. From these studies, it has emerged that cytokines, such as IL-1, TNF-α, TNF-β, and IFN-γ impair insulin secretion and, when added in combination of two or more, these cytokines are destructive to rodent and human β cell in whole islet preparation in vitro *(9)*. The combination of proinflammatory cytokines is implicated in increased Fas (CD95) and MHC class I and class II expression on β cells and increased expression of Fas and class I molecules has been reported in pancreatic tissue of recent-onset Type 1 diabetics *(8)*. Recently, in the NOD model, it was shown that diabetogenic T cell became FasL-positive in vivo and could kill cytokine sensitized β cells *(12)*.

It has been shown that activation of resident macrophages in rat islets by treatment of the islets with TNF-α and lipopolysaccharide (LPS) in vitro resulted in inhibition of insulin secretion; this was mediated by the intra-islet release of IL-1, followed by IL-1-induced expression of nitric oxide synthase (iNOS) in the β cells. Regarding the mechanisms by which the cytokines induce the insulin impairment and the β cell destruction, most evidence points to nitric oxide (NO) and/or free radicals produced in β cells exposed to the cytokines *(8,13)*.

In addition to direct cytotoxic actions of cytokines on islet β cells, cytokines may render β cells susceptible to destruction by islet-infiltrating T cells, such as MHC class I-restricted CD8[+] T cells. Despite the role of cytokines as mediators of β cell damage, suggested by in vitro experiments involving the systemic administration of these cytokines to NOD mice and BB rats, in vivo experiments showed that many of those cytokines (including IL-1, IL-2, TNF-α, TNF-β) are able to prevent diabetes development *(14–17)*.

The data available in the literature regarding the proinflammatory cytokine production capacity of diabetic patients are contrasting and not conclusive. An increased IL-1 production capacity and decreased IL-1 receptor antagonist/IL-1 ratio was demonstrated in peripheral blood mononuclear cells (PBMC) from newly diagnosed IDDM patients as compared to normal controls and long-standing IDDM patients. This proinflammatory imbalance in IDDM patients may be important in the pathophysiology of the β cell lysis *(18)* and the direct or indirect action of the proinflammatory cytokines on β cell destruction is vital to the understanding of the progression of Type 1 diabetes.

3. SERUM CYTOKINES AS A MARKER OF TH1/TH2 BIAS AND A DATA REINTERPRETATION

Several groups have investigated the presence of cytokines in the sera of Type 1 diabetes patients. The goal of this approach was to find evidence for Th1/Th2 bias or evidence of immune dysregulation. The presence of serum cytokines has been investigated in IDDM patients before and after the onset of the disease. These studies show that recently diagnosed IDDM patients had significantly higher levels of IL-2, IFN-γ, TNF-α, and IL-1 compared with normal controls, noninsulin-dependent Type 1 diabetes patients, and long-standing patients. In addition, the levels of macrophage-derived cytokines are consistently raised throughout the prediabetic period *(19)*. This finding is consistent with both the NOD mouse and BB rat models of diabetes in which the appearance of macrophages in the islets of Langherans was the first event warning of the onset of insulitis *(20)*. Other investigators have conflicting evidence in regard to TNF-α: Two groups report elevated serum TNF-α *(21,22)*, whereas other groups report lower levels of TNF-α in diabetic patients *(23)* or no change in serum TNF-α as compared to controls *(24)*. Elevated serum IFN-γ *(25)* or a Th1 bias *(26)* in new-onset Type 1 diabetics was also found.

We previously reported that in a group of long-term nonprogressors to Type 1 diabetes, enzyme-linked immunosorbant assay (ELISA) for IL-4 and IFN-γ detected cytokines in serum *(27)*. However, we and others *(28,29)* provide evidence for the identity of this activity in serum as heterophile antibody. Heterophile antibodies are antibodies that bind promiscuously to many different substrates including immunoglobulin and are known to cause false-positives in many two-site ELISAs *(30–32)*. Inclusion of fetal bovine serum (FBS) along with patient sera in ELISA inhibits the interference of the heterophile antibodies with the ELISA signal; or a positive signal with patient sera with mismatched coating and detection antibodies demonstrates the presence of heterophile antibody.

By these criteria of detection of heterophile antibodies, we examined prediabetic sera in more detail and found a percentage of sera (59/443) contain heterophile antibody. In addition, we show no evidence of serum IL-4 by IL-4 affinity column, IL-4 Western blot and MS/MS fragmentation spectra sequencing in one heterophile antibody-positive serum sample. Despite these data, we cannot exclude the presence of cytokine in every sera examined with the two pairs of antibodies used without further characterization. In addition, it is possible that not all heterophile antibodies are detectable with the pairs of antibodies we used. However, we demonstrate, by ELISA, affinity column, and Western blot for human immunoglobulin, that the heterophile antibody containing sera (as defined by the aforementioned criteria) do contain promiscuously, but not indiscriminantly, binding immunoglobulin *(33)*.

The presence of heterophile antibody in sera of at risk for Type 1 diabetes individuals has been found segregated in families and correlated with protection from Type 1 diabetes by the presence of the protective MHC allele DQB1*0602 *(28,29)*. In addition, serum heterophile antibodies were found to correlate with a genotype polymorphism in exon 1 of the costimulation molecule, CTLA4 *(29)*. Thus, the presence of heterophile antibodies may be a marker for a larger susceptibility or resistance phenotype in persons at risk for Type 1 diabetes.

Based on this information, we examined markers for two distinct groups of heterophile antibodies in a large population of first-degree relatives of patients with Type 1 diabetes who were positive for the autoantibodies islet cell antibody (ICA) and/or insulin autoantibody (IAA). We found that we could distinguish two (at least) groups of heterophile antibodies based on the other groups of antibodies (pair 1 and pair 2 on ELISA) reactive with the heterophile antibodies and we found that these two groups of heterophile antibodies correlated with either more rapid disease onset or delayed disease onset *(33)*.

We provide evidence that, in addition to autoantibody-disease markers, the presence of different heterophile antibodies in individuals with diabetes autoimmunity predict the disease course. Heterophile antibodies were detected in significantly higher numbers in patients with islet-cell autoantibodies as compared to the control population. Moreover, when the subjects were divided into three groups, disease incidence could be further stratified. Twenty-two individuals, whose serum was heterophile antibody-positive on pair 2 antibody ELISA (but negative on pair 1 antibody ELISA), had significantly higher incidence of developing diabetes after 5 yr, while 37 individuals, with heterophile antibody-positive on pair 1 ELISA (regardless of pair 2 ELISA result), had a significantly lower incidence of developing diabetes. The disease course correlated with binding of the serum heterophile antibodies was to either pair 1 or pair 2 monoclonal antibodies (MAbs) vs pair 2 antibodies alone (33). This suggests that different antibody crossreactivities with immunoglobulin are predictive of disease course. Attempts to identify the cognate antigen(s) for these protective anti-immunoglobulin antibodies are in progress.

A critical question remains as to what induces the circulating heterophile antibodies that can be associated with disease progression. Historically, heterophile antibodies have been sheep-cell agglutinins associated with mononucleosis *(34)*. High incidence has been reported among patients with autoimmune thrombocytopenia *(35)*. Thus, we postulate that the presence of certain classes of heterophile antibody represents evidence of previous immune responses that are linked, in the cases of protection, to the DQB1*0602 HLA haplotype.

It is provocative to speculate about the protective, destructive, or (auto)antigen reactive nature of heterophile antibodies in Type 1 diabetes, as rheumatoid factor is prevalent in arthritic joints and thought to contributre to pathogenesis *(36)*. The function of heterophile antibodies could include potentiation of T cell growth or promiscuous binding to growth receptors. Alternatively, autoreactive T cells of either Th type may influence the group of heterophile antibodies generated.

Because many investigators have examined patient sera for evidence of cytokine expression *(37–39)* in a variety of disorders other than diabetes (human immunodeficiency virus [HIV], multiple sclerosis [MS], and allergy), these data are presented as a cautionary example for reinterpretation of existing literature and to investigators who wish to examine serum for different factors. Further characterization of these heterophile antibodies groups (in correlation with susceptible and resistant MHC alleles, immune gene-related polymorphisms, and autoantibodies) could lead to better understanding diabetes autoimmunity and to new markers in Type 1 diabetes disease development and progression.

4. AUTOANTIBODY ISOTYPES AS A MEASURE OF CYTOKINE-MEDIATED ANTIBODY CLASS SWITCHING

It is well characterized in murine systems that Th1 vs Th2 responses are associated with antibody isotype class switches *(40)*. Although it is not as clear in humans, IgE and IgG4 have been associated with Th2 responses *(41)*. Petersen and colleagues in the Childhood Diabetes in Finland Study group have recently found a decrease in the Th2 immune response in new-onset patients and siblings as reflected in the GAD65 antibody-isotype profile *(42)*. Individuals at low risk had a GAD65 isotype profile that was more Th2-like and more matured (IgG1 > IgM). In agreement with this study, Bonfacio and colleagues found that auto-antibodies to GAD65 and IA-2 were generally of the IgG1 isotype and they also found that an IgG4 isotype response to insulin dominated in several patients but was not considered protective *(43)*. In another study, GAD autoantobodies were found to be more Th1-like in isotype *(26)*. From these few studies, the data suggest that the auto-antibodies produced in the course of Type 1 diabetes development are Th1-associated. More studies of this kind will be of great value in evaluating the role of cytokines in the autoimmune response in Type 1 diabetes. However, it has been reported that a low antibody response to GAD65 correlated with a vigorous T cell response to GAD65 and vice versa *(44)*. How the isotype of the autoantibody affects this response remains to be determined.

5. CELLULAR COMPONENT OF INFLAMMATORY INSULITIS

What are the antigens of importance in Type 1 diabetes and what evidence is there for T cell reactivity to these antigens? A large number of studies have been done to elucidate T cell function, but with conflicting results. What is known concerning autoreactive T cells in human Type 1 diabetes is discussed.

In patients with Type 1 diabetes, the majority of β cells in the islets of Langerhans have been destroyed and the remaining islets are abnormally small; this change is apparent at the time of disease onset or soon after *(45,46)*. Histological examination of diabetic pancreata shows an inflammatory infiltrate referred to as insulitis. This infiltrate consists of CD8$^+$ and CD4$^+$ T lymphocytes, B lymphocytes, macrophages, and NK cells *(10,47–49)*. There are greater numbers of CD8$^+$ T cells in insulitis infiltrates of patients with newly diagnosed disease who had died of diabetic ketoacidosis *(3)*. In the islets examined from the recent-onset patients, macrophages and lymphocytes identified in the insulitis infiltrate appeared to have an activated morphology. The number of macrophages per islet ranged from 10–21 and the number of T cells per islet ranged from 22–208. Immunohistochemical staining of the islet for IFN-γ producing cells showed frequency of IFN-γ$^+$ cells per islet ranging from 6–65 cells. The lymphocytes generally outnumbered the macrophages 10:1 in infiltrated islets *(48)*. This suggests an inflammatory environment in islets in patients with active disease. In another report that examined the islet-enriched fraction of autopsy pancreata from four new-onset patients (1–5 d after diagnosis) and one long term patient (21 yr), reverse transcription polymerase chain reaction (RT-PCR) analysis detected elevated IFN-α in all patients with disease, whereas IFN-γ was detected in controls as well as one of the new-onset patients *(11)*. Because tissue from new-onset patients is extremely limited, these studies serve as the basis for examining autoreactive T cells in human Type 1 diabetes.

6. SKEWED T CELL RECEPTOR (TCR) USAGE IN INSULTIS

One measurement of antigenic response by T cells is examination of TCR usage. Islet tissue from pancreatic graft biopsies of two new-onset patients were characterized for the repertoire of TCR cDNAs. Histological evaluation of these tissues showed that most of the T cells in inflammatory infiltrates were CD8$^+$TCR$\alpha\beta^+$ and CD4-CD8-TCR$\gamma\delta^+$ in both patients. As compared to 1/31 cDNAs derived from peripheral blood in the first patient, 19/26 insulitis derived sequences were Vβ3+ and 5/19 insulitis-derived sequences were Vα14$^+$. In the second patient, selective Jβ, but not Vβ, gene usage was seen and 19/29 sequences were Vα22$^+$ and 5/28 were Vα14$^+$. There was also restricted gene usage in TCR$\gamma\delta^+$ insulitis-derived cells as well; in patient 1, Vγ1, Vγ2, Vγ3, Vδ1, and Vδ2 were used and in patient 2, Vγ1, Vγ2, Vγ3, and Vδ1 were used *(50)*. In another case where pancreatic tissue from two patients was examined for TCR gene usage, a dominant enrichment for Vβ7 with unselected Vα-chain segments was seen; in addition, culture of lymphocytes from nondiabetics with diabetic isleT cell membrane preparation yielded Vβ7$^+$ T cell clones. This indicated a skewing of TCR usage in T cells in diabetic pancreata *(51)*. These data indicated a restricted usage of TCR genes in both TCR$\alpha\beta^+$ and TCR$\gamma\delta^+$ T cells and a restricted antigen recognition. What the antigen(s) might be is discussed in the next section.

7. AUTOREACTIVE T CELLS IN TYPE 1 DIABETES

There is a growing number of autoantigens implicated in the reactivity of T lymphocytes in human Type 1 diabetes (reviewed in refs. *3,46,52*). These antigens include GAD65, insulin, ICA69, insulinoma-associated IA-2ic tyrosine phosphatase protein (53), heat-shock protein 60 *(54,55)*, sulphatide *(56)*, carboxypeptidase H, and others *(52,57)*. The major proteins of interest as autoantigens are insulin and its precursors and GAD65.

8. IMPORTANT T CELL EPITOPES FOR INSULIN AND GAD65

The specific epitopes of insulin recognized by T cells in humans have been reported to be both in the A chain loop (A1-14/B1-16 peptide) and in the B chain (A16-A21/B10-B25) *(58)* and the HLA-DR molecules DR3,

DR4, and DR5 restricted reactivity to these peptides; here, synthetic peptides were used as antigen. An alternate approach is to stimulate PBMCs with whole antigen, in this case, proinsulin, and retest lines and clones with peptides; using this method the C-peptide between the A and B chains in proinsulin was found to be an epitope *(59)*. T cell hybridomas derived from HLA-DR4 (A1*0101, B1*0401) transgenic mice immunized with prepro-insulin or proinsulin were found to be reactive to this same epitope at the C-peptide/A-chain junction. In addition EBV-B cells (Epstein Barr virus transformed B cells) were found to process these epitope and T cells from HLA-DR4 individuals recognized this peptide *(60)*.

The recognition of epitopes in GAD65 by T cells is a complex issue. The peptides of the GAD65 protein have homology to pro-insulin *(61)* and a Coxsackie virus protein P2-C (PEVKEK) *(57)*. In both of these cases, the GAD peptides could stimulate T cell responses from peripheral blood. In a search for other GAD65 peptides recognized by T cells, 3 HLA-DR2 (B1*1601 or B1*1501) restricted peptides and 2 HLA-DR4 (B1*0401) peptides (one near in proximity to the homology region shared with the Coxsackie virus protein) were identified as naturally processed and presented peptides of GAD65 *(62)*. In addition, HLA-DQ8, expressed as a transgene in mice, was found to recognize at least four epitopes in GAD65 that contain a motif *(63)*. To add to the degeneracy of multiple peptides binding to HLA molecules, isolated HLA molecules from both protective and susceptible alleles could bind multiple peptides from both IA-2 and GAD65 *(64)*. The analysis of important T cell epitopes in Type 1 diabetes will be crucial for understanding the nature of the T cell response in this disease.

9. T CELL REACTIVITY IN TYPE 1 DIABETES

In spite of the identification of these important epitopes, the main question remains as to whether any of these proteins/peptides are specifically processed, presented, and recognized in Type 1 diabetes. Many studies have examined this question. Greater T cell reactivity was seen to GAD peptides and proinsulin in PBMC from at-risk subjects *(61)*; to GAD peptides in at-risk and new-onset patients *(57)*; or to whole islet proteins, GAD65, IA-2, or pancreatic digest in new-onset patients *(65)*. Greater reactivity to insulin was seen in new-onset patients and these patients had a lower requirement for insulin therapy *(66)*. Conversely, many studies have found no difference in T cell reactivity between individuals at-risk, new-onset, or normal controls for T cell reactivity to IA-2 *(67)*; GAD65 peptides including the PEVKEK peptide *(68)*; and insulin or pro-insulin *(69,70)*, though some alteration in T cell reactivity was seen in insulin treated patients.

These conflicting results prompted a workshop to standardize T cell assays in Type 1 diabetes. Standardized, blinded preparations of auto-antigens were sent to laboratories around the world and all laboratories used the same protocol for T cell reactivity (with some differences in serum sources). The outcome of this workshop was that no differences could be seen in T cell reactivity to any antigen between new-onset Type 1 diabetes patients and controls *(71)*. Future workshops will include different T cell assays, including measurement of T cell-secreted cytokines and assays examining different activation states of auto-antigen-reactive T cells *(72)*.

10. CYTOKINES AND T CELL RESPONSES TO AUTOANTIGEN

Only a very few studies have focused on the of cytokine secretion by autoreactive T cells in Type 1 diabetes. In stimulation of PBMC with the GAD65 peptide that includes the region of homology to the Coxsackie viral protein and examination of cytokines by RT-PCR, there was increased IFN-γ signal in 2/4 new-onset children and IL-4 mRNA was decreased in the Type 1 diabetics *(73)*. In a study that examined heat-shock protein 60 T cell responses from twins discordant for Type 1 diabetes, it was shown that amount of Th1-type cytokines did not differ between the groups, but IL-4 secretion was depressed. This was also true of the T cell response to mitogen *(74)*. Several reports indicated that the Th2-type response in Type 1 diabetics to mitogen is reduced *(75,76)*. These few data suggest that the Th-2 response in Type 1 diabetics is decreased and a general IL-4 secretion defect may occur in Type 1 diabetics.

11. ARE T CELLS IN TYPE 1 DIABETES DEFECTIVE?

Regardless of which antigen(s) T cells are reactive to in Type 1 diabetes, there is a body of literature that suggests that T cells in Type 1 diabetics have an inherent signaling defect. This defect is thought to involve IL-2 in that T cells from Type 1 diabetics produce less IL-2 than T cells from controls and Type 2 diabetics *(77)*. The IL-2 defect is also implicated in anergy of T cells; in order for diabetic T cells to proliferate to a variety of auto-antigens, exogenous IL-2 was required for response *(78,79)*. Interestingly, no exogenous IL-2 was required for T cell response to whole proteins such as proinsulin, but IL-2 was required for most peptide responses *(78)*. Another study suggested that the TCR/CD3 complex in diabetic T cells was defective in signaling because stimulation through the TCR/CD3 complex resulted in impaired proliferative response. In this case, IL-2 could not rescue the T cell response. This is despite normal surface expression of TCR, CD3, and CD25 and normal signaling through CD28 *(80)*.

12. NK T CELLS: DEFINITION AND RELATIONSHIP TO TYPE 1 DIABETES

Recent attention has focused on murine CD161$^+$ T cells as a potential immunoregulatory family important in determining the Th1/Th2 bias of CD4$^+$ Th cells *(81)*. In contrast to CD4$^+$/CD8$^+$ T cells, invariant CD1d-restricted T cells have the capacity, without priming, to rapidly secrete both IL-4 and IFN-γ within hours of TCR engagement. This suggests an important role in immunoregulation and possibly in Th1/Th2 differentiation *(82–85)*. Although the role of NK1 T cells in Th1/Th2 differentiation is under investigation, CD1 knockout mice lacking invariant Vα14Jα281 T cells exhibit alterations in anti-CD3-induced IL-4 secretion, though they are still capable of mounting a Th2 response *(86)*. As such, they are thought to be one early source of IL-4 important for subsequent Th2 responses *(81,85)*. Because various knockout mice lacking Vα14Jα281 NK1.1$^+$ T cells can still mount specific Th2 responses, other pathways must exist for the acquisition of this phenotype *(86–89)*.

Relatively high frequencies (up to 1.5%) of CD4-CD8-(DN) T cells are found in the peripheral blood *(90)*. Within this population, cells expressing invariant Vα24JαQ TCR α chains are preferentially paired with Vβ11, and to a lesser extent Vβ2, 3, 5, and 8 *(90,91)*. Human invariant Vα24JαQ T cells are homologous to the murine Vα14Jα281 NK1.1$^+$ T cell, which have a TCR α chain in which the Vα14 segment is rearranged to pair with Jα281 with no N-region diversity. Both human and murine invariant T cells are restricted by CD1d or CD1.1 molecules, respectively *(81,92)*. These proteins are Class I MHC-related molecules that contain glycolipid or phospholipid moieties in the antigen-binding groove *(93–98)*. There are families of DN T cells with conserved, but unidentified function. Several groups have reported human and murine NK T cells with similar phenotypic and functional properties. Murine CD1-restricted cells include CD4$^+$ Vα14$^+$ NK1.1 T cells *(99,100)* and Vα14$^-$ T cells *(101–103)*. In humans, Vα24$^+$Vβ11$^+$ NK T cells with N-region additions have been reported to be restricted by CD1d *(104)* and human CD4$^+$ Vα24-JαQ-Vβ11$^+$ T cells exhibited similar cytokine secretion and surface-marker expression as compared to NK T cells *(105)*. In addition, Vα24JαQ T cells with conservative amino acid substitutions for the serine at the C-terminus of the Vα24 segment were found to behave similarly to invariant NK T cells, whereas clones with nonconservative amino acid substitutions were unable to recognize CD1d *(106)*. Thus, variations of the invariant NK T cell exist and may represent populations of NK T cells with varying functions.

The tissue distribution of the NK T cell ligand, mouse CD1 and human CD1d, is complex. Mouse CD1 gene transcription has been detected in the thymus, liver, brain, spleen, and intestinal epithelial and CD1 protein has been detected on the surface of cortical thymocytes; intestinal epithelial cells; hematopoetic lineage cells, including constitutive expression on T and B cells; macrophages; and dendritic cells (DC) *(99–101,107,108)*. In various tissues, the protein may adopt different conformations as assessed by MAb reactivity and ability to differentially stimulate CD1d-reactive clones and hybridomas *(107,109,110)*. This may reflect the association of CD1 and tissue-specific ligands or masking/accessory molecules. The form and distribution of CD1d will influence the response of Vα24-JαQ T cells.

An important role for CD1d-restricted T cells has been demonstrated in regulating T cell responses to tumors and auto-antigens. CD1-dependent T cells were shown to be involved in antitumor immunity *(83,111,112)*. In the *lpr* model of systemic lupus erythematosus (SLE), the frequency of Vα14⁺ NK T cells was diminished before disease onset *(113)*. Augmentation of Vα14+ NK T cells by adoptive transfer of purified CD4⁻CD8⁻ cells enriched for IL-4 and little IFN-γ or IL-10 secetion prevented disease, whereas a CD4⁻CD8⁻ T cell population secreting IFN-γ and little IL-4 or injection anti-Vα14 antibody aggravated disease *(114)*. The development of diabetes in the NOD model was inhibited by the transfer of a thymocyte or splenic population enriched for the αβ DN T cell population *(115,116)*.

In the diabetes-prone BB rat, it has been found that there is a deficit in the number of RT6⁺ T cells, which are the homolog to the human NK T cell *(117)*. In fact, if T cells and NK T cells are included in the intragraft lymphoid tissues in whole pancreaticoduodenal transplant from Wistar Furth rats to BB rats, diabetes recurrence is prevented and it can be shown that the NK T cells in the graft proliferate and produce IFN-γ and IL-4 *(118–120)*.

There are a number of additional observations suggesting that invariant NK T cells may function in an important regulatory role in autoimmunity. In humans, the frequency of peripheral Vα24JαQ T cells was decreased in systemic sclerosis *(121)* and in rheumatoid synovium *(122)*. In humans with Type 1 diabetes, a decrease in the frequency of NK T cells in monozygotic twins discordant for IDDM was observed. Moreover, whereas the NK T cell clones from nondiabetic siblings secreted IL-4 and IFN-γ, the NK T cells from subjects with IDDM secreted IFN-γ but not IL-4 *(27)*. These alterations of NK T cell clones from identical twins discordant for Type 1 diabetes suggested that environmental events contributed to the alterations in cytokine secretion. The circulating frequencies of these cells were diminished in Type 1 diabetes and clones raised from such individuals lacked the ability to secrete IL-4 *(27)*. It will be of great interest to manipulate populations of NK T cells in islet transplant in disease models. Thus, CD1d-restricted T cells are implicated in the regulation of inflammatory processes at several levels, especially in Type 1 diabetes.

CD1d-restricted NK T cells with invariant TCR-α chains represent a potentially major functional population of T cells in humans. Unlike MHC class II restricted CD4⁺ T cells, NK T cells circulate in an activated state as evidenced by medium-affinity IL-2 receptors and rapidly secrete cytokines with TCR crosslinking *(123)*. This suggests that CD1d-restricted NK T cells have an important early function in regulating immune responses. The multi-functionality of CD1d restricted T cells is provocative; murine NK T cells have a profound role in the IL-12-mediated rejection of tumors *(111)*. Interestingly, it has been recently demonstrated that NK T cells are capable of killing CD1d-expressing dendritic cells (DC) *(124)*. Therefore, CD1d-restricted T cells may regulate key immune responses in autoimmune diseases and tumor rejection. The complex regulation of families of CD1d-restricted T cells by tissue-specific CD1d expression may greatly influence regulatory and inflammatory immune responses in autoimmune diseases, tumor rejection, and infection.

13. CONCLUDING REMARKS

In summary, cytokines are important in the pathogenesis of human Type 1 diabetes and for a Th1/Th2-biased response in human Type 1 diabetes. Proinflammatory and procytotoxic cytokines have profound effects on β-islet cell survival. The limited analysis of the isotypes of autoreactive antibodies suggests Th1 bias in the disease state. Examination of pancreatic tissue from new-onset subjects shows a role for the invading inflammatory lymphocytes in insulitis and their proinflammatory cytokines. However, the influence of cytokines secreted in the microenvironment and their influence on T cell function in humans is unclear, although there is limited data to suggest that Type 1 diabetic T cells are defective in IL-4 secretion. There may be signaling defects or states of T cell anergy to investigate in Type 1 diabetes. Better and more sensitive T cell assays must be established and the role of NK T cells must be investigated, especially in the transplant setting, so that we can understand the inflammatory process that destroys β-islet cells in Type 1 diabetes.

REFERENCES

1. She, J.-X. (1996) Susceptibility to type I diabetes:HLA-DQ and DR revisited. *Immunol. Today* **17,** 323–329.
2. Todd, J. A. (1999) From gemone to aetiology in a multifactorial disease, type 1 diabetes. *BioEssays* **21,** 164–174.
3. Atkinson, M. A. and Maclaren, N. K. (1994) The pathogenesis of insulin-dependent diabetes mellitus. *N. Eng. J. Med.* **331,** 1428–1436.
4. Lernmark, A. (1999) Selected culprits in type 1 diabetes β-cell killing. *J. Clin. Invest.* **104,** 1487–1489.

5. Verge, C. F., Gianani, R., Kawasaki, E., Yu, L., Pietropaolo, M., Jackson, R. A., et al. (1996) Prediction of type I diabetes in first-degree relatives using a combination of insulin, GAD, and ICA512bdc/IA-2 autoantibodies. *Diabetes* **45,** 926–933.

6. Charlton, B. and Lafferty, K. J. (1995) The Th1/Th2 balance in autoimmunity. *Curr. Opin. Immunol.* **7,** 793–798.

7. Liblau, R. S., Singer, S. M., and McDevitt, H. O. (1995) Th1 and Th2 CD4+ T cells in the pathogenesis of organ-specific autoimmune diseases. *Immunol. Today* **16,** 34–38.

8. Rabinovitch, A. (1998) An update on cytokines in the pathogenesis of insulin-dependent diabetes mellitus. *Diabetes Metabol. Rev.* **14,** 129–151.

9. Mandrup-Poulsen, T. (1996) The role of interleukin-1 in the pathogenesis of IDDM. *Diabetology* **39,** 1005–1029.

10. Foulis, A. K., Farquharson, M. A., and Meager, A. (1987) Immunoreactive alpha-interferon in insulin-secreting beat cells in type 1 diabetes mellitus. *Lancet* **ii,** 1423–1427.

11. Huang, X., Yuan, J., Goddard, A., Foulis, A., James, R. F. L., Lernmark, A., et al. (1995) Interferon expression in the pancreases of patients with type 1 diabetes. *Diabetes* **44,** 658–664.

12. Amrani, A., Verdaguer, J., Thiessen, S., Bou, S., and Santamaria, P. (2000) IL-1α, IL-1β, and IFN-γ mark B cells for Fas-dependent destruction by diabetogenic CD4+ T lymphcytes. *J. Clin. Invest.* **105,** 459–468.

13. Rabinovitch, A. and Suarez-Pinzon, W. L. (1998) Cytokines and their roles in pancreatic islet β-cell destruction and insulin-dependent diabetes mellitus. *Biochem. Pharmacol.* **55,** 1139–1149.

14. Seino, H., Takahashi, K., Satoh, J., Zhu, X. P., Sagara, M., Masuda, T., et al. (1993) Prevention of autoimmune diabetes with lymphotoxin in NOD mice. *Diabetes* **42,** 398–404.

15. Satoh, J., Seino, H., Shintani, S., Tanaka, S.-I., Ohteki, T., Masada, T., et al. (1990) Inhibition of type 1 diabetes in BB rats with recombinant human tumour necrosis factor-α. *J. Immunol.* **145,** 1395–1399.

16. Zielasek, J., Burkart, V., Naylor, P., Goldstein, A., Kiesel, U., and Kolb, H. (1990) Interleukin 2-dependent control of disease development in spontaneously diabetic BB rats. *Immunology* **69,** 209–214.

17. Jacob, C. O., Asiso, S., Michie, S. A., McDevitt, H. O., and Acha-Orbea, H. (1990) Prevention of diabetes in nonobese diabetic mice by tumour necrosis factor (TNF): similarities between TNFα and IL-1. *Proc. Natl. Acad. Sci. USA* **87,** 968–972.

18. Netea, M. G., Hancu, N., Blok, W. L., Grigorescu-Sido, P., Popa, L., Popa, V., and van der Meer, J. W. (1997) Interleukin 1 beta, tumour necrosis factor-alpha and interleukin 1 receptor antagonist in newly diagnosed insulin-dependent diabetes mellitus: comparison to long standing diabetes and healthy individuals. *Cytokine* **9,** 284–287.

19. Hussain, M. J., Peakman, M., Gallati, H., Lo, S. S. S., Hawa, M., Viberti, G. C., et al. (1996) Elevated serum levels of macrophage-derived cytokines precede and accompany the onset of IDDM. *Diabetology* **39,** 60–69.

20. Walker, R., Bone, A. J., Cooke, A., and Baird, D. J. (1988) Distinct macrophage subpopulations in pancreas of prediabetic BB/E rats: possible role for macrophages in the pathogenesis of IDDM. *Diabetes* **37,** 1301–1304.
21. Espersen, G. T., Mathiesen, O., Grunnet, N., and Jensen, S. D. (1993) Cytokine plasma levels and lymphocyte subsets in patients with newly diagnosed insulin-dependent (type 1) diabetes mellitus before and following initial insulin treatment. *APMIS* **101,** 703–706.
22. Cavallo, M. G., Pozzilli, P., Bird, C., Wadhwa, M., Meager, A., Visalli, N., et al. (1991) Cytokines in the sera from insulin-dependent diabetic patients at diagnosis. *Clin. Exp. Immunol.* **86,** 256–259.
23. Lorini, R., De Amici, M., d'Annunzio, G., Vitali, L., and Scaramuzza, A. (1995) Low serum levels of tumor necrosis factor-alpha in insulin-dependent diabetic children. *Hormone Res.* **43,** 206–209.
24. Mooradian, A. D., Reed, R. L., Meredith, K. E., and Scuderi, P. (1991) Serum level of tumor necrosis factor and IL-1α and IL-1β in diabetic patients. *Diabetes Care* **14,** 63–65.
25. Tovo, P. A., Cerutti, F., Palomba, E., Salomone, C., and Pugliese, A. (1984) Evidence of circulating interferon-gamma in newly diagnosed diabetic children. *Acta Paed. Scand.* **73,** 785–788.
26. Ng, W. Y., Thai, A. C., Lui, K. F., Yeo, P. P. B., and Cheah, J. S. (1999) Systemic levels of cytokines and GAD-specific autoantibody isotypes in Chinese IDDM patients. *Diabetes Res. Clin. Practice* **43,** 127–135.
27. Wilson, S. B., Kent, S. C., Patton, K. T., Orban, T., Jackson, R. A., Exley, M., et al. (1998) Extreme Th1 bias of invariant Vα24JαQ T cells in type 1 diabetes. *Nature* **391,** 177–181.
28. Redondo, M. J., Gottlieb, P. A., Motheral, T., Mulgrew, C., Rewers, M., Babu, S., et al. (1999) Heterophile anti-mouse immunoglobulin may interfer with cytokine measurements in patients with HLA alleles protective for type 1A diabetes. *Diabetes* **48,** 2166–2170.
29. She, J.-X., Ellis, T. M., Wilson, S. B., Wasserfall, C. H., Marron, M., Reimsneider, S., et al. (1999) Heterophile antibodies segregate in families and are associated with protection from type 1 diabetes. *Proc. Natl. Acad. Sci. USA* **96,** 8116–8119.
30. Boscato, L. M. and Stuart, M. C. (1986) Incidence and specificity of interference in two-site immunoassays. *Clin. Chem.* **32,** 1491–1495.
31. Boscato, L. M. and Stuart, M. C. (1988) Heterophilic antibodies: a problem for all immunoassays. *Clin. Chem.* **34,** 27–33.
32. Levinson, S. S. (1992) Antibody multispecificity in immunoassay interference. *Clin. Biochem.* **25,** 77–87.
33. Orban, T., Kent, S. C., Malik, P., Milner, J. D., Schuster, K., Jackson, R. A., et al. (2001) Heterophile antibodies indicate progression of autoimmunity in human type 1 diabetes mellitus before clinical onset. *Autoimmunity*, in press.
34. Nikoskelainen, J. and Hanninen, P. (1975) Antibody response to Epstein-Barr virus in infectious mononucleosis. *Infect. Immunity* **11,** 42–51.
35. Clofent-Sanchez, G., Laroche-Traiean, J., Lucas, S., Rispal, P., Pellegrin, J. L., Nurden, P., et al. (1997) Incidence of anti-mouse antibodies in thrombocytopenic patients with autoimmune disorders. *Human Antibodies* **8,** 50–59.

36. Carson, D. A., Chen, P. P., Fox, R. I., Kipps, T. J., Jirik, F., Goldfien, R. D., et al. (1987) Rheumatoid factor and immune networks. *Ann. Rev. Immunol.* **5,** 109–126.

37. Trotter, J. L., Damico, C. A., Trotter, A. L., Collins, K. G., and Cross, A. H. (1995) Interleukin-2 binding proteins in sera from normal subjects and multiple sclerosis patients. *Neurology* **45,** 1971–1974.

38. Senaldi, G., Peakman, M., Natoli, C., Hussain, M. J., Gallati, H., McManus, T., et al. (1994) Relationship between the tumour-associated antigen 90K and cytokines in the circulation of persons infected with human immunodeficiency virus. *J. Infect.* **28,** 31–39.

39. Ohshima, Y., Katamura, K., Miura, M., Mikawa, H., and Mayumi, M. (1995) Serum levels of interleukin 4 and soluble CD23 in children with allergic disorder. *Eur. J. Paed.* **154,** 723–728.

40. Abbas, A. K., Murphy, K. M., and Sher, A. (1996) Functional diversity of helper T lymphocytes. *Nature* **383,** 787–793.

41. Coffman, R. L., Lebman, D. A., and Rothman, P. (1993) Mechanism and regulation of immunolglobulin isotype switching. *Adv. Immunol.* **54,** 229–270.

42. Petersen, J. S., Kulmala, P., Clausen, J. T., Knip, M., Dyrberg, T., and the Childhood Diabetes in Finland Study Group. (1999) Progression to type 1 diabetes is associated with a change in the immunolglobulin isotype profile of autoantibodies to glutamic acid decarboxylase (GAD65). *Clin. Immunol.* **90,** 276–281.

43. Bonifacio, E., Scirpoli, M., Kredel, K., Fuchtenbusch, M., and Ziegler, A.-G. (1999) Early autoantibody responses in prediabetics are IgG1 dominated and suggest antigen specific regulation. *J. Immunol.* **163,** 525–532.

44. Harrison, L. C., Honeyman, M. C., DeAizpurua, H. J., Schmidli, R. S., Colman, P. G., Tait, B. D., et al. (1993) Inverse relation between humoral and cellular immunity glutamic acid decarboxylase in subjects at risk of insulin-dependent diabetes. *Lancet* **341,** 1365–1369.

45. Gepts, W. (1965) Pathological anatomy of the pancreas in juvenile diabetes mellitus. *Diabetes* **14,** 619–633.

46. Atkinson, M. A. and Maclaren, N. K. (1993) Islet cell autoantigens in insulin-dependent diabetes. *J. Clin. Invest.* **92,** 1608–1616.

47. Bottazzo, G. F., Dean, B. M., McNally, J. M., MacKay, E. H., Swift, P. G. F., and Gamble, D. R. (1985) In situ characterization of autoimmune phenoma and expression of HLA molecules in the pancreas in diabetic insulitis. *N. Engl. J. Med.* **313,** 353–360.

48. Foulis, A. K., McGill, M., and Farquharson, M. A. (1991) Insulitis in type 1 (insulin-dependent) diabetes mellitus in man-macrophages, lymphocytes, and interferon-γ containing cells. *J. Pathol.* **165,** 97–103.

49. Hanninen, A., Jalkanen, S., Salmi, M., Toikkannen, S., Nikolakaros, G., and Simell, O. (1992) Macrophages, T cell receptor usage, and endothelial cell activation in the pancreas at the onset insulin-dependent diabetes mellitus. *J. Clin. Invest.* **90,** 1901–1910.

50. Santamaria, P., Lewis, C., Jessurun, J., Sutherland, D. E. R., and Barbosa, J. J. (1994) Skewed T cell receptor usage junctional and heterogeneity among isletitis αβ and γδ T cells in human IDDM. *Diabetes* **43,** 599–606.

51. Conrad, B., Weidmann, E., Trucco, G., Rudert, W. A., Behboo, R., Ricordi, C., et al. (1994) Evidence for superantigen involvement in insulin-dependent diabetes mellitus aetiology. *Nature* **371,** 351–355.

52. Roep, B. O. (1996) T cell responses to autoantigens in IDDM. *Diabetes* **45,** 1147–1156.

53. Peakman, M., Stevens, E. J., Lohmann, T., Narendran, P., Dromey, J., Alexander, A., et al. (1999) Naturally processed and presented epitopes of the islet cell autoantigen IA-2 eluted from HLA-DR4. *J. Clin. Invest.* **104,** 1449–1451.

54. Abulafia-Lapid, R., Elias, D., Raz, I., Keren-Zur, Y., Atlan, H., and Cohen, I. R. (1999) T cell proliferative responses of type 1 diabetes patients and healthy individuals to human hsp60 and its peptides. *J. Autoimmunol.* **12,** 121–129.

55. Cohen, I. R. (1997) The Th1/Th2 dichotomy, hsp60 autoimmunity, and type 1 diabetes. *Clin. Immunol. Immunopath.* **84,** 103–106.

56. Buschard, K., Schloot, N. C., Kaas, A., Bock, T., Horn, T., Fredman, P., and Roep, B. O. (1999) Inhibition of insulin-specific autoreactive T cells by sulphatide which is variably expressed in beta cells. *Diabetology* **42,** 1212–1218.

57. Atkinson, M. A., Bowman, M. A., Campbell, L., Darrow, B. L., Kaufman, D. L., and Maclaren, N. K. (1994) Cellular immunity to a determinant common to glutamate decarboxylase and Coxsackie virus in insulin-dependent diabetes. *J. Clin. Invest.* **94,** 2125–2129.

58. Naquet, P., Ellis, J., Tibensky, D., Kenshole, A., Singh, B., Hodges, R., et al. (1988) T cell autoreactivtiy to insulin in diabetic and related non-diabetic individuals. *J. Immunol.* **140,** 2569–2578.

59. Semana, G., Gausling, R., Jackson, R. A., and Hafler, D. A. (1999) T cell autoreactivity to proinsulin epitopes in diabetic patients and healthy subjects. *J. Autoimmunol.* **12,** 259–267.

60. Congia, M., Patel, S., Cope, A. P., De Virgilis, S., and Sonderstrup, G. (1998) T cell epitopes of insulin defined in HLA-DR4 transgenic mice are derived from preproinsulin and proinsulin. *Proc. Natl. Acad. Sci. USA* **95,** 3883–3888.

61. Rudy, G., Stone, N., Harrison, L. C., Colman, P. G., McNair, P., Brusic, V., et al. (1995) Similar peptides from tewo beta cell autoantigens, proinsulin and glutamic acid decarboxylase, stimulate T cells of individuals at risk for insulin-dependent diabetes. *Mol. Med.* **1,** 625–633.

62. Endl, J., Otto, H., Jung, G., Dreisbusch, B., Donie, F., Stahl, P., et al. (1997) Identification of naturally processed T cell epitopes from glutamic acid decarboxylase presented in the context of HLA-DR alleles by T lymphocytes of recent onset IDDM patients. *J. Clin. Invest.* **99,** 2405–2415.

63. Herman, A. E., Tisch, R. M., Patel, S. D., Parry, S. L., Olson, J., Noble, J. A., et al. (1999) Determination of glutamic acid decarboxylase 65 peptides presented by the type 1 diabetes-associated HLA-DQ8 class II molecule identifies an immunogenic peptide motif. *J. Immunol.* **163,** 6275–6282.

64. Harfouch-Hammond, E., Walk, T., Otto, H., Jung, G., Bach, J. F., van Endert, P. M., et al. (1999) Identification of peptides from autoantigens

GAD65 and IA-2 that bind to HLA class II molecules predisposing to or protecting from type 1 diabetes. *Diabetes* **48**, 1937–1947.

65. Durinovic-Bello, I., Hummel, M., and Ziegler, A.-G. (1996) Cellular immune response to diverse islet cell antigens in IDDM. *Diabetes* **45**, 795–800.

66. Mayer, A., Rharbaoui, F., Thivolet, C., Orgiazzi, J., and Madec, A. M. (1999) The relationship between peripheral T cell reactivity to insulin, clinical remissions and cytokine production in type 1 (insulin-dependnt) diabetes mellitus. *J. Clin. Endocrin. Metabol.* **84**, 2419–2424.

67. Ellis, T. M., Schatz, D. A., Ottendorfer, E. W., Lan, M. S., Wasserfall, C., Salisbury, P. J., et al. (1998) The relationship between humoral and cellular immunity to IA-2 in IDDM. *Diabetes* **47**, 566–569.

68. Schloot, N. C., Roep, B. O., Wegmann, D. R., Yu, L., Wang, T. B., and Eisenbarth, G. S. (1997) T cell reactivity to GAD65 peptide sequences shared with Coxsackie virus protein in recent-onset IDDM, post-onset IDDM patients and control subjects. *Diabetology* **40**, 332–338.

69. Ellis, T. M., Jodoin, E., Ottendorfer, E., Salisbury, P., She, J. X., Schatz, D. A., et al. (1999) Cellular immune responses against proinsulin: no evidence for enhanced reactivity in individuals with IDDM. *Diabetes* **48**, 299–303.

70. Schloot, N. C., Roep, R. O., Wegmann, D., Yu, L., Chase, H. P., Wang, T., and Eisenbarth, G. S. (1997) Altered immune response to insulin in newly diagnosed compared to insulin-treated diabetic patients and healthy control subjects. *Diabetology* **40**, 562–572.

71. Roep, B. O., Atkinson, M. A., van Endert, P. M., Gottlieb, P. A., Wilson, S. B., and Sachs, J. A. (1999) Autoreactive T cell responses in insulin-dependent (type 1) diabetes mellitus. *J. Autoimmun.* **13**, 267–282.

72. Zhang, J., Markovic-Plese, S., Lacet, B., Raus, J., Weiner, H. L., and Hafler, D. A. (1994) Increased frequency of interleukin 2-responsive T cells specific for myelin basic protein and protolipid protein in peripheral blood and cerebrospinal fluid of patients with multiple sclerosis. *J. Exp. Med.* **179**, 973–984.

73. Karlsson, M. G. and Ludvigsson, J. (1998) Determination of mRNA expression for IFN-gamma and IL-4 in lymphocytes from children with IDDM by RT-PCR technique. *Diabetes Res. Clin. Practice* **40**, 21–30.

74. Kallman, B. A., Lampeter, E. F., Hanifi-Moghaddam, P., Hawa, M., Leslie, R. D., and Kolb, H. (1999) Cytokine secretion patterns in twins discordant for type 1 diabetes. *Diabetology* **42**, 1080–1085.

75. Rapoport, M. J., Mor, A., Vardi, P., Ramot, Y., Winker, R., Hindi, A., and Bistritzer, T. (1998) Decreased secretion of Th2 cytokines precedes up-regulated and delayed secretion of Th1 cytokines in activated peripheral blood mononuclear cells from patients with insulin-dependent diabetes mellitus. *J. Autoimmun.* **11**, 635–642.

76. Berman, M. A., Sandborg, C. I., Wang, Z., Imfeld, K. L., Zaldivar Jr., F., Dadufalza, V., and Buckingham, B. A. (1996) Decreased IL-4 production in new onset type 1 insulin-dependent diabetes mellitus. *J. Immunol.* **157**, 4690–4696.

77. Kaye, W. A., Adri, M. N., Soeldner, J. S., Rabinowe, S. L., Kaldany, A., Kahn, C. R., et al. (1986) Acquired defect in interleukin-2 production in patients with type 1 diabetes mellitus. *N. Engl. J. Med.* **315**, 920–924.

78. Dosch, H.-M., Cheung, R. K., Karges, W., Pietropaolo, M., and Becker, D. J. (1999) Persistent T cell anergy in human type 1 diabetes. *J. Immunol.* **163,** 6933–6940.

79. Miyazaki, I., Cheung, R. K., Gaedigk, R., Hui, M. F., Van der Meulin, J., Rajotte, R. V., et al. (1995) T cell activation and anergy to islet cell antigen in type 1 diabetes. *J. Immunol.* **154,** 1461–1469.

80. Nervi, S., Atlan-Gepner, C., Fossat, C., and Vialettes, B. (1999) Constitutive impaired TCR/CD3-mediated activation of T cells in IDDM patients co-exist with normal costimulation pathways. *J. Autoimmun.* **13,** 247–255.

81. Bendelac, A., Rivera, M. N., Park, H.-S., and Roark, J. H. (1997) Mouse CD1-specific NK1 T cells: development, specificity, and function. *Ann. Rev. Immunol.* **15,** 535–562.

82. Bendelac, A., Lantz, O., Quimby, M. E., Yewdell, J. W., Bennink, J. R., and Brutkiewicz, R. R. (1995) CD1 recognition by mouse NK1+ T lymphocytes. *Science* **268,** 863–865.

83. Tamada, K., Harada, M., Abe, K., Li, T., Tada, H., Onoe, Y., et al. (1997) Immunosuppressive activity of cloned natural killer (NK1.1+) T cells established from murine tumor-infiltrating lymphocytes. *J. Immunol.* **158,** 4846–4854.

84. Yoshimoto, T. and Paul, W. (1994) CD4+NK1.1+ T cells promptly produce interleukin 4 in response to in vivo challenge with anti-CD-3. *J. Exp. Med.* **179,** 1285–1295.

85. Yoshimoto, T., Bendelac, A., Watson, C., Hu-Li, J., and Paul, W. E. (1995) Role of NK1.1+ T cells in a Th2 response and in immunoglobulin E production. *Science* **270,** 1845–1847.

86. Brown, D. R., Fowell, D. J., Corry, D. B., Wynn, T. A., Moskowitz, N. H., Cheever, A. W., et al. (1996) β2-microglobulin-dependent NK1.1+ T cells are not essential for T helper cell 2 immune responses. *J. Exp. Med.* **184,** 1295–1304.

87. Smiley, S. T., Kaplan, M. H., and Grusby, M. J. (1997) Immunoglobulin E production in the absence of interleukin-4-secreting CD1-dependent cells. *Science* **275,** 977–979.

88. Mendiratta, S. K., Martin, W. D., Hong, S., Boesteanu, A., Joyce, S., and Van Kaer, L. (1997) *CD1d1* mutant mice are deficient in natural T cells that promptly produce IL-4. *Immunity* **6,** 469–477.

89. Chen, Y.-H., Chiu, N. M., Mandal, M., Wang, N., and Wang, C.-R. (1997) Impaired NK1+ T cell development and early IL-4 production in CD1-deficient mice. *Immunity* **6,** 459–467.

90. Porcelli, S., Yockey, C. E., Brenner, M. B., and Balk, S. P. (1993) Analysis of T cell antigen receptor (TCR) expression by human peripheral blood CD4-8- α/β T cells demonstrates preferential use of several Vβ genes and an invariant TCR α chain. *J. Exp. Med.* **178,** 1–16.

91. Porcelli, S., Gerdes, D., Fertig, A., and Balk, S. (1996) Human T cells expressing an invariant Vα24JαQ TCRα are CD4-negative and heterogeneous with respect to TCRβ expression. *Human Immunol.* **48,** 63–67.

92. Masuda, K., Makino, Y., Cui, J., Ito, T., Tokuhisa, T., Takahama, Y., et al. (1997) Phenotypes and invariant αβ TCR expression of peripheral Vα14+ NK T cells. *J. Immunol.* **158,** 2076–2082.

93. Joyce, S., Woods, A. S., Yewdell, J. W., Bennink, J. R., De Silva, A. D., Boesteanu, A., et al. (1998) Natural ligand of mouse CD1d1: cellular glycosylphosphatidylinositol. *Science* **279**, 1541–1544.

94. Kawano, T., Cui, J., Koezuka, Y., Toura, I., Kaneko, Y., Motoki, K., et al. (1997) CD1d-restricted and TCR-mediated activation of Vα14 NKT cells by glycosylceramides. *Science* **278**, 1626–1629.

95. Brossay, L., Chioda, M., Burdin, N., Koezuka, Y., Casorati, G., Dellabona, P., et al. (1998) CD1d-mediated recognition of an a-Galactosylceramide by natural killer T cells is highly conserved through mammalian evolution. *J. Exp. Med.* **188**, 1521–1528.

96. Spada, F. M., Koezuka, Y., and Porcelli, S. A. (1998) CD1d-restricted recognition of synthetic glycolipid antigens by human killer T cells. *J. Exp. Med.* **188**, 1529–1534.

97. Zeng, Z.-H., Castano, A. R., Segelke, B. W., Stura, E. A., Peterson, P. A., and Wilson, I. A. (1997) Crystal structure of mouse CD1: MHC-like fold with a large hydrophobic binding groove. *Science* **277**, 339–345.

98. Gumperz, J. E., Roy, C., Makowska, A., Lum, D., Sugita, M., Podrebarac, T., et al. (2000) Murine CD1d-restricted T cell recogition of cellular lipids. *Immunity* **12**, 211–221.

99. Chen, H. and Paul, W. (1997) Cultured NK1.1+CD4+ T cells produce large amounts of IL-4 and IFN-γ upon activation by anti-CD3 or CD1. *J. Immunol.* **159**, 2240–2249.

100. Bendelac, A. (1995) CD1: presenting unusual antigens to unusual T lymphocytes. *Science* **269**, 185,186.

101. Behar, S. M., Podrebarac, T. A., Roy, C. J., Wang, C. R., and Brenner, M. B. (1999) Diverse TCRs recognize murine CD1. *J. Immunol.* **162**, 161–167.

102. Cardell, S., Tangri, S., Chan, S., Kronenberg, M., Benoist, C., and Mathis, D. (1995) CD1-restricted CD4+ T cells in major histocompatibility complex class II-deficient mice. *J. Exp. Med.* **182**, 993–1004.

103. Chiu, Y.-H., Jayawardena, J., Weiss, A., Lee, D., Park, S.-H., Varsat-Dautry, A., and Bendelac, A. (1999) Distinct subsets of CD1d-restricted T cells recognize self-antigens loaded in different cellular compartments. *J. Exp. Med.* **189**, 103–110.

104. Exley, M., Garcia, J., Balk, S. P., and Porcelli, S. (1997) Requirements for CD1d recognition by human invariant Vα24JαQ+ NKR-P1A+ T cells. *J. Exp. Med.* **186**, 109–120.

105. Davodeau, F., Peyrat, M.-A., Necker, A., Dominici, R., Blanchard, F., et al. (1997) Close phenotypic and functional similarities between human and murine αβ T cells expressing invariant TCR-α chains. *J. Immunol.* **158**, 5603–5611.

106. Kent, S. C., Hafler, D. A., Strominger, J. L., and Wilson, S. B. (1999) Noncanonical Vα24JαQ T cells with conservative a chain CDR3 region amino acid substitutions are restricted by CD1d. *Human Immunol.* **60**, 1080–1089.

107. Park, S. H., Roark, J. H., and Bendelac, A. 1998. Tissue-specific recognition of mouse CD1 molecules. *J. Immunol.* **160**, 3128–3134.

108. Garboczi, D. N., Ghosh, P., Utz, U., Fan, Q. R., Biddison, W. E., and Wiley, D. C. (1996) Structure of the complex between human T cell receptor, viral peptide and HLA-A2. *Nature* **384**, 134–141.

109. Balk, S. P., Ebert, E. C., Blumenthal, R. L., McDermott, F. V., Wucherfennig, K. W., Landau, S. B., et al. (1991) Oligoclonal expansion and CD1 recognition by human intestinal intraepithelial lymphocytes. *Science* **253,** 1411–1415.

110. Blumberg, R. S., Terhorst, C., Bleicher, P., McDermott, F. V., Allan, C. H., Landau, S. B., et al. (1991) Expression of a nonpolymorphic MHC classI-like molecule, CD1D, by human intestinal epithelial cells. *J. Immunol.* **147,** 2518–2524.

111. Cui, J., Shin, T., Kawano, T., Sato, H., Kondo, E., Toura, I., et al. (1997) Requirement for Vα14 NKT cells in IL-12-mediated rejection of tumors. *Science* **278,** 1623–1626.

112. Nakamura, E., Kubota, H., Sato, M., Sugie, T., Yoshida, O., and Minato, N. (1997) Involvement of NK1+ CD4- CD8- αβ T cells and endogenous IL-4 in non-MHC-restricted rejection of embryonal carcinoma in genetically resistant mice. *J. Immunol.* **158,** 5338–5348.

113. Mieza, M. A., Itoh, T., Cui, J. Q., Makino, Y., Kawano, T., Tsuchida, K., et al. (1996) Selective reduction of Vα14+ NK T cells associated with disease development in autoimmune-prone mice. *J. Immunol.* **156,** 4035–4040.

114. Zeng, D., Dick, M., Cheng, L., Amano, M., Dejbakhsh-Jones, S., Huie, P., et al. (1998) Subsets of transgenic T cells that recognize CD1 induce or prevent murine lupus: role of cytokines. *J. Exp. Med.* **187,** 525–582.

115. Hammond, K. J. L., Poulton, L. D., Palmisano, L. J., Silveira, P. A., Godfrey, D. I., and Baxter, A. G. (1998) α/β-T cell receptor (TCR)+CD4-CD8- (NKT) thymocytes prevent insulin-dependent diabetes mellitus in nonobese diabetic (NOD)/Lt mice by the influence of interleukin (IL)-4 and/or IL-10. *J. Exp. Med.* **187,** 1047–1056.

116. Baxter, A. G., Kinder, S. J., Hammond, K. J. L., Scollay, R., and Godfrey, D. I. (1997) Association between αβTCR+CD4-CD8- T cell deficiency and IDDM in NOD/Lt mice. *Diabetes* **46,** 572–582.

117. Iwakoshi, N. N., Greiner, D. L., Rossini, A. A., and Mordes, J. P. (1999) Diabetes prone BB rats are severly deficient in natural killer T cells. *Autoimmunity* **31,** 1–14.

118. Tori, M., Ito, T., Yumiba, T., Ohkawa, A., Maeda, A., Sawai, T., et al. (1999) Proliferation of donor-derived NKR-P1A(+) TCR alpha beta (+) (NK T) cells in the nonrecurrent spontaneous diabetic BB rats transplanted with pancreaticoduodenal grafts of Wistar Furth donors. *Transplant. Proc.* **31,** 2741–2742.

119. Tori, M., Ito, T., Yumiba, T., Maeda, A., Sawai, T., Miyasaka, M., et al. (1999) Significant role of intragraft lymphoid tissues in preventing insulin-dependent diabetes mellitus recurrence in whole pancreaticoduodenal transplantation. *Microsurgery* **19,** 338–343.

120. Tori, M., Ito, T., Yumiba, T., Ohkawa, A., Maeda, A., Sawai, T., et al. (1999) IL-4 production in IDDM-nonrecurrent pancreas-transplanted BB rats with donor-derived NKR-P1A(+) TCR alpha beta (+) (NK T) cells, but not in IDDM-recurrent BB rats. *Transplant. Proc.* **31,** 1940,1941.

121. Sumida, T., Sakamoto, A., Murata, H., Makino, Y., Takahashi, H., Yoshida, S., et al. (1995) Selective reduction of T cells bearing invariant Vα24JαQ antigen receptor in patients with systemic sclerosis. *J. Exp. Med.* **182,** 1163–1168.

122. Maeda, T., Keino, H., Ashara, H., Taniguichi, M., Nishioka, K., and Sumida, T. (1999) Decreased TCR AV24AJ18(+) double-negative T cells in rheumatoid synovium. *Rheumatology* **38,** 186–188.

123. Vicari, A. P. and Zlotnik, A. (1996) Mouse NK1.1+ T cells: a new family of T cells. *Immunol. Today* **17,** 71–76.

124. Nicol, A., Nieda, M., Koezuka, Y., Porcelli, S., Suzuki, K., Tadokoro, K., et al. (2000) Dendritic cells are targets for human invariant V alpha 24+ natural killer T cell cytotoxic activity: an important immune regulatory function. *Exp. Hematol.* **28,** 276–282.

13

Cytokines in Human Rheumatoid Arthritis and Murine Models

Marie Wahren-Herlenius, Helena Erlandsson Harris, Per Larsson, and Lars Klareskog

1. INTRODUCTION

Rheumatoid arthritis (RA) is a disease that mainly, but not exclusively, affects diarthrodial joints with inflammation in the synovial tissue as an early manifestation. This synovial inflammation is commonly followed by a destruction of adjacent cartilage and bone, resulting in the typical erosions that constitute one of the diagnostic criteria for RA. Being a common and severe disease, the synovial inflammation in RA has been subject to a continuous analysis concerning specificity and regulation of immune and inflammatory reactions assumed to cause the inflammation and destruction. The synovial tissue and fluid are relatively readily accessible for detailed analysis, and in particular during recent years, the RA synovial inflammation has also constituted a "first case for analysis" when basic immunology has provided tools to analyze new molecular mechanisms in immunologic diseases in humans. This has contributed to the fact that some of the most interesting new concepts for immunotherapy in human immunologic disease have been tried most extensively in RA.

Two issues have constantly been in focus of investigations of the inflammation in RA: what causes the inflammation to be selective for joints, and what are the mechanisms responsible for regulating the inflammation, determining among other things its chronicity and destructivity? Classically, it has been assumed that selective T and/or B cell immunity account for the tissue specificity, whereas cytokines and other regulatory molecules would mainly determine the intensity and character of the inflammation, in similar ways in different target tissues. Both these concepts are, however, currently challenged. Concerning organ selectivity of the inflammation, there is

From: *Cytokines and Autoimmune Diseases*
Edited by: V. K. Kuchroo, et al. © Humana Press Inc., Totowa, NJ

increasing evidence that selective autoimmunity may not always be needed to cause arthritis; selective inflammation in joints can be caused by systemic challenges with nonimmunogenic adjuvants *(1)*, with antibodies reactive with ubiquitous antigens *(2)* as well as after systemic overexpression of tumor necrosis factor-α (TNF-α) *(3)*. Also, the contributions of various inflammatory molecules, particularly cytokines, in organ-specific inflammation may vary considerably between various tissue-specific inflammatory diseases.

Consequences of these more recent insights are obviously that expression and regulation of cytokines and other regulatory molecules need to be studied separately and in detail in inflammatory diseases affecting different organs, and that targeting of regulatory molecules may be more useful for selective immunotherapy than was earlier thought to be the case. Another evident implication is that experimental models being used to investigate pathogenesis and therapies for diseases like RA need to be scrutinized in detail concerning the expression and regulatory functions of molecules such as cytokines.

Against this background, the present chapter has as one of its major aims to describe in some detail the expression and known regulatory roles of major cytokines in RA on one hand, and in the most important animal models for RA on the other hand. To facilitate the understanding of the complex networks, the cytokines are tentatively divided into pro- and inflammatory cytokines, and cytokines with both properties.

2. CYTOKINES IN RHEUMATOID ARTHRITIS

Studies aimed at understanding the role of various cytokines in the pathogenesis of RA are faced with a number of difficulties. First, it is not known to which extent the clinical conditions that are defined under the name RA make use of similar or dissimilar patterns of cytokines during the development of synovitis. Thus, both descriptive and more analytical studies need to be performed in a relatively large number of patients with varying disease courses. This notion is examplified by the recent finding from our own laboratory of large variations between individual patients concerning the expression of TNF-α in the inflamed synovium *(4)*, which indicates that considerable differences may exist between patients concerning the dependence on TNF-α in the pathogenesis.

Second, both descriptive and analytical studies need to be performed at different stages of disease development as the relative role of different cytokines may vary significantly between different stages of disease, which has been shown to be the case in animal models of RA. This is emphasized by the fact that the cellular composition of the pannus tissue developing at

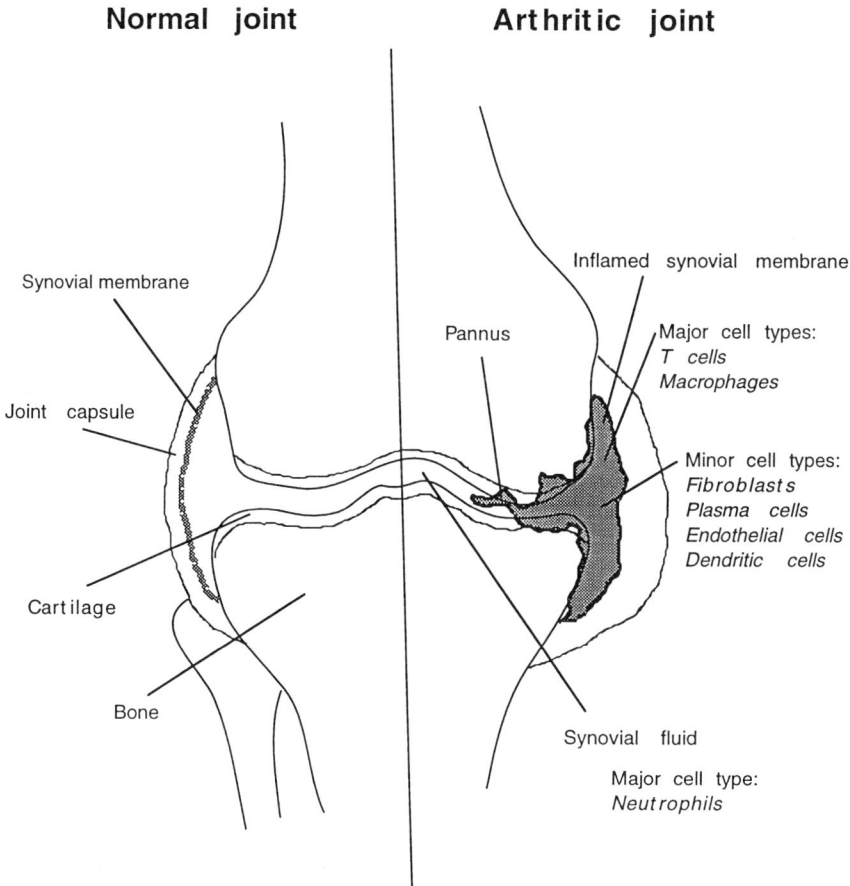

Fig. 1. Schematic illustration of the joint. The cartilage surface is smooth in the normal joint (*left*). In the rheumatic joint (*right*) the cartilage surface is covered by pannus containing mainly T cells and macrophages, but also fibroblasts, plasma cells, and dendritic cells. Angiogenesis is seen. The synovial fluid contains mainly neutrophils.

later stages of disease differs from the cellular composition within synovial villi (Fig. 1). There is also clear evidence from experimental animal studies that chronicity of disease may be regulated by genes that do not necessarily influence susceptibility to disease or severity of early phases of the disease. Studies therefore should include analysis of synovial biopsies taken at various stages of disease in order to permit an understanding of its dynamics.

Third, hypotheses on the pathogenetic and functional role of various cytokines are mainly formed from descriptive studies on the expression of these cytokines in inflamed tissue at various, often late phases of disease and from functional in vitro studies on synovial cells. However, any such hypothesis needs to be verified in vivo. In order to do so, one is in most cases obliged to use animal models with similarities to the human situation in the aspects that are to be investigated. An interesting example was the hypothesis that T cells and T cell cytokines were of less importance in RA, based on the findings of relative paucity of T cell-derived cytokines as opposed to monokines in the rheumatoid synovitis. Subsequently, however, it was demonstrated that similar relationships between few cells producing T cell-derived cytokines and many cells producing monokines could be observed in collagen-induced arthritis (CIA) in mice, where it had earlier been unambigously demonstrated that T cells are necessary for the disease to develop *(5)*.

Most importantly for pathogenetically oriented research in RA, possibilities for in vivo verification of pathogenetic principles are now becoming available in humans with the introduction of targeted therapies directed against both particular cells and distinct cytokines. The new possibilities given to analyze pathogenetic questions during use of targeted therapies such as TNF-blockade will be discussed in a separate section.

2.1. Expression and Function of Individual Cytokines

2.1.1. Proinflammatory Cytokines

2.1.1.1. TNF-α

TNF-α is a macrophage- and T cell-derived cytokine with multiple pro-inflammatory effects. It was early shown to be present in relatively large amounts in the synovial fluid of RA patients *(6)*. Subsequently, it has been shown both that the presence of TNF-α in synovial-joint biopsies may vary considerably between different patients, and that presence of TNF-α is most marked close to the site where the bone and cartilage destruction takes place, i.e., in the pannus region. Polymorphic alleles of TNF-α exist, but no disease association with any particular allele has yet been demonstrated *(7–9)*.

TNF-α has a central role in cytokine networks by regulating other proinflammatory cytokines; interleukin-1 (IL-1), IL-6, and granulocyte-macrophage colony-stimulating factor (GM-CSF) *(10–12)*. In addition, TNF-α upregulates expression of adhesion molecules on vascular endothelial cells and is chemotactic for monocytes and neutrophils, leading to accumulation of the inflammatory cells in the synovium. TNF-α stimulates collagenase and prostaglandin E production, induces cartilage and bone destruction in cell cultures *(13)*, and can activate osteoclasts *(14)*. Interestingly, the hyporesponsiveness of synovial T cells has been reported to depend at least partially on chronic TNF-α signaling *(15)*.

Levels of the soluble TNF-α receptor are increased in the inflamed RA joint *(16)*. These receptors function as natural inhibitors of TNF-α, binding the soluble cytokine and thereby blocking its interaction with cell-surface receptors. The amount of soluble TNF receptors detected in RA joints has been estimated to have the capacity of blocking approximately half of the TNF-α activity *(17)*.

2.1.1.2. IL-1

The proinflammatory cytokine IL-1 exists in two forms, IL-1α and -β. They bind to the same receptor and have similar activities. IL-1 expressed in RA synovium is synthesized mainly by macrophages and fibroblasts and to some extent by neutrophils *(18–20)*, and production of IL-1 by cultured synovial cells has been detected in vitro *(21)*. IL-1α is not detected in synovial fluid or plasma *(22,23)*, since it is secreted poorly from the cells. IL-1β is the main secreted form.

One of the proinflammatory effects of IL-1 in RA is to induce prostaglandin E and collagenase production in synovial cells *(24)*. Stimulation of proteoglycan, glycosaminoglycan synthesis, and matrix metalloproteinase-1 (MMP-1) expression has been reported *(25–27)*, and an important role for IL-1 in the pathogenesis of RA seems to be its promotion of bone resorbtion *(28)*. In synoviocytes IL-1 also upregulates the expression of other cytokines such as GM-CSF *(29)* and IL-6 *(11)*. In addition, IL-1 increases expression of collagen types I and III in chondrocytes *(30)* and induces fever and production of acute-phase proteins.

A natural inhibitor of IL-1, the IL-1 receptor antagonist (IL-1ra) can be detected in the joints of patients with RA *(31,32)*. IL-1ra is homologous to IL-1α and IL-1β with a high affinity for the membrane bound IL-1 receptor and acts through competitive binding *(33)*. However, because IL-1 activates the cell at very low receptor occupancy, a 10- to 100-fold excess of IL-1ra is needed to block the effects of IL-1 *(34)*, and levels of IL-1ra in RA are around one- to fourfold excess.

2.1.1.3. IL-6

IL-6 is produced by T cells, fibroblasts, and macrophages. Most IL-6 is produced by macrophages in RA *(35,36)*. It possesses proinflammatory properties and augments many actions directly induced by IL-1 and TNF-α.

High levels of IL-6 are present in synovial fluid of patients with RA, and serum levels of IL-6 in RA correlate with markers assessing disease activity such as acute-phase proteins *(22,37,38)*. IL-6 is also produced by synovial cells in vitro *(11)*. IL-6 can stimulate B cell proliferation and immunoglobulin production, properties that might be of importance for rheumatoid factor secretion in the synovium. IL-6 also enhances acute-phase protein secretion by the liver and can induce osteoclast differentiation from hematopoietic precursors *(39)*.

2.1.1.4. IL-8

Expression of IL-8 has been identified in RA *(40)*, and cells producing IL-8 localizes to the synovial membrane and cartilage-pannus junction *(41)*.

2.1.1.5. GM-CSF

GM-CSF can be detected in rheumatoid joints. Cultured synovial macrophages also produce GM-CSF *(12,29,42)*. GM-CSF activates macrophages to produce proinflammatory cytokines and can induce differentiation of myeloid cells, whereby the number of mature macrophages in the inflamed synovium increases *(43)*. Addition of anti-GM-CSF monoclonal antibodies (MAbs) to synovial-tissue cultures downregulates human leukocyte antigen DR (HLA-DR) expression by monocytes. This can be interpreted as GM-CSF contributing to the increased expression of MHC class II molecules by synovial macrophages *(44)*.

2.1.1.6. IL-15

In the rheumatoid joint, IL-15 is expressed by synovial-lining cells, macrophages, fibroblasts, and within lymphocytic aggregates *(45)*. In RA, locally produced IL-15 can recruit and activate synovial T cells and induce monocyte-derived TNF-α production *(46)*. Levels of IL-15 correlate with TNF-α activity, and have been shown to be necessary to maintain the production of TNF-α in culture *(46)*.

IL-15 can induce T cell proliferation, and because little IL-2 is present in the rheumatoid joint IL-15 might be an important local T cell mitogenic factor.

2.1.1.7. IL-16

IL-16 has been recorded in synovial fluid from RA patients and IL-16 transcripts demonstrated in the synovial membrane. *In situ* hybridization has revealed IL-16 mRNA-expressing cells in the lining layer of rheumatoid synovial tissue. In the sublining area, only scattered cells positive for IL-16 transcripts could be detected, mainly located adjacent to blood vessels *(47)*.

IL-16 has chemoattractant properties *(48,49)* and can induce migration of CD4[+] cells into sites of inflammation *(50,51)*. Evidence exists that IL-16 uses the CD4 molecule as its receptor. IL-16 stimulates expression of the IL-2 receptor and MHC class II molecules on resting cells *(51)*. An inhibitory effect of IL-16 on CD3/TCR-mediated lymphocyte activation has also been described *(52,53)*. These seemingly contradictory functions of IL-16 may in fact add to the understanding of the pathopysiological findings in RA as a complex disease in which anergy and inflammation occur at the same time.

2.1.1.8. IL-17

The T cell-derived cytokine IL-17 is produced at high levels in RA synovium *(54)*. Around 1% of the T cells express IL-17, comparable to results with IFN-γ *(55)*. Th1 and Th0 cells derived from RA synovial tissue produce IL-17 in vitro *(56)*. Its production is downregulated by IL-4 and IL-13 *(57)*. IL-17 contributes to the inflammatory conditions in the rheumatoid joint by stimulating production of proinflammatory cytokines such as IL-6, IL-1, and TNF-α *(58)*.

2.1.1.9. IL-18

IL-18 is localized primarily to lymphocytic aggregates in the RA synovia, where it is produced mainly by activated macrophages *(59)*. Significant IL-18 levels can be detected in synovial fluid of RA joints. IL-18 has been demonstrated to induce IFN-γ production together with IL-12 or IL-15 and to independently promote GM-CSF and nitric oxide (NO) production by synovial tissues in vitro. IL-18 also induces TNF-α synthesis by macrophages in synovial cultures *(59)*.

IL-18 inhibits osteoclast formation in vitro, independent of IFN-γ production, an effect that can be abolished by addition of neutralizing antibodies to GM-CSF *(60)*.

2.1.2. Anti-Inflammatory Cytokines

2.1.2.1. IL-10

IL-10 is primarily produced by monocytes and macrophages, but T and B cells also secrete IL-10 after activation. IL-10 has potent anti-inflammatory effects on both T cells and monocyte function. It inhibits T cell proliferation, downregulates antigen-presenting cells (APCs), and accessory-cell function of macrophages *(61–64)*. IL-10 also decreases the production of several pro-inflammatory cytokines by human monocytes in vitro *(63)*.

In the rheumatoid joint, IL-10 is produced locally by synovial monocytes *(65–68)*. IL-10 can be detected in RA synovial fluid, where levels are higher than in serum *(69)*. It is also spontaneously secreted by cultured synovial cells *(65,67,70)*.

IL-10 can shift the balance of IL-1 and IL-1ra production by synoviocytes, favoring IL-1ra production *(71)*. Production of IL-10 by synovial monocytes appears to inhibit local IFN-γ production *(72)*. Addition of recombinant IL-10 to synovial-cell cultures downregulates production of IL-1β and TNF-α and prevents cartilage degradation *(65,70,71,73)*. IL-10 also decreases expression of HLA-DR on synovial fluid macrophages and decreases proliferation of synovial fluid T cells *(70)*.

The anti-inflammatory effects of IL-10 have been further demonstrated by addition of anti-IL-10 antibodies to synovial cell cultures, yielding increased production of the proinflammatory cytokines TNF-α, IL-1β, GM-CSF, and IFN-γ *(65,70)*.

2.1.2.2. IL-4

IL-4 is produced by activated Th2 cells, and was initially reported as absent or expressed in low levels in synovial fluid of RA patients *(74)*. However, in some but not all synovial samples, IL-4 mRNA expression has been detected *(55,75)*. IL-4 was recently also reported to be produced locally in RA synovial biopsies *(76)*, and could also be detected in synovial fluid from RA patients *(77)*, where the number of IL-4 producing mononuclear cells (MNCs) is increased as compared to peripheral blood *(69)*. Also, increased serum levels of IL-4 have been reported in RA patients compared to healthy controls *(78)*. Taken together these findings may be interpreted as challenging the view of RA as a Th1 mediated disease.

IL-4 has anti-inflammatory activity *(79)* and has been shown to inhibit production of proinflammatory cytokines *(80,81)*. IL-4 can shift the balance of IL-1 and IL-1ra production by synoviocytes, in favor of IL-1ra production *(71,82)*. On the other hand, both IL-4 and IL-13 enhance the monocyte MHC II expression *(82)*. IL-4 has also been demonstrated to decrease bone resorption in vitro *(83)*.

2.1.2.3. IL-13

IL-13 shares many of the anti-inflammatory effects of IL-4, and is 30% identical at the protein level. The main producers of IL-13 are activated T cells in the RA synovium. Exogenously applied IL-13 downregulates TNF-α and IL-1β production by synovial-fluid MNCs in vitro *(77,82)*. IL-13, like IL-4 inhibits bone resorption in vitro *(84)*.

2.1.3. Cytokines with Both Anti- and Proinflammatory Properties

2.1.3.1. TGF-β

High levels of transforming growth factor-β (TGF-β) have been measured in synovial fluid and are produced by cultured synovial cells in vitro *(74,85,86)*. TGF-β expression is localized mainly to the synovial lining of synovial membranes, but has also been detected in sublining regions and at the cartilage-pannus junction *(85,87)*.

TGF-β possesses immunoregulatory properties and inhibits lymphocyte proliferation *(88)*. TGF-β can also induce collagen mRNA expression and inhibit collagenase mRNA expression by cultured synoviocytes *(85)*. TGFβ1 appears to be the most important TGF-β cytokine in rheumatoid synovitis *(87,89–91)*. In primary articular chondrocyte cultures, IL-1β induces TGFβ3 protein synthesis but reduces that of TGFβ1 and TGFβ2 isoforms *(91)*. TGF-β is also angiogenic, exerting its effect via recruitment of macrophages, which in turn secrete angiogenic factors acting on endothelial cells *(74,92–94)*. At higher concentrations TGF-β inhibits the angiogenic potential of other factors, revealing its bifunctional role in angiogenesis *(95)*.

2.1.3.2. IL-12

IL-12 promotes IFN-γ production and the generation of Th1 cells. Expression of IL-12 has been detected in rheumatoid joints *(96)*, where it is produced by infiltrating macrophages and synovial lining cells *(97)*.

2.1.3.3. IFN-γ

IFN-γ is a T cell-derived cytokine that can be detected at the mRNA level in RA joints, though protein levels are low *(55,75,98)*. Approximately 1 out of 300 CD3$^+$ T cells in RA synovium expresses IFN-γ mRNA as detected by *in situ* hybridization *(55)*, though there is considerable interpatient variability *(76)*.

In addition to being a potent macrophage activator, IFN-γ directs development of naive T cells into proinflammatory Th1 cells and can induce HLA-DR expression on monocytes. However, anti-IFN-γ antibodies cannot inhibit HLA-DR upregulating activity of synovial fluid. In conjuction with the low levels found in RA tissues, this indicates that IFN-γ may not be the main macrophage-activating factor in RA *(98)*.

2.2. Questions Evolving from Analysis of Cytokine Expression in Human RA

Descriptive studies of the cytokine expression in human RA raises a number of questions. High expression of fibroblast- and macrophage-derived cytokines such as TNF-α, IL-1, IL-6, GM-CSF, and TGF-β is detected in many patients (Fig. 2); cytokines produced by T cells are more scarcely described, even though T cells represent a large proportion of the inflammatory cells invading the synovia. The results from different studies are, however, often in part contradictory, probably reflecting the range of variability between patients and stages of disease. Thus, animal models are essential to answer questions such as the relative importance of T cells and macrophages, and their relevance in different stages of disease, including initial arthritis-inducing events. In addition, such models can increase the understanding of how the cytokine network operates, how it is balanced, and how it can be favorably manipulated.

3. CYTOKINE EXPRESSION IN ANIMAL MODELS OF RA

3.1. Conceptually Different Models

Several experimental models for arthritis have been defined and developed as means of answering the questions arisen from studies in RA patients.

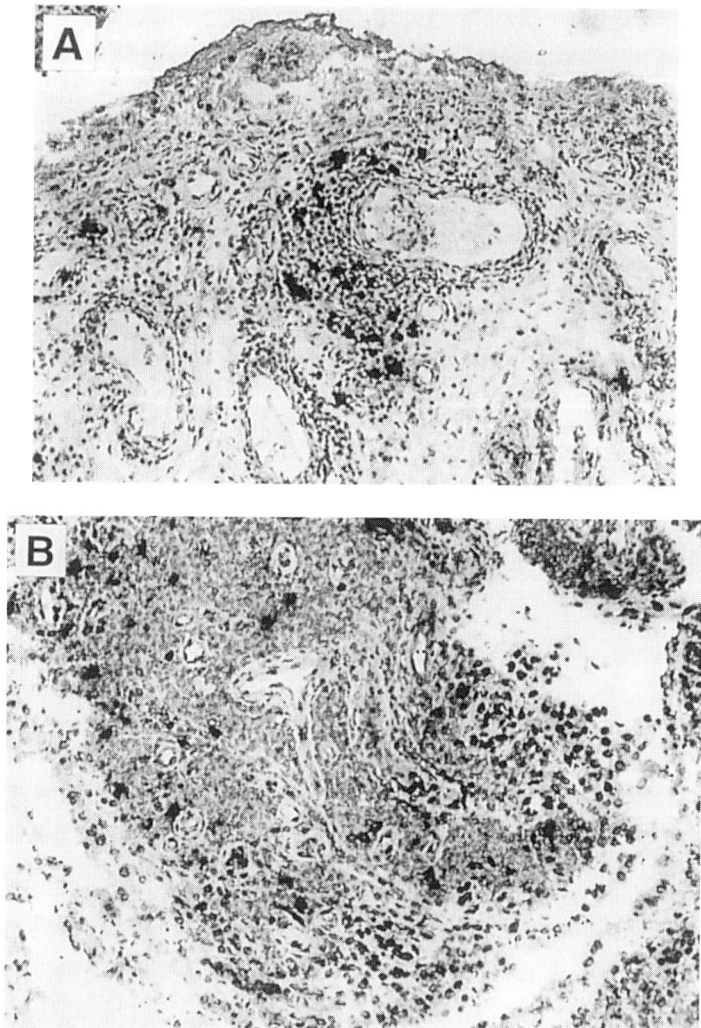

Fig. 2. (A) TNF-α producing cells in a cryopreserved synovial-membrane biopsy specimen arthroscopically obtained from an RA patient. Cells producing TNF-α are detected in the sublining layers in focal infiltrates of mononuclear cells, here clustering around a blood vessel in a perivascular aggregate. Intracellular staining to verify local production was performed after fixation with paraformaldehyde and permeabilization with saponin. Photo: Ann-Kristin Ulfgren. **(B)** IL-1β producing cells in human synovia from a patient with RA biopsised via arthroscopy. Staining of cryosections reveals profuse IL-1β production in the pannus in this patient. Note that the number of cytokine producing cells, including IL-1β and TNF-α, can differ substantially between patients. Photo: Ann-Kristin Ulfgren.

Arthritis models exist in rats, mice, rabbits, and monkeys. They can be divided into models with spontaneously developing disease, induced diseases, and genetically modified models. Most commonly used are the models of induced diseases in rodents (*see* Table 1).

The vast number of experimental rodent models for arthritis, and the different ways that they are provoked, may all reflect various aspects of rheumatoid disease. Many features are similar among the different models, but differences also exist, a significant aspect being that not all models develop chronic disease. It is therefore of importance when comparing results between RA and experimental models to be aware of the experimental model used, and the general features of that particular model. Depending on which aspect of the arthritogenic process one wants to study, care must be taken in chosing the most suitable model.

The role of a certain cytokine as arthritis-promoting can be studied in detail in mice knocked-out for the actual cytokine gene or its receptor. Similarly, transgenic animals with constant overexpression of a certain cytokine are useful tools in dissecting arthritogenic mechanisms *(3)*.

Apart from the models mentioned earlier and in Table 1, the susceptibility of various cytokine/cytokine-receptor knockout mice for induced arthritis has been tested, and are of importance in elucidating the role of a particular cytokine in arthritis development. Later, some experimental models for arthritis that we consider to have been of great impact for the field will be discussed briefly, and then the role of different cytokines in different models will be indicated.

3.1.1. Collagen- and Adjuvant-Induced Arthritides

Adjuvant-induced arthritides and cartilage-antigen-induced arthritides are conceptually different models of RA. Both are T cell dependent *(99,100)* and major histocompatibility complex (MHC)-linked *(101,102)*, features which they share with human RA, and hence are well-suited for studies of T cell dependence and MHC-linkage. The influence of a joint-specific T cell response can be addressed in strains of rats resistant to oil-induced arthritis but susceptible to cartilage antigen-induced arthritis. The lack of a defined antigen responsible for the T cell response in adjuvant arthritides makes it difficult to understand whether cartilage specificity exists in these models or not. The fact however, that substances with adjuvantic properties can cause T cell dependent and MHC-restricted arthritis is worth considering as a possible disease-inducing mechanism in humans as well as in experimental animals. Cytokines expressed in cartilage-antigen-induced and adjuvant-induced arthritis are mainly of a Th1 pattern with high levels of proinflammatory monokines, another feature shared with human RA. On the other hand, a Th2

Table 1
Murine Models for Arthritis

Group division	Experimental model	Type of inocculum	Models in mice	Ref.	Models in rat	Ref.
Spontaneously developing models		Not applicable	NZB/KN Biozzi MRL lpr/lpr DBA/1 males	(180) (181) (182) (183)	No	
Models induced with:						
(a) Infectious agents	Staph. Aureus	Live bacteria	Yes	(184)	Yes	(195)
	Yersinia	Live bacteria	Yes	(185)	Yes	(196)
	Mycobacteria	Live bacteria	Yes	(186)	Yes	(186)
(b) Non-infectious bacterial compunds	Adjuvant-induced	Heat-killed myco-bacteria + mineral oil	No (only if co-treatment with anti-IL-4 Ab)	(187)	Yes	(197)
	LPS-induced	Lipopolysaccharide	No		Yes	(198)
	Streptococcal cell wall-induced	Fragmented strepto-coccal cell walls	Yes	(188)	Yes	(199)
(c) Adjuvants	Oil-induced	Mineral oil (FIA)	No		Yes	(1)
	Pristane-induced	Pristane oil	Yes	(189)	Yes	(102)
	Avridine-induced	Synthetic	No		Yes	(200)
	Squalene-induced	Endogenous mammalian lipid	No		Yes	(198,201)
(d) Systemic + intra-articular antigen-injection		Methylated BSA	Yes	(190)	Yes	(202)

(e) Cartilage antigen	Collagen II-induced	Collagen II + adjuvant	Yes	(191)	Yes	(104)
	Collagen IX-induced	Collagen IX + adjuvant	Yes	(192)	No
	Collagen XI-induced	Collagen XI + adjuvant	Yes	(192)	Yes	(203)
	Cartilage oligomeric matrix protein (COMP)-induced	COMP + adjuvant	No		Yes	(204)
	Proteoglycan-induced	Proteoglycan + adjuvant	Yes	(193)	No
	Cartilage glycoprotein 39	Cartilage glycoprotein 39 + adjuvant	Yes	(194)	No
(f) Other	Mercuric chloride-induced	Mercuric chloride	No		Yes	(103)
Genetically modified animals developing spontaneous arthritis	TNF-α transgene	Not applicable	Yes	(3)	No
	HLA B27 transgene		Yes	(205)	Yes	(207)
	K/B×N(+g)		Yes	(2)	No
	T cell leukemia virus type I transgene		Yes	(206)	No
	IL-1ra knockout		Yes	(123)	No

cytokine production can also promote arthritis, as demonstrated in the model of mercuric chloride-induced arthritis in Brown Norwegian (BN) rats *(103)*.

First described by Trentham et al. in 1977 *(104)*, CIA is probably the most commonly used experimental model for RA. Collagen-induced arthritis can be induced in both rats and mice with heterologous collagen type II, and in one rat strain, Dark Agonti (DA) rats, homologous collagen type II can be used resulting in a true autoimmune model *(105)*. TNF-α is the dominant cytokine in CIA and anti-TNF-α treatment ameliorates CIA *(106,107)*. Despite the well-established T cell dependence in CIA, T cell-derived cytokines are rarely found in the inflamed joints *(5,108)*.

3.1.2. TNF-α Transgenic and TNF-α Knockout Mice

Mice transgenic for the human TNF-α gene and with a constant overexpression of TNF-α have been reported to develop a severe and erosive arthritis *(3,109)*. Few T cells can be detected in the joints of these mice, and the arthritis is probably not T cell dependent since transgenic mice backcrossed to RAG knockouts, which lack functional lymphocytes, develop arthritis *(110)*. A transgenic mouse with only cell-surface bound TNF-α also develops arthritis, indicating that there is no strict need for TNF-α secretion in arthritis development *(111)*. Though the model is not suited for studies of etiologic factors for human RA owing to its lack of T and B cell dependence, these results indicate that TNF-α production induces arthritogenic inflammation. However, the findings that TNF-α p55 receptor knockout mice are susceptible to CIA and TNF-α –/– mice to mycoplasma-induced arthritis *(112)* implies that TNF-α is not essential for arthritis, as it can still develop in animals deprived of TNF-α.

3.1.3. K/BxN Mice

A recent model for arthritis in K/BxN mice has been reported *(2)*. Spontaneous development of chronic, erosive arthritis in mice transgenic for a rearranged TCR recognizing bovine RNase 41-61 peptide crossed onto mice with a NOD background was demonstrated. With the NOD MHC haplotype Ag7 the transgenic TCR recognizes glucose-6-phosphate isomerase, a glycolytic enzyme. Thus, systemic autoimmunity to a ubiquitously expressed self-antigen was demonstrated to lead to joint-specific inflammation. Later the arthritis was proven to be both T and B cell dependent. Once initiated by T cells, pathology is driven almost entirely by immunoglobulins *(113)*. By polymerase chain reaction (PCR), high levels of TNF-α mRNA were detected in synovial fluid, and by enzyme-linked immunosorbent assay (ELISA) high levels of IL-6 were found.

3.2. Proinflammatory Cytokines

The models reflecting most of the human RA features including T cell and MHC-dependence are the collagen- and adjuvant-induced arthritides, and the description of cytokine expression in models of RA has therefore mainly been concentrated to these models.

3.2.1. TNF-α

It is well-established that TNF-α is a mediator of pathology in arthritis. TNF-α is reported to be the most abundant cytokine in CIA *(5,108)*, and is strongly expressed in synovia during the acute phase of antigen-induced arthritis *(114)*. The role of TNF-α in the pathogenesis of CIA in mice has been investigated by administration of the cytokine or its antibody. TNF-α given systemically increased both incidence and disease severity, while anti-TNF-α antibody protected against the development of CIA *(106)*. Several other studies have recorded that anti-TNF-α antibodies given therapeutically will ameliorate joint disease in rodents *(115–117)*. Analogous results have been obtained using IgG-TNF-receptor fusion protein. Mice carrying a modified human TNF-α transgene, as mentioned earlier, develop an erosive arthritis. The arthritis can be prevented with anti-human TNF-α antibody *(3)*.

3.2.2. IL-1

In CIA, IL-1β has been detected in synovial tissues. Compared to TNF-α, the expression of IL-1β occurred later in the disease process *(108)*. Earlier studies have revealed that injection of recombinant human IL-1β can increase the incidence and cause an earlier onset of CIA *(118,119)*. Furthermore, it has been reported that daily administration of a high dose IL-1 receptor antagonist prevented the development of disease, whereas a low dose reduced the incidence and delayed onset *(120)*. It has also been demonstrated that the combination of anti-IL-1α and anti-IL-1β given therapeutically was highly effective in established disease, reducing both inflammation, and cartilage destruction *(121)*. More recently, it was reported that anti IL-1α/β treatment ameliorated both early and full-blown disease; however, the most profound suppression was observed with anti-IL-1β *(122)*. In Streptococcal cell-wall-arthritis, IL-1 has been proposed to play a major role in cartilage destruction while TNF-α affects joint swelling. IL-1 receptor antagonist-deficient mice of a Balb/cA background have been demonstrated to spontaneously develop chronic arthritis, whereas IL-1 receptor antagonist-deficient mice on C57BL/6J background did not develop pathology *(123)*.

3.2.3. IL-2

Antibodies given prophylactically against the IL-2 receptor have proven effective in suppressing CIA *(124)*. This was demonstrated by the fact that disease incidence became lower and disease itself less severe. Though these results are interesting, they must be interpreted in relation to the findings of Müssener et al., who reported that in mice with CIA, no IL-2 expression could be detected in joints at any investigated time-point *(5)*.

3.2.4. IL-6

One report states that IL-6 is heavily expressed together with TNF-α and IFN-γ in synovia during the acute phase of antigen-induced arthritis in mice. This correlates with results from murine CIA, where IL-6 was expressed in a similar pattern to TNF-α. Mihara et al. demonstrated that IL-6 suppressed the development of adjuvant arthritis in rats when administered from the time of adjuvant injection *(125)*. The role of IL-6 in antigen-induced arthritis has also been investigated using IL-6 knockout mice *(126)*. In these mice a more severe cartilage proteoglycan depletion was apparent compared to that seen in normal mice, thus indicating an important role for IL-6 in suppressing the arthritic insult on cartilage *(127)*. CIA has also been induced in IL-6 knockout mice, which resulted in delayed onset and reduced severity of disease *(128)*.

3.2.5. GM-CSF

In a recent study it has been demonstrated that mice treated systemically with GM-CSF 20–25 d after collagen type II immunization had a consistently greater incidence and more rapid onset of disease *(129)*.

3.2.6. IL-15

A profound suppression of the development of CIA was achieved by administration of soluble IL-15 receptor α-chain into DBA/1 mice *(130)*.

3.2.7. IL-17

Increased levels of IL-17 mRNA have been reported in lymph nodes of rats with adjuvant arthritis. No expression in synovial membranes, however, could be detected *(131)*.

3.2.8. IL-18

Coadministration of IL-18 to mice at the same time as immunization with collagen type II/Freund's incomplete adjuvant increased the incidence of arthritis *(132)*.

3.3. Anti-Inflammatory Cytokines

3.3.1. IL-4

No expression of IL-4 mRNA has been detected in draining lymph nodes of rats with either CIA or oil-induced arthritis *(133)*, nor has IL-4 been detected in arthritic limbs of mice with CIA *(5)*. In Streptococcal cell wall-induced arthritis in rats, it has been reported that sustained treatment with IL-4 suppressed the chronic, but not the acute phase of disease *(134)*. A recent study has demonstrated that IL-4 alone did not provoke any effect, and that IL-10 only slightly suppressed CIA. A more pronounced amelioration was observed with the combination of IL-4 and IL-10, both at onset and in established disease *(135)*. However, another recent study demonstrated that systemic administration of IL-4 alone, using vector cells engineered to secrete this protein, significantly reduced incidence and severity of CIA *(136)*.

3.3.2. IL-10

IL-10 treatment of rats and mice with CIA has been recorded to suppress both incidence and the inflammatory process, whereas anti-IL-10 has been reported to trigger the onset and increase the severity of murine CIA. In the IL-10-treated rats, a shift in the IgG2a/IgG1 ratio of anti-collagen antibodies suggests an induction of a Th2 response in these animals *(137–139)*. Similarly, mice infected with an adenovirus construct containing a viral IL-10 gene showed lower incidence and decreased severity of CIA. This effect could be inhibited by treatment with anti-IL-10 antibodies *(140)*.

3.3.3. IL-13

The anti-inflammatory effects of IL-13 on CIA have been explored using systemic administration of IL-13 via injections of vector cells transfected with IL-13 gene-transfected cells (136). With this experimental setup, the arthritis was attenuated.

3.4. Cytokines with Both Anti- and Proinflammatory Properties

3.4.1. TGF-β

Investigation of the expression of precursor TGF-β isoforms in arthritic synovia of rats with CIA reveals an abundant expression of all three isoforms, and the expression increases with time after immunization. It was proposed that TGFβ1 and TGFβ2 might have an active role in the fibrotic changes occurring at later stages of CIA (141). Results obtained in functional in vivo studies of TGF-β are contradictory. It has been reported that local injection of TGFβ1 or TGFβ2 into footpads of normal collagen-immunized rats induced arthritis or accelerated its onset *(89,142,143)*, whereas systemic administration of TGFβ1 had a protective effect on experimental arthritis in rodents *(106,144,145)*. In other words, the effect of TGF-β appears to depend on the route of administration.

3.4.2. IL-12

It has been reported that IL-12 can both suppress and enhance autoimmune disease depending on the adjuvant *(146)*, dose *(147)*, and time *(122)* of administration. In the absence of mycobacteria in the adjuvant (Freund's incomplete adjuvant) the incidence of murine CIA in DBA/1 mice is low (max 30%), whereas immunization with collagen type II in Freund's incomplete adjuvant plus IL-12 or collagen type II in Freund's complete adjuvant results in severe arthritis with an incidence of 100% *(146)*. In contrast, prophylactic systemic administration of high doses of IL-12 ameliorates CIA in DBA/1 mice immunized with collagen type II in Freund's complete adjuvant *(147)*. In another study, the potential role of IL-12 at the onset of arthritis has been evaluated *(148)*. Interestingly, this report indicates that IL-12 has a stimulatory role in early arthritis development, whereas it has a suppressive role in the established phase of CIA. Finally, the role of IL-12 in CIA has also been evaluated in IL-12-deficient mice of the DBA/1 genetic background *(149)*. The data presented in this study demonstrated that both the incidence and severity of disease was reduced in mice unable to produce biologically active IL-12.

3.4.3. IFN-γ

In rats immunized with collagen type II, IFN-γ mRNA could be detected in draining lymph nodes *(133)*. In mice with CIA IFN-γ is expressed in the synovia during early stages of clinical disease. At later stages, the expression has vanished *(5)*. IFN-γ has also been reported to be heavily expressed in synovia during the acute phase of antigen-induced arthritis in mice *(114)*. Opposing effects on CIA have been described for IFN-γ treatment, disease-promoting as well as disease-limiting. Local injection of IFN-γ into the foot-pads of collagen type II-immunized mice accelerates the the onset and increases the severity of the disease *(150)*. Conversely, therapeutic as well as prophylactic treatment with high doses of systemically administred IFN-γ ameliorates CIA *(151)*. A disease-limiting role for endogenous IFN-γ in CIA has been inferred from studies in which anti-IFN-γ treatment was associated with more severe arthritic lesions *(152)*. In another study it was reported that the outcome of anti-IFN-γ treatment in CIA depends on the time of administration, early treatment being associated with reduced severity and late treatment being associated with aggravation of disease *(153)*. Similar complex results have also been reported in adjuvant arthritis *(151,154)*. Interestingly, in two studies it was demonstrated that an accelerated CIA develops in DBA/1 mice lacking IFN-γ receptors *(155,156)*, whereas in another study it was demonstrated that mice lacking interferon regulatory factor-1 develop a less severe arthritis *(157)*. IFN-γ knockout mice were recently reported to have enhanced susceptibility to CIA, an effect that was entirely dependent on IL-12 *(158)*.

3.4.4. IL-5

IL-5 could not be detected in arthritic limbs of mice with CIA *(5)*.

3.5. Concluding Remarks Concerning Cytokine Expression in Animal Models for RA

Arthritis can be induced in a variety of ways in experimental animals, and all of the models mimic human disease in some respect. Most commonly studied is collagen type II arthritis, which can be induced in both rats and mice. This model has several features in common with RA, including MHC-linkage and T cell dependence. In a specific rat strain, DA rats, CIA even becomes chronic if induced by rat collagen type II.

Analyzing the cytokine expression in these models, expression of TNF-α and IL-1 has been demonstrated, findings similar to those in many RA patients. The TNF-α transgenic mouse has been pivotal in understanding that TNF-α might play a central role in development of arthritis, contributing to the rapid development of TNF-α blocking therapies. In addition, IL-1 has been demonstrated to have important arthritogenic properties, with emphasis on joint destruction. Molecules where inhibitory effects on arthritis have been observed are IL-6, IL-10, and IL-4. These understandings and indications may be used for designing novel approaches in treating RA as described later.

4. NEW CYTOKINE-BASED THERAPEUTIC STRATEGIES IN RA

4.1. Specific vs General Therapies

An ideal treatment of RA would be aimed at affecting only disease-inducing cells, and the issue of antigen-specific and autoreactive T cells harboring disease-inducing capacity has been extensively addressed in immunologically oriented rheumatologic research. However, such treatment is presently not an option in human disease, because eventual autoreactive and clonally expanded T cells remain elusive and our knowledge of the pathogenic mechanisms operating at the apex of the disease pyramid is still limited. The design of most novel emerging treatments for diseases such as RA is therefore directed to more general targets of the inflammatory cascade, even though some disease-specificity of cytokines can be distinguished. The disadvantage, owing to their general anti-inflammatory as well as immunoregulatory effects of such treatments, may be induction of systemic immunosuppression and dysregulation leading to side effects such as infections, malignancies, and autoimmunity.

4.2. Therapeutic Strategies

Several ways exist to influence the inflammation causing arthritis by either inhibiting proinflammatory cytokine effects or enhancing anti-inflammatory effects. They include: (1) blocking or neutralizing MAbs directed to the cytokine or its receptor; (2) other exogenous receptor antagonists; (3) cytokine receptor constructs that competitively inhibit the binding of the cytokine to its receptor; (4) molecules that inhibit intracellular signal transduction; and (5) molecules that inhibit cytokine synthesis.

4.3. Cytokine-Based Therapies

Two major achievements have been combined in order to design new strategies for the treatment of RA. First, with increased understanding of the pathophysiology of the inflamed synovial tissue, the inflammatory cells infiltrating the synovial membrane and their secreted products have been identified *(159)*. High-affinity cell-surface receptors as well as secreted receptors capable of binding cytokines indicate a sophisticated regulation of the inflammatory response within the joint tissue and constitute additional potential targets for treatment *(33)*. Second, it is now possible to design hybrid, humanized, or fully human MAbs as well as recombinant cytokines and cytokine-receptor proteins, which may be used for treatment of patients.

4.3.1. TNF-α Inhibition

TNF-α blocking therapy has been demonstrated to effectively suppress the disease activity in many patients with RA. Key findings that led to the choice of TNF-α inhibition as a therapeutic approach was that TNF-α among other proinflammatory cytokines, was produced in excess in the rheumatic joint; TNF-α being produced mainly by macrophages close to areas of cartilage destruction *(160)*, and that blocking of TNF-α in cultures of synovial cells in vitro also caused inhibition of futher production of other proinflammatory molecules such as IL-1 *(161)*. Also, the TNF-α transgenic mouse *(3)* demonstrated development of spontaneous, chronic, and erosive arthritis. Administration of TNF-α blocking antibody could inhibit the development of the joint inflammation in animals with CIA *(106,162)*.

4.3.2. Anti-TNF-α MAbs and TNF-α Receptor Fusion Proteins

A number of clinical trials using TNF-α blocking antibodies in RA have been published. Most trials have enrolled patients with established and active disease. These patients have also been considered more or less refractory to conventional treatment.

The chimeric mouse/human MAb cA2/infliximab is a high-affinity IgG antibody. Good tolerability and clinical improvement was demonstrated in initial studies of patients with refractory RA *(163)*. Significant efficacy compared to placebo has been demonstrated *(164)* and a dose-dependent relationship found. Though higher doses had better effect, the improvement was transient and therefore cA2 infusions repeatedly for extend periods combined with methotrexate therapy has been tried. The results demonstrate that concurrent methotrexate treatment enhances and prolongs clinical response to cA2 *(165,166)*. No increase of severe side effects such as infections, malignancies, or development of lupus-like autoimmune disease was observed, though an increase in mild upper-respiratory airway infections was reported. However, regarding more severe long-term side-effects, the length of the observation period and the number of patients so far treated are not enough to definitely exclude the possibility that TNF-α blocking therapy might increase the risk of, e.g., neoplastic disease.

Soluble TNF receptors (sTNF-R) consist of the shed extracellular portion of TNF receptors. Both the p55 and the p75 sTNFR have been detected in the synovial tissue of the arthritic joint. A recombinant human TNFR Fc fusion protein p75 dimer (rhu sTNFR:Fc/etanercept) has been used in experimental arthritis. It both prevents development and suppresses established CIA in mice *(167)*, and is now being evaluated in clinical trials *(168–170)*. The results demonstrate significant improvement, comparable with that observed in the trials of TNF-α blocking antibodies.

Even though the downregulation of synovial TNF-α formation by systemic anti-TNF-α therapy was recently demonstrated *(171)*, some patients benefit more from the treatment than other. This might be explained by the observed inter-patient variability in intra-articular TNF-α expression *(4)*.

4.3.3. Interleukin-1 Inhibition

IL-1 has been demonstrated to be an important mediator of joint inflammation and destruction in both human and animal arthritis models. The efficacy of IL-1ra in refractory RA has been studied *(172)*. A significant response was observed, although the results on signs and symptoms of arthritis were less impressive than with TNF blockade. However, there was a significant slowing of radiological progression of disease. IL-1ra was well-tolerated in most patients and no major adverse events were observed.

Synovial biopsies from a small cohort of patients participating in the study were obtained demonstrating a reduction in the total number of sublining layer-infiltrating macrophages and T cells, together with a downregulation of the adhesion molecules E-selectin and VCAM-1 *(173)*.

4.3.4. IL-10 Treatment

IL-10 has anti-inflammatory and immunoregulatory properties and suppresses the release of proinflammatory cytokines. In humans, IL-10 induces a depression of monocyte functions. Recombinant human IL-10 has been used in a trial of healthy volunteers demonstrating inhibition of IL-1 and TNF-α production induced by endotoxin *(174)*. rhu IL-10 is currently being tested in RA and a dose-finding study has been completed (175), but so far solid results on efficacy in clinical trials are lacking.

4.3.5. IL-6 Treatment

IL-6 is a proinflammatory cytokine inducing an acute-phase response characterized by an increase of acute-phase protein levels in the blood. High levels of IL-6 are found in the synovial fluid of RA patients, and it correlates with disease activity. In an open study of five patients with RA, administration of murine anti-IL-6 MoAb for 10 d *(176)* was well-tolerated and induced a transient clinical improvement in all patients. Randomized placebo-controlled trials to assess the effectiveness of blocking IL-6 in RA are still lacking.

4.4. Gene Therapy

The emerging concept of gene therapy as a future option for the treatment of RA will only briefly be addressed in this chapter. For a more thorough review of the arguments in favor of gene therapy in experimental and human arthritis *see* refs. *177,178.* Gene therapy has been aimed at transfecting genes, either ex vivo or in vivo, of key inflammatory molecules such as sTNFR (p55 or p75), IL-1ra, or IL-10. Another approach has been to downregulate the production of proinflammatory cytokines via the transcription factor NF-κB, which is essential for transcription of many proinflammatory cytokine-genes. This has been achieved by the use of double-stranded DNA decoys, overexpression of inhibitory protein IκBα, and the application of antisense oligonucleotides complementary to the initiation sites of translation. The problems of local delivery and intracellular uptake of these NF-κB-inhibitory molecules need to be solved before they may be used in human trials, because systemic delivery can be suspected to lead to severe adverse reactions.

Gene therapy has been demonstrated as effective in inhibiting or ameliorating inflammation in experimental models of arthritis. Virally mediated vectors have been used for transfection either ex vivo or in vivo. This induces a transient gene transcription as well as protein synthesis and excretion. A pioneering clinical trial in RA of ex vivo gene transfer to autologous synoviocytes engineered using a retrovirus vector to secrete IL-1ra locally in the joint is under way *(179).*

5. SUMMARY

Many cytokines appear to contribute to the Th1-driven autoimmune disease RA. Based on our current knowledge of the invading inflammatory cells of the rheumatic synovial membrane and their secreted products, new therapies for RA have been developed. Blocking therapies against TNF-α and IL-1 have been successful in experimental models of arthritis and in human RA. Because many other cytokines as well as cytokine-receptor molecules are involved in the inflammatory process leading to joint inflammation and destruction in RA, new blocking therapies directed to other molecules than TNF-α and IL-1 will be of great interest.

REFERENCES

1. Kleinau, S., Erlandsson, H., Holmdahl, R., and Klareskog, L. (1991) Adjuvant oils induce arthritis in the DA rat. I. Characterization of the disease and evidence for an immunological involvement. *J. Autoimmun.* **4,** 871–880.
2. Kouskoff, V., Korganow, A.-S., Duchatelle, V., Degott, C., Benoist, C., and Mathis, D. (1996) Organ-specific disease provoked by systemic autoimmunity. *Cell* **87,** 811–822.
3. Keffer, J., Probert, L., Cazlaris, H., Georgopoulos, S., Kaslaris, E., Kioussis, D., and Kollias, G. (1991) Transgenic mice expressing human tumor necrosis factor: a predictive genetic model of arthritis. *EMBO J.* **10,** 4025–4031.
4. Ulfgren, A.-K., Gröndal, L., Lindblad, S., Khademi, M., Johnell, O., Klareskog, L., and Andersson, U. (2000) Interindividual and intraarticular variation of proinflammatory cytokines in rheumatoid arthritis: potential implication for RA therapy. *Ann. Rheum. Dis.* **59,** 439–447.
5. Müssener, Å., Litton, M. J., Lindroos, E., and Klareskog, L. (1997) Cytokine production in synovial tissue of mice with collagen-induced arthritis. *Eur. J. Immunol.* **107,** 485–493.
6. Saxne, T., Palladino, M. A., Heinegård, D., Talal, N., and Wollheim, F. A. (1988) Detection of tumor necrosis factor alpha but not tumor necrosis factor β in rheumatoid arthritis synovial fluid and serum. *Arthritis Rheum.* **31,** 1041–1045.
7. Wilson, A. G., de Vries, N., Pociot, F., di Giovine, F. S., van der Putte, L. B., and Duff, G. W. (1993) An allelic polymorphism within the human tumor necrosis factor alpha promotor region is strongly associated with HLA A1, B8, and DR3 alleles. *J. Exp. Med.* **177,** 557–560.
8. Brinkman, B. M., Giphart, M. J., Verhoef, A., Kaijzel, E. L., Naipal, A. M., Daha, M. R., et al. (1994) Tumor necrosis factor alpha-308 gene variants in relation to major histocompatibility complex alleles and Felty's syndrome. *Human Immunol.* **41,** 259–266.
9. Brinkman, B. M., Huizinga, T. W., Kurban, S. S., van der Velde, E. A., Schreuder, G. M., Hazes, J. M., et al. (1997) Tumor necrosis factor alpha gene polymorphisms in rheumatoid arthritis: association with susceptibility to, or severity of, disease? *Br. J. Rheumatol.* **36,** 516–521.
10. Brennan, F. M., Chantry, D., Jackson, A. M., Maini, R. N., and Feldman, M. (1989) Cytokine production in culture by cells isolated from the synovial membrane. *J. Autoimmun.* **2,** 177–186.
11. Guerne, P.-A., Zuraw, B. L., Vaughan, J. H., Carson, D. A., and Lotz, M. (1988) Synovium as a source of interleukin-6 *in vitro*. Contributions to local and systemic manifestation of arthritis. *J. Clin. Invest.* **83,** 585–592.

12. Haworth, C., Brennan, F. M., Chantry, D., Turner, M., Maini, R. N., and Feldmann, M. (1991) Expression of granulocyte-macrophage colony-stimulating factor in rheumatoid arthritis: regulation by tumor necrosis factor-alpha. *Eur. J. Immunol.* **21,** 2575–2579.

13. Dayer, J. M., Beutler, B., and Cerami, A. (1985) Cachectin/tumor necrosis factor stimulates collagenase and prostaglandin E2 production by human synovial cells and dermal fibroblasts. *J. Exp. Med.* **162,** 2163–2168.

14. Bertolini, D. R., Nedwin, G. E., Bringman, T. S., Smith, D. D., and Mundy, G. R. (1986) Stimulation of bone resorption and inhibition of bone formation *in vitro* by human tumor necrosis factors. *Nature.* **319,** 516–518.

15. Lai, N. S., Lan, J. L., Yu, C. L., and Lin, R. H. (1995) Role of tumor necrosis factor-alpha in the regulation of activated synovial T cell growth: down-regulation of synovial T cells in rheumatoid arthritis patients. *J. Immunol.* **25,** 3243–3248.

16. Cope, A. P., Aderka, D., Doherty, M., Engelmann, H., Gibbons, D., Jones, A. C., et al. (1992) Increased levels of soluble tumor necrosis factor receptors in the sera and synovial fluid of patients with rheumatic diseases. *Arthritis Rheum.* **35,** 1160–1169.

17. Brennan, F. M., Gibbons, D. L., Cope, A. P., Katsikis, P., Maini, R. N., and Feldmann, M. (1995) TNF inhibitors are produced spontaneously by rheumatoid and osteoarthritis synovial joint cell cultures: evidence of feedback control of TNF action. *Scand. J. Immunol.* **42,** 158–165.

18. Fontana, A., Hengartner, H., Weber, E., Fehr, K., Grob, P. J., and Cohen, G. (1982) Interleukin-1 activity in the synovial fluid of patients with rheumatoid arthritis. *Rheumatol. Int.* **2,** 49–53.

19. Firestein, G., Alvaro-Garcia, J., and Maki, R. (1990) Quantitative analysis of cytokine gene expression in rheumatoidarthritis. *J. Immunol.* **144,** 3347–3353.

20. Quale, J. A., Adams, S., Bucknall, R. C., and Edwards, S. W. (1995) Interleukin-1 expression by neutrophils in rheumatoid arthritis. *Ann. Rhem. Dis.* **54,** 930–933.

21. Miyasaka, N., Sato, K., Goto, M., Sasano, M., Natsuyama, M., Inoue, K., and Nishioka, K. (1988) Augmented interleukin-1 production and HLA-DR expression in the synovium of rheumatoid arthritis patients. Possible involvement in joint destruction. *Arthritis Rheum.* **31,** 480–486.

22. Holt, I., Cooper, R. G., Denton, J., Meager, A., and Hopkins, S. J. (1992) Cytokine inter-relationships and their association with disease activity in arthritis. *Br. J. Rheumatol.* **31,** 725–733.

23. McNiff, P. A., Stewart, C., Sullivan, J., Showell, H. J., and Gabel, C. A. (1995) Synovial fluid from rheumatoid arthritis patients contains sufficient levles of IL-1β and IL-6 to promote production of serum amyloid A by Hep3B cells. *Cytokine* **7,** 209–219.

24. Dayer, J.-M., de Rochemonteix, B., Burrus, B., Demczuk, S., and Dinarello, C. A. (1986) Human recombinant interleukin 1 stimulates collagenase and prostaglandin E2 production by human synovial cells. *J. Clin. Invest.* **77,** 645–648.

25. Yaron, I., Meyer, F. A., Dayer, J. M., and Yaron, M. (1987) Human recombinant interleukin-1 beta stimulates glycosaminoglycan production in human synovial fibroblast cultures. *Arthritis Rheum.* **30,** 424–430.

26. McCachren, S. S., Greer, P. K., and Niedel, J. E. (1989) Regulation of human synovial fibroblast collagenase messenger RNA by interleukin-1. *Arthritis Rheum.* **32,** 1539–1545.

27. Arner, E. C. and Pratta, M. A. (1989) Independent effects of interleukin-1 on proteoglycan breakdown, proteoglycan synthesis, and prostaglandin E2 release from cartilage in organ culture. *Arthritis Rheum.* **32,** 288–297.

28. Gowen, M., Wood, D. D., Ihrie, E. J., McGuire, M. K. B., and Russell, G. G. (1983) An interleukin-1 like factor stimulates bone resorption *in vitro.* *Nature.* **306,** 378–380.

29. Alvaro-Gracia, J. M., Zvaifler, N. J., Brown, C. B., Kaushansky, K., and Firestein, G. S. (1991) Cytokines in chronic inflammatory arthritis. IV. Analysis of the synovial cells involved in granulocyte-macrophage colony-stimulating factor production and gene expression in rheumatoid arthritis and its regulation by IL-1 and tumor necrosis factor-alpha. *J. Immunol.* **146,** 3365–3371.

30. Goldring, M. B., Birkhead, J., Sandell, L. J., Kimura, T., and Krane, S. M. (1988) Interleukin 1 suppresses expression of cartilage-specific types II and IX collagens and increases types I and III collagens in human chondrocytes. *J. Clin. Invest.* **82,** 2026–2037.

31. Firestein, G. S., Berger, A. E., Tracey, D. E., Chosay, J. G., Chapman, D. L., Paine, M. M., et al. (1992) IL-1 receptor antagonist protein production and gene expression in rheumatoid arthritis and osteoarthritis synovium. *J. Immunol.* **149,** 1054–1062.

32. Deleuran, B. W., Chu, C. Q., Field, M., Brennan, F. M., Katsikis, P., Feldmann, M., and Maini, R. N. (1992) Localization of interleukin-1alpha, type 1 interleukin-1 receptor and interleukin-1 receptor antagonist in the synovial membrane and cartilage/pannus junction in rheumatoid arthritis. *Br. J. Rheumatol.* **31,** 801–809.

33. Arend, W. P. and Dayer, J.-M. (1990) Cytokines and cytokine inhibitors or antagonists in rheumatoid arthritis. *Arthritis Rheum.* **33,** 305–315.

34. Firestein, G., Boyle, D. L., Yu, C., Paine, M. M., Whisenand, T. D., Zvaifler, N. J., and Arend, W. P. (1994) Synovial interleukin-1 receptor antagonist and interleukin-1 balance in rheumatoid arthritis. *Arthritis Rheum.* **37,** 644–652.

35. Waage, A., Kaufmann, C., Espevik, T., and Husby, G. (1989) Interleukin-6 in synovial fluid from patients with arthritis. *Clin. Immunol. Immunopathol.* **50,** 394–398.

36. Field, M., Chu, C.-Q., Feldmann, M., and Maini, R. N. (1991) Interleukin-6 localisation in the synovial membrane in rheumatoid arthritis. *Rheumatol. Int. Clin. Exp. Invest.* **11,** 45–50.

37. Bardwaj, N., Snathanam, U., Lau, L. L., Tatter, S. B., Ghrayed, J., Rivelis, M., et al. (1989) IL-6/IFN-β2 in synovial effusions of patients with rheumatoid arthritis and other arthritides: identification of several isoforms and studies of cellular sources. *J. Immunol.* **143,** 2153–2159.

38. Houssiau, F. A., Devogelaer, J.-P., van Damme, J., Nagant de Deuxchaisnes, C., and van Snick, J. (1988) Interleukin-6 in synovial fluid and serum of patients with rheumatoid arthritis and other inflammatory arthritides. *Arthritis Rheum.* **31,** 784–788.

39. Jilka, R. L., Hangoc, G., Girasole, G., Passeri, G., Williams, D. C., Abrams, J. S., et al. (1992) Increased osteoclast development after estrogen loss: mediation by interleukin-6. *Science.* **257,** 88–91.

40. Brennan, F. M., Zachariae, C. O. C., Chantry, D., Larsen, C. G., Turner, M., Maini, R. N., et al. (1990) Detection of interleukin-8 biologic activity in synovial fluids from patients with rheumatoid arthritis and production IL-8 mRNA by isolated synovial cells. *Eur. J. Rheumatol.* **20,** 2141–2144.

41. Deleuran, B., Lemche, P., Kristensen, M., Chu, C. Q., Field, M., Jensen, J., et al. (1994) Localization of IL-8 in the synovial membrane and cartilage-pannus junction in rheumatoid arthritis. *Scand. J. Rheumatol.* **23,** 2–7.

42. Firestein, G. S., Xu, W.-D., Townsend, K., Broide, D., Alvaro-Gracia, J., Glasebrook, A., et al. (1988) Cytokines in chronic inflammatory arthritis I. Failure to detect T cell lymphokines (interleukin 2 and interleukin 3) and presence of makrophage colony-stimulating factor (CSF-1) and a novel mast cell growth factor in rheumatoid synovitis. *J. Exp. Med.* **168,** 1573–1586.

43. Hamilton, J. A. (1993) Rheumatoid arthritis: opposing actions of haemopoietic growth factors and slow-acting anti-rheumatic drugs. *Lancet* **342,** 536–539.

44. Alvaro-Gracia, J. M., Zvaifler, N. J., and Firestein, G. S. (1989) Cytokines in chronic inflammatory arthritis IV. Granulocyte/macrophage colony-stimulating factor-mediated induction of class II MHC antigen on human monocytes: possible role in rheumatoid arthritis. *J. Exp. Med.* **170,** 865–875.

45. McInnes, I. B., Al-Mughales, J., Field, M., Leung, B. P., Huang, F. P., Dixon, R., et al. (1996) The role of interleukin-15 in T cell migration and activation in rheumatoid arthritis. *Nature Med.* **2,** 175–182.

46. McInnes, I. B., Leung, B. P., Sturrock, R. D., Field, M., and Liew, F. Y. (1997) Interleukin-15 mediates T cell-dependent regulation of tumor necrosis factor-alpha production in rheumatoid arthritis. *Nature Medicine.* **3,** 189–195.

47. Franz, J. K., Kolb, S. A., Hummal, K. M., Lahrtz, F., Neidhart, M., Aicher, W. K., et al. (1998) Interleukin-16, produced by synovial fibroblasts, mediates chemoattraction for CD4+ T lymphocytes in rheumatoid arthritis. *Eur. J. Immunol.* **28,** 2661–2671.

48. Berman, J. S., Cruikshank, W. W., Center, D. M., Theodore, A. C., and Beer, D. J. (1985) Chemoattractant lymphokines specific for the helper/inducer T-lymphocyte subset. *Cell. Immunol.* **95,** 105–112.

49. Cruikshank, W. W., Berman, J. S., Theodore, A. C., Bernardo, J., and Center, D. M. (1987) Lymphokine activation of C4+ T lymphocytes and monocytes. *J. Immunol.* **138,** 3817–3823.

50. Center, D. M., Kornfeld, H., and Cruikshank, W. W. (1996) Interleukin 16 and its function as a CD4 ligand. *Immunol. Today.* **17,** 476–481.

51. Cruikshank, W. W., Center, D. M., Nisar, N., Wu, M., Natke, B., Theodore, A. C., and Kornfeld, H. (1994) Molecular and functional analysis of a

lymphocyte chemoattractant factor: association of biologic function with CD4 expression. *Proc. Natl. Acad. Sci. USA* **91,** 5109–5113.

52. Theodore, A. C., Center, D. M., Nicoll, J., Fine, G., Kornfeld, H., and Cruikshank, W. W. (1996) CD4 ligand IL-16 inhibits the mixed lymphocyte reaction. *J. Immunol.* **157,** 1958–1964.

53. Cruikshank, W. W., Lim, K., Theodore, A. C., Cook, J., Fine, G., Weller, P. F., and Center, D. M. (1996) IL-16 inhibition of CD3-dependent lymphocyte activation and proliferation. *J. Immunol.* **157,** 5240–5248.

54. Chabaud, M., Fossiez, F., Taupin, J. L., and Miossec, P. (1998) IL-17 enhances the effects of IL-1 on IL-6 and LIF production by rheumatoid arthritis synoviocytes. *J. Immunol.* **161,** 409–414.

55. Simon, A. K., Seipelt, E., and Sieper, J. (1994) Divergent T cell cytokine patterns in inflammatory arthritis. *Proc. Natl. Acad. Sci. USA* **91,** 8562–8566.

56. Aarvak, T., Chabaud, M., Miossec, P., and Natvig, J. B. (1999) IL-17 is produced by some proinflammatory Th1/Th0 cells but not by Th2 cells. *J. Immunol.* **162,** 1246–1251.

57. Chabaud, M., Durand, J. M., Buchs, N., Fossiez, F., Page, G., Frappart, L., and Miossec, P. (1999) Human interleukin-17. A T cell-derived proinflammatory cytokine produced by the rheumatoid synovium. *Arthritis Rheum.* **42,** 963–970.

58. Fossiez, F., Djossou, O., Chomarat, P., Flores-Romo, L., Ait-Yahia, S., Maat, C., et al. (1996) T cell interleukin-17 induces stromal cells to produce proinflammatory and hemtopoietic cytokines. *J. Exp. Med.* **183,** 2593–2603.

59. Gracie, J. A., Forsey, R. J., Chan, W. L., Gilmour, A., Leung, B. P., Greer, M. R., et al. (1999) A proinflammatory role for IL-18 in rheumatoid arthritis. *J. Clin. Invest.* **104,** 1393–1401.

60. Horwood, N. J., Udagawa, N., Elliott, J., Grail, D., Okamura, H., Kurimoto, M., et al. (1998) Interleukin-18 inhibits osteoclast formation via T cell production of granulocyte macrophage colony-stimulating factor. *J. Clin. Invest.* **101,** 595–603.

61. Yssel, H., de Waal Malefyt, R., Roncarolo, M.-G., Abrams, J. S., Lahesmaa, R., Spits, H., and de Vries, J. E. (1992) IL-10 is produced by subsets of human CD4+ T cell clones and peripheral blood T cells. *J. Immunol.* **149,** 2378–2384.

62. Fiorentino, D. F., Zlotnik, A., Vieira, P., Mosmann, T. R., Howard, M., Moore, K. W., and O'Garra, A. (1991) IL-10 acts on the antigen-presenting cell to inhibit cytokine production by Th1 cells. *J. Immunol.* **146,** 3444–3451.

63. de Waal Malefyt, R., Abrams, J., Bennett, B., Fidgor, C. G., and de Vries, J. E. (1991) Interleukin 10 (IL-10) inhibits cytokine synthesis by human monocytes: an autoregulatory role of IL-10 produced by monocytes. *J. Exp. Med.* **174,** 1209–1220.

64. Vieira, P., de Waal Malefyl, R., Dang, M. N., Johnson, K. E., Kastelein, R., Fiorentino, D. F., et al. (1991) Isolation and expression of human cytokine synthesis inhibitory factor cDNA clones: homology to Epstein-Barr virus open reading frame BCRFI. *Proc. Natl. Acad. Sci. USA* **88,** 1172–1176.

65. Katsikis, P. D., Chu, C. Q., Brennan, F. M., Maini, R. N., and Feldmann, M. (1994) Immunoregulatory role of interleukin 10 in rheumatoid arthritis. *J. Exp. Med.* **179,** 1517–1527.

66. Chomarat, P., Banchereau, J., and Miossec, P. (1995) Differential effects of interleukin 10 and 4 on the production of interleukin-6 by blood and synovium monocytes in rheumatoid arthrtis. *Arthritis Rheum.* **38,** 1046–1054.

67. Cush, J. J., Splawski, J. B., Thomas, R., McFarlin, J. E., Schulze-Koops, H., Davis, L. S., et al. (1995) Elevated interleukin-10 levels in patient with rheumatoid arthritis. *Arthritis Rheum.* **38,** 94–104.

68. Llorente, L., Richaud-Patin, Y., Fior, R., Alcocer-Varela, J., Wijdenes, J., Fourrier, B. M., et al. (1994) *In vivo* production of interleukin-10 by non-T cells in rheumatoid arthritis, Sjögren's syndrome and systemic lupus erythematosus. *Arthritis Rheum.* **37,** 1647–1655.

69. Rönnelid, J., Berg, L., Rogberg, S., Nilsson, A., Albertsson, K., and Klareskog, L. (1998) Production of T cell cytokines at the single-cell level in patients with inflammatory arthritides; enhanced activity in synovial fluid compared to blood. *Br. J. Rheumatol.* **37,** 7–14.

70. Isomäki, P., Luukkainen, R., Saario, R., Toivanen, P., and Punnonen, J. (1996) Interleukin-10 functions as an anti-inflammatory cytokine in rheumatoid synovium. *Arthritis Rheum.* **39,** 386–395.

71. Chomarat, P., Vannier, E., Dechanet, J., Rissoan, M. C., Banchereau, J., Dinarello, C. A., and Miossec, P. (1995) Balance of IL-1 receptor antagonist/IL-1β in rheumatoid synovium and its regulation by IL-4 and IL-10. *J. Immunol.* **154,** 1432–1439.

72. Chomarat, P., Rissoan, M.-C., Banchereau, J., and Miossec, P. (1993) Interferon gamma inhibits interleukin-10 production by monocytes. *J. Exp. Med.* **177,** 523–527.

73. van Roon, J. A. G., van Roy, J. A. M., Gmelig-Meyling, F. H. J., Lafeber, F. P. J. G., and Bijlsma, W. J. (1996) Prevention and reversal of cartilage degradation in rheumatoid arthritis by interleukin-10 and interleukin-4. *Arthritis Rheum.* **39,** 829–835.

74. Miossec, P., Naviliat, M., D'Angeac, A., Sany, J., and Banchereau, J. (1990) Low levels of interleukin-4 and high levels of transforming growth factor-β in rheumatoid synovitis. *Arthritis Rheum.* **33,** 1180–1187.

75. Chen, E., Keystone, E. C., and Fish, E. N. (1993) Restricted cytokine expression in rheumatoid arthritis. *Arthritis Rheum.* **36,** 901–910.

76. Ulfgren, A.-K., Lindblad, S., Klareskog, L., Andersson, J., and Andersson, U. (1995) Detection of cytokine producing cells in the synovial membrane from patients with rheumatoid arthritis. *Ann. Rheum. Dis.* **54,** 654–661.

77. Isomäki, P., Luukkainen, R., Toivanen, P., and Punnonen, J. (1996) The presence of interleukin-13 in rheumatoid synovium and its anti-inflammatory effects on synovial fluid macrophages from patients with rheumatoid arthritis. *Arthritis Rhem.* **39,** 1693–1702.

78. Rivas, D., Mozon, L., Zamorano, J., Gayo, A., Torre-Alonso, J. C., Rodriguez, A., and Gutierrez, C. (1995) Upregulated expression of IL-4 receptors and increased levels of IL-4 in rheumatoid arthritis patients. *J. Autoimmun.* **8,** 587–600.

79. Gautam, S., Tebo, J. M., and Hamilton, T. A. (1992) IL-4 suppresses cytokine gene expression induced by IFN-gamma and/or IL-2 in murine peritoneal macrophages. *J. Immunol.* **148,** 1725–1730.

80. Miossec, P., Briolay, J., Dechanet, J., Wijdenes, J., Martinez-Valdez, H., and Banchereau, J. (1992) Inhibition of the production of proinflammatory cytokines and immunoglobulins by interleukin-4 in an *ex vivo* model of rheumatoid arthritis. *Arthritis Rheum.* **35,** 874–883.

81. te Velde, A. A., Huijbens, R. J., Heije, K., de Vries, J. E., and Figdor, C. G. (1990) Interleukin-4 (IL-4) inhibits secretion of IL-1β, tumor necrosis factor alpha, and IL-6 by human monocytes. *Blood* **76,** 1392–1397.

82. de Waal Malefyt, R., Figdor, C. G., Huijbens, R., Mohan-Peterson, S., Bennett, B., Culpepper, J., et al. (1993) Effects of IL-13 on phenotype, cytokine production, and cytotoxic function of human monocytes. Comparison with IL-4 and modulation by IFN-gamma or IL-10. *J. Immunol.* **151,** 6370–6381.

83. Miossec, P., Chomarat, P., Dechanet, J., Moreau, J. F., Roux, J. P., Delmas, P., and Banchereau, J. (1994) Interleukin-4 inhibits bone resorption through an effect on osteoclasts and proinflammatory cytokines in an ex vivo model of bone resorption in rheumatoid arthritis. *Arthritis Rheum.* **37,** 1715–1722.

84. Onoe, Y., Miyaura, C., Kaminakayashiki, T., Nagai, Y., Noguchi, K., Chen, Q. R., et al. (1996) IL-13 and IL-4 inhibit bone resorption by supressing cyclooxygenase-2-dependent prostaglandin synthesis in osteoblasts. *J. Immunol.* **156,** 758–764.

85. Lafyatis, R., Thompson, N. L., Remmers, E. F., Flanders, K. C., Roche, N. S., Kim, S. J., et al. (1989) Transforming growth factor-beta production by synovial tissues from rheumatoid patients and streptococcal cell wall arthritic rats. *J. Immunol.* **143,** 1142–1148.

86. Taketazu, F., Kato, M., Gobl, A., Ichijo, H., ten Dijke, P., Itoh, J., et al. (1994) Enhanced expression of TGF-βs and TGF-β type II receptor in the synovial tissues of patients with rheumatoid arthritis. *Lab. Invest.* **70,** 620–630.

87. Chu, C. Q., Field, M., Abney, E., Zheng, R. Q., Allard, S., Feldmann, M., and Maini, R. N. (1991) Transforming growth factor-β1 in rheumatoid synovial membrane and cartilage/pannus junction. *Clin. Exp. Immunol.* **86,** 380–386.

88. Wahl, S. M., McCartney-Francis, N., and Mergenhagen, S. E. (1989) Inflammatory and immunomodulatory roles of TGF-beta. *Immunol. Today* **10,** 258–261.

89. Fava, R. A., Olsen, N. J., Postlewaithe, A. E., Broadley, K. N., Davidson, J. M., Nanney, L. B., et al. (1991) Transforming growth factor beta 1 (TGF-beta 1) induced neutrophil recruitment to synovial tissues: implications for TGF-beta-driven synovial inflammation and hyperplasia. *J. Exp. Med.* **173,** 1121–1132.

90. Goddard, D. H., Grossman, S. L., Williams, W. V., Weiner, D. B., Gross, J. L., Eidvoog, K., and Dasch, J. R. (1992) Regulation of synovial cell growth. Coexpression of transforming growth factor beta and basic fibroblast growth factor by cultured synovial cells. *Arthritis Rheum.* **35,** 1296–1303.

91. Villinger, P. M., Kusari, A. B., ten Dijke, P., and Lotz, M. (1993) IL-1 beta and IL-6 selectivity induce transforming growth factor-beta isoforms in human articular chondrocytes. *J. Immunol.* **151,** 3337–3344.

92. Fava, R., Olsen, N., Keshi-Oja, J., Moses, H., and Pincus, T. (1989) Active and latent forms of transforming growth factor beta activity in synovial effusions. *J. Exp. Med.* **169,** 291–296.

93. Lotz, M., Kekow, J., and Carson, D. A. (1990) Transforming growth factor-beta and cellular immune responses in synovial fluids. *J. Immunol.* **144,** 4189–4194.

94. Wahl, S. M., Allen, J. B., Wong, H. L., Dougherty, S. F., and Ellingsworth, L. R. (1990) Antagonistic and agonistic effects of transforming growth factor-beta and IL-1 in rheumatoid synovium. *J. Immunol.* **145,** 2514–2519.

95. Colville-Nash, P. R. and Scott, D. L. (1992) Angiogenesis and rheumatoid arthritis: pathogenic and therapeutic implications. *Ann. Rheum. Dis.* **51,** 919–925.

96. Bucht, A., Larsson, P., Thorne, C., Pisa, P., Smedegård, G., Keystone, E. C., and Grönberg, A. (1996) Expression of interferon-gamma (IFN-gamma), IL-10, IL-12 and transforming growth factor beta (TGF-beta) mRNA in synovial fluid cells from patients in the early and late phases of rheumatoid arthritis (RA). *Clin. Exp. Immunol.* **103,** 357–367.

97. Sakkas, L. I., Johanson, N. A., Scanzello, C. R., and Platsoucas, C. D. (1998) Interleukin-12 is expressed by infiltrating macrophages and synovial lining cells in rheumatoid arthritis and osteoarthritis. *Cell. Immunol.* **188,** 105–110.

98. Firestein, G. S. and Zvaifler, N. J. (1987) Peripheral blood and synovial fluid monocyte activation in inflammatory arthritis II. Low levels of synovial fluid and synovial tissue interferon suggests that gamma-interferon is not the primary macrophage activating factor. *Arthritis Rheum.* **30,** 864–871.

99. Taurog, J. D., Sandberg, G. P., and Mahowald, M. L. (1983) The cellular basis of adjuvant arthritis. II. Characterization of the cells mediating passive transfer. *Cell. Immunol.* **80,** 198–204.

100. Holmdahl, R., Goldschmidt, T. J., Kleinau, S., Kvick, C., and Jonsson, R. (1992) Arthritis induced in rats with adjuvant oil is a genetically restricted, alpha-beta T cell dependent autoimmune disease. *Immunology* **76,** 197–202.

101. Griffiths, M. M., Eichwald, E. J., Martin, J. H., Smith, C. B., and DeWitt, C. W. (1981) Immunogenetic control of experimental type II collagen-induced arthritis I. Susceptibility and resistance among inbred strains of rats. *Arthritis Rheum.* **24,** 781–789.

102. Vingsbo, C., Sahlstrand, P., Brun, J. G., Jonsson, R., Saxne, T., and Holmdahl, R. (1996) Pristane-induced arthritis. *Am. J. Pathol.* **149,** 1675–1683.

103. Kiely, P. D., Thiru, S., and Oliveira, D. B. (1995) Inflammatory polyarthritis induced by mercuric chloride in the Brown Norway rat. *Lab. Invest.* **73,** 284–293.

104. Trentham, D. E., Townes, A. S., and Kang, A. H. (1977) Autoimmunity to type II collagen: an experimental model of arthritis. *J. Exp. Med.* **146,** 857–868.

105. Larsson, P., Kleinau, S., Holmdahl, R., and Klareskog, L. (1990) Homologous type II collagen-induced arthritis in rats. Characterization of the disease and demonstration of clinically distinct forms of arthritis in two strains of rats after immunization with the same collagen preparation. *Arthritis Rheum.* **33,** 693–701.

106. Thorbecke, G. J., Shah, R., Leu, C. H., Kuruvilla, A. P., Hardison, A. M., and Palladino, M. A. (1992) Involvement of endogenous tumor necrosis fac-

tor alpha and transforming growth factor beta during induction of collagen type II arthritis in mice. *Proc. Natl. Acad. Sci. USA* **89,** 7375–7379.

107. Åkerlund, K., Erlandsson Harris, H., Tracey, K. J., Wang, H., Fehniger, T., Klareskog, L., et al. (1999) Anti-inflammatory effects of a new tumor necrosis factor-alpha (TNF-alpha) inhibitor (CNI-1493) in collagen-induced arthritis (CIA) in rats. *Clin. Exp. Immunol.* **115,** 32–41.

108. Marinova-Mutafchieva, L., Williams, R. O., Mason, L. J., Mauri, C., Feldmann, M., and Maini, R. N. (1997) Dynamics of proinflammatory cytokine expression in the joints of mice with collagen-induced arthritis (CIA). *Clin. Exp. Immunol.* **107,** 507–512.

109. Butler, D. M., Malfait, A. M., Mason, L. J., Warden, P. J., Kollias, G., Maini, R. N., et al. (1997) DBA/1 mice expressing the human TNF-alpha transgene develop a severe, erosive arthritis: characterization of the cytokine cascade and cellular composition. *J. Immunol.* **159,** 2867–2876.

110. Kollias, G., Douni, E., Kassiotis, G., and Kontoyiannis, D. (1999) On the role of tumor necrosis factor and receptors in models of multiorgan failure, rheumatoid arthritis, multiple sclerosis and inflammatory bowel disease. *Immunol. Rev.* **169,** 175–194.

111. Georgopoulos, S., Plows, D., and Kollias, G. (1996) Transmembrane TNF is sufficient to induce localized tissue toxicity and chronic inflammatory arthritis in transgenic mice. *J. Inflamm.* **46,** 86–97.

112. Edwards, K. C., Chlipala, E. S., Dinarello, C. A., Reznikov, L. L., Moldawer, L. L., and Bendele, A. (1999) Clinical and histopathological characterization of arthritis in male and female tumor necrosis factor-a knock-out (TNF-alpha-/-) and membrane bound TNF-alpha transgenic (TNF-alpha TgA86) mice injected with *Mycoplasma pulmonis* or *Mycoplasma arthritidis*. *Arthritis Rheum.* **42,** S120.

113. Matsumoto, I., Staub, A., Benoist, C., and Mathis, D. (1999) Arthritis provoked by linked T and B cell recognition of a glycolytic enzyme. *Science* **286,** 1732–1735.

114. Hersmann, G. H., Kriegsmann, J., Simon, J., Huttich, C., and Brauer, R. (1998) Expression of cell adhesion molecules and cytokines in murine antigen-induced arthritis. *Cell Adhes. Commun.* **6,** 69–82.

115. Piguet, P. F., Grau, G. E., Vesin, C., Loetscher, H., Gentz, R., and Lesslauer, W. (1992) Evolution of collagen arthritis in mice is arrested by treatment with anti-tumour necrosis factor (TNF) antibody or recombinant soluble TNF receptor. *Immunology* **77,** 510–514.

116. Williams, R. O., Mason, L. J., Feldmann, M., and Maini, R. (1994) Synergy between anti-CD4 and anti-tumour necrosis factor in the amelioration of established collagen-induced arthritis. *Proc. Natl. Acad. Sci. U.S.A.* **91,** 2762–2766.

117. Williams, R. O., Feldmann, M., and Maini, R. I. (1992) Anti-tumor necrosis factor ameliorates joint disease in murine collagen-induced arthritis. *Proc. Natl. Acad. Sci. USA* **89,** 9784–9788.

118. Hom, J. T., Bendele, A. M., and Carlson, D. G. (1988) *In vivo* administration with IL-1 accelerates the development of collagen-induced arthritis in mice. *J. Immunol.* **141,** 834–841.

119. Hom, J. T., Gliszczynski, V. L., Cole, H. W., and Bendele, A. M. (1991) Interleukin 1 mediated acceleration of type II collagen-induced arthritis: effects of anti-inflammatory or anti-arthritic drugs. *Agents Actions.* **33,** 300–309.

120. Wooley, P. H., Whalen, J. D., Chapman, D. L., Berger, A. E., Richard, K. A., Aspar, D. G., and Staite, N. D. (1993) The effects of an interleukin-1 receptor antagonist protein on type II collagen-induced arthritis and antigen-induced arthritis in mice. *Arthritis Rheum.* **36,** 1305–1314.

121. van den Berg, W. B., Joosten, L. A., Helsen, M., and van de Loo, F. A. (1994) Amelioration of established murine collagen-induced arthritis with anti-IL-1 treatment. *Clin. Exp. Immunol.* **95,** 237–243.

122. Joosten, L. A. B., Helsen, M. M. A., van de Loo, F. A. J., and van den Berg, W. B. (1996) Anticytokine treatment of established collagen type II-induced arthritis in DBA/1 mice. A comparative study using anti-TNFalpha, anti-IL-1β, and IL-1ra. *Arthritis Rheum.* **39,** 797–809.

123. Horai, R., Saijo, S., Tanioka, H., Nakae, S., Sudo, K., Okahara, A., et al. (2000) Development of chronic inflammatory arthropathy resembling rheumatoid arthritis in interleukin 1 receptor antagonist-deficient mice. *J. Immunol.* **191,** 313–320.

124. Banerjee, S., Wei, B. Y., Hillman, K., Luthra, H. S., and David, C. S. (1988) Immunosuppression of collagen-induced arthritis in mice with an anti-IL-2 receptor antibody. *J. Immunol.* **141,** 1150–1154.

125. Mihara, M., Ikuta, M., Koishihara, Y., and Ohsugi, Y. (1991) Interleukin 6 inhibits delayed-type hypersensitivity and the development of adjuvant arthritis. *Eur. J. Immunol.* **21,** 2327–2331.

126. Van de Loo, F. A., Kuiper, S., van Enckevort, F. H., Arntz, O. J., and van den Berg, W. B. (1997) Interleukin-6 reduces cartilage destruction during experimental arthritis. A study in interleukin-6 deficient mice. *Am. J. Pathol.* **151,** 177–191.

127. Ohshima, S., Saeki, Y., Mima, T., Sasai, M., Nishioka, K., Nomura, S., et al. (1998) Interleukin 6 plays a key role in the development of antigen-induced arthritis. *Proc. Natl. Acad. Sci. USA* **95,** 8222–8226.

128. Sasai, M., Saeki, Y., Ohshima, S., Nishioka, K., Mima, T., Tanaka, T., et al. (1999) Delayed onset and reduced severity of collagen-induced arthritis in IL-6 knock-outs. *Arthritis Rheum.* **42,** 1635–1643.

129. Campell, I. K., Bendele, A., Smith, D. A., and Hamilton, J. A. (1997) Granulocyte-macrophage colony stimulating factor exacerbates collagen-induced arthritis in mice. *Ann. Rheum. Dis.* **56,** 364–368.

130. Ruchatz, H., Leung, B. P., Wei, X. Q., McInnes, I. B., and Liew, F. Y. (1998) Soluble IL-15 receptor alpha-chain administration prevents murine collagen-induced arthritis: a role for IL-15 in development of antigen-induced immunopathology. *J. Immunol.* **160,** 5654–5660.

131. Bush, K. A., Walker, J. S., and Kirkham, B. W. (1999) Interleukin-17, interferon gamma and tumor necrosis factor mRNA is increased in adjuvant arthritis. *Arthritis Rheum.* **42,** S119.

132. Leung, B. P., Esfanderi, E., Liew, F. Y., and McInnes, I. B. (1999) Interleukin-18 (IL-18) promotes collagen-induced arthritis in DBA/1 mice. *Arthritis Rheum.* **42,** S121.

133. Müssener, Å., Klareskog, L., Lorentzen, J. C., and Kleinau, S. (1995) TNF-alpha dominates cytokine mRNA expression in lymphoid tissues of rats developing collagen- and oil-induced arthritis. *Scand. J. Immunol.* **42,** 128–134.

134. Allen, J. B., Wong, H. L., Costa, G. L., Bienkowski, M. J., and Wahl, S. M. (1993) Suppression of monocyte function and differential regulation of IL-1 and IL-1ra by IL-4 contribute to resolution of experimental arthritis. *J. Immunol.* **151,** 4344–4351.

135. Joosten, L. A., Lubberts, E., Durez, P., Helsen, M. M., Jacobs, M. J., Goldman, M., and van den Berg, W. B. (1997) Role of interleukin 4 and interleukin 10 in murine collagen-induced arthritis. Protective effect of interleukin 4 and interleukin 10 treatment on cartilage destruction. *Arthritis Rheum.* **40,** 249–260.

136. Bessis, N., Biossier, M. C., Ferrara, P., Blankenstein, T., Fradelizi, D., and Fournier, C. (1996) Attenuation of collagen-induced arthritis in mice by treatment with vector cells engineered to secrete interleukin-13. *Eur. J. Immunol.* **26,** 2399–2403.

137. Walmsley, M., Katsikis, P. D., Abney, E., Parry, S., Williams, R. O., Maini, R. N., and Feldmann, M. (1996) Interleukin-10 inhibition of the progression of established collagen-induced arthritis. *Arthritis Rheum.* **39,** 495–503.

138. Persson, S., Mikulowska, A., Narula, S., O´Garra, A., and Holmdahl, R. (1996) Interleukin-10 suppresses the development of collagen type II-induced arthritis and ameliorates sustained arthritis in rats. *Scand. J. Immunol.* **44,** 607–614.

139. Tanaka, Y., Otsuka, T., and Hotokebuchi, T. (1996) Effect of IL-10 on collagen-induced arthritis in mice. *J. Clin. Invest.* **95,** 2868–2876.

140. Apparailly, F., Verwaerde, C., Jacquet, C., Auriault, C., Sany, J., and Jorgensen, C. (1998) Adenovirus-mediated transfer of viral IL-10 gene inhibits murine collagen-induced arthritis. *J. Immunol.* **160,** 5213–5220.

141. Müssener, Å., Funa, K., Kleinau, S., and Klareskog, L. (1997) Dynamic expression of transforming growth factor-betas (TGF-β) and their type I and type II receptors in the synovial tissue of arthritic rats. *Clin. Exp. Immunol.* **107,** 112–119.

142. Allen, J. B., Manthey, C. L., Hand, A. R., Ohura, K., Ellingsworth, L., and Wahl, S. M. (1990) Rapid onset synovial inflammation and hyperplasia induced by transforming factor beta. *J. Exp. Med.* **171,** 231–247.

143. Cooper, W. O., Fava, R. A., Gates, C. A., Cremer, M. A., and Townes, A. S. (1992) Acceleration of onset of collagen-induced arthritis by intra-articular injection of tumour necrosis factor or transforming growth factor beta. *Clin. Exp. Immunol.* **89,** 244–250.

144. Brandes, M. E., Allen, J. B., Ogawa, Y., and Wahl, S. M. (1991) Transforming growth factor beta 1 suppresses acute and chronic arthritis in experimental animals. *J. Clin. Invest.* **87,** 1108–1113.

145. Kuruvilla, A. P., Shah, R., Hochwald, G. M., Liggitt, H. D., Palladino, M. A., and Thorbecke, G. J. (1991) Protective effect of transforming growth factor beta 1 on experimental autoimmune diseases in mice. *Proc. Natl. Acad. Sci. USA* **88,** 2918–2921.

146. Germann, T., Szeliga, J., Hess, H., Störkel, S., Podlaski, F. J., Gately, M. K., et al. (1995) Administration of interleukin 12 in combination with type II collagen induces severe arthritis in DBA/1 mice. *Proc. Natl. Acad. Sci. USA* **92,** 4823–4827.
147. Hess, H., Gately, M. K., Rude, E., Schmitt, E., Szeliga, J., and Germann, T. (1996) High doses of interleukin-12 inhibit the development of joint disease in DBA/1 mice immunized with type II collagen in complete Freund's adjuvant. *Eur. J. Immunol.* **26,** 187–191.
148. Joosten, L. A., Lubberts, E., Helsen, M. M., and van den Berg, W. B. (1997) Dual role of IL-12 in early and late stages of murine collagen type II arthritis. *J. Immunol.* **159,** 4094–4102.
149. McIntyre, K. W., Shuster, D. J., and Gillooly, K. M. (1996) Reduced incidence and severity of collagen-induced arthritis in interleukin-12-deficient mice. *Eur. J. Immunol.* **26,** 2933–2938.
150. Mauritz, N. J., Holmdahl, R., Jonsson, R., Van der Meide, P. H., Scheynius, A., and Klareskog, L. (1988) Treatment with gamma-interferon triggers the onset of collagen arthritis in mice. *Arthritis Rheum.* **31,** 1297–1304.
151. Nakajima, H., Takamori, H., Hiyama, Y., and Tsukada, W. (1990) The effect of treatment with interferon-gamma on type II collagen-induced arthritis. *Clin. Exp. Immunol.* **81,** 441–445.
152. Williams, R. O., Williams, D. G., Feldmann, M., and Maini, R. N. (1993) Increased limb involvement in murine collagen-induced arthritis following treatment with anti-interferon-gamma. *Clin. Exp. Immunol.* **92,** 323–327.
153. Boissier, M. C., Chiocchia, G., and Bessis, N. (1995) Biphasic effect of interferon-gamma in murine collagen-induced arthritis. *Eur. J. Immunol.* **25,** 1184–1190.
154. Jacob, C. O., Holoshitz, J., Van der Meide, P., Strober, S., and McDewitt, H. O. (1989) Heterogeneous effects of interferon-gamma in adjuvant arthritis. *J. Immunol.* **142,** 1500–1505.
155. Manoury-Schwartz, B., Chiocchia, G., and Bessis, N. (1997) High susceptibility to collagen-induced arthritis in mice lacking IFN-gamma receptors. *J. Immunol.* **158,** 5501–5506.
156. Vermiere, K., Heremans, H., van den Putte, M., Huang, S., Billiau, A., and Matthys, P. (1997) Accelerated collagen-induced arthritis in IFN-gamma receptor deficient mice. *J. Immunol.* **158,** 5507–5513.
157. Tada, Y., Ho, A., Matsuyama, T., and Mak, T. W. (1997) Reduced incidence and severity of antigen-induced autoimmune diseases in mice lacking interferon regulatory factor-1. *J. Exp. Med.* **185,** 231–238.
158. Ortmann, R. A. and Shevach, E. M. (1999) Enhanced susceptibility to collagen-induced arthritis in cytokine deficient mice. *Arthritis Rheum.* **42,** S122.
159. Brennan, F. M. and Feldmann, M. (1992) Cytokines in autoimmunity. *Curr. Opin. Immunol.* **4,** 754–759.
160. Feldmann, M., Brennan, F. M., and Maini, R. I. (1996) Role of cytokines in rheumatoid arthritis. *Ann. Rev. Immunol.* **14,** 397–440.
161. Brennan, F. M., Chantry, D., Jackson, A., Maini, R., and Feldmann, M. (1989) Inhibitory effect of TNF-alpha antibodies on synovial cell interleukin-1 production in rheumatoid arthritis. *Lancet* **2,** 244–247.

162. Williams, R. O., Feldmann, M., and Maini, R. I. (1992) Anti-tumour necrosis factor ameliorates joint disease in murine collagen-induced arthritis. *Proc. Natl. Acad. Sci. USA* **89,** 9754–9788.

163. Elliot, M., Maini, R. I., Feldmann, M., Long-Fox, A., Charles, P., Katsikis, P., et al. (1993) Treatment of rheumatoid arthritis with chimeric monoclonal antibodies to tumour necrosis factor alpha. *Arthritis Rheum.* **36,** 1681–1690.

164. Elliot, M., Maini, R. I., Feldmann, M., Kalden, J. R., Antoni, C., Smolen, J. S., et al. (1994) Randomized double-blind comparison of chimeric monoclonal antibody to tumor necrosis factor alpha (cA2) versus placebo in rheumatoid arthritis. *Lancet* **344,** 1105–1110.

165. Maini, R. I., Breedveld, F. C., Kalden, J. R., Smolen, J. S., Macfarlane, J. D., Antoni, C., et al. (1998) Therapeutic efficacy of multiple intravenous infusions of anti-tumor necrosis factor alpha monoclonal antibody combined with low-dose weekly methotrexate in rheumatoid arthritis. *Arthritis Rheum.* **41,** 1552–1563.

166. Maini, R., St Clair, E. W., Breedveld, F., Furst, D., Kalden, J., Weisman, M., et al. (1999) Infliximab (chimeric anti-tumour necrosis factor alpha monoclonal antibody) versus placebo in rheumatoid arthritis patients receiving concomitant methotrexate: a randomised phase III trial. ATTRACT Study Group. *Lancet* **354,** 1932–1939.

167. Wooley, P. H., Dutcher, J., Widmer, M. B., and Gillis, S. (1993) Influence of a recombinant human soluble tumor necrosis factor receptor antagonist protein on type II collagen-induced arthritis in mice. *J. Immunol.* **11,** 6602–6607.

168. Moreland, L. W., Margolies, G. R., Heck, L. W., Saway, A., Blosch, C., Hanna, R., and Koopman, W. J. (1996) Recombinant soluble tumor necrosis factor receptor (p80) fusion protein: toxicity and dose finding trial in refractory rheumatoid arthritis. *J. Rheumatol.* **23,** 1849–1855.

169. Moreland, L. W., Baumgartner, S. W., Schiff, M. H., Tindall, E. A., Fleischmann, R. M., Weaver, A. L., et al. (1997) Treatment of rheumatoid arthritis with a recombinant human tumor necrosis factor receptor (p75)-Fc fusion protein. *N. Engl. J. Med.* **337,** 141–147.

170. Weinblatt, M. E., Kremer, J. M., Bankhurst, A. D., Bulpitt, K. J., Fleischmann, R. M., Fox, R. I., et al. (1999) A trial of etanercept, a recombinant tumor necrosis factor receptor Fc fusion protein, in patients with rheumatoid arthritis receiving methotrexate. *N. Engl. J. Med.* **340,** 253–259.

171. Ulfgren, A.-K., Andersson, U., Engström, M., Klareskog, L., Maini, R., and Taylor, P. Systemic anti-TNFalpha therapy in rheumatoid arthritis downregulates synovial TNFalpha formation. *Submitted.*

172. Bresnihan, B., Alvaro-Garcia, J. M., Cobby, M., Doherty, M., Domljan, Z., Emery, P., et al. (1998) Treatment of rheumatoid arthritis with recombinant human interleukin-1 receptor antagonist. *Arthritis Rheum.* **41,** 2196–2204.

173. Cunnane, G., Madigan, A., and FitzGerald, O. (1996) Treatment with recombinant human Interleukin-1 receptor antagonist (rhIL-1ra) may reduce synovial infiltration in rheumatoid arthritis. *Arthritis Rheum.* **39,** S245.

174. Chernoff, A. E., Granowitz, E., Shapiro, L., Vannier, E., Lonnemann, G., Angel, J. B., et al. (1995) A randomized, controlled trial of IL-10 in humans. *J. Immunol.* **154,** 5492–5499.

175. Maini, R. N., Paulus, H., Breedveld, F. C., Moreland, L. W., St. Clair, E. W., Russell, A. S., et al. (1997) rHUIL10 in subjects with active rheumatoid arthritis: a phase I and cytokine response study. *Arthritis Rheum.* **40,** S224.

176. Wendling, D., Racador, E., and Widjenes, J. (1993) Treatment of severe rheumatoid arthritis by anti-interleukin 6 monoclonal antibodies. *J. Rheumatol.* **20,** 259–262.

177. Wallis, W. J., Furst, D., Strand, V., and Keystone, E. (1998) Biological agents and immunotherapy in rheumatoid arthritis. *Rheum. Dis. Clin. North Am.* **24,** 537–565.

178. Robbins, P. D., Evans, C. H., and Chernajovsky, Y. (1998) Gene therapy for rheumatoid arthritis. *Springer Semin. Immunopathol.* **20,** 197–209.

179. Ghivizzani, S. C., Kang, R., Muzzonigro, T., Whalen, J., Watkins, S. C., Herndon, J. H., et al. (1997) Gene therapy for arthritis - treatment of the first three patients. *Arthritis Rheum.* **40,** S223.

180. Nakamura, K., Kashiwazaki, S., Takagishi, K., Tsukamoto, Y., Morohoshi, Y., Nakano, T., and Kimura, M. (1991) Spontaneous degenerative polyarthritis in male New Zealand black/kn mice. *Arthritis Rheum.* **34,** 171–179.

181. Bouvet, J.-P., Couderc, J., Bouthillier, Y., Franc, B., Ducailar, A., and Mouton, D. (1990) Spontaneous rheumatoid-like arthritis in a line of mice sensitive to collagen-induced arthritis. *Arthritis Rheum.* **33,** 1716–1722.

182. Theofilopoulos, A. N. and Dixon, F. J. (1985) Murine models of systemic lupus erythematosus. *Adv. Immunol.* **37,** 269–390.

183. Nordling, C., Karlsson-Parra, A., Jansson, L., Holmdahl, R., and Klareskog, L. (1992) Characterization of a spontaneously occuring arthritis in male DBA/1 mice. *Arthritis Rheum.* **35,** 717–722.

184. Bremell, T., Lange, S., Svensson, L., Jennishe, E., Gröndahl, K., Carlsten, H., and Tarkowski, A. (1990) Outbreak of spontaneous staphylococcal arthritis and osteoarthritis in mice. *Arthritis Rheum.* **33,** 1739–1744.

185. Hill, J. L., Yong, Z., Laheji, K., Kono, D. H., and Yu, D. T. (1987) Experimental animal models of Yersinia infection and Yersinia-induced arthritis. *Contr. Microbiol. Immunol.* **9,** 228–232.

186. Cole, B. C. and Cassell, G. H. (1979) Mycoplasma infections as models of chronic joint inflammation. *Arthritis Rheum.* **22,** 1375–1381.

187. Yoshino, S., Murata, Y., and Ohsawa, M. (1998) Successful induction of adjuvant arthritis in mice by treatment with a monoclonal antibody against IL-4. *J. Immunol.* **161,** 6904–6908.

188. van den Broek, M. F., van den Berg, W. B., van den Putte, L. B. A., and Severijnen, A. J. (1988) Streptococcal cell wall-induced arthritis and flare-up reaction in mice induced by homologous or heterologous cell walls. *Am. J. Pathol.* **133,** 139–149.

189. Potter, M. and Wax, J. S. (1981) Genetics of susceptibility to pristane-induced plasmacytomas in Balb/cAn: reduced susceptibility in Balb/cJ with a brief description of pristane-induced arthritis. *J. Immunol.* **127,** 1591–1595.

190. Staite, N. D., Richard, K. A., Aspar, D. G., Franz, K. A., Galinet, L. A., and Dunn, C. J. (1990) Induction of an acute erosive monoarticular arthritis in mice by interleukin-1 and methylated bovine serum albumin. *Arthritis Rheum.* **33,** 253–260.

191. Courtenay, J. S., Dallman, M. J., Dayan, A. D., Martin, A., and Mosedale, B. (1980) Immunization against heterologous type II collagen induces arthritis in mice. *Nature* **283,** 666–668.

192. Boissier, M.-C., Chiocchia, G., Ronziere, M.-C., Herbage, D., and Fournier, C. (1990) Arthritogenicity of minor cartilage collagens (type IX and XI) in mice. *Arthritis Rheum.* **33,** 1–8.

193. Glant, T. T., Mikecz, K., Arzoumanian, A., and Poole, A. R. (1987) Proteoglycan-induced arthritis in Balb/c mice. Clinical features histopathology. *Arthritis Rheum.* **30,** 201–212.

194. Verheijden, G. F. M., Rijnders, A. W. M., Elewaut, J. H., de Keyser, F., Veys, E., Boots, A. M., Coenen-de-Roo, C. J. J., van Staveren, C. J., Miltenburg, A. M. M., Meijerink, J. H., and Bos, E. (1997) Human cartilage glycoprotein-39 as a candidate autoantigen in rheumatoid arthritis. *Arthritis Rheum.* **40,** 1115–1125.

195. Wiedermann, U., Tarkowski, A., Bremell, T., Hanson, L. A., Kahu, H., and Dahlgren, U. I. (1996) Vitamin A deficiency predisposes to staphylococcus aureus infection. *Infect. Immun.* **64,** 209–214.

196. Gaede, K., Mack, D., and Heesemann, J. (1992) Experimental Yersinia enterocolitica infection in rats: analysis of the immune response to plasmide-encoded antigens of arthritis-susceptible Lewis rats and arthritis resistant fischer rats. *Med. Microbiol. Immunol.* **181,** 165–172.

197. Pearson, C. M. (1956) Development of arthritis, periarthritis and periostitis in rats given adjuvants. *PSEBM* **91,** 95–101.

198. Lorentzen, J. C. and Klareskog, L. (1999) Identification of arthritogenic adjuvants of self and foreign origin. *Scand. J. Immunol.* **49,** 45–50.

199. Cromartie, W. J., Craddock, J. G., Schwab, J. H., Anderle, S., and Yang, C. (1977) Arthritis in rats after systemic injection of streptococcal cells or cell walls. *J. Exp. Med.* **146,** 1585–1602.

200. Chang, Y.-H., Pearson, C. M., and Abe, C. (1980) Adjuvant polyarthritis IV. Induction by a synthetic adjuvant: Immunologic, histopathologic, and other studies. *Arthritis Rheum.* **23,** 62–71.

201. Yoshino, S. (1996) Oral administration of type II collagen suppresses non-specifically induced chronic arthritis in rats. *Biomed. Pharmacother.* **50,** 24–28.

202. Gondolf, K. B., Batsford, S., Lässle, G., Curschellas, E., and Mertz, A. (1991) Handling of cationic antigens in the joint and induction of chronic allergic arthritis. *Virchows Arch. B Cell Pathol.* **60,** 353–363.

203. Morgan, K., Evans, H. B., Firth, S. A., Smith, M. N., Ayad, S., Weiss, J. B., and Holt, P. J. L. (1983) 1-alpha-2-alpha-3-alpha collagen is arthritogenic. *Ann. Rheum. Dis.* **42,** 680–683.

204. Carlsén, S., Hansson, A.-S., Olsson, H., Heinegård, D., and Holmdahl, R. (1998) Cartilage oligomeric matrix protein (COMP)-induced arthritis in rats. *Clin. Exp. Immunol.* **114,** 477–484.

205. Kahre, S. D., Hansen, J., Luthra, H. S., and David, C. S. (1996) HLA-B27 heavy chains contribute to spontaneous inflammatory disease in B27/human microglobulin (β2m) double transgenic mice with disrupted mouse β2m. *J. Clin. Invest.* **98,** 2746–2755.

206. Iwakura, Y., Saijo, S., Kioka, Y., Nakayama-Yamada, J., Itagaki, K., Tosu, M., et al. (1995) Autoimmunity induction by human T cell leukemia virus type 1 in transgenic mice that develop chronic inflammatory arthropathy resembling rheumatoid arthritis in humans. *J. Immunol.* **155,** 1588–1598.

207. Breban, M., Férnandez-Sueiro, J. L., Richardson, J. A., Hadavand, R. R., Maika, S. D., Hammer, R. E., and Taurog, J. D. (1996) T cells, but not thymic exposure to HLA-B27, are required for the inflammatory disease of HLA-B27 transgenic rats. *J. Immunol.* **156,** 794–803.

14

Systemic Lupus Erythematosus

Amy E. Wandstrat and Edward K. Wakeland

I. INTRODUCTION

Systemic lupus erythematosus (SLE) is considered to be the prototypic systemic autoimmune disorder. SLE is a chronic, inflammatory, multisystemic disorder of connective tissue characterized by involvement of the skin, joints, kidneys, and serosal membranes. SLE occurs in the general population at a rate of approx 1/2000 *(1)*. It is believed that individuals at risk for the disease are genetically predisposed but that induction of the disease requires an environmental trigger; that is, activation of SLE results from a combination of environmental triggers in the context of a susceptible genetic background.

Proof that genetic factors play a role in SLE is evidenced by a 10–16% incidence recurrence rate within families *(2)*. Further evidence that genetics play a role in this disease comes from twin studies where a 24–57% concordance rate has been found for monozygotic twins vs a 2–5% concordance rate for dizygotic twins *(2)*. This genetic component can be quantitated using λs, which is defined as the risk of recurrence for siblings as compared to that in the general population. A λs 1 indicates no genetic contribution, whereas the λs of fully-penetrant single gene Mendelian diseases such as cystic fibrosis are on the order of 500 *(3)*. The λs for SLE has been estimated to be in the range of 20–40, which indicates that more than one gene is involved in SLE pathogenesis and that genetic susceptibility is incompletely penetrant. This is comparable to other complex autoimmune disorders such as insulin-dependent type I diabetes (IDDM, $\lambda s = 15$) and multiple sclerosis (MS, $\lambda s = 20$) *(1)*. Unlike Mendelian diseases wherein one gene has a large impact on phenotype, susceptibility in multifactoral traits such as SLE stems from the combined impact of several contributing genes with low pentrance (e.g., the λs of the insulin gene in IDDM = 1.3). As a result, identifying the

From: *Cytokines and Autoimmune Diseases*
Edited by: V. K. Kuchroo, et al. © Humana Press Inc., Totowa, NJ

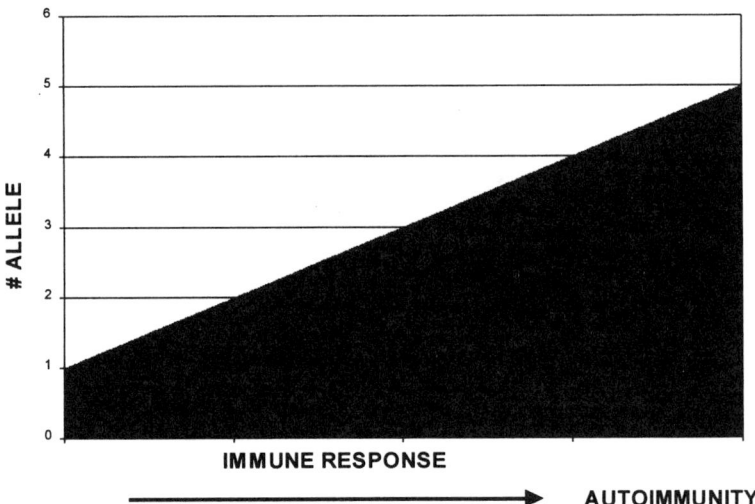

Fig. 1. The graph illustrates a potential scenario in the development of autoimmunity. In it, alleles that strengthen autoimmune response are found in combination, but too many of these immune-enhancing alleles reach an unknown threshhold level of immune response resulting in an autoimmune response.

genes involved in SLE has proven difficult owing to the fact that genes involved in complex traits can act with one another (epistasis) or independently (additivity).

It is possible that selection against the alleles that contribute to the disease is low and that many disease alleles are relatively common. Given the complex checks and balances that regulate activation in the immune system, one can envision that some alleles predisposing for autoimmune disease may serve to enhance the efficiency of immune responses to exogenous antigens. These alleles may actually be selected for (and therefore common) within the general population. These alleles may only be deletereous when they are in combinations that cause such a substantial increase in immune response that the immune system becomes dysregulated, allowing the presence of autoreactive T and B cells to slip into the immune system (Fig. 1).

Further complicating the SLE story is the presence of a strong gender bias in disease penetrance. SLE occurs in females 8–9 times as often as men and frequently develops in settings in which sympathoadrenomedullary and gonadal hormone levels are changing (e.g., during pregnancy, postpartum period, menopause, and estrogen administration). In addition, disease activity is worse in the morning, improves during the day and worsens at night suggesting that neuroendocrine immune mechanisms are also involved in disease pathophysiology *(4)*.

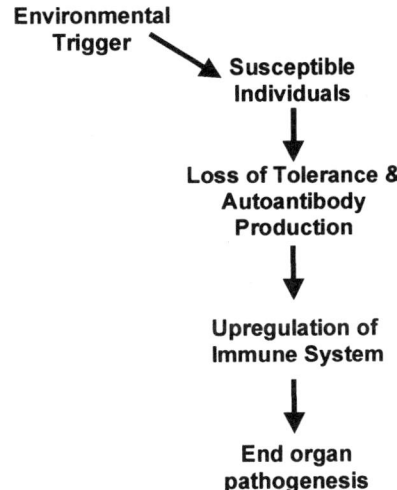

Fig. 2. A diagram of the biological pathways operating in SLE pathogenesis.

Although genetic predisposition is a dominant feature of SLE, disease expression is clearly dependent on some type of environmental trigger. The requirement for an environmental trigger makes logical sense in the context of autoimmune disease as the immune system has evolved to respond to external stimulus. In response to foreign antigen, the immune system undergoes dramatic proliferation and expansion. Prolonged periods of immune response to environmental triggers such as ultraviolet (UV) light or viral infection *(5)* may also serve to cause the immune system to become dysregulated. This, in turn, may again allow for autoreactive T and B cells to slip into the population and begin SLE disease progression. Pathogenesis of SLE appears to be a three-stage process with loss of tolerance and autoantibody production, a generalize upregulation and/or dysregulation of the immune system, and finally end organ-tissue destruction mediated by direct autoantibody binding and/or deposition of immune complexes *(6)* (Fig. 2).

2. IDENTIFYING GENES INVOLVED IN SLE IN HUMANS

2.1. Association Studies

Although the genes that mediate SLE are currently unknown, alleles from some immunologically relevant genes, especially in the major histocomaptibility complex (MHC), have been reported to be associated with the disease *(7)*. Association studies have inherent problems in that the presence of linkage disequillibrium complicates the identification of etiological alleles *(8)*. These type of studies also assume an *a priori* hypothesis that a particular candidate gene is involved in the disease process, and therefore such studies are unable to investigate contributions from genes not directly involved in the immune system. Nonetheless, these types of studies have revealed some interesting findings and a few of the more intriguing associations will be discussed more fully later.

2.1.1. MHC

An association between Class II MHC alleles and SLE has been described by numberous investigators *(7)*. Association studies, and more recently linkage studies, have linked the MHC, located on 6p11-21 in humans and chromosome 17 in mice with susceptibility to SLE in both humans and animal models *(9–12)*. The Class II HLA (human leukocyte antigens) -DR2 and -DR3 alleles separately confer a 2–3 greater risk for SLE in Caucasian populations, whereas HLA-DR2 and HLA-DR7 are associated with SLE susceptibility in African-American populations *(13)*. Although these associations support a role for HLA region polymorphisms, the identity of the true susceptibility gene for SLE in HLA is unclear. There are several alleles at adjacent loci that are in disequillibrium with DR3. These genes include Hsp70-2 *(14)*, the prolactin gene *(15)*, and a TNF-α promoter polymorphism *(16–18)*, all of which could potentially impact susceptibility. Located on chromosome 14, the presence of Hsp70-2 has been found to be more closely associated with SLE in African-American populations than DR3. In British populations, alleles of the prolactin gene are more closely associated. On the other hand, the G to A point mutation at position −308 in the TNF-α promoter has been associated with increased risk in both populations and in the African-American population, that risk is independent of the DR3 haplotype. The effect of the TNF-α promoter polymorphism may be a downstream effect as TNF is also involved in apoptosis and *Tnfr1* and *Tnfr2* knockout mice do not appear to be predisposed to autoimmunity.

2.1.2. Classic Complement Component Pathway

An association between members of the complement components and SLE has been well documented so we will only briefly mention the findings of these studies here. Deficiencies in complement components C1q, C2, and C4 have all been found in lupus patients *(13)*. Complete deficiency of C1q results in lupus greater than 90% of the time indicating that these genes can play a powerful role in susceptibility *(19)*. *C1q*-deficient mice have been generated by means of homologous recombination to disrupt the first exon of the gene *(20)*. High titers of ANA were detected in 54% of the *C1q*-deficient mice, compared to 33% in age-matched controls. At 8 mo of age, 25% develop severe crescenic glumerulonephritis (GN), characterized by the presence of immune deposits and multiple apoptotic cell bodies in injured glomeruli *(21)*. One hypothesis suggests that there may be a defect in the clearance of apoptotic cells in the *C1q*-deficient mice. *C1q* may therefore play a role in binding apoptotic cells and promoting their physiological clearance *(21)*. Complete deficiency of C2 is relatively common in the population with an allele frequency of approx 1%. Absence of C2 results in lupus roughly 33% of the time and accounts for approx 3% of all lupus patients *(22)*. Deficiency of C4 also appears to cause lupus in approx 75% of these individuals *(23,24)*. Also notable here is the finding that alleles or haplotypes that result in the production of lower levels of serum mannose-binding protein has been associate with lupus in African-American and Spanish populations *(25–27)*. Mannose-binding protein is an opsinin that directly binds to the surface of bacteria and activates complement.

Although these complement components are clearly involved in the pathogenesis of SLE in certain deficient individuals, they account for a very small percentage of the overall incidence of lupus in the general population. Nonetheless, the powerful impact of specific deficiencies on susceptibility indicate that the complement pathway strongly impacts at least one pathway to disease susceptibility.

2.1.3. Fc Receptors

Located along 1q21-q23, alleles of the Fc receptors have been associated with SLE and several human linkage studies have found linkage of this region in SLE populations *(10–12,28)*. Intensively studied, FcγRI, FcγRII, and FcγRIII are expressed in a variety of cell types and bind IgG-containing immune complexes with distinct affinities *(29)*. Two common alleles, H131 and R131, of FcγRIIA, show distinct association patterns with SLE and LN (lupus nephritis). Substitution of a histidine (H) at amino acid 131 causes an increased affinity for IgG2 compared to that when arginine (R) is encoded and correlates with a higher association with lupus, especially LN in African-American and Korean populations *(30)*. Findings that the distribution of FcγRIIIA alleles differs in SLE patients when compared to that in the normal population have also been reported. When valine (V) is encoded at amino acid 176 instead of phenylalanine (F), this natural killer (NK) cell receptor has a higher binding affinity for IgG1 and IgG3 *(31)*. Additionally, alleles that fail to express a cell surface product of FcγRIIIB have been found in a few lupus patients *(32,33)*.

2.2. Linkage Studies

A classic approach to identify candidate genes for a particular disease involves linkage analysis via "identity by descent," whereby regions of genetic susceptibility are found to be shared by affected family members in comparison to unaffected family members. To date, four large linkage studies have been performed for SLE using sib-pair analyses methods *(10–12,34)*. In the study by Gaffney et al. *(11)*, the test population was mainly Caucasian (84/105 families) and strongest linkage was found to the MHC region on 6p11-p21. Screening a second cohort of 82 SLE sib-pair families, Gaffney et al. *(34)* found strongest linkage at 7p22. In the Moser et al. *(10)* study, the test population was almost equally divided between African-American (55/94 families) and European-American (31/94 families) populations and the strongest linkage was reported at 1q23. The final study also reported strongest linkage along chromosome 1 at 1q44 with their test population divided between Caucasian (37/80 families) and Mexican-American (43/80 families) populations *(12)*. Linkage was reported at several other regions. Regions that were identified in at least two of the studies were 1p36, 1q23-q24, 1q41-q44, 2q21-q32, 6p11-21 (MHC), 14q21-q23 (Hsp70-2), 16q13, 20p12-p13, and 20q11-q13 *(10–12)*. Several of these regions will be discussed in more detail later.

2.2.1. Chromosome 1 Candidate Genes

Several potential candidate genes are located within the 1q21-q23 region in humans. As discussed earlier, polymorphisms in Fc receptor genes have been found to be associated with lupus susceptibility in case-control studies. Another gene located near this region on human chromosome 1 is the APT1LG1 gene, which encodes Fas ligand. As will be discussed in detail later, disruption of the Fas-Fas ligand pathway has been shown to potentiate systemic autoimmunity in animal models *(35)*. Unfortunately, human studies have revealed no abnormality in the expression or function of the Fas apoptosis pathway in lupus patients. In a screen of 75 SLE patients, only 1 patient was found with a defect in the Fas ligand, APT1LG1, and none with a defect in Fas *(36)*. It is therefore believed that these genes are associated with SLE in only a small portion of patients.

Serum amyloid P component (SAP) is another gene located along chromosome 1q21-23. Recent studies demonstrate that mice carrying a targeted gene disruption of *Sap* spontaneously exhibit many of the autoimmune phenotypes commonly associated with SLE *(37)*. The functional role of *Sap* in degradation and removal of nuclear chromatin is disrupted in these mice, which may, in turn, cause the production of antinuclear autoantibodies (ANA).

Using a different approach, Tsao et al. *(38)* utilized information from murine linkage studies implicating susceptibility loci *Sle1/Nba2/Lbw7* on murine chromosome 1 to search for linkage in the likely syntenic human chromosome region 1q31-q42. They identified an approx 5 cM region in 1q41-q42 estimated to contain 150 genes that was later confirmed in all three of the linkage studies discussed earlier. Three candidate genes were further characterized, ADPRT, TGFβ2, and HLX1. Only ADPRT, a zinc-finger DNA binding protein that is involved in cellular proliferation, differentiation, and repair showed lower than normal levels of activity and allelic distortion in patients with SLE. An 85 bp polymorphism in the promoter region was found to be preferentially transmitted to affected offspring, primarily in Caucasian populations. Notably, however, autoimmune phenotypes characteristic of lupus have not been reported in *ADPRT* knockout mice.

2.2.2. Other Regions

Although regions on chromosomes 2, 16, and 20 were also reported as being linked to SLE, there is no strong candidate genes known to lie in these regions. The region along chromosome 16 at 16q13 is a 35cM region that has been linked to several autoimmune diseases including Crohn's, Blau, psoriasis, IDDM, and asthma *(13)*. Chromosome 2q21-33 includes several immunologically functional genes including CD26, CD28, Ly-family lymphocytic antigens, and CTLA-4. CTLA-4 binds to the B7 costimulatory molecules on APCs and plays a role in downregulating lymphocyte activation. Knockout mice develop a lymphoproliferative autoimmune disease *(39,40)*. On the other hand, regions along chromosome 20 are relatively devoid of genes known to have an immunological impact, although CD40 does lie in 20q11-q13 and is thought to be involved in B cell activation *(41)*.

3. MOUSE MODELS OF SLE

Several mouse models are available for SLE; including the MRL mouse, which is an admixture of LG/J, AKR/J, and C3H/Di backgrounds; the BXSB mouse, which is an inbreed of C57BL/6J (B6) and SB/Le backgrounds; and the New Zealand hybrid, which is an F1 of New Zealand Black (NZB) and New Zealand White (NZW) backgrounds *(8)*. Gene identification in mice can potentially translate directly to disease gene identification in humans owing to the high degree of synteny between the two genomes *(42)*. The MRL and BXSB mice carry single gene mutations that accelerate their lupus-like disease. These mutations are either rarely found in human populations, as is the case for the MRL-*lpr* mutation in the Fas gene and discussed earlier, or do not result in disease that mimics the human, as is the case for the BXSB Y-linked *Yaa* mutation that results in a more severe phenotype in males than females *(43)*. The New Zealand hybrid model develops lupus-like disease that resembles that seen in human patients and several studies have mapped non-MHC loci linked with nephritis and/or antibody production in this model. Figure 3 summarizes those regions involved in SLE that have been identified in these mouse models and underscores the complexity of the genetic component in autoimmune disease. Combinations of the genes in Fig. 3 have been shown to both facilitate or suppress the SLE phenotype.

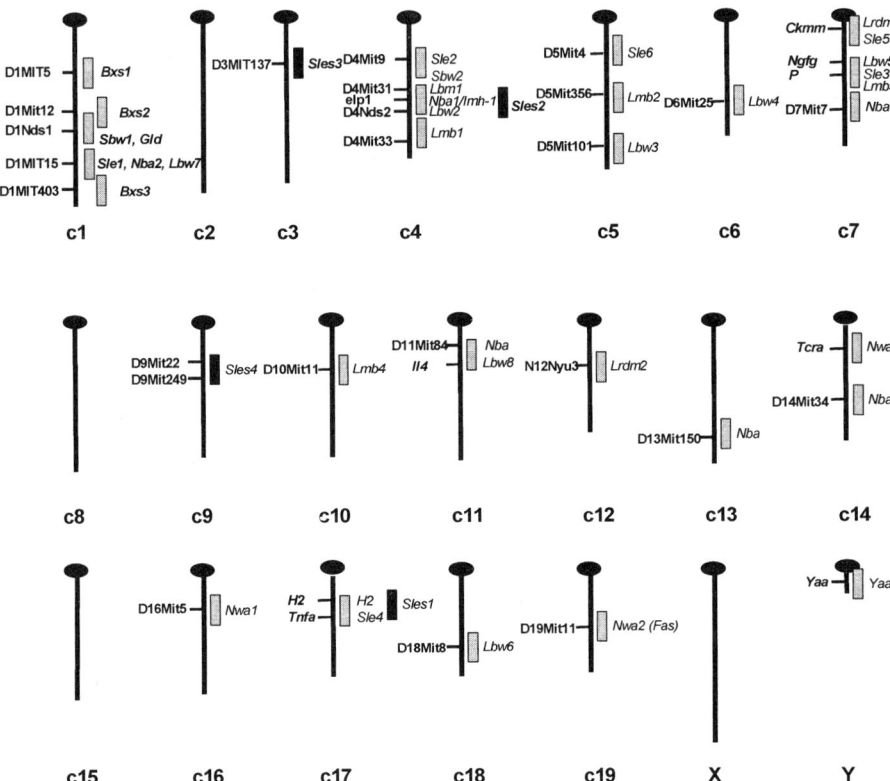

Fig. 3. A summary of genetic regions that are involved in murine SLE pathogenesis as identified by linkage analysis using a number of mouse models.

In the next few sections, we will explore how to dissect genetic contribution in a complex trait and how to identify distinct biological pathways that contribute to SLE pathogenesis and characterize their interactions using the NZM2410 mouse model as an example.

3.1. Genetic Dissection of a Complex Trait

Genome-wide scans initially linked genomic segments from chromosomes 1,4, and 7 to SLE in several NZW- or NZB-derived mouse strains *(9,44–50)*. Our lab has used the powerful tool of congenic strain derivation to analyze the functional impact of each individual region. A congenic strain is one wherein a chromosomal region of interest is moved from one mouse strain background to another. In our example, regions from chromosome 1, 4, and 7 in the NZM2410 mouse strain were segregated via a breeding strategy onto the C57BL/6J mouse background, a strain that does not exhibit any

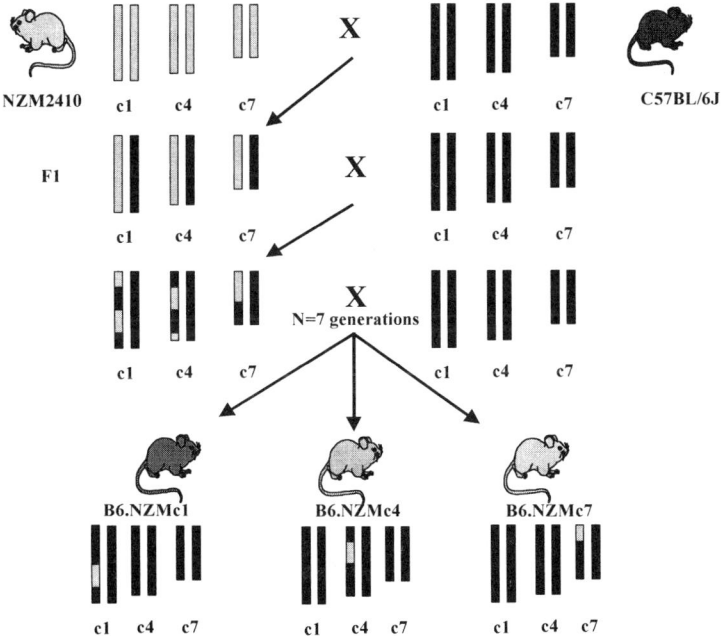

Fig. 4. An illustration of congenic strain construction. In this example, SLE susceptibility regions identified by linkage analysis in the NZM2410 strain are moved onto the SLE-resistant C57BL/6J background strain.

of the autoimmune phenotypes (Fig. 4). Successive backcross matings allows the segregation of only the region of interest to be NZM2410-derived. Subsequent matings allow the congenic interval to be further narrowed *(9)* and the functional properties to be determined for each region *(51,52)*. In the case of *Sle1*, an NZW-derived interval along murine chromosome 1 that we segregated against a B6 background, congenic-strain production has revealed the presence of more than one gene that confers autoantibody production. For two of the *Sle1* genes, *Sle1a* and *Sle1b*, the NZW-derived interval has been narrowed to regions <0.1 cM and recombinants that may help to further narrow these regions continue to be generated. Currently, we have derived congenic strains for *Sle1-3*, NZW-derived intervals along murine chromosome 1, 4, and 7, and are in the process of deriving congenic strains for additional susceptibility loci (*Sle5* and *Sle6*) as well as several suppressive loci (*Sles1-4*).

3.2. Phenotypic Assessment

A key criterion for identifying the genes that contribute to complex disease lies in being able to identify the component phenotypes that each contributes to the disease. Careful analysis of the component phenotype also enables the researcher to narrow the interval by excluding congenic regions that have no phenotypic impact. *Sle1-3* have been carefully studied in our lab and their component phenotypes have been well-documented *(51–55)*. *Sle1* mediates the loss of tolerance to nuclear antigens producing high titers of IgG ANA but only minimal nephritis *(53)*. *Sle2* leads to higher levels of polyclonal IgM antibody production indicative of polyclonal/polyreactive B cell activation *(54)*. *Sle3* affects CD4$^+$ T cells causing polyclonal IgG antibody production, reduces activation-induced cell death in CD4$^+$ T cells, and can cause the development of severe lupus nephritis *(55)*. More recent studies have described the component phenotypes for *Sle5* and *Sle6*. Located at the telomeric end of chromosome 7, *Sle5* triggers loss of tolerance to nuclear autoantigens like *Sle1*. Originating from the NZB strain, *Sle6* is located on chromosome 5 and is strongly associated with lupus nephritis and only weakly associated with humoral autoimmunity much like *Sle3 (50)*.

Another interesting aspect of congenic-strain manipulation and phenotypic assessment has been demonstrated by our ability to identify suppressors of these component phenotypes. In our mouse model system, the majority of the *Sle* genes originate from the NZW strain, a surprising result as NZW fails to develop any significant autoimmunity *(50)*. This suggested that the NZW strain contained not only genes that cause autoimmunity but also genes that suppress autoimmune phenotypes. F1 hybrids from a cross between the congenic strain containing *Sle1* (B6.NZMc1) and the NZW strain yielded progeny that developed severe autoimmunity and lupus nephritis, indicating that homozygosity for *Sle1* is essential for the development of autoimmune disease, as F1 hybrids from B6 X NZW crosses are phenotypically normal. Suppressor loci were identified by analyzing progeny from a (B6.NZMc1 X NZW)F1 X NZW backcross. Four epistatic modifiers, designated *Sles 1-4*, were then identified in a genomic scan using linkage analysis *(50)*. *Sles 1-4* are sufficient to account for the suppression of autoimmune phenotypes in the NZW strain. These results illustrate not only the complexity of SLE disease but also the advantage of using congenic-strain dissection to accurately map genes that impact complex disease phenotypes.

3.3. Functional Pathways in SLE Disease Progression

The validation of component phenotypes as distinct elements contributing to a complex disease is a crucial process in congenic dissection. Our approach to this issue has been to create a series of bi- and tricongenic mouse strains and assess the ability of combining congenic intervals to reconstruct SLE pathogenesis. Our results indicate that a triple congenic strain carrying

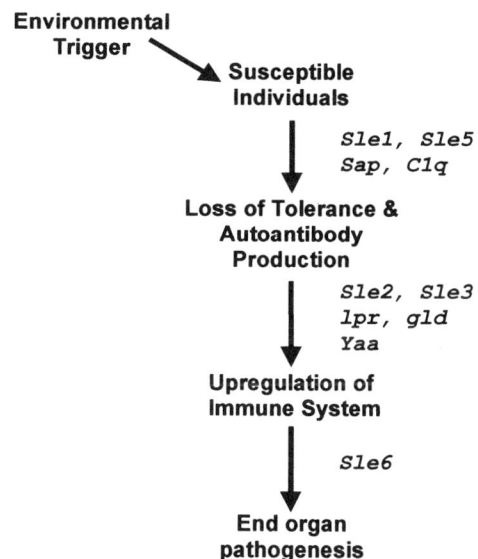

Fig. 5. A diagram of the biological pathways of SLE pathogenesis and identification of genes that contribute to each pathway.

Sle1, *Sle2*, and *Sle3* on the resistant B6 genome is sufficient to account for the complete lupus-nephritis phenotype seen in the NZM2410 mouse strain *(56)*. Bicongenic strains carrying *Sle1* with either *Sle2 (56)*, *Sle3 (52,57)*, or the BXSB-derived autoimmune accelerating gene *Yaa*, develop humoral autoimmunity with variably penetrant GN, resulting in fatal nephritis. This yields important information about the requirement for *Sle*1 because when *Sle2*, *Sle3*, or *Yaa* are combined in a biocongenic strain, these mice do not develop fatal lupus nephritis *(56)*. These results suggest that *Sle*1 is essential for the development of the disease and indicates that its functional pathway lies upstream to that of *Sle2* or *Sle3*. Currently, our working model of the disease involves the interaction of three different pathways (Fig. 5).

The first pathway contains genes such as *Sle1*, *Sap*, *C1q*, and possibly *Sle5 (52,53)*. These genes trigger the loss of immune tolerance to nuclear autoantigens and at least in the case of *Sle1* are essential for the initiation of the autoimmune cascade. Genes in this pathway need to interact with genes from other pathways such as *Sle2* and *Sle3* to mediate a truly pathogenic response. *Sle2 (54)* and *Sle3 (52,55)* are in the second genetic pathway and impact disease pathogenesis by enhancing the autoimmune response and causing a generalized immune upregulation and/or dysregulation. Genes such as *lpr (58)*, *gld* (58), and *Yaa (43)* would also be included in this path-

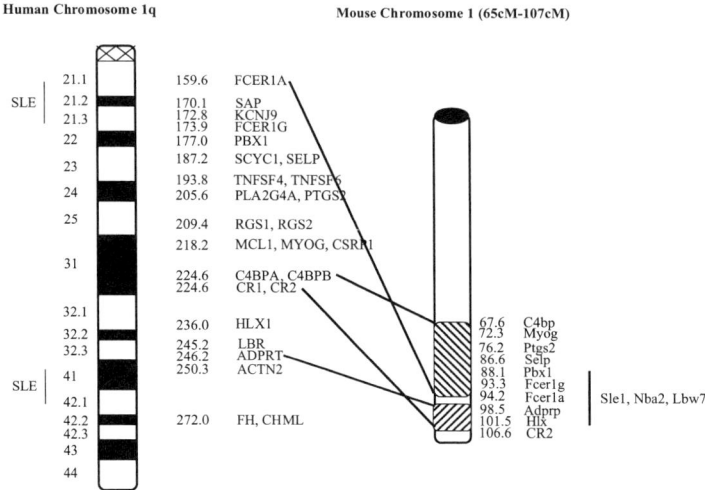

Fig. 6. Diagram of the syntenic relationship between murine chromosome 1 and human chromosome 1q.

way. These genes do not create an autoimmune phenotype in resistant genomes but greatly enhance the disease phenotype in genomes when combined with genes, such as those in the first pathway, that cause loss of tolerance and autoantibody production. The final pathway mediates end organ damage. Genes in this pathway are likely to be genes such as *Sle6*, which impacts the development of GN but has little or no effect on autoantibody production *(50)*.

4. DRUG THERAPY AND GENETIC INTERVENTION

Although unraveling the complex genetics involved in SLE has proven to be a long, painstaking process, there are several lines of evidence that indicate that these efforts will yield valuable strategic targets for disease intervention. First, identification of *Sle1* in the mouse may be of significant importance in understanding human disease. *Sle*1 lies in a region of the murine chromosome that is syntenic to human 1q21-q44. As discussed earlier, this region has been detected repeatedly in both human and mouse studies as having several, separate, putative genetic linkages (Fig. 6). Evidence from NZM bi and tricongenic mouse strains indicates that *Sle1* is a key element of the SLE pathogenic cascade. The fact that *Sle1* is essential for disease pathogenesis makes it an attractive target for therapeutic intervention. Also epistatic modifiers can suppress *Sle1 (50)*. The finding that epistatic modifiers exist in mouse models has significant implications for the human as one would expect that these types of modifiers would also exist in human populations. Although suppressive modifiers will complicate linkage studies aimed at identifying susceptibility genes, identification of genes with suppressive abilities may reveal, either directly or indirectly, strategies for gene and/or drug therapies that either mimic the suppressive function or act on the functional pathway that the modifiers impact. The finding that *Sles1-4* can completely ameliorate SLE disease pathogenesis, even in the presence of potent susceptibility genes such as *Sle1*, *Sle2*, *Sle3*, and *Sle6*, underscores the profound effect that epistasis can have on the expression of fatal lupus. Understanding the genes and genetic pathways involved in SLE may ultimately provide completely effective therapies for the treatment of SLE.

REFERENCES

1. Kotzin, B. L. (1996) Systemic lupus erythematosus. *Cell* **85,** 303–306.
2. Arnett, F. C. (1997) The genetics of human lupus, in *Dubois' Lupus Erythematosus* (Wallace, D. C. and Hahn, B. eds.), Williams and Wilkins, Baltimore, MD, pp. 77–117.
3. Landers, E. S. and Schork, N. J. (1994) Genetic dissection of complex traits. *Science* **265,** 2037–2048.
4. Wilder R.L. (1995) Neuroendocrine-immune system interactions and autoimmunity. *Annu. Rev. Immunol.* **13,** 307–338.
5. Foster, M. H. (1999) Relevance of systemic lupus erythematosus nephritis animal models to human disease. *Sem. Nephr.* **19,** 12–24.
6. Wakeland, E. K., Morel, L., Mohan, C., and Yui, M. (1997) Genetic dissection of lupus nephritis in murine models of SLE. *J. Clin. Immunol.* **17,** 272–281.
7. Schur, P. (1995) Genetics of systemic lupus erythematosus. *Lupus* **4,** 425–437.
8. Vyse, T. J. and Kotzin, B. L. (1998) Genetic susceptibility to systemic lupus erythematosus. *Annu. Rev. Immunol.* **16,** 261–292.
9. Morel, L., Rudofsky, U. H., Longmate, J. A., Schiffenbauer, J., and Wakeland, E. K. (1994) Polygenic control of susceptibility to murine systemic lupus erythematosus. *Immunology* **1(3),** 219–229.
10. Moser, K. L., Neas, B. R., Salmon, J. E., Yu, H., Gray-McGuire, C., Asundi, N., et al. (1998) Genome scan of human systemic lupus erythematosus: evidence for linkage on chromosome 1q in African-American pedigrees. *Proc. Natl. Acad. Sci. USA* **95,** 14,869–14,874.
11. Gaffney, P. M., Kearns, G. M., Shark, K. B., Ortmann, W. A., Selby, S. A., Malmgren, M. L., et al. (1998) A genome-wide search for susceptibility genes in human systemic lupus erythematosus sib-pair families. *Proc. Natl. Acad. Sci. USA* **95,** 14,875–14,879.
12. Shai, R., Quismorio Jr., F., Li, L. Kwon, O. J., Morrison, J., Wallace, D. J., et al. (1999) Genome-wide screen for systemic lupus erythematosus susceptibility genes in multiplex families. *Human Mol. Genet.* **8,** 639–644.
13. Harley, J. B., Moser, K. L., Gaffney, P. M., and Behrens, T. W. (1998) The genetics of human systemic lupus erythematosus. *Curr. Opin. Immunol.* **10,** 690–696.

14. Jarjour, W., Reed, A. M., Gauthier, J., Hunt, S., and Winfield, J. B. (1996) The 8.5-kb PsfI allele of the stress protein gene, Hsp70-2. An independent risk factor for systemic lupus erythematosus in African-Americans? *Human Immunol.* **45,** 59–63.

15. Brennan, P., Hajeer, A. H., Ong, K. R., Worthington, J., John, S., Thompson, W., et al. (1997) Alleleic markers close to prolactin are associated with HLA-DRB1 susceptibility alleles among women with rheumatoid arthritis and systemic lupus erythematosus. *Arthritis Rheum.* **40,** 1383–1386.

16. Rudwaleit, M., Tikly, M., Khamashta, M. A., Gibson, K., Klinke, J., Hughes, G., et al. (1996) Interethnic differences in the association of tumor necrosis factor promoter polymorphisms with systemic lupus erythematosus. *J. Rheumatol.* **23,** 1725–1728.

17. Hajeer, A. H., Worthington, J., Davies, E. J., Hillarby, M. C., Poulton, K., and Ollier, W. E. (1997) TNF microsatellite a2, b3 and d2 alleles are associated with systemic lupus erythematosus. *Tissue Antigens* **49,** 222–227.

18. Sullivan, K. E., Wooten, C., Schmeckpeper, B. J., Goldman, D., and Petri, M. (1997) A promoter polymorphism of tumor necrosis factor a associated with systemic lupus erythematosus in African-Americans. *Arthritis Rheum.* **40,** 2207–2211.

19. Reid, K. B. M. (1993) Deficiency of the first componenet of human complement, in *Immunodeficiencies* (Rosen, F. S. and Seligman, M., eds.), Harwood Academic Publishers, Philadelphia, PA, pp. 283–293.

20. Petry F., McClive P.J., Botto M., Morley B.J., Morahan G., and Loos M. (1996) The mouse C1q genes are clustered on chromosome 4 and show conservation of gene organization. *Immunogenetics* **43,** 370–376.

21. Botto, M., Dell'Agnola, C., Bygrave, A. E., Thompson, E. M., Cook, H. T., Petry, F., et al. (1998) Homozygous C1q deficiency causes glomerulonephritis associated with multiple apoptotic bodies. *Nature Gen.* **19,** 56–59.

22. Provost, T. T., Arnett, F. C., and Reichlin, M. (1983) Homozygous C2 deficiency, lupus erythematosus and anti-Ro(SS-A) antibodies. *Arthritis Rheum.* **26,** 1279–1282.

23. Fielder, A. H. L., Walport M.J., Batchelor, J. R., Rynes, R. I., Black, C. M., Dodi, I. A., et al. (1983) Family study of the major histocompatibility complex in patients with systemic lupus erythematosus: importance of null alleles of C4A and C4B in determining disease susceptibility. *Brit. Med. J.* **286,** 425–428.

24. Davies, E. J., Steers, G., Ollier, W. E., Grennan, D. M., Cooper, D. M., Hay, E. M., and Hillarby, M. C. (1995) Relative contributions of HLA-DQA and complement C4A loci in determining susceptibility to systemic lupus erythematosus. *Br. J. Rheumatol.* **34,** 221–225.

25. Davies, E. J., Snowden, N., Hillarby, M. C., Cathy, D., Grennan, D. M., Thompson, W., and Ollier, W. E. (1995) Mannose-binding protein gene polymorphism in systemic lupus erythematosus. *Arthritis Rheum.* **38,** 110–114.

26. Sullivan, K. E., Wooten, C., Goldman, D., and Petri, M. (1996) Mannose-binding protein polymorphism in black patients with systemic lupus erythematosus. *Arthritis Rheum.* **39,** 2046–2051.

27. Davies, E. J., The L.S., Ordi-Ros, J., Snowden, N., Hillarby, M. C., Hajeer, A., et al. (1997) A dysfunctional allele of the mannose binding protein gene

associates with systemic lupus erythematosus in a Spanish population. *J. Rheumatol.* **24,** 485–488.

28. Tsao, B. P., Cantor, R. M., Kalunian, C., Chen, C. J., Badsha, H., Singh, R., et al. (1997) Evidence for linkage of a candidate chromosome 1 region to human systemic lupus erythematosus. *J. Clin. Invest.* **99,** 725–731.

29. Gibson, A., Wu, J., Edberg, J. C., and Kimberly, R. P. (1999) Fcgamma receptor polymorphisms: insights into pathogenesis, in *Lupus: Molecular and Cellular Pathogenesis* (Kammer, G. and Tsokos, G. C., eds.), Human Press, Totowa, NJ, pp. 557–573.

30. Parren, P., Warmerdam, P., Boeije, J., Boeije, L .C., Arts, J., Westerdaal, N. A., Vlug, A., et al. (1992) On the interaction of IgG subclasses with the low affinity FcGammaIIA. *J. Clin. Invest.* **90,** 1537–1546.

31. Wu, J., Bansal, V., Arnett, F. C., Reveille, J. D., Ginzler, E. M., Gourley, M. F., et al. (1997) The FcgammaRIIIA 176F/V polymorphism associates with the SLE phenotype in Caucasians and African Americans. *Arthritis Rheum.* **40,** S316.

32. Clark, M., Liu, L., Clarkson, S., Ory, P., and Goldstein, I. (1990) An abnormality of the gene that encodes neutrophil Fc receptor III in a patient with systemic lupus erythematosus. *J. Clin. Invest.* **86,** 341–346.

33. Enenkel, B., Jung, D., and Frey, J. (1991) Molecular basis of IgG Fc receptor III defect in a patient with systemic lupus erythematosus. *Eur. J. Immunol.* **21,** 659–663.

34. Gaffney P.M., Ortmann W.A., Selby, S. A., Shark, K. B., Ockenden, T. C., Rohlf, K. E., et al. (2000) Genome screening in human systemic lupus erythematosus: results from a second Minnesota cohort and combined analyses of 187 sib-pair families. *Am. J. Human Genet.* **66,** 547–556.

35. Nagata, S. and Suda, T. (1995) Fas and Fas ligand: lpr and gld mutations. *Immunol. Today* **16,** 39–43.

36. Wu, J., Wilson, J., Xiang, L., Schur, P. H., and Mountz, J. D. (1996) Fas ligand mutation in a patient with systemic lupus erythematosus and lymphoproliferative disease. *J. Clin. Invest.* **98,** 1107–1113.

37. Bickerstaff, M. C., Botto, M., Hutchinson, W. L., Herbert, J., Tennent, G. A., Bybee, A., et al. (1999) Serum amyloid P component controls chromatin degradation and prevents antinuclear autoimmunity. *Nature Med.* **5,** 694–697.

38. Tsao, B. P., Cantor, R. M., Grossman, J., Shen, N., Teophilov, N. T., Wallace, D. J., et al. (1999) PARP alleles within the linked chromosomal region are associated with systemic lupus erythematosus. *J. Clin. Invest.* **103,** 1135–1140.

39. Waterhouse, P., Penninger, J. M., Timms, E., Wakeman, A., Shahinian, A., Lee, K. P., et al. (1995) Lymphoproliferative disorders with early lethality in mice deficient in Ctla-4. *Science* **270,** 985–988.

40. Tivol, E. A., Borriello, F., Schweitzer, A. N., Lynch, W. P., Bluestone, J. A., and Sharpe, A. H. (1995) Loss of CTLA-4 leads to massive lymphoproliferation and fatal multiorgan tissue destruction, revealing a critical negative regulatory role of CTLA-4. *Immunology* **3,** 541–547.

41. Wortis, H. H., Teutsch, M., Huger, M., Zheng, J., and Parker, D. C. (1995) B-cell activation by cross-linking of surface IgM or ligation of CD40 involves alternative signal pathways and results in different b-cell phenotypes. *Proc. Natl. Acad. Sci. USA* **92,** 3348.

42. Nadeau, J. (1989) Maps of linkage and synteny homologies between mouse and man. *Trends. Genet.* **5,** 82–86.
43. Izui, S., Merino, R., Fossati, L., and Iwamoto, M. (1994) The role of the Yaa gene in lupus syndrome. *Intl. Rev. Immunol.* **11,** 211–230.
44. Drake, C. G., Rozzo, S. J., Hirschfeld, H. F., Smarnworawong, N. P., Palmer, E., and Kotzin, B. K. (1995) Analysis of the NZB contribution to lupus-like renal disease: Multiple genes that operate in a threshhold manner. *J. Immunol.* **154,** 2441–2447.
45. Rozzo, S. J., Vyse, T. J., Drake, C. G., and Kotzin, B. L. (1996) Effect of genetic background on the contribution of New Zealand Black loci to autoimmune lupus nephritis. *Proc. Natl. Acad. Sci. USA* **93,** 15,164–15,168.
46. Vyse, T. J., Rozzo, S. J., Drake, C. G., Izui, S., and Kotzin, B. L. (1997) Control of multiple autoantibodies linked with a lupus nephritis susceptibility locus in New Zealand black mice. *J. Immunol.* **158,** 5566–5574.
47. Kono, D. H., Burlingame, R. W., Owens, D. G., Kuramochi, A., Balderas, R. S. Balomenos, D., and Theofilopoulos, A. N. (1994) Lupus susceptibility loci in New Zealand mice. *Proc. Natl. Acad. Sci. USA* **91,** 10,168–10,172.
48. Drake, C. G., Babcok, S. K., Palmer, E., and Kotzin, B. K. (1994) Genetic analysis of the NZB contribution to lupus-like autoimmune disease. *Proc. Natl. Acad. Sci. USA* **91,** 4062–4065.
49. Vyse, T. J., Drake, C. G., Rozzo, S. J., Roper, E., Izui, S., and Kotzin, B. L. (1996) Genetic linkage of IgG autoantibody production in relation to lupus nephritis in New Zealand hybrid mice. *J. Clin. Invest.* **98,** 1762–1772.
50. Morel, L., Tian, X.-H., Croker, B. P., and Wakeland, E. K. (1999) Epistatic modifiers of autoimmunity in a murine model of lupus nephritis. *Immunology* **11,** 131–139.
51. Morel, L., Yu, Y., Blenman, K. R., Caldwell, R. A., and Wakeland, E. K. (1996) Production of congenic mouse strains carrying SLE-susceptibility genes derived from the SLE-prone NZM/Aeg2410 strain. *Mamm. Genome* **7,** 335–339.
52. Morel, L., Mohan, C., Croker, B. P., Tian, X.-H., and Wakeland, E. K. (1997) Functional dissection of systemic lupus erythematosus using congenic mouse strains. *J. Immunol.* **158,** 6019–6028.
53. Mohan, C., Alas, E., Morel, L., Yang, P., and Wakeland, E. K. (1998) Genetic dissection of SLE pathogenesis: *Sle1* on murine chromosome 1 leads to a selective loss of tolerance to H2A/H2B/DNA subnucelosomes. *J. Clin. Invest.* **101,** 1362–1372.
54. Mohan, C., Morel, L., Yang, P., and Wakeland, E. K. (1997) Genetic dissection of SLE pathogenesis: *Sle2* on murine chromosome 4 leads to B-cell hyperactivity. *J. Immunol.* **159,** 454–465.
55. Mohan, C., Yu, Y., Morel, L., Yang, P., and Wakeland, E. K. (1999) Genetic dissection of SLE pathogenicity: *Sle3* on murine chromosome 7 impacts T cell activation, differentiation, and cell death. *J. Immunol.* **162,** 6492–6502.
56. Morel, L., Croker, B. P., Blenman, K. R., Mohan, C., Huang, G., Gilkeson, G., and Wakeland, E. K. (2000) Genetic reconstitution of systemic lupus erythematosus immunopathology with polycongenic murine strains. *Proc. Natl. Acad. Sci. USA* **97,** 6670–6675.

57. Mohan, C., Morel, L., Yang, P., Watanabe, H., Croker, B., Gilkeson, G., and Wakeland, E. K. (1999) Genetic dissection of lupus pathogenesis: a recipe for nephrophilic autoantibodies. *J. Clin. Invest.* **103,** 1685–1695.
58. Cohen, P. L. and Eisenberg, R. A. (1991) Lpr and gld: Single gene models of systemic autoimmunity and lymphoproliferative disease. *Annu. Rev. Immunol.* **9,** 243–269.

15
Myasthenia Gravis

Premkumar Christadoss and Elzbieta Goluszko

1. INTRODUCTION

Myasthenia gravis (MG) is a classical antibody-mediated autoimmune disease involving the neuromuscular junction (NMJ). Antibodies to nicotinic acetylcholine receptors (AChR), with or without complement activation, destroy the AChR at the NMJ, leading to neuromuscular-transmission defect, and culminating in muscle weakness and fatigue. Anti-AChR antibodies of all IgG isotypes are detected in the serum of approx 85% of MG patients. Approximately 70% of MG patients have hyperplastic thymus and 15% have thymoma. Whether the thymic pathology seen in MG is a consequence or the cause of MG is not known. The factors (e.g., infection) that trigger the autoimmune response to AChR remain obscure. However, human leukocyte antigen-DQ gene (*HLA-DQ*), tumor necrosis factor-α (*TNF*-α) and -β, interleukin-1β (*IL-1*β), or *IL-10* polymorphisms have been associated with MG *(1–7)*. Although these polymorphisms are associated with MG, they do not provide a direct genetic or immunological evidence for specific gene(s) involved in the initiation and perpetuation of autoimmune MG. The experimental autoimmune MG (EAMG) in mice is a reliable animal model that mimics human MG in most of the clinical and immunopathological aspects *(8)*. The mouse model of EAMG has already given us an enormous insight into the genetic, cellular, and molecular mechanisms involved in EAMG pathogenesis *(8)*. To understand the role of specific cytokines involved in the afferent (antigen-processing, presentation of peptides, and T-B cognate interaction) and efferent (B cell activation, differentiation, and production of pathogenic anti-AChR antibodies) limbs of an autoimmune response to AChR, one should first understand the contribution of T and B cells, and major histocompatibility complex (MHC) and T

From: *Cytokines and Autoimmune Diseases*
Edited by: V. K. Kuchroo, et al. © Humana Press Inc., Totowa, NJ

cell receptor (*TCR*) genes in the development of EAMG. In the first section of this review, the genes, cells, and molecules involved in EAMG pathogenesis will be discussed. The role of specific cytokines implicated in human MG pathogenesis will be explored in the second section. Recent findings related to the crucial role of proinflammatory cytokines involved in the autoimmune response to AChR and in the development of clinical EAMG, utilizing specific cytokine or cytokine-receptor gene knockout mice will be discussed in detail in the final section. The chapter will conclude by introducing a subject on combination immunotherapy.

2. GENES, CELLS, AND MOLECULES INVOLVED IN EAMG PATHOGENESIS

For the past two decades, studies in our laboratory have been devoted to identifying the MHC and *TCR* genes, T and B cell population, and AChR pathogenic T cell epitopes involved in EAMG pathogenesis. The immune-response gene at the *H-2A* region determined EAMG susceptibility in mice with H-2^b haplotype *(9)*. The *H-2A* region also influenced both the cellular and humoral immune response to AChR *(9–11)*. MHC class II β-chain mutation with three altered amino acids partially prevented, and MHC class II gene deficiency completely prevented the development of cellular and humoral immune response to AChR and clinical EAMG *(12,13)*. CD4 cell depletion by antibody or *CD4* gene-targeted mutation suppressed anti-AChR antibody production and EAMG development *(14,15)*, thus demonstrating a crucial role of MHC class II-restricted CD4 cells in the production of pathogenic anti-AChR antibodies by AChR-reactive B cells. However, MHC class I-restricted CD8 cells do not play a significant role, because MHC class I gene deficiency in β2*m* gene knockout mice did not influence the development of clinical EAMG *(16)*. MHC class II-restricted AChR-reactive CD4 cells are also activated in patients with MG *(17)*. A dominant T cell epitope has been mapped within AChR α-subunit regions 146–162, and neonatal or adult tolerance to this T cell epitope suppressed EAMG development *(18)*. In both mouse EAMG and human MG, there was a lack of usage of highly restricted AChR-specific TCR genes *(19,20)*. The μ gene KO mice deficient in B cells failed to generate anti-AChR antibodies and were completely resistant to the development of EAMG, thus providing evidence for anti-AChR antibodies produced by B cells as mediator of pathogenesis *(21,22)*. The prevention of clinical EAMG, despite the presence of anti-AChR antibodies in C5-deficient mice, implicated the crucial role of complement in EAMG pathogenesis *(23)*. Also, the CD28-B7 and CD40L-CD40 costimulatory signals are required during the primary immune response to AChR *(24)*.

3. CYTOKINES IN HUMAN MG

3.1. Cytokine Gene Polymorphisms in MG

3.1.1. TNF Polymorphism

Genes for TNF are arranged in the central region of MHC. In the *TNF-α* gene, the presence of allele *2*, *A2* is associated with higher inducible levels of TNF-α. In female Swedish Caucasian patients with early onset of MG and thymic hyperplasia *TNF-α 308 A2/A2* genotype frequency was significantly increased, while the genotype *A1/A1* frequency was decreased compared to that in healthy individuals *(3,25)*. It was suggested that the impact of *TNF-α-308 A2* allele may result in disregulation of the immune system in patients with thymic hyperplasia and early onset of the disease. MG patients having thymoma and titin antibody were more often homozygous for the *TNFA*T1* and *TNFB*2* alleles. In early-onset MG with absence of titin antibodies correlated with the presence of *TNFA*T2* and *TNFB*1* alleles *(4)*. In another study of MG patients with thymic hyperplasia, a positive association with the *TNFB*1* allele and phenotype and a negative association with the *TNFB*2/2* genotype was observed. In MG patients with thymoma, a positive association with the *TNFB*2/2* genotype and a negative association with the *TNFB*1* allele and *1/2* genotype was found *(5)*.

3.1.2. IL-1β Polymorphism

In Swedish Caucasian MG population, the frequencies of the *IL-1β* genotype *A2/A2* and the allele *2* were increased, whereas that of genotype *A1/A1* decreased. Also the *IL-1β* Taq I restriction fragment length polymorphism (RFLP) allele 2 plays a more important role in patients negative for HLA-B8 *(6)*.

3.1.3. IL-10 Polymorphism

Huang et al. demonstrated a novel genetic association of MG to IL-10 gene on *1q 31-32*. MG patient carrying *IL-10.G* allele *134* had higher serum AChR antibodies, whereas those with normal thymic histology carried *IL-10 R allele 112*, suggesting a differential role for *IL-10* in MG subgroups. The authors speculate that patients with *IL-10* allele *134* or genotype *134/136* might have higher inducible IL-10 secretion in vivo when the individual encounters the autoantigen and elicits the autoimmune response, leading to augmented production of anti-AChR antibodies *(7)*.

The aforementioned polymorphisms of *TNF*, *IL-1β*, and *IL-10* observed in MG patients merely associate these polymorphisms to MG. Does the mere inheritance of a high secretory type (e.g., TNF-α) in an individual predispose to MG? We predict that the presence of a high secretory type (e.g.,

TNF-α) could promote the initiation of disease in concert with other factors (e.g., *HLA-DQ*, infection) or promote an already existing disease.

3.2. Cytokine mRNA Expression in Blood Mononuclear Cells in MG Patients

Cytokine mRNA expression were enumerated in mononuclear cells (MNC) derived from MG patients after *in situ* hybridization with labeled complementary DNA oligonucleotide probes for *IFN-γ*, *IL-4*, and *TGF-β*. Elevated numbers of cells expressing IFN-γ and IL-4 mRNA were observed in MG patients, compared to patients with a noninflammatory neurological diseases and healthy controls. TGF-β positive cells were also elevated in MG patients *(26)*. However, similar mRNA expression of cytokine-positive MNC were observed in patients with other inflammatory neurological diseases *(26)*. Also, there was no association between numbers of cytokine-positive blood MNC and severity of MG.

These studies fail to provide a clear-cut picture on how specific cytokines contribute to MG pathogenesis. The role of specific cytokines, before, during, and after induction of MG could be explored using the animal models of MG.

4. CYTOKINES IN ANIMAL MODELS OF MG

4.1. The Role of IFN-γ

The ectopic expression of proinflammatory T helper (Th)$_1$ cytokine IFN-γ in the NMJ of mice generated a humoral IgG response to an unidentified antigen within the motor end plate, resulting in an MG-like syndrome *(27)*. In human MG, does IFN-γ directly destroy AChR at the NMJ? IFN-γ, like IFN-α, may regulate the expression of AChR at the NMJ *(28)*, but logically may not be involved in the direct destruction of AChR in MG patients. To demonstrate a direct genetic evidence for the involvement of IFN-γ in the development of EAMG, Balaji et al. tested the requirement of IFN-γ in the development of AChR-induced EAMG. *IFN-γ* gene knockout (*IFN-γ* knockout) in (129/SVEV × C57BL6) F2 mice and wild-type (129/SVJ × C57BL6) F2 mice were immunized with AChR in CFA and assessed for clinical and immunopathological manifestations of EAMG. *IFN-γ* knockout mice were completely resistant to the development of clinical EAMG *(29)*. Compared to the wild-type mice, the *IFN-γ* knockouts in the 129 background had a dramatic reduction in the anti-AChR antibodies, including the IgG$_1$ and IgG$_{2a}$ isotypes. However, AChR-primed lymph node cells from *IFN-γ* knockout mice exhibited no suppression of lymphocyte proliferative response to AChR and its dominant α146–162 peptide. The lack of suppression of T cell proliferative response to AChR and dominant α146–162 peptide in *IFN-γ* knockout mice was not surprising, because IFN-γ has been suggested to be an anti-proliferative cytokine. However, suppression of anti-AChR antibody of the IgG_1 isotype was surprising because IFN-γ has not been shown to promote IgG_1 class switching, and is mainly involved in IgG_{2a} class switching. Therefore, we studied the effect of IFN-γ deficiency in the C57BL/6 background (B6.*IFN-γ* knockout). Only a partial suppression of clinical EAMG was observed in B6.*IFN-γ* knockout mice, and specifically IgG_{2a} anti-AChR antibody production was suppressed (Deng et al., in preparation). One should note that B6 mice have a deletion of IgG_{2a} gene and carry an alternate isotype IgG_{2c}. The small amount of anti-IgG_{2a} anti-AChR antibody we detect in B6 mice is presumably owing to cross reactivity between antibodies to IgG_{2a} and IgG_{2c} isotypes. The contribution of IFN-γ in EAMG development was further complemented by the observation of lower incidence of clinical EAMG in IFN-γ receptor-deficient mice *(30)* with reduction in the IgG_{2a} and IgG_3 anti-AChR antibody isotypes.

4.2. Role of IL-12

IL-12 is a key regulatory cytokine that promotes differentiation of naive T cells into Th_1 cells. AChR-immunized *IL-12* gene (p40) knockout mice had suppressed production of serum anti-AChR antibodies of IgG_{2a} and IgG_3 isotypes. AChR-primed IL-12 knockout mice also showed suppressed IFN-γ production after in vitro stimulation with AChR *(31)*. *IL-12 p35* knockout mice demonstrated lower incidence and later onset of clinical EAMG, and significantly lower anti-AChR IgG_{2a} isotypes. The AChR-specific lymphocytes of *IL-12 p35$^{-/-}$* mice could produce IFN-γ independent of IL-12 p35 deficiency (Goluszko et al., in preparation).

4.3. Role of IL-4

IL-4 deficiency in B6 mice failed to prevent clinical EAMG. Although anti-AChR antibody levels in AChR-immunized B6.*IL-4* knockout mice is similar to wild type B6 mice, the anti-AChR IgG_1 isotype was reduced *(32)*. Moreover, the lymphocyte proliferative response to AChR and α146–162 peptide were similar in B6 and IL-4 knockout mice. In another study, Karachunski et al. *(33)* reported a slight increase in the incidence of clinical EAMG in IL-4-deficient mice, compared to wild-type B6 mice. However, data from both the laboratories confirm that IL-4 does not facilitate the development of EAMG in B6 mice *(32,33)*. *IL-4* gene polymorphism was also not observed in human MG patients *(34)*, thus supporting the findings in EAMG.

IFN-γ and IL-12, the classical Th1 (cell-mediated) cytokine, facilitated the development of antibody-mediated EAMG. Further, the cellular in vitro immune response to AChR is well-preserved in *IFN*-γ knockout and *IFN*-γ receptor knockout mice. IL-4, the classical Th2 (humoral-mediated) cytokine, failed to facilitate the development of antibody-mediated EAMG. The facilitative effect of IFN-γ and IL-12 (Th1) and the lack of facilitative effect of IL-4 (Th2), in a classical antibody-mediated EAMG, contradict the currently held dogma that Th1 cytokines are responsible for cell-mediated and Th2 cytokines for humoral-mediated phenomena. Each cytokine is produced by numerous cell types and have a plethora of functions. Therefore, the classification of cytokines to Th_1 and Th_2 would not fit well in every system of study, especially those done in vivo.

4.4. Role of IL-10

IL-10 has been shown to suppress T cell-immune responses and augment B cell production of antibodies *(35,36)*. To analyze the precise role of IL-10 in EAMG pathogenesis, we have studied the immune response in *IL-10* gene knockout (IL-10 knockout) mice in B6 background after immunization with AChR in CFA. AChR-immune *IL-10* knockout mice are less susceptible to the induction of EAMG compared to B6 mice. However, AChR-immunized *IL-10* knockout mice have an augmented AChR-specific T cell response and IFN-γ production and no reduction in anti-AChR antibody level *(37)*.

4.5. Role of TNF and Lymphotoxins

TNF polymorphism has been observed in MG patients *(3–6)*, and TNF-α- and LT-stimulate B and T cells and can modulate MHC class II expression *(38–41)*. TNF-α and LT-α/β also play a critical role in the development of lymph nodes (LN) and germinal centers in spleen and LN *(42–47)*. Because of the aforementioned reasons and a significant number of MG patients have hyperplastic thymus containing germinal centers, we hypothesized that TNF and/or LT could be involved in MG pathogenesis. To test this hypothesis, we screened for EAMG in *TNF-R p55*- and *p75*-deficient ($p55^{-/-}p75^{-/-}$) mice in the B6 background. The biological effects of TNF-α and LT-α are transmitted through membrane-bound TNF-R p55 and TNF-R p75 receptor molecules. Therefore, *TNF-R $p55^{-/-}p75^{-/-}$* mice are defective in TNF-α and LT-α signaling. *TNF-R*-deficient mice do not show any obvious abnormalities in lymphoid organs, as well as T and B cell compartments. The *TNFR $p55^{-/-}p75^{-/-}$* mice were resistant to the development of clinical EAMG and the resistance was associated with reduced serum levels of IgG, IgG_1, IgG_{2a}, and IgG_{2b} anti-AChR antibody isotypes. However, the IgM anti-AChR antibody isotype was not reduced in TNF-R $p55^{-/-}p75^{-/-}$ mice, suggesting defective anti-AChR IgG class switching. The cellular immune response to AChR and dominant α146–162 peptide was suppressed in TNF-R $p55^{-/-}$

p75$^{-/-}$ mice (Goluszko et al., submitted). LT-α deficiency completely protected B6 mice from developing clinical EAMG. AChR immunized LT-α deficient mice are capable of mounting a primary IgM anti-AChR antibody response, but are less capable of switching to the pathogenic anti-AChR IgG isotypes *(48)*.

4.6. Role of IL-6

IL-6 promotes B cell maturation and activation, differentiation, and IgG antibody isotype switching *(49)*. IL-6 also upregulates MHC class II expression *(50)*. Further, MG patients thymic epithelial cells overproduce IL-6, and therefore, IL-6 could be involved in thymic hyperplasia and germinal-center formation *(51)*. To provide a direct genetic evidence for a critical role of IL-6 in EAMG, *IL-6* gene knockout (IL-6 knockout) mice in B6 background were evaluated for EAMG pathogenesis. *IL-6* knockout mice developed normally, and only 17% of AChR-immunized *IL-6* knockout mice developed clinical EAMG, compared to 83% of wild -type B6 mice (Deng et al., in preparation). A reduction in the anti-AChR antibody response was observed in *IL-6* knockout mice. IL-6 deficiency suppressed anti-AChR antibody of IgG$_1$ and IgG$_2$ isotypes, but failed to influence the early IgM anti-AChR immune response, suggesting defective IgG class switching. AChR and α146–162 peptide-specific lymphocyte response and IFN-γ and IL-10 production were suppressed in *IL-6* knockout mice, suggesting a possible regulatory role of IL-6 on AChR-specific IFN-γ and IL-10 production (Deng et al., in preparation).

4.7. IFN-α Suppresses EAMG Development

IFN-α treatment after immunization with AChR, or administered after established clinical EAMG, either prevented or induced significant remission of clinical EAMG. *(52,53)*. The remission after IFN-α treatment was associated with a reduction of CD4 cells and anti-AChR antibodies of IgG$_1$ and IgG$_{2b}$ isotypes. It is possible that IFN-α treatment reduced the MHC class II expression or costimulatory molecule activation. IFN-α also has a direct enhancing effect on AChR expression in rat myotubes in cultures *(28)*.

4.8. AChR- or Peptide-Specific Tolerance Modulate Cytokine Production

High-dose systemic tolerance with α146–162 in complete Freund's adjuvant (CFA) induced determinant spread (infectious tolerance) by downregulating IL-2, IFN-γ, and IL-10, and partially suppressed EAMG *(54)*, without immune deviation. Even after oral tolerance with α146–162 peptide IL-2, IFN-γ, and IL-10 were suppressed *(55)*. Oral tolerance with AChR

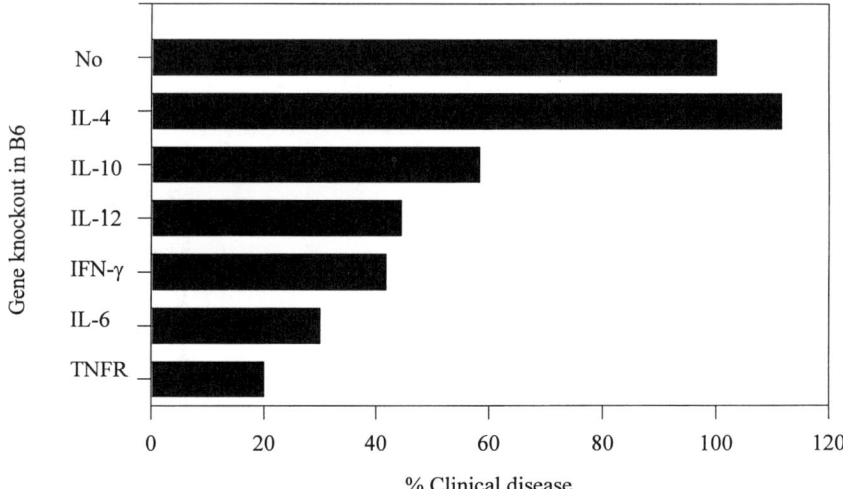

Fig. 1. The hierarchy of the involvement of TNF and IL-6 in EAMG pathogenesis. Incidence of EAMG in cytokine-gene knockout mice is expressed as relative percentage of mice with clinical disease compared to maximum clinical incidence achieved in wild-type B6 mice. Data represent mean of three independent experiments for IFN-γ, two independent experiments for IL-10 and IL-12, and one experiment for IL-6 and TNFR gene knockout mice. The % clinical disease calculated using the formula:

$$\frac{\text{\% KO mice with disease}}{\text{\% of B6 with disease}} \times 100$$

downregulated IFN-γ and IL-4 and upregulated TGF-β *(56)*. Either oral or nasal tolerance with recombinant AChR α-subunit down regulated Th1 cytokines *(57,58)*. However, nasal tolerance with AChR α-subunit peptides or AChR tolerance downregulated Th1 and upregulated Th2 cytokines *(59,60)*. Whether the above antigen-specific tolerance could reverse the established disease is yet to be seen.

5. CONCLUSION

The hierarchy of the involvement of TNF, IL-6, IFN-γ, IL-12, and IL-10 in EAMG pathogenesis is illustrated in Fig. 1. TNF and IL-6 top the list of the cytokines that are crucial for the development of cellular and humoral immune response to AChR and the development of clinical EAMG. IFN-γ, IL-12, and IL-10 also contribute to the development of clinical EAMG, however, in the absence of one of these cytokines, significant numbers of mice still could develop EAMG owing to a possible compensatory effect of other cytokines (e.g., TNF, IL-6) involved in the disease. IL-4 is not involved in EAMG pathogenesis in B6 mice. Most of the cytokines or their receptor knockout studies are performed in B6 background, and therefore the role of cytokines studied will apply only for this background. All these cytokine knockout mice developed normally and have an intact immune system. In the future, the findings derived from cytokine gene knockout mice should be complemented with findings from in vivo neutralization or augmentation of specific cytokines during the development of EAMG. TNF and IL-6 could act both in the afferent and efferent limb of an autoimmune response to AChR; and its effect on B cell activation, differentiation, and class switching would significantly influence the outcome of disease. Therefore, therapeutic blockade of TNF and/or IL-6 might significantly control the ongoing disease. This form of nonspecific therapy could be instituted for a temporary period of time, followed by maintenance therapy with antigen-specific tolerance (e.g., high-dose T cell epitope tolerance).

ACKNOWLEDGMENT

Our studies reported in this review were supported by grants from NIH, Muscular Dystrophy Association, Association Francaise Contre les Myopathies, Myasthenia Gravis Foundation of America, Sealy Foundation, and James W. McLaughlin Foundation.

REFERENCES

1. Bell, J., Rassenti, L., Smoot, S., Smith, K., Newby, C., Hohlfeld, R., et al. (1986) HLA-DQ beta-chain polymorphism linked to myasthenia gravis. *Lancet* **1,** 1058–1060.
2. Hjelmstrom, P., Giscombe, R., Lefvert, A. K., Pirskanen, R., Kockum, I., Landin-Olsson, M., et al. (1996) Polymorphic amino acid domains of the HLA-DQ molecule are associated with disease heterogeneity in myasthenia gravis. *J. Neuroimmunol.* **65,** 125–131.
3. Hjelmstrom, P., Peacock, C. S., Giscombe, R., Pirskanen, R., Lefvert, A. K., Blackwell, J. M., et al. (1998) Polymorphism in tumor necrosis factor genes associated with myasthenia gravis. *J. Neuroimmunol.* **88,** 137–143.
4. Skeie, G. O., Pandey, J. P., Aarli, J. A., and Gilhus, N. E. (1999) TNFA and TNFB polymorphisms in myasthenia gravis. *Arch. Neurol.* **56,** 457–461.
5. Zelano, G., Lino, M. M., Evoli, A., Settesoldi, D., Batocchi, A. P., Torrente, I., et al. (1998) Tumour necrosis factor beta gene polymorphisms in myasthenia gravis. *Eur. J. Immunogenet.* **25,** 403–408.
6. Huang, D., Pirskanen, R., Hjelmstrom, P., and Lefvert, A. K. (1998) Polymorphisms in IL-1beta and IL-1 receptor antagonist genes are associated with myasthenia gravis. *J. Neuroimmunol.* **81,** 76–81.

7. Huang, D. R., Zhou, Y. H., Xia, S. Q., Liu, L., Pirskanen, R., and Lefvert, A. K. (1999) Markers in the promoter region of interleukin-10 (IL-10) gene in myasthenia gravis: implications of diverse effects of IL-10 in the pathogenesis of the disease. *J. Neuroimmunol.* **94,** 82–87.

8. Christadoss, P., Poussin, M., and Deng, C. (2000) Animal models of myasthenia gravis. *Clini. Immunol.* **94,** 75–87.

9. Christadoss P., Lennon V. A., Krco C. J., Lambert E. H, and David C. S. (1981) Genetic control of autoimmunity to acetylcholine receptors: role of Ia molecules. *Ann N Y Acad Sci,* **377,** 258-277.

10. Christadoss, P., Lennon, V. A., and David, C. (1979) Genetic control of experimental autoimmune myasthenia gravis in mice. I. Lymphocyte proliferative response to acetylcholine receptors is under H-2-linked Ir gene control. *J. Immunol.* **123,** 2540–2543.

11. Christadoss, P., Lennon, V. A., Krco, C. J., and David, C. S. (1982) Genetic control of experimental autoimmune myasthenia gravis in mice. III. Ia molecules mediate cellular immune responsiveness to acetylcholine receptors. *J. Immunol.* **128,** 1141–1144.

12. Christadoss, P., Lindstrom, J. M., Melvold, R. W., and Talal, N. (1985) Mutation at I-A beta chain prevents experimental autoimmune myasthenia gravis. *Immunogenetics* **21,** 33–38.

13. Kaul, R., Shenoy, M., Goluszko, E., and Christadoss, P. (1994) Major histocompatibility complex class II gene disruption prevents experimental autoimmune myasthenia gravis. *J. Immunol.* **152,** 3152–3157.

14. Christadoss, P. and Dauphinee, M. J. (1986) Immunotherapy for myasthenia gravis: a murine model. *J. Immunol.* **136,** 2437–2440.

15. Zhang, G. X., Xiao, B. G., Bakhiet, M., van der Meide, P., Wigzell, H., Link, H., et al. (1996) Both CD4+ and CD8+ T cells are essential to induce experimental autoimmune myasthenia gravis. *J. Exp. Med.* **184,** 349–356.

16. Shenoy, M., Kaul, R., Goluszko, E., David, C., and Christadoss, P. (1994) Effect of MHC class I and CD8 cell deficiency on experimental autoimmune myasthenia gravis pathogenesis. *J. Immunol.* **153,** 5330–5335.

17. Hohlfeld, R., Conti-Tronconi, B., Kalies, I., Bertrams, J., and Toyka, K. V. (1985) Genetic restriction of autoreactive acetylcholine receptor-specific T lymphocytes in myasthenia gravis. *J. Immunol.* **135,** 2393–2399.

18. Shenoy, M., Oshima, M., Atassi, M. Z., and Christadoss, P. (1993) Suppression of experimental autoimmune myasthenia gravis by epitope- specific neonatal tolerance to synthetic region alpha 146-162 of acetylcholine receptor. *Clin. Immunol. Immunopathol.* **66,** 230–238.

19. Wu, B., Shenoy, M., Goluszko, E., Kaul, R., and Christadoss, P. (1995) TCR gene usage in experimental autoimmune myasthenia gravis pathogenesis. Usage of multiple TCRBV genes in the H-2b strains. *J. Immunol.* **154,** 3603–3610.

20. Melms, A., Oksenberg, J. R., Malcherek, G., Schoepfer, R., Muller, C. A., Lindstrom, J., et al. (1993) T-cell receptor gene usage of acetylcholine receptor-specific T-helper cells. *Ann. NY Acad. Sci.* **681,** 313,314.

21. Dedhia, V., Goluszko, E., Wu, B., Deng, C., and Christadoss, P. (1998) The effect of B cell deficiency on the immune response to acetylcholine receptor

and the development of experimental autoimmune myasthenia gravis. *Clin. Immunol. Immunopathol.* **87**, 266–275.

22. Li, H., Fu-Dong, S., Bing, H., Bakheit, M., Wahren, B., Berglof, A., et al. (1998) Experimental autoimmune myasthenia gravis induction in B cell-deficient mice. *Intl. Immunol.* **10**, 1359–1365.

23. Christadoss, P. (1988) C5 gene influences the development of murine myasthenia gravis. *J. Immunol.* **140**, 2589–2592.

24. Shi, F. D., He, B., Li, H., Matusevicius, D., Link, H., and Ljunggren, H. G. (1998) Differential requirements for CD28 and CD40 ligand in the induction of experimental autoimmune myasthenia gravis. *Eur. J. Immunol.* **28**, 3587–3593.

25. Huang, D. R., Pirskanen, R., Matell, G., and Lefvert, A. K. (1999) Tumour necrosis factor-alpha polymorphism and secretion in myasthenia gravis. *J. Neuroimmunol.* **94**, 165–171.

26. Link, J., Navikas, V., Yu, M., Fredrikson, S., Osterman, P. O., and Link, H. (1994) Augmented interferon-gamma, interleukin-4 and transforming growth factor-beta mRNA expression in blood mononuclear cells in myasthenia gravis. *J. Neuroimmunol.* **51**, 185–192.

27. Gu, D., Wogensen, L., Calcutt, N. A., Xia, C., Zhu, S., Merlie, J. P., Fox, H. S., et al. (1995) Myasthenia gravis-like syndrome induced by expression of interferon gamma in the neuromuscular junction. *J. Exp. Med.* **181**, 547–557.

28. Andre, P., Brauns, S., Passaquin, A. C., Coupin, G., Barthaleyns, T., Warker, J. M., et al. (1988) Rat interferon enhances the expression of acetylcholine receptors in rat myotubes in culture. *J. Neurosci. Res.* **19**, 297.

29. Balasa, B., Deng, C., Lee, J., Bradley, L. M., Dalton, D. K., Christadoss, P., et al. (1997) Interferon gamma (IFN-gamma) is necessary for the genesis of acetylcholine receptor-induced clinical experimental autoimmune myasthenia gravis in mice. *J. Exp. Med.* **186**, 385–391.

30. Zhang, G. X., Xiao, B. G., Bai, X. F., van der Meide, P. H., Orn, A., and Link, H. (1999) Mice with IFN-gamma receptor deficiency are less susceptible to experimental autoimmune myasthenia gravis. *J. Immunol.* **162**, 3775–3781.

31. Moiola, L., Galbiati, F., Martino, G., Amadio, S., Brambilla, E., Comi, G., et al. (1998) IL-12 is involved in the induction of experimental autoimmune myasthenia gravis, an antibody-mediated disease. *Eur. J. Immunol.* **28**, 2487–2497.

32. Balasa, B., Deng, C., Lee, J., Christadoss, P., and Sarvetnick, N. (1998) The Th2 cytokine IL-4 is not required for the progression of antibody- dependent autoimmune myasthenia gravis. *J. Immunol.* **161**, 2856–2862.

33. Karachunski, P. I., Ostlie, N. S., Okita, D. K., and Conti-Fine, B. M. (1999) Interleukin-4 deficiency facilitates development of experimental myasthenia gravis and precludes its prevention by nasal administration of CD4+ epitope sequences of the acetylcholine receptor. *J. Neuroimmunol.* **95**, 73–84.

34. Huang, D., Xia, S., Zhou, Y., Pirskanen, R., Liu L., and Lefvert, A. K. (1998) No evidence for interleukin-4 gene conferring susceptibility to myasthenia gravis. *J. Neuroimmunol.* **92**, 208–211.

35. Berg, D. J., Leach, M. W., Kuhn, R., Rajewsky, K., Muller, W., Davidson, N. J., et al. (1995) Interleukin 10 but not interleukin 4 is a natural suppressant of cutaneous inflammatory responses. *J. Exp. Med.* **182**, 99–108.

36. Ishida, H., Muchamuel, T., Sakaguchi, S., Andrade, S., Menon, S., and Howard, M. (1994) Continuous administration of anti-interleukin 10 antibodies delays onset of autoimmunity in NZB/W F1 mice. *J. Exp. Med.* **179,** 305–310.

37. Poussin, M. A., Goluszko, E., Houghes, T., Duchiella, S. I., and Christadoss, P. (2000) Suppression of experimental autoimmune myasthenia gravis in IL10 gene-disrupted mice is associated with reduced B cell and serum cytotoxicity on mouse cell line expressing AChR. *J. Neuroimmuno.* **111,** 152.

38. Jelinek, D. F. and Lipsky, P. E. (1987) Enhancement of human B cell proliferation and differentiation by tumor necrosis factor-alpha and interleukin 1. *J. Immunol.* **139,** 2970–2976.

39. Sung, S. S., Bjorndahl, J. M., Wang, C. Y., Kao, H. T., and Fu, S. M. (1988) Production of tumor necrosis factor/cachectin by human T cell lines and peripheral blood T lymphocytes stimulated by phorbol myristate acetate and anti-CD3 antibody. *J. Exp. Med.* **167,** 937–953.

40. Watanabe, Y. and Jacob, C. O. (1991) Regulation of MHC class II antigen expression. Opposing effects of tumor necrosis factor-alpha on IFN-gamma-induced HLA-DR and Ia expression depends on the maturation and differentiation stage of the cell. *J. Immunol.* **146,** 899–905.

41. Pujol-Borrell, R., Todd, I., Doshi, M., Bottazzo, G. F., Sutton, R., Gray, D., et al. (1987) HLA class II induction in human islet cells by interferon-gamma plus tumour necrosis factor or lymphotoxin. *Nature* **326,** 304–306.

42. De Togni, P., Goellner, J., Ruddle, N. H., Streeter, P. R., Fick, A., Mariathasan, S., et al. (1994) Abnormal development of peripheral lymphoid organs in mice deficient in lymphotoxin [see comments]. *Science* **264,** 703–707.

43. Pasparakis, M., Alexopoulou, L., Episkopou, V., and Kollias, G. (1996) Immune and inflammatory responses in TNF alpha-deficient mice: a critical requirement for TNF alpha in the formation of primary B cell follicles, follicular dendritic cell networks and germinal centers, and in the maturation of the humoral immune response [see comments]. *J. Exp. Med.* **184,** 1397–1411.

44. Matsumoto, M., Mariathasan, S., Nahm, M. H., Baranyay, F., Peschon, J. J., and Chaplin, D. D. (1996) Role of lymphotoxin and the type I TNF receptor in the formation of germinal centers. *Science* **271,** 1289–1291.

45. Matsumoto, M., Fu, Y. X., Molina, H., and Chaplin, D. D. (1997) Lymphotoxin-alpha-deficient and TNF receptor-I-deficient mice define developmental and functional characteristics of germinal centers. *Im°munol. Rev.* **156,** 137–144.

46. Ettinger, R., Mebius, R., Browning, J. L., Michie, S. A., van Tuijl, S., Kraal, G., et al. (1998) Effects of tumor necrosis factor and lymphotoxin on peripheral lymphoid tissue development. *Intl. Immunol.* **10,** 727–741.

47. Chaplin, D. D. and Fu, Y. (1998) Cytokine regulation of secondary lymphoid organ development. *Curr. Opin. Immunol.* **10,** 289–297.

48. Goluszko, E., Hellstrom, P., Deng, C., Ruddle, N., and Christadoss, P. (2001) Lymphotoxin alpha deficiency completely protects B6 mice from developing clinical experimental autoimmune myasthenia gravis. *J. Neuroimmunol.* **113,** 109.

49. Taga, T. and Kishimoto, T. (1997) Gp130 and the interleukin-6 family of cytokines. *Annu. Rev. Immunol.* **15,** 797–819.

50. Yang, T. H., Aosai, F., Norose, K., Ueda, M., and Yano, A. (1996) Differential regulation of HLA-DR expression and antigen presentation in Toxoplasma

gondii-infected melanoma cells by interleukin 6 and interferon gamma. *Microbiol. Immunol.* **40,** 443–449.

51. Cohen-Kaminsky, S., Devergne, O., Delattre, R. M., Klingel-Schmitt, I., Emilie, D., Galanaud, P., et al. (1993) Interleukin-6 overproduction by cultured thymic epithelial cells from patients with myasthenia gravis is potentially involved in thymic hyperplasia. *Eur. Cytokine Netw.* **4,** 121–132.

52. Shenoy, M., Baron, S., Wu, B., Goluszko E., and Christadoss, P. (1995) IFN-alpha treatment suppresses the development of experimental autoimmune myasthenia gravis. *J. Immunol.* **154,** 6203–6208.

53. Deng, C., Goluszko, E., Baron, S., Wu, B., and Christadoss, P. (1996) IFN-alpha therapy is effective in suppressing the clinical experimental myasthenia gravis. *J. Immunol.* **157,** 5675–5682.

54. Wu, B., Deng, C., Goluszko, E., and Christadoss, P. (1997) Tolerance to a dominant T cell epitope in the acetylcholine receptor molecule induces epitope spread and suppresses murine myasthenia gravis. *J. Immunol.* **159,** 3016–3023.

55. Baggi, F., Andreetta, F., Caspani, E., Milani, M., Longhi, R., Mantegazza, R., Cornelio, F., and Antozzi, C. (1999) Oral administration of an immunodominant T-cell epitope downregulates Th1/Th2 cytokines and prevents experimental myasthenia gravis. *J. Clin. Invest.* **104,** 1287–1295.

56. Ma, C. G., Zhang, G. X., Xiao, B. G., Wang, Z. Y., Link, J., Olsson, T., et al. (1996) Mucosal tolerance to experimental autoimmune myasthenia gravis is associated with down-regulation of AChR-specific IFN-gamma-expressing Th1-like cells and up-regulation of TGF-beta mRNA in mononuclear cells. *Ann. NY Acad. Sci.* **778,** 273–287.

57. Barchan, D., Asher, O., Tzartos, S. J., Fuchs, S., and Souroujon, M. C. (1998) Modulation of the anti-acetylcholine receptor response and experimental autoimmune myasthenia gravis by recombinant fragments of the acetylcholine receptor. *Eur. J. Immunol.* **28,** 616–624.

58. Barchan, D., Souroujon, M. C., Im, S. H., Antozzi, C., and Fuchs, S. (1999) Antigen-specific modulation of experimental myasthenia gravis: nasal tolerization with recombinant fragments of the human acetylcholine receptor alpha-subunit. *Proc. Natl. Acad. Sci. USA* **96,** 8086–8091.

59. Ma, C. G., Zhang, G. X., Xiao, B. G., Link, J., Olsson, T., and Link, H. (1995) Suppression of experimental autoimmune myasthenia gravis by nasal administration of acetylcholine receptor. *J. Neuroimmunol.* **58,** 51–60.

60. Karachunski, P. I., Ostlie, N. S., Okita, D. K., and Conti-Fine, B. M. (1997) Prevention of experimental myasthenia gravis by nasal administration of synthetic acetylcholine receptor T epitope sequences. *J. Clin. Invest.* **100,** 3027–3035.

III

CYTOKINES AND AUTOIMMUNITY: A SYNTHESIS

16
Cytokines in Autoimmune Disease

Vijay K. Kuchroo and Lindsay B. Nicholson

1. INTRODUCTION

Cytokines play an important role in the induction and regulation of autoimmune diseases. They mediate the expansion and differentiation of T helper (Th) cells to generate autoantigen-reactive pathogenic or protective effectors, they help self-reactive B cells to produce autoantibodies, and they also participate in mediating tissue damage in the target organ. Cytokines also control tissue tolerance and "immune-privilege" and prevent the propagation of inflammation in a number of organs. In addition, in concert with the selectin and intergrin molecules, cytokines control the trafficking and homing of self-reactive cells to target organs. Simply put, cytokines form a central coordinating network of soluble effector molecules and this plays a crucial role at every step of development of autoimmune disease: in the generation of pathogenic (or protective) effectors, in the trafficking of pathogenic cells to the target organ, and in mediating tissue damage or tissue tolerance in the target organ.

Of all the cells of the immune system, self-reactive CD4$^+$ T cells play perhaps the most important role in both induction and regulation of autoimmune diseases. How do these CD4$^+$, Th cells mediate their pathogenic and protective effects in an autoimmune disease? This question is probably best answered by the paradigm initially proposed by Mossman and colleagues, that naive Th cells differentiate following activation into distinct functional subgroups, which are characterized by their pattern of cytokine secretion (Part I). Originally it was hypothesized that upon activation this differentiation of Th cells was into two different pathways, T helper 1 (Th1) and T helper 2 (Th2). We now know that this classification is oversimplified, because other distinct Th subsets like Th helper 3 (Th3) and T regulatory 1

From: *Cytokines and Autoimmune Diseases*
Edited by: V. K. Kuchroo, et al. © Humana Press Inc., Totowa, NJ

(Tr1) have also been identified, and some effector Th cells have mixed patterns of cytokine secretion that do not clearly fall into either one of the described Th subsets. Nevertheless, this classification of Th subsets, each producing distinct sets of cytokines, has provided a framework within which one can understand how self-reactive cells can develop into either pathogenic or protective effectors. Furthermore, work with transgenic T cells has conclusively shown that cells with identical T cell receptors (TCRs) have the potential to differentiate to different phenotypes and that these cells can have different effects on autoimmunity depending on their state of differentiation.

Based on initial observations, it was proposed that upon activation with cognate ligand naive Th cells differentiate into Th1 cells which secrete interleukin-2 (IL-2) and interferon-γ (IFN-γ), activate macrophages and elicit delayed-type hypersensitivity (DTH) reactions or Th2 cells that produce IL-4, IL-10, and IL-13, are important for IgE production and suppress cell-mediated immunity. The cytokines produced by each subset act as their own autocrine growth factors but crossregulate the other subset's development and function. This model has been successfully applied to explain a number of immune phenomena in vivo. Interestingly studies of single cells have shown little or no evidence for coordinate expression of cytokine genes, whereas studies of the plasticity of Th phenotypes have shown that in vitro, chronic antigen exposure leads to more stable polarization than does short term culture. This suggests two important constraints of the model. Th cell "phenotype" is best analyzed at a population level rather than at a cellular level, and polarized phenotypes are likely to be most relevant in chronic diseases such as autoimmunity.

This book has been divided into three major sections: The first section includes chapters that summarize the basic concepts of T cell activation, expansion, and differentiation including the role of antigen, costimulatory molecules, and transcription factors in cytokine-gene expression. This section also includes a chapter on chemokines and chemokine receptors, which are crucial for trafficking and homing of self-reactive cells into tissues. In the second section of the book, we have included chapters on how cytokines play a role in mediating tissue damage in autoimmune disease. Because basic mechanisms of activation and expansion of self-reactive T cells in lymph nodes are the same, but the target organ involved in each disease is unique, this leads to some common concepts with respect to the induction of autoreactive cells but then to different pathologies and outcomes in the effector phase, because the end-organ involved in each disease is different. In view of this, a section on the role of cytokines in the induction and regulation of several major autoimmune diseases including diabetes, multiple sclerosis (MS), rheumatoid arthritis (RA), uveitis, myasthenia gravis (MG), and systemic lupus erythromatosis (SLE) (including their animal models) have been included. It is hoped that basic scientists involved in studying cytokine biology will benefit from the clinical chapters listing the profound effects of various cytokines on the induction and regulation of autoimmune diseases. Conversely, the clinical scientist studying autoimmune diseases could gain from the chapters discussing how effector cells that regulate or mediate autoimmune diseases attain different cytokine phenotypes. In this chapter, we will try to bring together the essence of each chapter presented in the two preceding sections, and to synthesize a comprehensive understanding of the current state of knowledge on the role of cytokines in the induction of autoimmune disease.

2. T CELL DIFFERENTIATION AND GENERATION OF PATHOGENIC AND PROTECTIVE EFFECTORS OF AUTOIMMUNE DISEASE

Before a T cell-mediated autoimmune disease develops, the immune response goes through a number of discrete steps: The self-reactive T cells have to undergo activation, expansion and differentiation; traffic to the target organ; and get reactivated there before they mediate tissue damage. The four essential features that contribute to the pathogenicity of an autoreactive T cell are: (1) the nature of the target antigen, (2) epitope specificity, (3) cytokine profile, and (4) expression of appropriate surface molecules (e.g., adhesion molecules, chemokine receptors (for trafficking), and death receptors (like FasL).

In the case of antibody-mediated diseases, such as SLE, MG, and some forms of RA, the expansion of both CD4$^+$ T cells, and self-reactive B cells, which produce pathogenic antibody of an appropriate isotype, are necessary for the induction of disease. The isotype of the antibody is perhaps the defining feature of whether an antibody can mediate pathology, and this again is controlled by the cytokine help that self-reactive B cells receive during expansion and differentiation. Thus, the cytokine profile that an autoreactive T cell attains during expansion and differentiation is crucial for the outcome of an autoimmune response; if a T cell acquires a cytokine profile that is directly pathogenic and/or helps autoreactive B cells to produce pathogenic antibodies, this will result in tissue damage and the induction of autoimmune disease. On the other hand, if during expansion of autoreactive T cells, the T cells develop a cytokine profile that is nonpathogenic, these cells will not generate a pathogenic T cell response, and may even protect the organ from tissue damage and prevent the development of autoimmune disease. One important distinction that can be drawn from the work discussed in this book is the difference between cytokines as a marker of phenotype and cytokines as mediators of inflammation and tissue injury. In most cases, differentiation to a Th1 phenotype is closely associated with pathogenicity, but the elaboration of specific Th1 cytokines by effector cells is not found to be necessary for the development of disease.

In experimental autoimmune models, the phenotype of T cells that induce disease (and protection) has been exhaustively studied but the data in human autoimmune disease is limiting simply because the pathogenic effects of T cells cannot be tested. In a number of experimental and human autoimmune diseases, Th1 cells that produce IL-2 and IFN-γ have been implicated as pathogenic effectors, but in other autoimmune diseases there are indications that the autoimmune disease is mediated by Th2 cells, which produce IL-4, IL-10, and IL-13. In addition to Th1 and Th2 cells, in a number of instances cells that produce predominantly transforming growth factor-β (TGF-β) (Th3) or IL-10 (Tr1) have been implicated in protection from autoimmune disease. Therefore a question central to our understanding of autoimmunity is how does a Th precursor (Thp) cell acquire a cytokine profile during expansion and differentiation? If one understands the basic mechanisms that control T cell differentiation, this may provide us with avenues to modulate cytokine phenotype and prevent tissue damage and autoimmunity, and even promote protection against autoimmune disease. Besides the genetic makeup of the individual, T cell differentiation is affected by a number of factors: cytokines themselves, cell-surface receptors including costimulatory molecules, and route, dose and type of antigen (*see* Fig. 1).

3. ROLE OF CYTOKINES AND TRANSCRIPTION FACTORS

Cytokines are the most dominant factors affecting T cell differentiation. The best understood initiators of Th cell differentiation are the cytokines IL-12 and IL-4, which may be present early in an immune response, following activation of the innate immune system by conserved microbial structural elements (proteins, polysaccharides, or lipids). Microbial pathogens induce IL-12 production from macrophages and dendritic cells (DC) and the Th1

Fig. 1. Overview of the role of cytokines in the development and regulation of autoimmune disease. **(A)** In the draining lymph node antigen specific naive precursor Th cells are activated in a microenvironment which determines how they differentiate. Signals from a diverse array of receptors, which detect both soluble factors and the state of cell surface receptors on APCs and other cells in the microenvironment, are integrated and initiate an explosive period of growth and differentiation. **(B)** Differentiated effector T cells traffic to the target organ where they act on and

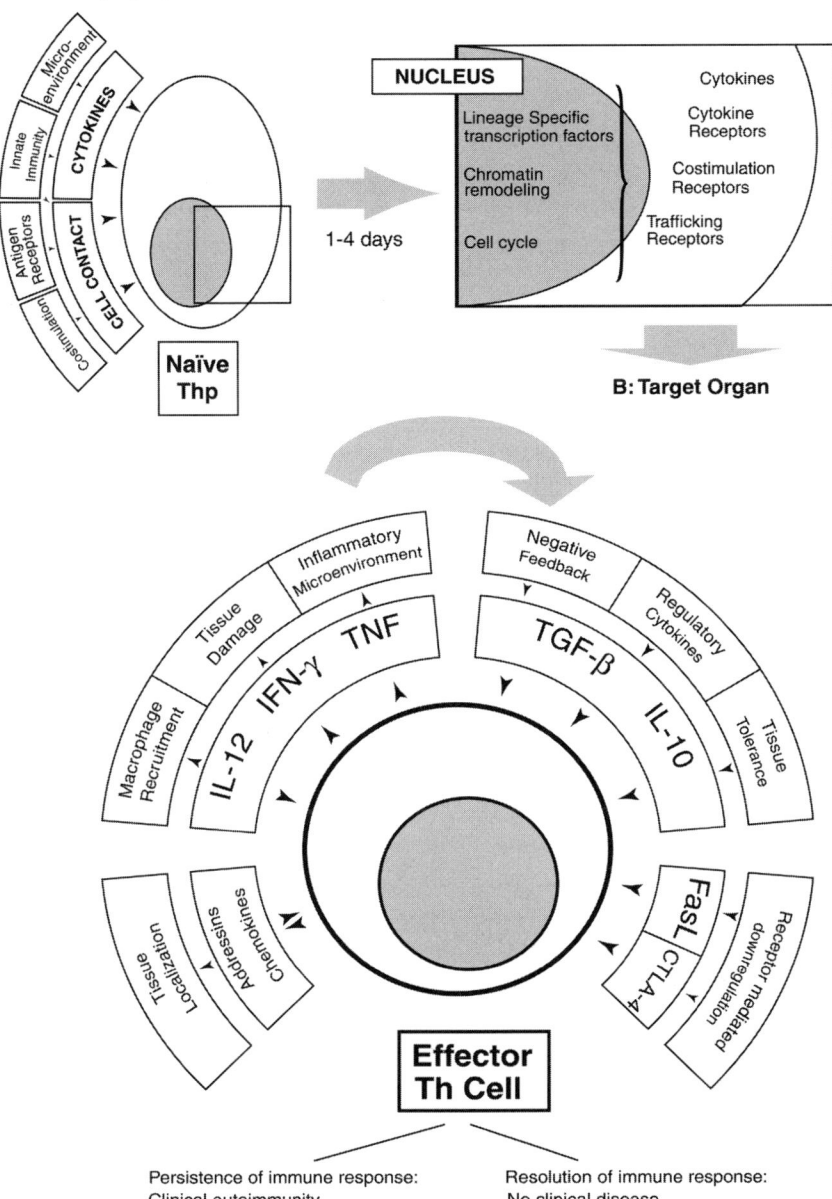

A: Draining Lymph Node

NUCLEUS

Lineage Specific transcription factors

Chromatin remodeling

Cell cycle

1-4 days

Cytokines

Cytokine Receptors

Costimulation Receptors

Trafficking Receptors

Naïve Thp

B: Target Organ

Inflammatory Microenvironment

Negative Feedback

Tissue Damage

Regulatory Cytokines

Macrophage Recruitment

TNF

IFN-γ

IL-12

TGF-β

IL-10

Tissue Tolerance

Tissue Localization

Addressins

Chemokines

FasL

CTLA-4

Receptor mediated downregulation

Effector Th Cell

Persistence of immune response: Clinical autoimmunity

Resolution of immune response: No clinical disease

Fig. 1. *(continued)* are acted upon by the microenvironment. Proinflammatory cytokines promote recruitment of macrophages and cell death, but may also be important in inducing downregulatory mechanisms which limit the immune response and tissue damage. Where the immune response resolves, this is clinically silent. When it persists, autoimmune disease ensues. The mechanisms proposed by this figure are supported by experimental data, however the exact nature of these complex interactions remain to be elucidated.

cytokine IFN-γ from Thp cells, and this promotes their differentiation along the Th1 pathway. On the other hand, IL-4 promotes differentiation of Thps along the Th2 pathway. One source of IL-4 may be NK 1.1 T cells that express markers of both αβT cells and natural killer (NK) cells and recognize lipids or glycolipids. These cells produce a burst of IL-4 following activation and are believed to be an initial source of the IL-4 that promotes Th2 differentiation (*see* Part I, Chapter 5 by Exley and Wilson). Therefore signals from the environment are integrated to induce a cytokine milieu that will regulate patterns of gene transcription.

The ligation of cytokine receptors on the surface of T cells by IL-4 and IL-12 acts in concert with TCR-derived signals to induce specific transcription factors necessary for the differentiation of T cells. IL-12 induces STAT-4 (signal transducer and activators of transcription) following ligation of IL-12 receptor in Thp cells, which in turn is crucial for the induction of IFN-γ production. IL-4 induces STAT-6 following ligation of the IL-4 receptor on Thp, which helps transcription of the IL-4 gene. However the STAT transcription factors do not act alone but in combination with TCR-derived signals, and through the process of chromatin remodeling, which opens specific cytokine loci (*see* Part I, Chapter 1 by Rengarajan and Glimcher and Section I, Chapter 2 by Shannon and Holloway).

In Thp cells, cytokine genes are generally inactive and are found on condensed chromatin, containing unmodified histones and densely methylated DNA. Cellular activation results in acetylation of histones and demethylation of DNA, leading to locus opening and transcriptionally competent genes. The chromatin structure thus plays a very important role in the regulation of gene expression by changing in a cell-type specific fashion, with alterations in the chromatin structure of individual cytokine loci making them accessible to transcription factors. Comparison of the chromatin structure associated with the genes for the Th1 cytokine IFN-γ and the Th2 cytokine IL-4 in naive and differentiated Th1 and Th2 cells has revealed that there is tissue-specific chromatin remodeling. In Th2 cells, which express IL-4, the IL-4 locus was found to be accessible and open, whereas the IFN-γ locus displayed a closed configuration. The converse was true for Th1 clones, which had an open IFN-γ but not IL-4 locus. Thus, naive T cells do not have an accessible configuration for either gene, but upon differentiation specific loci become accessible. One important property of chromatin remodeling is that gene accessibility is inheritable by daughter cells. This provides a mechanism whereby phenotype is maintained through multiple cell divisions. As proposed in Part I, Chapter 1, this chromatin remodeling plays an important role in accessibility, communication, and epigenetic imprinting and memory.

Transcription of cytokine genes requires a cooperative and synergistic action of multiple ubiquitous and cytokine promoter-specific *trans*-activating elements to promote gene transcription. Whereas some transcription factors like NFAT, AP-1, and NF-κB induce the transcription of multiple cytokine genes, recent identification of specific transcription factors that are restricted in their expression in Th1 and Th2 cells and that induce transcription of either IL-4 or IFN-γ has provided a molecular basis for understanding T cell differentiation. c-maf, a proto-oncogene, was found to be selectively upregulated, upon crosslinking of the TCR, during the course of Th2 but not Th1 differentiation. c-maf strongly transactivates IL-4 but not IL-5 or IL-10 transcription. GATA-3, a second transcription factor identified as Th2-specific, increases transcription of most of the Th2 cytokines including IL-4, IL-5, IL-10, and IL-13. Induction of GATA-3 is dependent on STAT6. Both GATA-3 and c-maf may remodel chromatin and increase IL-4 locus accessibility for the TCR-derived transcription factors. Expression of T-bet, a member of the T-box family of transcription factors that regulate many developmental processes, strongly correlates with the expression of IFN-γ in Th1 and NK cells. T-bet has a profound effect on IFN-γ production, in that when overexpressed it significantly transactivates the IFN-γ promoter, whereas retroviral transduction of T-bet into primary, developing, and fully polarized Th2 cells induces IFN-γ secretion and represses IL-4 and IL-5 production. T-bet may also repress GATA-3 and GATA-3 may repress T-bet expression during Th2 development. The relative predominance of T-bet and GATA-3 may serve to control the fate of naive Th-cell commitment to a specific subset (*see* Part I, Chapter 1 by Rengarajan and Glimcher). In summary, transcription-factor regulation and chromatin remodeling provide the molecular machinery to drive and maintain T cell differentiation by cytokines.

4. ROLE OF ANTIGEN

Although nonantigen specific factors (e.g., cytokines) are the dominant T cell polarizers in tissue culture, it is clear that the nature of TCR ligands (peptide/major histocompatibility complex [MHC] complex) and quantity and quality of TCR signaling also influences Th polarization. For many years, it was generally assumed that activation of T cells was an all-or-none phenomenon: When peptide/MHC fit with the TCR was sufficient and significant, the T cell responded by proliferation and effector function (cytokine release or cell killing). However, if the interaction of peptide/MHC complex with the TCR did not reach this threshold, the peptide/MHC complex was ignored and no signals were generated. This view was challenged with the observation that altered peptides (variant ligands; also called altered peptide ligands or APLs) made by single amino acid substitutions at the TCR contact residues of the agonist ligands could evoke some but not all T cell functions.

It was found that different cytokine patterns could be obtained from the same T cell activated with different ligands, suggesting that each cytokine may have different thresholds for induction and therefore that the pattern of cytokine induction may have a hierarchical organization. This in turn may effect T cell differentiation, depending on the affinity of interaction of the ligand for the TCR in the Thp. The identification of APLs that antagonize, anergize, or partially activate T cell clones has allowed one to reanalyze the ability of TCR ligands to affect T cell differentiation.

The biological rationale for this complexity is not well-understood. One possible explanation arises from the realization that a single TCR has the potential to productively engage many different peptide ligands. If in a lifetime, a T cell encounters more that one activating ligand, especially if one of these ligands is derived from a pathogen and the other is an autoantigen, being able to respond differently to each could be advantageous. On the other hand, there is evidence that in chronic infections, rapidly mutating viruses can exploit the existence of TCR peptide antagonists to inhibit effector $CD8^+$ T cells, which is unlikely to be of benefit to the host. Understanding the significance and role of T cell-APL interactions in vivo remains an interesting challenge.

In vitro, one fruitful approach has been the use of altered peptide is with different affinities for MHC. In these experiments, altering amino-acids that effect MHC binding but that preserve residues that contact TCR allowed the generation of a family of myelin basic protein (MBP) Ac1-9 derivatives with IC_{50} values across a six-log concentration range. Immunization with low-affinity peptide resulted in an immune response that was skewed towards the production of Th2 cytokines, whereas using the high affinity ligand increased the frequency of IFN-γ producing cells in vivo. Thus, manipulating the level of display of peptide MHC can influence the phenotype of the T cell response and this is consistent with data from experiments using naive T cells expressing a transgenic TCR that antigen concentration influences the phenotype of the resulting T cell population. It is also possible that changes in the pattern of T cell differentiation with different MHC alleles may occur by a similar mechanism. From these results, it appeared that low amounts of peptides or partial agonists favored IL-4 production, whereas relatively high peptide concentrations or superagonists ligands favored IFN-γ production (*see* Part I, Chapter 3 by Itoh and Germain).

The hierarchical organization of each individual effector cytokine and threshold of activation required to induce a specific cytokine is likely to play a major role in dictating the functional response and outcome of T cell differentiation. How does this hierarchical organization result in the induction of distinct cytokines from a naive or a fully polarized cell? Partial phosphorylation of the CD3-z chain has been seen in T cells encountering altered ligands and developing into Th2 cells, whereas full phosphorylation was seen when naive and differentiated Th1 cells bearing the same TCR were activated with the agonist ligand. A number of reports suggest that TCR signaling in established Th2 cells more closely resembles the pattern of activation seen with partial agonists including little or no detectable TCR-associated protein phosphorylation, and limited activation/phosphorylation of Fyn, Lck, ZAP-70, or PLC-γ1. In addition, Th2 cells without lck activity still have an ability to make Th2 cytokines. Similarly, calcium elevations in Th2 cells are transient and of lower amplitude than those seen with Th1 cells with the same TCR and using the same ligand. Thus, not only does the partial pattern of signaling favor the generation of Th2 cells, but these Th2 cells also show a restricted pattern of signaling, whereas Th1 cells with the same TCR show a full phosphorylation pattern and downstream second messengers. If IFN-γ requires a stronger signal than IL-4 production, then weak signaling will induce IL-4 and reinforce the Th2 phenotype. In contrast, a more robust signaling would be necessary to induce IFN-γ, and the IFN-γ production would promote further Th1 differentiation by inducing IL-12 from macrophages. The strong signals necessary for IFN-γ production would surpass the threshold necessary for IL-4 production and both locus opening and selective induction of transcription factors necessary for IFN-γ production, which repress IL-4 production (like T-bet) would then maintain the Th1 phenotype (*see* Part I, Chapter 3 by Itoh and Germain). This model does not however explain the observations that in a number of studies, Th2 development has been shown to require more potent signals. It is not clear how to reconcile these apparently opposite findings, but the organization of thresholds required for the induction of IL-4 vs IFN-γ in naive vs fully polarized cells may differ, which could explain such opposite results.

5. CELL-SURFACE RECEPTORS AND COSTIMULATORY MOLECULES

Interventions targeted at blocking various cell surface molecules (e.g., B7 and CD4) have been shown to affect T cell phenotype and the development of disease in a number of models. These effects could be either because of changes in the overall strength of signal, or because signals from costimulators have qualitative effects on T cell differentiation. The CD28/CTLA-4-B7-1/B7-2 costimulation pathway is one of the important influences on cytokine balance and affects T cell differentiation. In vivo CTLA4-Ig, which blocks B7-1 and B7-2 interactions, prevented the development of experimental autoimmune encephalomyelitis (EAE) and increased expression of Th2 cytokines in the target organ, suggesting a role for this pathway in differentially affecting Th1/Th2 cytokine balance. The role of B7-1 and B7-2 in Th differentiation has been intensively studied. In vitro studies using Chinese hamster ovary (CHO) cell transfectants expressing B7-1 or B7-2 suggested that B7-1 and B7-2 may have a distinct capacity to induce Th1 and Th2 cells. The administration of anti-B7-1 and B7-2 antibodies also suggested that blocking these molecules in vivo affected the development of autoimmunity and T cell differentiation. Whereas B7-1 induced Th1 responses, B7-2 directed Th2 responses. This was confirmed in a number of studies, but it was not seen in all systems. However, using B7-1- and B7-2-deficient antigen-presenting cells (APCs) from B7 knockout mice, it was later concluded that B7-1 and B7-2 both contribute to Th1 and Th2 cytokine production, but with a greater role for B7-2 in IL-4 induction. The signals induced by B7-1 and B7-2 into T cells are also distinct and how they contribute to differentiation has not been directly evaluated (*see* Part I, Chapter 4 by Buhlmann and Sharpe). Another means by which B7s may regulate cytokine production is by their expression on T cells. In vitro studies using TCR transgenic T cells cocultured with peptide and wild-type APCs, found that the B7-1 deficient T cells produced more IL-4 and less IFN-γ than the wild-type T cells under the same conditions, suggesting that B7-1 expression on T cells regulates IL-4 production. This costimulatory pathway is discussed in detail in Chapter 4 by Buhlmann and Sharpe.

Like CD28, inducible costimulatory molecule (ICOS), a closely related member of the CD28 family, also has positive costimulatory activity, enhancing proliferation and cytokine production. However, it has several properties that are distinct in that it is rapidly induced following activation and does not stimulate IL-2 but superinduces IL-10. Another member of the B7 family called B7-H1 (which is distinct from B7-H), which serves as a ligand for PD-1 also costimulates T cell proliferation and produces IL-10 in the presence of IL-2. The function of B7h-ICOS and B7-H1 interactions in Th differentiation is currently being actively investigated and how blocking these pathways may affect the development of autoimmune disease is an ongoing area of interest.

6. ROLE OF INNATE IMMUNE SYSTEM

Increasing evidence suggests that there is a close collaboration between the innate and adaptive immune system in that activation of the innate immune system influences the outcome of the immune responses of the adaptive immune system both in terms of expansion and differentiation of T cell clonotypes and the development of autoimmune diseases. NK cells and NK T cells are part of the innate immune system that help shape responses in the adaptive immune system. During the last decade, a unique family of CD1d-reactive T cells have been identified and these play an important role in the regulation of immune responses, affect T cell differentiation, and affect peripheral tolerance. This subset of CD1-d reactive T cells was called NK-T cells because they were found to express the surface markers for both $\alpha\beta$TCR and NK cells. Although their function is not clearly understood, their imbalance or dysfunction correlates with pathogenesis in many T cell-mediated autoimmune diseases. The NK1.1 T cells are restricted by the CD1-d molecule, express an invariant rearrangement of the TCR (Vα14, Jα281, and Vβ8) and are present at a very high frequency (0.5–1%) in thymus and spleen. Human NK 1.1 T cells have a homologous invariant TCR rearrangement expressing Vα24JαQ. These cells have been shown to recognize microbial glycolipid antigens in the context of CD1-d and the compound a-galactosylcermide (a-galcer) obtained from marine sponges activates both human and mouse NK1.1 T cells. The cells are able to secrete a burst of IL-4 and IFN-γ in response to activation with mitogenic stimulation without prior IL-4 priming. The capacity of unprimed NK1.1 T cells to produce large quantities of IL-4 rapidly is believed to provide an early source of IL-4 for Th2 differentiation and thus plays an important role in Th phenotype development. In addition NK1.1 T cells can efficiently lyse CD1-d expressing DC. Because DC1 are important in the induction of Th1 cells, the lysis of the DC1s by the NK1.1 cells may play a significant part in a negative feedback loop limiting the induction of Th1 responses (*see* Part I, Chapter 5 by Exley and Wilson).

Loss or diminished frequency of CD1-d restricted T cells correlates with the development of autoimmunity in both mice and humans. In the SJL and nonobese diabetic (NOD) mouse strains, which are highly susceptible to EAE and type 1 diabetes, there is a striking decrease or a functional defect in the NK T cells. The decrease in the NK1.1 T cells in SJL mice is owing to a mutation in the promoter of CD161 (NK 1.1) resulting in lower expression of the protein. In NOD mice, the quantitative defect is associated with the reduced ability of these T cells to produce IL-4, IL-10, and IFN-γ following stimulation, and disease in the NOD mouse can be prevented by adoptive transfer of CD1d-restricted T cells. Furthermore administration of a-GalCer in NOD mice protects them from developing diabetes. A defective function in the CD1d-restricted T cells is also associated with the development of type-1 diabetes in humans. Analysis of NK1.1 T cells in monozygotic twins that were discordant for insulin-dependent diabetes mellitus (IDDM), showed that $V\alpha24J\alpha Q$ T cells were present at higher frequencies in the nonprogressors when compared to the diabetics. Furthermore, the $V\alpha24J\alpha Q$ T cells from the diabetic sibling showed loss of IL-4 and maintenance of IFN-γ responses, thus exhibiting a Th1 bias. In contrast, NK1.1 T cells form nonprogressive siblings and normal volunteers produced both IL-4 and IFN-γ following activation. The loss of $V\alpha24J\alpha Q$ T cells or reduction in their frequencies in the circulation or in the target tissues has been observed in a number of other autoimmune diseases, including RA and MS (*see* Part I, Chapter 5 by Exley and Wilson and Part II, Chapter 12 by Kent, Viglietta, and Hafler). In addition to NK1.1 T cells, IL-12 or IL-10 produced by macrophages upon interaction with microbial elements will direct T cell differentiation in the adaptive immune system.

Another group of soluble mediators that are very important in the regulation of immune responses are the chemokines. Upon expansion and differentiation, autoreactive T cells produce different chemokines and also acquire cell-surface expression of chemokine receptors that allow them to egress from lymph nodes and promote their trafficking to sites of inflammation and into target organs. As naive cells differentiate and expand, both Th1 and Th2 cells lose the expression of CCR7, which allows them to home to lymph nodes, and this promotes their exit from lymph nodes. In addition, Th1 and Th2 cells acquire different patterns of expression of chemokine receptors in that Th1 cells express CXCR3, which is the receptor for the chemokine IP-10. In contrast, Th2 cells upregulate CCR3, CCR4, and CCR8 chemokine receptors which are the receptors for the chemokines eotaxin, MDC, and I309, respectively. The loss of the CCR7 chemokine receptor and selective expression of other chemokine receptors allows the differentiated T cells to egress lymph nodes and traffic to sites of inflammation or target tissues where the ligands for these receptors are found in high concentrations. In contrast to T cells, activated DC downregulate CCR1 and CCR5 chemokine receptors to egress from sites of inflammation and upregulate CCR7 to target their trafficking to lymph nodes, where they present antigens to lymphocytes, which then expand and differentiate. The spatial and temporal chemokine production by various cell types and expression of specific chemokine receptors by effector cells is an important regulatory mechanism in controlling the trafficking of leukocytes and in the pathogenesis of autoimmune diseases and tissue injury (*see* Part I, Chapter 7 by Ransohoff and Karpus).

7. ROLE OF CYTOKINES IN TISSUE INJURY AND TISSUE TOLERANCE

After expansion and differentiation in the lymph node, autoreactive T cells home to their specific target tissue where they can promote tissue damage or protect the organ from autoimmunity. The pathogenic and protective properties of these lymphocytes are defined by their phenotype. However the role that individual cytokines play in the target tissue is more variable. For antibody-mediated disease, cytokines largely provide help and control antibody-isotype switching during the induction and expansion phase of the B cell response. The ability of an autoantibody to fix complement, and mediate antibody-dependent cellular cytotoxicity (ADCC) may then determine whether it is pathogenic and can mediate tissue injury.

As shown in the chapters in Part II of this book, Th1 cells and/or their cytokines are strongly implicated in the induction of a number of autoimmune diseases and tissue injury. Surprisingly, this is also true in a number of antibody-mediated autoimmune diseases (e.g., SLE and MG) which have a strong component of Th1 autoimmune response. However, this is not say that Th2-cells cannot induce autoimmune diseases or that Th2 dependent antibody cannot mediate tissue damage. For example, in uveitis induced in IFN-$\gamma^{-/-}$ mice, and in encephalitis induced in immunocompromised mice by the transfer of MBP-specific Th2 cells, tissue damage still arises, but the underlying pathology is strikingly different from what is seen in disease induced in normal mice.

The phenotype of pathogenic T cells in mice has been best-studied in experimental models of organ-specific autoimmune diseases, particularly induced models of MS (like EAE) and spontaneous models of disease, especially type I diabetes in the NOD mouse. In most cases, autoreactive T cells capable of mediating organ-specific autoimmune disease fell exclusively into the Th1 subset (*see* Part II, Chapter 8 by Segal and Shevach). In several adoptive transfer studies in disease models, including EAE in SJL and B10.PL mice, diabetes in NOD mice, and uveitis in Lewis rats and in mice, it has been shown that disease can be transferred by autoantigen-specific Th1 or Tc1 cells, which produce IFN-γ, TNF-α, and/or lymphotoxin. On the other hand, in these models Th2 cells with the same antigenic specificity lose their ability to induce disease and in some cases protect hosts form the development of disease and tissue destruction.

By analyzing cytokine expression in different inflamed target tissues, it has been shown that there is often an increased expression of Th1 cytokines both in experimental autoimmune diseases and also in biopsy specimens from patients with such diseases as RA, Crohn's disease, type 1 diabetes, and MS. However, the microenvironment is an extremely complex mixture of different cytokines, and to address the question of whether a candidate cytokine is directly pathogenic, investigators have generally either examined its effects on different cell types in vitro, blocked the action of the cytokine with antibodies in vivo, overexpressed the cytokine by transgenesis in vivo in a general or tissue specific fashion, or removed the cytokine by generating the disease in an animal model in which the cytokine gene has been knocked out. One important observation that arises from these studies is that cytokines, although they can be directly toxic, are often not the ultimate mediators of tissue destruction, which is carried out by the macrophages that they activate. A second point is that even though the development of disease depends on T cells that are differentiated under conditions that lead to a Th1 phenotype, the effector cytokines that are critical to tissue destruction may be different in different diseases. An example is the difference in the effect that TNF blockade has in the treatment of RA, where it is a very effective treatment for disease (*see* Part II, Chapter 13 by Wahren-Herlenius et al.), and MS where it has been reported to exacerbate disease (*see* Part II, Chapter 11 by Weiner).

The reason for these differences may lie in the different responses of the target tissue following an influx of inflammatory lymphocytes. Sites of profound immunological privilege such as the eye enjoy a very different microenvironment compared with organs such as the gut, which have an enormous exposure to both environmental antigens as well as to the circulation. The target tissues may also display different patterns of sensitivity to the cytokine environment; for example, bone and cartilage may be damaged more by cytokines that activate bone resorption compared to oligodendrocytes being more damaged by direct cytotoxicity.

Issues of tissue tolerance are highlighted in chapters (*see* Part II, Chapter 8 by Segal and Shevach and Chapter 9 by Caspi). The eye employs both cytokine-mediated and cell contact-mediated strategies to regulate the impact of inflammatory lymphocytes. Because occular tissues express FasL, resident APCs can signal infiltrating cells to undergo apoptosis. Activated lymphocytes are eliminated by a process that triggers IL-10 production, and antigen-bearing cells that have ingested lymphocytes that have undergone apoptosis appear to be involved in the induction of regulatory lymphocytes, a process that can result in generalized tolerance to subsequent antigen challenge. Some of these interactions are believed to take place in the spleen. In addition to these cell contact-dependent mechanisms, privileged organs are bathed in fluids such as the aqueous humor (AH) of the eye and the cerebrospinal fluid (CSF) in the brain, which maintain relatively high levels of regulatory cytokines and other soluble factors such as TGF-β2 and IL-1RA, which can both inhibit lymphocyte function, and promote immune deviation, which is itself immunoregulatory. Biological fluids derived from immune-privileged sites alter the properties of conventional APCs and induce immune deviation towards a Th2 phenotype. Therefore, some tissues maintain a very high "barrier to entry" to the development of immune-mediated inflammation, and this leads to immune privilege by virtue of the generation of a specialized microenvironment.

Such mechanisms are not, of course, unique to these specific tissues. Both TGF-β, and also IL-10, have been shown to have an important role in regulating inflammation in a number of different models of autoimmune disease. It has been shown in vitro that these cytokines act primarily on APCs, suppressing the secretion of IL-12 and the expression of MHC class II and costimulatory molecules. The importance of these cytokines can also be inferred by studies of the impact of their presence and absence in a diverse number of animal models of disease. Furthermore, the observation that the genetic deletion of IFN-γ can exacerbate autoimmune disease, for example EAE, may be because in the absence of this Th1 cytokines there is inefficient induction of the counter-regulatory cytokine IL-10.

8. THE ROLE OF CYTOKINES IN THE THERAPY OF AUTOIMMUNE DISEASE

Understanding the biology of cytokines has at least two applications to the treatment of autoimmune disease. The first is as a marker for disease and therefore as a surrogate marker for disease progression and to monitor the efficacy of therapy. Cytokines that alter with changes in the general levels of inflammation can be measured in the circulation where they reflect disease activity. Also by monitoring changes in cytokines following different therapies, it may be possible to infer a mechanism of action for the therapy. For example, the effectiveness of cyclophosphamide in the treatment of MS may be related to its ability to induce immune deviation and increase IL-4 and TGF-β (*see* Part II, Chapter 11 by Weiner). It is clearly important to assess the impact of potential therapies on cytokine regulation in autoimmune-disease models because this may give clues as to its likely effectiveness in patients.

The second area in which understanding cytokine biology is critical is in identifying targets for specific intervention. There are at least two approaches to exploiting what we now know about the role of cytokines in autoimmune disease with the goal of designing specific therapy. The first approach is to target one or a few effector cytokines, with the aim of inhibiting tissue damage in the target organ. The second is to enhance normal mechanisms of immunoregulation. This has the potential advantage that is can inhibit both the recruitment and expansion of new antigen-specific pathogenic T cell clones from the naive Thp pool, and also that by bystander suppression it can downregulate inflammation within the target organ.

The most successful example of therapy of the first kind is the use of treatments that inhibit TNF-α in RA. Both anti-TNF antibodies and soluble TNF receptor (TNF-R) have been evaluated in clinical trials, and studies with antibodies have proven this treatment to be efficacious. This is also the case with IL-1RA (receptor antagonist), a natural inhibitor of IL-1 (*see* Part II, Chapter 13 by Wahren-Herlenius et al.). On the other hand, as discussed earlier, in MS anti-TNF therapy exacerbates disease, illustrating that efficacy in one autoimmune disease does not ensure effectiveness in all autoimmune diseases.

Regulatory cytokines can also be used directly as therapy. In animal models of autoimmunity, it has been shown that treatment with Th2 cytokines can ameliorate disease, both when these cytokines are given directly and also when the are administered by engineering expression of Th2 cytokines in cells that then traffic to the target organ (*see* Part II, Chapter 10 by Bettelli and Nicholson). These studies are aimed at overcoming problems of toxicity, which are known to arise with systemic administration of cytokines, and it is hoped that local delivery may overcome problems of systemic toxicity. At present it remains unclear how these approaches will be applied successfully in patients.

Exploiting normal mechanisms of immunoregulation to treat autoimmune disease is a more elegant, but also a more ambitious, approach to therapy. Because it enhances the normal working of the immune system, it should be specific and selective in its actions. However, there are several potential problems that have not yet been overcome. The first barrier to success is that we do not yet understand regulatory mechanisms in any detail. Although there is now persuasive evidence implicating TGF-β and IL-10 as downmodulators of immune responses, it is not clear how these cytokines can be induced in a specific and targeted way. The second problem is that, although in animal models it has been possible to define with some precision how disease is initiated, and to prevent this by many different approaches, patients do not present themselves for therapy until after the disease state is established. Successful treatment must therefore deal with an established autoimmune response and also the concomitant target organ damage. Therefore, although in animal models IL-12 provides an extremely effective target for early intervention which prevents the development of autoimmune disease (*see* Part II, Chapter 8 by Segal and Shevach), it may be a less useful target in patients with established disease.

Two treatments for MS that have proven effective and whose mechanisms of action include effects on cytokines are treatment with glatiramer acetate (copaxone) and treatment with IFN-β. For both these therapies, there is evidence that they are associated with the induction of a Th2 immune response, and part of their benefit may arise from the immune deviation of an established pathological response and/or the generation of a crossreactive regulatory response to autoantigen (*see* Part II, Chapter 11 by Weiner).

Another therapy directed at manipulating normal immunoregulatory mechanisms is the induction of oral tolerance. This seeks to exploit the experimental observation that feeding protein antigens can lead to a state of unresponsiveness to subsequent immunization with antigen plus adjuvant. In animals, this occurs through multiple mechanisms, including apoptosis, at high antigen concentrations, and the induction of regulatory Th3 cells occurs at low antigen concentrations. In the clinic, this therapy has been applied to a number of different autoimmune diseases including MS, RA, and type 1 diabetes. Although there have been a number of encouraging studies on small numbers of patients, the efficacy of this treatment has not been established by large clinical trials. Effective use of this therapy may need more sophisticated techniques to assess which patients will benefit from treatment, or alternatively require the development of adjuvants to therapy that will increase efficacy.

Another technique that has benefit in animal models is the administration of APLs, which are mutants derived from the cognate peptide ligand by changing TCR contact residues. These analogs can block the development of autoimmune diseases such as EAE by inducing regulatory-cell populations that secrete Th2 cytokines and that crossreact with the cognate peptide. They are generally most effective when given before disease develops or at the time it is induced; however, there is data that they can induce regulation of an ongoing autoimmune response. Two recently reported clinical trials of APLs in MS have shown that their administration to patients can have a measurable effect on the various immunological parameters such as T cell crossreactivity and cytokine production. However, there was no evidence of clinical benefit in these trials and in some case the suggestion that APLs may induce exacerbation of disease. This underlines the heterogenous nature of immune responses in an outbred human population.

In animal models, it is clear that targeting costimulatory pathways can inhibit disease by altering patterns of cytokine secretion. Most studies have investigated targeting signals transmitted into the T cell via the receptors CD28 and CTLA-4 (CD152) following ligation by their counter-receptors CD80 and CD86. It has been shown that altering costimulation can shift cytokine profile and that in animal models this can both reduce or exacerbate clinical disease. Treatment with soluble CTLA4Ig has been reported as being effective in ameliorating psoriasis. Therefore, such manipulations can have therapeutic benefit in patients, and the range and application of these therapies will likely increase in the next few years.

9. SUMMARY

Cytokines provide a network of effector molecules that connect cells of the immune system and cells of different target tissues in an intricate web of responses. Many of the most significant interactions in this network occur in microenvironments that may be isolated from the general circulation, that may have unique tissue-specific properties, and therefore in which immune cells of identical function may have very different effects. It is clear that this network is comprised of numerous checks and balances that limit or permit tissue damage under subtly different circumstances. In many cases, the outcome may relate to how positive feedback for the secretion of specific cytokines becomes established.

In autoimmune disease, pathology seems to be induced predominantly by T cells that have developed in environments that promote Th1 differentiation, even though Th1 effector cytokines such as IFN-γ and TNF-α have clearly been shown to be redundant to the development of disease. In experimental models, it has been shown that blocking IL-12 is almost always effective in preventing disease. However, how much of this effectiveness depends on intervening when disease is being induced remains to be determined. IL-10 and TGF-β are both powerful immunoregulatory cytokines, which may be exploited in therapy in the future. One elusive goal with these cytokines is developing techniques to target their delivery in a tissue-specific fashion. This ambition reaches its apex with aspirations towards antigen/organ-specific immunomodulatory therapy. It is clear that achieving this goal will require an intimate understanding of the complex interplay between immune cells, the tissue microenvironment, and the network of cytokines that links the two.

Index

407